Managing Health Care Demand

Scott MacStravic
Principal
Demand Engineering
Golden, Colorado

Gary Montrose
President
Ashby • Montrose & Company
Denver, Colorado

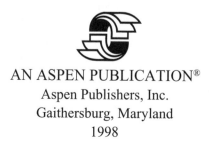

AN ASPEN PUBLICATION®
Aspen Publishers, Inc.
Gaithersburg, Maryland
1998

The authors have made every attempt to ensure the accuracy of the information herein. However, appropriate information sources should be consulted, especially for new or unfamiliar procedures. It is the responsibility of every practitioner to evaluate the appropriateness of a particular opinion in the context of actual clinical situations and with due considerations to new developments. Authors, editors, and the publisher cannot be held responsible for any typographical or other errors found in this book.

Library of Congress Cataloging-in-Publication Data

MacStravic, Robin E. Scott.
Managing health care demand/Robin E. Scott MacStravic, Gary
Montrose.
p. cm.
Includes bibliographical references and index.
ISBN 0-8342-0927-6 (hardcover)
1. Medical care—Utilization. 2. Medical care—Cost control.
3. Consumer behavior. 4. Health promotion. 5. Managed care
programs (Medical care) I. Montrose, Gary. II. Title.
[DNLM: 1. Health Services Needs and Demand—organization &
administration. 2. Managed Care Programs—organization &
administration. 3. Health Promotion—organization & administration.
W 84.1 M175m 1998]
RA410.6.M33 1998
362.1'04258'068—DC21
DNLM/DLC
for Library of Congress
97-47204
CIP

Orders: (800) 638-8437
Customer Service: (800) 234-1660

About Aspen Publishers • For more than 35 years, Aspen has been a leading professional publisher in a variety of disciplines. Aspen's vast information resources are available in both print and electronic formats. We are committed to providing the highest quality information available in the most appropriate format for our customers. Visit Aspen's Internet site for more information resources, directories, articles, and a searchable version of Aspen's full catalog, including the most recent publications: **http://www.aspenpub.com**
Aspen Publishers, Inc. • The hallmark of quality in publishing
Member of the worldwide Wolters Kluwer group.

Editorial Resources: Bill Fogle
Library of Congress Catalog Card Number: 97-47204
ISBN: 0-8342-0927-6

Printed in the United States of America

1 2 3 4 5

Table of Contents

Foreword

When a new breed of animal appears, it takes a while for people to agree about what it is. We classify it by its looks. We take the mutt and look for similarities to its purebred origins. We try and place it within the context of the familiar. We argue about whether it is truly new or whether it really is just a new label on an old friend (or enemy). What we like we attribute to being a descendant of our favorite lineage. What we dislike we attribute to flaws in either the genetics or the upbringing of the creature. It takes a while for us to see the new arrival as a unique entity—certainly a creation that combines all of its environment and origins—but a new and unique arrival nonetheless.

On the many occasions when I have had the opportunity to talk or write about the notion of "Demand Management" since 1993, I have watched as a variety of purebred owners claimed or denied paternity of the mutt. Depending on the purebred of choice, the new field has been claimed as (or as not) the offspring of Health Promotion, Utilization Review, Prevention, patient advocacy, decision-making theory, nurse advisory lines, and CQI. Consistently, audiences asked what demand management "really" was, hoping to put it in a familiar category that would help them decide if the animal was friendly or dangerous. Some would make a quick decision about Demand Managements' true breed—"it's really UR"—and accept or reject the concept accordingly. Others waited to see who wanted to own the new breed—"oh, this is a managed care strategy"—and made a decision based on their opinion about the owners. In both cases, the reactions produced some unfair results. First, people looking at this new creature were inevitably influenced by strong preconceptions about its parents or its sponsors. And second, everything about the new creature was lumped into a single category of good or bad, worthwhile or not. Few of us saw its unique possibilities or the complex aspects of its character.

As one of the people who has been quite fond of (and quite intrigued by the possibilities of) this Demand Management creature since its appearance, the response of the health care profession has been at various times frustrating, amusing and inspiring. To push the analogy even farther: we have seen some efforts to drive the new breed to extinction, because it threatens to wipe out other traditional breeds. We have seen organizations join the Demand Management parade by dressing up any old animal to look like the new breed. We have seen wonderful new litters of demand management tools born in places that have never heard of the breed and couldn't care less what they are called. One way or another, the little mutt caused quite a stir.

But slowly and steadily awareness has grown. People have started seeing the creature itself, instead of just labeling the category to which it might belong. And demand management has its attractive features. The elements of Demand Management have such a natural appeal that we eventually have to notice. Something feels right about having patients more involved in and informed about their own care. Something looks right when accurate information becomes accessible and available at the time a person needs it. Something sounds right when individuals are asked to take part in their own health management and care. When we step away from suspicions about who is trying to take (or who might lose) control of care delivery, the premise works. Patients have been missing in many of our equations. When we add them to the formula many positive things can happen. Something is intuitively right about providing health care this way.

Unfortunately, what feels intuitively so right and seems so appealing hasn't succeeded consistently in practice. In some cases interventions work beautifully to benefit the health of patients while reducing the cost of care. In others, the intervention sits idle and has little effect at all. Proponents sing the praises of the former, while skeptics stake their position on the latter. For those standing between the extremes, lessons continue to trickle in. It seems nothing is universally effective, because the process isn't perfect and the dynamics aren't sufficiently well understood. We still need to learn more about how to market such services. We still need to learn how to encourage and promote new roles for patients and providers. We need to examine the mechanisms of delivering and receiving support. We still need better measurement of and better data about its impact.

The question remains: Is this new breed merely a guiding companion for the patient, or can it be a beast of burden to help ease the increasing load placed on our providers. Could it even, perhaps, be a shepherd for moving the entire care system? Maybe now we can begin to see the possibilities with open minds.

Students of Demand Management will be encouraged by the work and thinking in this book. It takes such a broad view of demand, and the management thereof, that narrow characterizations become inadequate. It presents the complexity and diversity of care-seeking and care delivery among the purebreds as well as the cross-breeds. Because of its breadth and depth, the reader can no longer see demand management as any single endeavor, within an single profession, or having any single intention. The incentives are multifaceted and the challenges considerable.

Advocates and doubters alike will probably find their positions changed by this book. Or at least modified. The authors provide openings and opportunities for many groups previously excluded by some of the earlier Demand Management dogma. The authors provide perspective and rationale for everyone: the community, the provider, the employer, the insurer, the hospital, the occupational health system, the family, and the individual. They provide an incredibly thorough review of where we've been, and they propose creative structures and mechanisms to describe where we are and could be going. It will instantly become a valued resource for those wanting to understand the discipline and adopt some of its useful tools. Almost certainly, it will also become a launching site for even more substantive and educated debates about the particulars of who should own, manage, create, and deliver demand-related services.

The release of this text signifies a significant step in the evolution of the "demand-side" movement. The book demonstrates a need for structured guidance in the field, acknowledges a documentable history of progress, and suggests a future market for its concepts and tools. The release of this text shows that the new animal has emerged with an identity beyond its family and background, one that has characteristics worth considering. It seems there might actually be a new breed of care.

Wendy D. Lynch, Ph.D.
Lynch Consulting, Ltd.
Lakewood, Colorado

Preface

Despite all the rhetoric about change in the healthcare industry over the past two decades, the actual system of care and service delivery remains remarkably untouched. Managed care, once thought to be the panacea for runaway costs, now appears to be stalled, unable to stem a new wave of pent-up industry-wide cost pressures.

Healthcare consumers continue to be frustrated with the inability of the healthcare system to respond to their individual health care needs, and the levels of service remain dismal. Consumers are seeking out substitutes and alternatives to traditional providers and health plans in ever increasing numbers. Many healthcare organizations have begun to respond to their challenges by implementing a variety of consumer-focused demand management programs. Such programs, designed to "empower" consumers have thus far either been too generic to be useful, too restrictive, or poorly coordinated with the rest of the care delivery system.

Physicians too, are increasingly frustrated with managed care-imposed systems, including consumer-direct nurse call center services, feeling as if they are being left out of the patient service equation. Piecemeal care management programs have disrupted the patient-physician relationship and so far have contributed little in the way of system-wide quantifiable improvements in cost, service, or quality.

The concept of better managing consumer demand, or truly satisfying consumers' unique health needs has extraordinary potential to achieve outstanding levels of service and clinical quality at lower cost, where correctly implemented. Experts estimate that in the US alone, avoidable care expenditures well exceed 200 billion dollars annually. Demand Management, an old economics term, has been widely and effectively used in other industries for years. A relatively new concept in healthcare, first defined in the literature by thought leaders such as Wendy Lynch PhD, who authored the foreword for this new book, it focuses on the largely unrecognized demand side of the classic supply-demand equation. Demand Management in healthcare means anticipating what individual consumers need to know in order to make the best decisions to achieve optimum potential health status. Demand Management is, or should be at its foundation, consumer-centric; where the individual controls decision-making for personal or family health, and is recognized as able to take the right actions if given the right options, information, resources and support. When people are given the right information and advice, and helped to implement their choices, the outcome is far more likely to be higher quality care, lower cost, and satisfied consumers, according to a growing body of research findings and practical experience.

MacStravic and Montrose provide a critical starting point for a consumer-focused healthcare industry in its infancy. Until now, there has been no single authoritative and comprehensive text describing the entire discipline of demand management in healthcare. As such, the authors have delivered an important and much needed set of guidelines supported by exhaustive research and original thinking, to articulate a broad new perspective on demand management. They have tackled an extremely difficult challenge in trying to provide a framework around the complexities of integrated health, disease, decision and demand management. By challenging traditional thinking, the authors have detailed a vision for demand management that goes far beyond the nurse call center to a much broader population management and community oriented perspective. They explicitly describe the many systemic interdependencies necessary for providers, health plans and others to improve consumer health and care management as a business discipline and public service. Their vision of demand management is consumer focused yet provider supported, with an emphasis on shared responsibility and shared decision making. They offer consumer engagement strategies that are segmented, targeted, and tailored to individuals' needs, readiness levels, and capabilities.

The vision in this book reflects the evolution of early demand management, (the first generation) which included self-care guidebooks and nurse advice and triage, serving primarily as a marketing tool; not as a sophisticated care management process to achieve targeted and measurable cost, service and quality outcomes. This is important because most current demand management programs have been unable to demonstrate substantive and sustainable bottom-line results. Overall use by plan members has been dismally low, and there is little evidence of use by those members most likely to benefit. Toward this end, the authors have introduced the bold notion of "continuous demand improvement" that challenges the industry to more rigorously measure and monitor demand management interventions against explicit strategic, economic, clinical, and consumer satisfaction objectives.

Though demand management has enormous power and potential, to achieve the expected benefits, the discipline must exist within an even broader new care delivery paradigm, a critical piece of a broader model for Integrated Health Management as we have described in "Changing Healthcare." This Andersen Consulting model recognizes a shifting paradigm toward active consumer engagement which places the individual at the center of the universe with the tools, information and incentives to facilitate better care coordination and more appropriate use of healthcare resources. MacStravic and Montrose expand upon this theme, of liberating the consumer, enabling him or her to express and realize unique healthcare needs and preferences. Demand management is truly about satisfying such needs, thereby minimizing avoidable health risks, reducing inappropriate utilization, improving service and ultimately the quality of life.

As the authors pointedly note, the prevailing use of the term demand management is not only unfortunate, but insufficient and inaccurate. The term 'management' leaves providers and consumers with the impression that someone is doing something to them that will restrict their access to necessary healthcare resources. Demand management is really more appropriately termed health management or care management, and must be thought of in a much broader customer service context in order to fully deliver on its full potential value. Imagine, for example, a health industry common practice where a person calling for health advice, schedules a follow-up visit with the appropriate care provider, obtains pre-authorization for the visit concurrently, is reminded of immunization needs of her two children, and is then offered the opportunity to coordinate the children's visits with her own physician visit! This kind of service is becoming commonplace in other industries, yet it is far beyond the capabilities of most healthcare organizations today.

At Andersen Consulting we have the opportunity to work with leading edge companies, across different industry sectors to define the consumer-corporate "moment of value". Readers with backgrounds in today's customer service industries will resonate with our experience: where consumers encounter mass-produced yet highly customized service with the touch of a few keypad buttons, on demand, available 24 hours a day.

Expectations for similar levels of service within healthcare are growing rapidly. The financial services industry is perhaps the best example of where these types of robust customer service solutions are fundamentally changing the ways consumers and businesses interact. While once banking was done completely through in-person visits to the local branch, consumers can now bank by telephone, drive-through ATM's or bank over the Internet. Through any of these consumer-selected channels, information is now easily accessed and routine transactions processed efficiently, accurately and in a highly confidential manner.

While healthcare and banking are certainly not identical, the use of multichannel networks to offer wide and consistent access to highly personal service will be extremely attractive to consumers seeking routine healthcare advice, information, and care support. It is also interesting to note that organizations such as General Electric, Fidelity, and several large banks, entertainment, telecommunication and media corporations which have developed the technology platforms necessary to support highly customized customer relationship management, are giving serious consideration to leveraging these capabilities into the healthcare marketplace. This type of catalytic event may someday drive a sea change across the healthcare industry.

MacStravic and Montrose recognize the potential for industry-wide transformation, and provide a detailed roadmap for those organizations courageous enough to embark early on such a journey. As with any transformational change however, the journey is not without risk. In dealing with these issues the authors take a page out of our Business Integration and Enterprise Transformation play books, by providing both a blueprint for a long term demand management vision, as well as a practical migration strategy which enables short-term benefits that will help mitigate risk along the way.

We have had the opportunity to work with one of the authors (GM) and are gratified to find strong agreement on the application of consumer-focused service delivery and care management solutions. Even more important, we share the same very exciting vision for enterprise-wide demand management done correctly. Our collective point of view, validated by extensive client work and a deep understanding of multiple service industries, is that comprehensive demand management program will help reaffirm the best out of the physician-patient relationship (moment of value), improving overall provider productivity, and individual and population health, while positively impacting financial performance, and long term customer retention.

MacStravic and Montrose explore what will be necessary to achieve this value proposition. Their analysis of industry experience to date, research synthesis from hundreds of pilot studies, and fresh thinking coincides with our view that for demand management to succeed on a large scale five essential elements must be present, all enabled by a comprehensive information infrastructure and an integrated technology platform. First, segmentation of the population to enable mass customization within a demand management program is essential. A one-size-fits-all strategy can not be effective. Grouping members with similar decision-making styles enables the development of targeted interventions more likely to achieve the behavior change necessary for improved health. Second, the integration of multiple channels is an essential prerequisite to a comprehensive demand management solution. While the call center is an important method for accessing limited urgent care support services, it must sit within a broader care construct. In addition to the office or clinic, other channels such as the internet, web TV, video-conferencing, and community kiosks will provide low cost easy access, delivering a consistent experience, interactive exchanges necessary for effective care management and new levels of individualized service.

We have seen the rise of personal banking through all sorts of channels where a consumer can make a transaction over the phone, the internet, or at a kiosk. Robust telephony and database infrastructures makes instantaneous skills-based routing to different care specialists anywhere in the country or around the world now technically feasible. In the not-too-distant future, healthcare consumers will be directed, over video-enabled web TV sets, to the most appropriate medical personnel to get answers or treatment advise based upon prerecorded health data, and their own level of self-efficacy. A hesitant Spanish-speaking mother communicating with an automated call center will be quickly identified, and electronically routed to a Spanish-speaking nurse with appropriate expertise in neonatal medicine, and other culturally relevant issues.

Third, programs and services will be integrated as never before. Currently, a consumer accesses one phone number for diabetes management, another for nurse advice services and yet another for pre-authorizations, claims and billing information. Uncoordinated systems result in case managers, business managers, and disease managers unintentionally offering conflicting information and advice. Only a common infrastructure can help provide a one stop shopping experience for both healthcare consumers and providers.

Fourth, for key stakeholders, especially physicians, demand management programs will be integrated with clinical management solutions. This necessitates that discrete data elements be incorporated from the electronic patient record and communicated amongst physicians, hospitals, employers, government agencies, and allied health providers. Care teams will operate system-wide, managing lifetime care plans tailored to each individual's needs and resources.

Fifth, opportunities for active learning from captured data will be better leveraged. With a multi-channel infrastructure, valuable information currently inaccessible will be utilized to anticipate population and individual health needs to help avoid unnecessary crises. The challenge is to use such information for both continuous program enhancements and adjusting care plans at the individual level. Information related to care delivery "best practices" will also be automatically communicated early to providers and consumers, an essential feature of overall population health management.

Finally, and most important, these components will be integrated into an enterprise-wide framework ensuring that key processes are aligned, that enabling technology is operating, and the environment supports employee behavior change necessary to operate within an integrated health and demand management paradigm.

Although this book is lengthy and far reaching, do not be intimidated. The authors have been sensitive enough to provide an innovative navigator tool in the beginning of the book which will help guide both the experienced and novice reader to appropriate sections of the book. Make use of this resources as a strategic planning guide and ongoing reference book to get the most value out of the information and concepts within the book. The authors offer definitions and context for the variety of terms loosely used currently in the health management arena. They offer a vocabulary for the dialog and debate so essential to develop demand management to a level that will produce the tremendous benefits that we believe are possible and inevitable.

Demand management is a whole new business discipline. MacStravic and Montrose bring to this book tremendous experience and insight to the emerging consumer-focused demand management industry. While not everyone is going to agree with all their concepts, the authors have done a commendable job of breaking down a vast and extremely intricate subject into easily understandable components. They have taken "loose notions" about empowering consumers and behavior change and have provided us with a useful set of tools that for many years to come will be the seminal resource for future research, graduate training, and business needs. This book, though three years in the making, presents ideas that are truly revolutionary. The authors are once again already at work preparing a variety of provider readiness assessment and implementation tools for those organizations which recognize the competitive advantage to be gained by deeply understanding the full potential of their current demand management efforts; enabling their leadership to implement the new consumer paradigm.more comprehensively, more strategically and more effectively. Those industry leaders who recognize the vast untapped opportunities presented here will, we believe, gain in market advantage, those who do not will be destined to be followers, likely to reap far less of the rewards of cost saving and customer loyalty waiting to be harvested.

Andersen Consulting Health Services Practice

James B. Hudak
Global Managing Partner
Health Services

Kurt H. Miller
Managing Partner
Global Care Delivery and Medical Management Solutions Team

Michael Eliastam, MD, MPP, FACP
Physician Director
Medical Management Solutions Team

Acknowledgments

Many of our colleagues have contributed to this book in a variety of ways. We will mention a few, and apologize to any we may have overlooked. Donald E. L. Johnson, Editor and Publisher of Health Care Strategic Management, Englewood, CO and long a major player in the health care publishing industry was responsible for introducing us and suggesting our collaboration. Dean Coddington, of Moore, Fisher, Coddington in Denver, CO, one of the foremost strategic consultants in health care and a well-known author himself, was one of the first to encourage the writing of this book. Jack Bruggeman, of Aspen Publishers, and Steve LaRose, editor of *Inside Preventive Care,* provided both encouragement and advice early in its development.

Catharyn Baird provided much of the initial research, and supplied ideas and editorial assistance throughout. Carol Jeanotilla turned our rough ideas for the book's graphic exhibits into a highly creative reality. And Wendy Lynch, Ph.D., offered a vast number of insightful comments and suggestions as a reviewer of the manuscript. While responsibility for the final content rests entirely with us, we feel they have added greatly to the quality of this project.

Introduction

The title of this book reflects what has come to be the accepted term for a wide variety of efforts aimed at controlling or "curbing" health care utilization for the benefit of payers and providers at risk. While managing "utilization" has been used chiefly to describe efforts by payers to control providers, managing "demand" can apply to both providers and consumers, since both influence how much care is demanded.

DEMAND?

A number of terms have been used by others to address similar challenges. Integrated lifestyle management,[1] personal[2] and personalized[3] health management have been used to describe the challenge of improving the health of populations to reduce their use of health care. Disease prevention and management[4] could easily cover the same challenge, since "prevention" can logically include health promotion and risk reduction as well as primary prevention, and "disease" can include both injuries and adverse pregnancy outcomes to be prevented.

Total health management (owned by Adventist Health Systems Sunbelt, Orlando, FL) and care management[5] have been used to describe phone triage and counseling programs used to inform consumers of choices available when needing care. Demand management (owned by Health Decisions International, Golden, CO) has been trademarked as a specific product combining self-care and triage counseling services aimed at consumers and what they do once motivated by symptoms. Since many programs aimed at controlling demand employ call centers and because call centers can be used for outbound health risk assessment, health promotion, disease self-management, and related purposes, this term could also cover the entire scope of functions aimed at influencing the factors that drive consumer demand for health care.[6]

We have chosen to focus the book's title on demand as opposed to health, utilization, or disease, though all three are so closely related that the distinction is often imperceptible. We will address health promotion and risk reduction as essential components of any effort to manage demand and disease self-management as well. We will include employee health and the demand for occupational health and disability services as well as the health and demand of general consumers.

MANAGEMENT?

We have concerns, however, about the use of the term management when thus applied. Managing providers, certainly physicians, has long been likened to herding cats. Professionals in health care, particularly when they are not employees, but independent contractors, tend to bridle at the idea of being managed (i.e., controlled or manipulated) by nonphysicians or physician administrators in distant offices. Physicians, in particular, resent having others dictate what they can and cannot do and say and complain that they cannot give as high quality care to patients under managed care as they can under indemnity insurance.[7] They risk losing the trust and respect of patients whenever they are perceived as being managed by payers.

The idea of "managing" consumers seems even more inappropriate. Managers rely on power, authority, or, ideally, leadership skills. They attempt to exert their will over people in their own organizations, over whom they have an accepted authority. But by what right do they rule over consumers? Health insurers and managed care plans are supposed to *serve* consumers, arguably their ultimate customers.[8] One does not *manage* customers; at best one tries to *market* to them successfully to attract, influence, satisfy, and retain them.

Management typically has a simple rule about *choice*: "My way or the highway!" It aims to achieve general compliance with the one right way to do things. Yet the very future of *managed* care is said to be in doubt, at least partly because it has not offered customers enough well-informed choice.[9] A marketing paradigm at least recognizes the importance of choice, both as a means of promoting the likelihood that consumers will find *something* they like and as a value in itself, a degree of control versus coercion. *Management* is simply the wrong paradigm for influencing consumer behavior, except perhaps in law enforcement.[10]

Throughout this book we use the term demand improvement to describe what we think is the real challenge—improving both the health and care-seeking behaviors of consumers. And we employ something more like a marketing paradigm (ie, one in which sponsors and practitioners of demand improvement attempt to deliver value to consumers as a primary aim, as opposed to focusing exclusively on maximizing their own value). Cutting costs has always been the easier path to short-term financial success, while improving value is the more difficult, but ultimately more rewarding business strategy.[11]

In our paradigm, demand *improvement* means improving the health and quality of life of consumers first, with many more considerations than just the quantity of health care utilization and expenditures. It delivers value to consumers by empowering them to better manage their own health, illnesses, and injuries and to make the most informed choices about necessary health care. We treat the savings to sponsors that successful demand improvement initiatives have been shown to produce as well-deserved rewards for delivering improved consumer value, rather than as the sole aim and chief justification for such initiatives.

We are convinced that had such a paradigm been used from the beginning by payers, particularly by managed care organizations (MCOs), the years of health maintenance organization (HMO) bashing by consumer champions, media, lawyers, and legislators would have been avoided. We believe that payers and providers at financial risk can achieve at least as much success in dealing with that risk by focusing on delivering improved value to consumers as they have through attempts to control providers and manage demand.

We also prefer the idea of *improving* demand because it clearly denotes a concern with the *quality* of demand as well as quantity. And it implies a willingness to continuously strive to do better, where "management" aims primarily at compliance—now. We hope that continuous demand improvement becomes as widely recognized and practiced in health care as are continuous quality improvement and process improvement.[12]

This book will focus on improving health and demand through positively influencing *consumer* behavior. While we recognize the pivotal role that *providers* can play in influencing consumers' health-risk behaviors and their demand for and use of health services, we are convinced that utilization management is better applied to providers, though it has had its failures as well as successes. We will discuss the role of providers only as helpful and potentially powerful supporters of improvements in consumer behavior.[13]

While our primary focus will be on delivering value to consumers as a precondition for successful demand improvement, we will also address other stakeholders who stand to benefit therefrom. Employers, providers, governments, and health plans can all gain much more than cost savings through properly targeted, planned, and implemented demand improvement initiatives. We will regularly point out where such added gains are possible and where they have been documented.

Because so many stand to gain so much from successful demand improvement, including consumers themselves, we address this book to the wide variety of individuals and organizations who should consider sponsoring, initiating, or participating in specific efforts. We will discuss examples of a variety of physicians' and nurses' initiatives, as well as efforts by governments, hospitals, employers, unions, health plans, and community organizations. We hope all potential sponsors and participants will approach the idea of improving demand with an open mind and particularly that they will be open to the idea of cooperating with each other in specific efforts.

HOW THE BOOK IS ORGANIZED

This book in organized into five parts. Part I introduces demand improvement, defining and delineating what it involves, contrasting it to largely problematic provider- or supply-focused efforts, and pointing out both logical reasons for improving demand and documented evidence of its results. For readers already familiar with the full scope of demand improvement, and particularly those convinced of its worth, this part may be superfluous and could be skimmed. We recommend reading Chapter 2, however, in order to become familiar with the definitions of terms and specific approach we take to the subject throughout the book.

Part II offers a variety of underpinnings for successful demand improvement initiatives and outlines fundamental ways of thinking about and preparing for both strategic and programmatic planning for such initiatives. For readers already comfortable with systems thinking and consumer behavior-change models and with the information and communications foundations for influencing consumer behavior, the first four chapters in this part may also be skimmed. Readers can select which ones of these they wish to learn more about, though we recommend that all read the last chapter in Part II on demand improvement strategy.

Part III introduces what we feel is a complete set of demand improvement tactics, any one of which might be appropriate for specific initiatives, depending on circumstances. Each tactic is worthy of a book of its own, and each has been the subject of books by others. We discuss them as options to consider in the specific context of their potential use in improving health and demand. We recommend this part to all readers considering specific initiatives, if only to acquaint themselves with tactical options they may not have tried or considered in the past. On the other hand, for readers interested chiefly in the strategic aspects of demand improvement and remote from program planning and implementation, this part may be skipped or kept for later reference use.

Part IV covers the particulars of planning specific initiatives, beginning with a recommended planning format and ending with a chapter on evaluation. It is aimed chiefly at those who are charged with planning or implementation at the program level. Readers already confident in their planning, implementation, and evaluation skills may find the content all too familiar, but we believe there are some "wrinkles" that apply particularly to demand improvement that will offer value to all readers in our coverage of these topics.

Part V addresses each of the four domains we include in demand improvement, with a separate and well-referenced chapter on each. Each of these chapters contains many examples of a variety of initiatives implemented by a variety of sponsors. Where strategic planners are focused on one or two of these domains, or even on one or two types of initiatives in one domain, they may choose to reserve for later reading the sections and chapters devoted to other initiatives. We recommend that readers at least skim all four chapters for the full scope of the four domains to become familiar with all the possibilities that may apply to their situation, as well as their most immediate challenges. We feel these chapters should be useful references for subsequent strategic and tactical thinking. And we strongly recommend the last chapter in this part as a source of suggestions for the future development of demand improvement thinking and action in general.

A "NAVIGATOR"

One of the reviewers of the original manuscript reminded us that this book is much too long and detailed for many readers. Moreover, by attempting to cover virtually everything that a wide variety of readers might be interested in learning about the subject, it runs the risk of being too elementary for some and redundant for many experienced readers. She suggested we provide the equivalent of an Internet Navigator as a guide to particular categories of readers on what they should focus on now versus what they might skim or reserve for later reference.

We can hardly customize our advice to every possible type of reader, but two key reader characteristics may help focus their selective attention: (1) strategic versus programmatic interest or responsibility; and (2) familiar versus unfamiliar with the field of demand (management) improvement. While we cannot offer software for readers' use, we do offer a recommended list of parts and chapters (a "Navigator") for each of four categories of readers: A. Strategic Sophisticates; B. Strategic Newcomers; C. Programmatic Sophisticates; and D. Programmatic Newcomers.

We can only estimate where the greatest interest and value might lie for these four segments of readers, but we hope that our "Navigator" will enable most readers to focus on the sections they will find most interesting and relevant, given their backgrounds and responsibilities. In addition to this overall guide, we recommend that readers look through the introductions to each part and each chapter for further help in deciding where they might gain the greatest benefit. Readers whose background and experience have given them great familiarity with a particular chapter topic may find it reasonable to skim or skip discussions that would otherwise fit their interests and responsibilities.

We have identified separate chapters as warranting one of three labels in the Navigator. One label indicates that the chapter is optional for the designated reader segment, useful for reference, perhaps. Another denotes the chapter is recommended, though individual readers may rate specific chapters lower or higher in relevance depending on their individual backgrounds and responsibilities. A third identifies those chapters we feel are essential to any reader's understanding of the discipline of demand improvement and most likely to offer new information and insights.

We hope this guide will at least suggest better options than trying to wade through everything in the book in order to discover specific content of particular interest. Obviously we feel each chapter offers something of value to a significant number of readers or we would not have included it. We suggest that readers might make a first run through focusing on the topics of immediate relevance, reserving other "optional" and "useful" chapters for later reading and reference.

KNOWLEDGE NAVIGATOR

X = Optional
✳ = Useful
○ = Essential

Chapters		Have Strategic Experience	New to Strategic Level	Have Program Experience	New to Programming Level
Pt. I	1	X	○	✳	○
	2	○	○	○	○
	3	X	○	X	✳
	4	X	○	X	✳
	5	✳	○	✳	○
Pt. II	6	✳	✳	✳	✳
	7	✳	✳	✳	✳
	8	X	✳	✳	○
	9	X	✳	✳	○
	10	✳	○	X	✳
Pt. III	11	X	X	✳	○
	12	X	X	✳	○
	13	X	X	✳	○
	14	X	X	✳	○
	15	X	X	✳	○
Pt. IV	16	✳	✳	✳	○
	17	X	✳	✳	○
	18	✳	○	✳	○
	19	✳	○	✳	○
	20	○	○	○	○
Pt. V	21	✳	○	✳	○
	22	✳	○	✳	○
	23	✳	○	✳	○
	24	✳	○	✳	○
	25	○	○	○	○

NOTE THAT PART V CHAPTERS 21–24 MAY BE READ SELECTIVELY BASED ON STRATEGIC OR PROGRAMMATIC INTEREST IN ONE DOMAIN OR COMPONENT(S) THEREOF AMONG THE FOUR DEMAND IMPROVEMENT DOMAINS.

REFERENCES

1. J. Bensky and P. Reynolds, "Keeping Them Well," *Health Systems Review* 29, no. 2 (1996):20–24.

2. I. Lazarus, "Putting Personal Health Management on the Line," *Managed Healthcare* 7, no. 7 (1997):53, 54, 58

3. "PHM '97: Personalized Health Management" (Conference sponsored by IBC Group, Southborough, MA, November 17–19, 1997, Beverly Hills, CA).

4. T. Hughes, et al., "The Role of Population Research in Disease Prevention and Management," *Disease Management & Health Outcomes* 1, no. 1 (1997):42–48.

5. C. Appleby, "Speed Dialing," *Hospitals & Health Networks,* 20 May 1997, 58–60.

6. G. Montrose, "Demand Management May Help Stem Costs," *Health Management Technology* February 1995, 18, 21.

7. "Currrents—Managed Care," *Hospitals & Health Networks,* 5 September, 1997, 27–28.

8. D. Beckham, "The Most Important Day," *Healthcare Forum Journal* 39, no. 3 (1996):84–89.

9. R. Herzlinger, *Market-Driven Health Care—Who Wins, Who Loses in the Transformation of America's Largest Service Industry* (Reading, MA: Addison-Wesley, 1997).

10. S. MacStravic, "Managing Demand in Health Care: The Wrong Paradigm," *Managed Care Quarterly* 5, no. 4 (Autumn 1997):8–17.

11. J. Brandon and D. Morris, *Just Don't Do It! Challenging Assumptions in Business* (New York, NY: McGraw-Hill, 1997), 235–255.

12. S. MacStravic, "Remarketing Healthcare: CDI = Continuous Demand Improvement," *The Alliance Report,* March/April 1996, 4, 6, 8, 9, 13.

13. G. Montrose and T. Sullivan, "Demand Management Presents Healthy Opportunities for Physicians," *Journal of Medical Practice Management* 13, no. 4 (1998): 187–190.

PART I

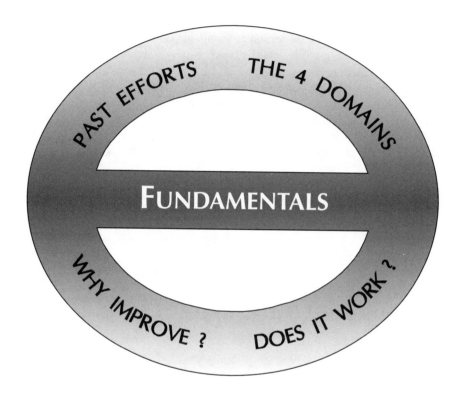

The purpose of Part I is to introduce and justify the pursuit of demand improvement. For those readers already familiar with the full variety of programs aimed at improving consumer health and care-seeking behavior—and already convinced of their efficacy and worth—this part may be superfluous. For those with room left to learn and for those who are undecided about focusing on consumers rather than providers in managing utilization, this part is strongly recommended.

Chapter 1 defines the concept of demand improvement as improving consumer health and care-seeking behavior. Chapter 2 describes the four categories of initiatives that constitute methods for improving demand, emphasizing the wide variety of possibilities available to payers and providers at risk. Chapter 3 identifies past utilization management efforts that have focused on controlling providers or restricting consumers, noting the limitations, risks, and occasional disasters that have accompanied such efforts.

Chapter 4 incorporates an array of arguments in favor of improving consumer demand for health care, in addition to or instead of controlling its supply. Chapter 5 supplements and supports these arguments with evidence from hundreds of studies and case examples where consumer health and care-seeking behaviors have been improved, with resulting value delivered to payers and providers who sponsored initiatives and to consumers themselves.

Part I provides both the vocabulary and dynamics that should make possible an understanding and informed consideration of the potential for improving consumer health care demand. It is offered as the foundation for the balance of the book, which focuses on how to plan, implement, and evaluate specific initiatives to improve consumer health and care-seeking behavior for the benefit of all concerned.

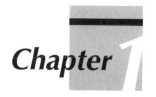

Chapter 1

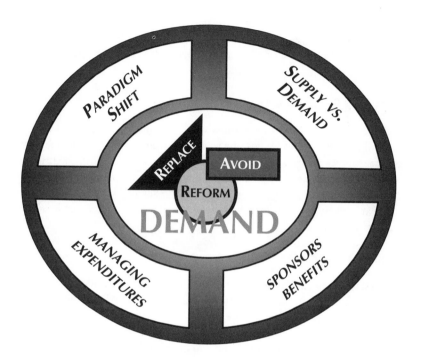

In this chapter we define the basic focus of the book and relate it to other approaches used in the fundamental challenge of controlling health care utilization. We will point out the essential differences between our approach to that challenge and other approaches employed in the past, contrasting reactive and proactive, demarketing and remarketing, gatekeeper and gateway, provider and consumer, rights and responsibilities, management and marketing, reduction and improvement, and barrier and benefit aspects of such approaches.

It is our contention that reforming health care at the national level and that managing health care utilization and expenditures at the health plan, employee group, or community level can be carried out in optimal fashion only when consumers are a major, if not primary, focus of efforts. In this chapter we will introduce our reasons for focusing on improving *consumer demand for* health services, where consumers make the greater difference, as the complement to controlling providers' *supply* or *delivery* of services, the provider role. In the other chapters in Part I we will continue to justify our position.

MANAGING HEALTH CARE EXPENDITURES

In economic terms there are but three ways to manage the costs of health care: (1) control the amounts and types of services utilized, (2) control the quantity and types of resources used in providing those services, or (3) control the prices paid for such resources. Managers in health care payer and provider organizations have been doing as much as they know how in the latter two approaches; this book focuses exclusively on the first and on the effects that consumer behaviors have on utilization of services.[1]

Avoiding the Avoidable

The first challenge in optimizing consumer demand for health care is to avoid or prevent as much of consumer demand for care as possible. By promoting health, fitness, and wellness, we can reduce the susceptibility of populations to disease and injury. By preventing disease and injury through reductions in risky behavior and lifestyles and through improvements in immunization and safety, we can further reduce the number of occasions in a population where health care is needed and likely to be demanded. By empowering those with chronic conditions to manage those conditions better so as to reduce or prevent acute crises, we can further avoid the demand for health care.

There are widely varying estimates, some ranging as high as 50% to 70%, as to the proportion of symptoms, disease, and injury now affecting populations, conditions that could be avoided if everyone behaved in a perfectly healthy manner.[2] It is difficult to estimate the probabilities of reforming everyone's behavior, of course, so the proportion of need that can actually be eliminated is probably a good deal lower. If any significant reduction in demand-driving conditions can be achieved, then use of services should automatically be reduced, except for the use of wellness, risk reduction, and preventive services themselves.

Replacing the Replaceable

Once disease symptoms arise or injuries occur, consumers have two basic choices: deal with them on their own or seek the attention of the health care system. It is estimated that 80% to 90% of all symptoms and problems that arise are dealt with by consumers and their caregivers, without any professional involvement.[3] If that proportion can be increased, it will automatically lessen demands on the system. If consumers, as patients and caregivers, can be empowered to deal appropriately and effectively with more such situations themselves, then use of and expenditures for health care will decline.

Consumers can replace providers as sources of needed care in acute settings, such as cooperative (coop) care units in hospitals. Patients and their caregivers can reduce the extent of professional care needed at home as well. Well-trained parents can enable earlier discharge of newborns with problems. Family members can help keep elderly parents out of nursing homes. If the full potential of consumers' ability to manage their own chronic conditions can be realized, dramatic reductions in the need for professional help can be achieved.

Reforming the Reformable

Whatever success we can achieve in preventing health problems and the need for services and in replacing professional services with consumers' own efforts, there will still remain a substantial amount of morbidity for which professional health care is the appropriate response. The challenge is to reform the quantity, quality, and timing of consumer demand, once care is required, so that unnecessary and inappropriate services are not used while necessary and appropriate services are used. Estimates as high as $200 billion a year have been made as to the extent of unnecessary and inappropriate utilization.[4]

Reforming demand means increasing consumers' use of some services, especially of preventive and early detection services and perhaps of alternative medicine and outpatient care, while decreasing the use of others. The net result, according to most observers, would be a significant reduction in the total quantity of services used and particularly in the total burden of health care expenditures.

The probability of eliminating all unnecessary and inappropriate utilization may be low, but significant improvements in use and reductions in costs are clearly achievable. As will be described in Chapter 5, dramatic improvements in health and reductions in risk (avoided demand), increases in symptom self-care and disease self-management (replaced demand), as well as significant reductions in inappropriate health care utilization and expenditures (reformed demand) have been achieved by many health plans, employers, and providers.

QUANTIFYING EFFECTS

The combined effect of avoiding the avoidable, replacing the replaceable, and reforming the reformable can be estimated in quantitative terms. Purely for illustration, let us say that the average number of health problems encountered in a given population is 50 each year (counting everything: e.g., scrapes and bruises, headaches and fever, heart attacks and cancers). If that number could be reduced to 40, a 20% drop, there should follow a 20% reduction in health care utilization and expenditures, all other things being equal. (It is possible, of course, that the 10 problems avoided will be less serious than the 40 remaining, so that dollar savings may be less than 20%, though they might also be more.)

If the current proportion of unavoided problems that consumers cope with successfully, without professional services, is 80%, and if this proportion can be increased to 85%, a further reduction in demand should result. While an increase from 80% to 85% is a small relative *increase*, the *replacement* impact is from the original 20% requiring professional attention to 15%, or a 25% replacement of demand. If both 20% of all problems were avoided and 25% of demand were replaced by self-care, the total savings in demand could be 40%! Remaining demand would be 15% of the 40 incidents for a total of 6, or 60% of the original amount. (In this case it is likely that the problems where professional care is replaced by self-care would be less serious, so savings most likely would be less than 25% in dollar terms, but this is only an illustration.)

For demand reform, since both quality and quantity are involved, no such simple calculations are possible. However, if the net dollar effect of reform were a reduction of one sixth (16.67%) in average *expenditures* for necessary and appropriate demand (e.g., from $480 to $400 per case), then reducing unnecessary and inappropriate utilization would save another 16.67% in health care expenditures for a total reduction of 50%. Original expenses per person were for 50 "events," of which 10 cases required professional care at an average cost of $480 per case, or $4,800 per person. After all improvements, expenses would be for 40 "events," of which only 6 cases require care at an average cost of $400 per case, or $2,400 per person (Fig 1–1).

Whether the incidence of problems can truly be reduced by 20%, the proportion handled by consumers increased to 85%, and the costs per case reduced by 16.67% is a question to be addressed by sponsors relative to each population at risk. Sponsors may decide to aim for improvements only through avoiding problems, through replacing demand with self-care, through demand reform, or through some combination of the three. (See Chapter 10 for discussion of strategic investment options.)

Because there are costs for the interventions needed to prevent health problems from occurring, for empowering consumers to increase the proportion of problems they handle on their own, and for reforming the patterns of care that consumers demand once in the system, the *net* savings to sponsors from such interventions would be less than illustrated. The challenge is to select interventions that promise and deliver significant positive returns on the investment, not merely demand improvements per se.

Figure 1–1 Dollar Improvements

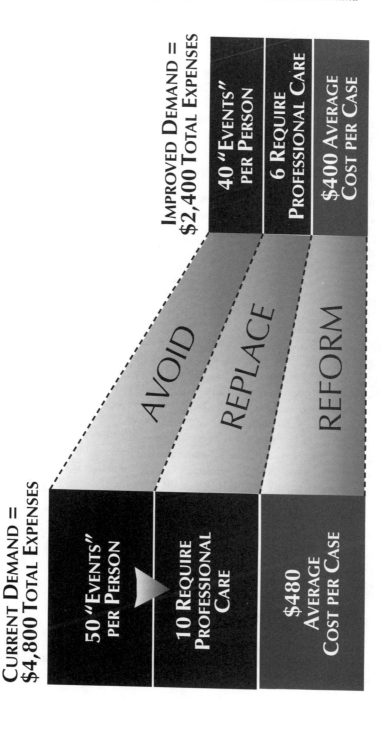

CURRENT DEMAND =
$4,800 TOTAL EXPENSES

50 "EVENTS"
PER PERSON

10 REQUIRE
PROFESSIONAL
CARE

$480
AVERAGE
COST PER CASE

AVOID

REPLACE

REFORM

IMPROVED DEMAND =
$2,400 TOTAL EXPENSES

40 "EVENTS"
PER PERSON

6 REQUIRE
PROFESSIONAL CARE

$400 AVERAGE
COST PER CASE

In any given population the proportions of preventable problems, replaceable demand, and unnecessary and inappropriate utilization will be unique. Each must be approached separately to determine where the greatest potential for improvement lies. It may turn out that the unavoidable and necessary/appropriate demand that remains is more expensive on average than what was avoided, replaced, and reformed, so that total savings are somewhat less. The challenge is to pick the best opportunities and make the most of them.

UTILIZATION = DEMAND × SUPPLY

In any services industry, utilization is a function of both providing (supplying) and consuming (demanding) services, the result of the joint influences of consumers and providers. In some health care situations (e.g., when the consumer is unconscious in an emergency) the provider all but completely dictates what services are used. In others (e.g., for cosmetic surgery and most preventive care) the consumer is the primary determinant. The focus of this book is on the consumer's role in determining the utilization of services, specifically on how to improve both consumers' health and demand behaviors so as to optimize their use of services in terms of value to themselves and to all affected stakeholders.

In this book we will address improving the health, utilization, and expenditure parameters of populations, including methods to better manage the use of services and efforts aimed at improving health/reducing risks, but focusing on consumer, rather than provider behaviors. The terms quality management and utilization management have long been applied to efforts that focus on the behavior of providers; demand improvement deals with consumers.

This does not mean that we will ignore providers; they are powerful, usually essential, partners in improving consumer health and demand behavior. It only means that we will not address how to get providers to "supply" or deliver better or less care; we will cover providers only as influencers on the demands of consumers. (See Chapter 3 for a discussion of "supply-side" efforts aimed at providers.)

In focusing exclusively on consumers, their health, and their use of health care, we are proposing that significant shifts be made in thinking about, planning, and executing specific initiatives aimed at managing utilization. Each of these shifts is advantageous in improving both the effectiveness and efficiency of efforts for improving the use of health services.

SHIFT 1: FROM REACTIVE TO PROACTIVE

The health care system has traditionally been an illness and injury system, geared to treating those whose acute or chronic conditions need medical attention. It has chiefly been a reactive system rather than a proactive one. Limited though significant attention has been given to preventing illness and injury; however, more of that attention has come through public health agencies than from private health plans and providers.

The limited attention given by providers to health rather than disease may be partially attributable to fee-for-service (FFS) financing; providers under FFS payment systems receive revenue based on how much care they provide. And after all, totally doing away with disease and injury would do away with hospitals and physicians as well. Another reason may be the way physicians are trained; once they have invested so much time and energy in learning complex diagnostic and treatment skills, they are committed to using those skills. Most preventive care can be rendered by nonphysicians and is not considered intellectually challenging by most physicians. Reducing health-risky behavior by patients can take a lot of time, and physicians tend to be poorly paid for counseling and similar "cognitive" services as compared to diagnosis and treatment.

Health plans, particularly those with the label health *maintenance* organizations, would seem logical sponsors of proactive efforts aimed at reducing the need for reactive health services. In many cases they have been, but their time-limited commitment to specific enrollees also limits the value they derive from prevention and promotion. With turnover among commercial plan enrollees as high as 20% per year, and usually higher among Medicare and Medicaid enrollees, there is little incentive for health plans to make investments in prevention, where they have long-term payoff.

Preventive services are often not sought by consumers. Consumers may be unaware of the dangers they face or of the prevention available for them. They may perceive themselves to be at such low risk that immunization seems too much trouble. They may feel that it is their right to live life to the fullest, with the health system responsible for fixing whatever problems result. In many cases consumers gain from illness and use of health services (e.g., time off from school or work, disability leave, and payments).

Consumers may not be convinced that their behavior will make a real difference to their health or need for care. They may not accept the idea that it is their responsibility to manage their own health and use of services, particularly when health insurance absolves them of financial responsibility for their transgressions. They may feel that the immediate and sure pleasure of a risky behavior outweighs the threatened, but only probable, distant pain of its long-term consequences.

An early purpose and necessity in managing consumption of health care is to move from a reactive to a proactive mode. This means not only moving the health care/provider system but consumers as well. It requires thinking upstream from the problems we are used to treating and looking for causes and interventions that may well be outside the traditional medical model. Reducing avoidable use of emergency medical services may include reducing the incidence of violence in society, for example. Reducing the incidence of disease and injury may involve psychological, social, and spiritual interventions, as well as medical. Healthy communities programs, sponsored by a variety of governmental, community, and health organizations, have taken such a broad view of the challenge.[5]

SHIFT 2: FROM DEMARKETING TO REMARKETING

The use of demarketing is an accepted approach to reducing demand in managed care.[6] It has been defined as using the marketing mix of product/benefits, price/costs, place/convenience, and promotion/advertising to reverse the normally desired effect (i.e., to *discourage* consumer purchasing or behavior instead of the traditional focus of marketing on *encouraging* consumer demand).[7] Demarketing can include:

- making a given product (e.g., drugs, tobacco) or the use of a particular service appear unattractive, offering little or no benefit—"product" focus;
- making a product or service extremely expensive to purchase (e.g., by increasing taxes on tobacco) or creating an image of the product/service as dangerous/harmful, painful, or embarrassing, e.g., requiring employees to pay more for indemnity as opposed to managed care health insurance—"price" focus;
- making a risky product or untested service difficult to obtain, hard to find, perhaps illegal to purchase or sell—"place" focus; and
- eliminating its advertising or "depromoting" its use by describing its dangers, lack of benefit, high costs and risks, poor availability or access, such has been done with tobacco—"promotion" focus

Through any combination of such tactics, demarketers may be able to reduce consumer demand.

Demarketing has been recommended as a response to the pattern of overuse of health services that threatens the Canadian health system.[8] It has been used by health plans to discourage abuse of emergency department (ED) care by making access more difficult (e.g., requiring plan preapproval of ED visits before covering the costs of care; imposing additional costs through copayment). Plans have demarketed long stays in the hospital after normal delivery by requiring providers to get permission for stays longer than 24 hours. They have depromoted use of extremely expensive treatments (e.g., bone marrow transplants) by insisting that physicians not mention their availability.

Unfortunately demarketing does not work particularly well in health care. When consumers feel the need and desire for some health service, simply frustrating their desire and discouraging them from using specific services is likely to leave them feeling both angry and underserved. Requiring preapproval before allowing use of emergency medical care when consumers perceive an emergency need generates resentment; it was a major factor in the demise of one HMO.[9] Attempts to demarket longer maternity stays have produced major public scandals and legislation guaranteeing 48-hour stays for normal delivery in many states. Health plans have been accused of imposing "gag rules" on physicians, a practice assailed by practically everybody, and a popular basis for managed care "bashing."[10]

The sensible alternative to demarketing can be termed "remarketing." Instead of *discouraging* use of a given product or service, *encourage* the use of a better option. In the case of emergency medical care, phone triage services are designed to promote self-care, to reduce callers' anxiety so they won't feel impelled to obtain immediate care, and to redirect callers to the best option for their circumstances, not to impose a barrier. Maternity programs can promote shorter stays by offering home care after discharge and enabling the mother to get needed rest and the baby to be professionally monitored. Consumers can be helped to make the most appropriate choice among alternative treatments rather than be kept ignorant about those treatments the health plan would rather not pay for.[11]

Aside from any ethical questions about the proper way to guide consumer use of health services, demarketing is likely to have negative long-term consequences on the success of health plans. Once consumers feel aggrieved by efforts to make care less accessible or more expensive or by policies that deprive them of useful information or reasonable options, they may disenroll from the plan, lobby their legislatures, or otherwise voice their displeasure to friends, employers, and unions. Few health plans can afford to constantly overcome high turnover among members; fewer still desire more legislative intervention in their affairs.

SHIFT 3: FROM GATEKEEPER TO GATEWAY

Many managed care plans rely on physicians serving as gatekeepers in controlling use of health services. Each member's primary physician is supposed to deliver all appropriate primary care and to consider carefully the need for any secondary or tertiary (i.e., specialist or subspecialist) services. By and large, physicians have mixed feelings about this role; primary physicians may prefer serving as coordinator and facilitator of their patients' use of services, whereas having to police such use for financial reasons conflicts with their role as patient advocates. Many seem to object particularly to being referred to as gatekeepers in the media or health plan literature.

Instead of striving to keep their patients' use of care in check, primary physicians can, by influencing patient behavior, be *advocates* for their patients' better health and *enablers* of their choosing the best care options. In effect, primary physicians can become gateways to improved quality of life and to patients' competent, confident management of their own health and health service use.

The unpopularity of the gatekeeper role among physicians is becoming recognized, as is its disadvantage in marketing to consumers. Many health plans are now promoting benefit plan options that permit direct access to specialists without having to go through the primary physician. Enabling providers to function as gateways versus gatekeepers will surely have distinct marketing advantages for health plans and provider systems.

SHIFT 4: FROM PROVIDER TO CONSUMER POWER

By reengineering the processes through which consumers select sources of health care and make health choices, power can be redistributed from providers to consumers. Rather than assuming providers can fix any problem, consumers take responsibility for managing their own health. Rather than waiting to discover what providers decide should be done, consumers learn about treatment options and become active partners in making choices that fit their own values.

Many providers have trouble with this concept. As highly trained professionals, they see themselves as uniquely qualified to evaluate their patients' health needs and to recommend proper treatment. Consumers normally lack the education and experience to make informed decisions about complex medical issues. It is bad enough when nonphysicians make health plan decisions in authorizing care; at least they do it full time and have some training. How can consumers be expected to have the expertise and objectivity demanded in most situations?

The challenge is to enable as well as empower consumers to make the best health behavior choices and to participate fully in choosing treatments. To do so they must have access to the information they need in ways they can understand at the times and places when they can use it. They must be encouraged to ask the right questions and raise the right issues when options are discussed. They must be given the information, education, and training they need to play their role well in each circumstance. Providers and payers must play a crucial role as educators and guides to information and training sources. Otherwise they will not realize the full potential of consumers as partners in managing their own health and in making the most appropriate health care decisions.

A host of information technologies are available to providers and payers to aid in enabling consumers to assume a new and expanded role in health management and care decision making. In addition to traditional communications, new interactive video and multimedia technologies, the Internet and its access to providers and consumers all over the world, simulations and virtual reality training techniques can enable consumers to make the best use of their new power. (See Chapter 9 for discussion of Technology.)

Experience has clearly shown that consumers who play an active role as partners with their physicians are more satisfied with their physician and health care in general.[12] As active participants in making treatment decisions, they are less at risk to sue for malpractice if something goes wrong.[13] Providers may not all welcome yielding power to consumers, but they will benefit from it, nonetheless.

SHIFT 5: FROM RIGHTS TO RESPONSIBILITIES

Along with a shift to consumer power comes a shift in roles and responsibilities. In the past consumers and their champions have fought for patient and consumer rights in the form of legislation that institutionalized consumer entitlement to basic health care. Despite decades of argument, the United States is near the bottom of industrialized countries in ensuring access to health care for all its citizens. The country has decided it cannot afford to continue paying for all the care that insured consumers demand and that providers deliver in an unmanaged system, to say nothing of additional care that presently uninsured consumers might demand if universal insurance coverage were achieved.

While the country clearly had in mind great social benefit when it gradually and incrementally increased public entitlement to health care, this created rights without corresponding responsibilities. Eliminating so many of the out-of-pocket costs of health care to consumers made them all but indifferent to what providers were ordering and to the effects their own behavior had on the costs of health care. If consumers could be taxed the precise amount by which their health expenditures exceed what they would be if they were responsible health citizens and prudent consumers of care, there would most likely be a lot more healthy consumers and a lower federal budget deficit.

It may be financially as well as politically impossible to create a system in which consumers pay for their irresponsibility regarding health, but it is possible to do a better job of promoting personal health responsibility. Along with greater power in making health care decisions comes greater responsibility for the consequences of those decisions. With greater access to the best information on the consequences of lifestyle choices, to programs promoting healthy lifestyles and appropriate treatment choices, consumers gain greater ownership in the consequences of their decisions.

Ultimately improving consumer health behaviors means improvement by consumers (i.e., self-improvement). Providers and payers can educate, offer incentives, and use marketing and a variety of tactics to influence consumer decisions and behavior, but the results are up to consumers themselves. Any effort aimed at improving consumer behavior may sound manipulative, but lifestyle decisions are always in the hands of consumers. Informing, educating, and training consumers to be active partners in making treatment choices enables *them* to better manage *their* demand.

SHIFT 6: FROM MANAGEMENT TO MARKETING

Both management and marketing are approaches to getting others to do what we want them to. Management normally aims at controlling the behavior of employees, perhaps of distributors or franchisees with whom it has formal partnerships. It typically relies on power and authority, occasionally on charismatic leadership to achieve its influence on behavior. It is poorly suited to improving the behavior of consumers who can easily terminate their relationship with providers or health plans, for example, or sabotage the efforts of their employers if they do not feel like being managed when it comes to health care.

Management also promises and delivers rewards and punishments and normally expects total compliance with orders and requests. Even when dealing with others outside the organization, such as suppliers, where formal authority is unavailable, managers can use their power as customers to influence behaviors, having available the implied threat of taking their business elsewhere.

Marketers have no power or authority; they aim to get people to *want* to behave the way marketers want them to by seeing to it that consumers will be and perceive themselves to be better off by complying. Marketers rely on the appeal of an exchange of value; consumers buy products and services in exchange for the benefits they gain from the experience. To alter behavior marketers arrange for consumers to gain more in doing so than they give up by switching from the former behavior.

Managers tend to employ an inside-out, me-first approach: "This is what I want them to do; how can I ensure that they do it?" Or: "This is what I want them not to do; how can I ensure that they don't do it?" They may issue orders, make rules, and establish policies and procedures clarifying what it is that employees are to do. Health plans have issued rules restricting what members can demand or requiring them to obtain approvals to do so. They have promoted shorter lengths of stay by "punishing" patients who stay longer by not paying for such stays.

Marketers try an outside-in approach: "This is what they want; how can I arrange for them to get it in a manner whereby I make a profit?" Where managers expect virtually perfect compliance, marketers are delighted if they can convert a small percentage of consumers to a different product or brand. They recognize that consumers differ widely in what they want, so perfect compliance is out of the question. They recognize the significant and lasting value of loyal customers, so aim at lasting and mutually satisfying relationships with consumers as opposed to control and restrictions for short-term savings.

Management may well succeed in making it difficult for consumers to use unnecessary or inappropriate services. Making rules and providing sanctions are well suited to such purposes. Clearly "managing" care has significantly reduced health care expenditures and has made HMOs popular among payers as compared to traditional indemnity insurance. Management typically has greater impact in a shorter time when it works. And the use of restrictions and penalties can produce immediate and significant reductions in health care demand and expenditures.

But when it comes to promoting the use of advantageous services, such as prevention, disease monitoring, and early detection, management has little in its arsenal to attract consumers. Marketing may well be suspect as a device for improving demand because of its traditional emphasis on promoting consumption, but when it comes to advantageous services, this is clearly what is intended.

And if health plans or employers wish to promote healthier lifestyles, both health-promoting behaviors such as exercise and good nutrition and sickness/injury-reducing behaviors such as not smoking and safe driving, management has little to offer. Employers may forbid smoking on the job or require the use of safety equipment at work, but how do they promote smoking cessation among employees outside work, or among dependents and retirees? How can health plans improve the health behaviors of their members through management tactics?

Despite their different approaches, management and marketing share the ability to offer incentives. Managers can promise and deliver *extrinsic* rewards, both financial incentives and psychosocial recognition, to those who comply with their requests or achieve organizational objectives. And these have proven successful in many specific initiatives aimed at consumer behavior improvements.

Marketers can complement management's extrinsic rewards by offering intrinsic benefits as well. They can strive to make the desired behavior more rewarding in itself (e.g., by making an exercise program more fun). They can work on eliminating physical and mental barriers to better behaviors, such as by offering free memberships to a nearby health club or special exercise programs designed for seniors or pregnant women.

This is not to say that managers are limited to the management paradigm when confronting the challenge of improving consumer behavior. They are increasingly employing more marketing-like approaches even to employees, such as contests and competitions to make work more fun. The key issue is whether marketers or managers aim to deliver consumer value as well as derive gains for themselves.

It is the necessity and ultimate worth of delivering value to customers, as a means to both entice initial exchanges and to build lasting relationships, that marks the essential contribution of the marketing paradigm. Old-fashioned management approaches aimed at control and restriction of consumers may have had short-term advantages but have produced a wide range of long-term disasters.

The challenge is to devise an optimum combination of management and marketing approaches, combining the commitment to influence a high proportion of all consumers—in a given employee, enrollee, patient, or community population—with a realization of the centrality of satisfying and maintaining good relations with consumers, as well as with other stakeholders (physicians, hospitals, and employers as well as health plans and community organizations). As will be discussed in Chapter 3, the blind adoption of management versus marketing tactics can have disastrous results.[14]

SHIFT 7: FROM REDUCTION TO REFORM

Early efforts at influencing consumer demand and virtually all efforts aimed at controlling provider delivery of health services were aimed at and evaluated in terms of *reductions* in utilization. Since expenditure reductions were the driving force behind such efforts, this is hardly surprising, but it is short-sighted and unfortunate.

Reducing consumer demand through deductibles, copayment, precertification, and similar demarketing or authoritarian management approaches may have reduced demand but did so indiscriminately. Consumers have failed to obtain preventive services and have delayed or avoided necessary care as well as unnecessary services, and this has often resulted in higher costs later on, when conditions worsened. It has also resulted in declining public confidence in managed care and in providers serving as advocates for their patients. (For more information, see Chapter 3.)

Wellness, health promotion, prevention, and health-risk reduction programs are designed to prevent avoidable expenditures, as well as to improve consumer health and quality of life. Empowering consumers to better manage their own health and chronic conditions can be a big cost saver, in addition to its benefits for consumers. It would be a mistake, however, to aim simply for reductions in utilization, without aiming simultaneously for improvement in both patterns of demand and consumer quality of life and clinical outcomes.

Continuous demand improvement should join continuous quality improvement as requisite competencies and perpetual goals for health care payers and providers alike. Demand reform efforts should aim for increasing the percentage of the cases in which consumers get the right care at the right time in the right place. In one example this meant arranging for the employer to pay for home care for a pregnant woman threatened with premature delivery, even though home care was not a covered benefit, because it improved the outcome for the patient and reduced costs to the employer.[15]

Evaluation of programs to improve consumer demand for health care must address the *quality* as well as *quantity* of health services utilization. Are consumers getting the care they need, particularly prevention and early detection? Are they getting care at the optimal time for health, quality of life, and financial impact? Are they getting it from the sources best able to deliver the right care? Are they satisfied with the care they get and the procedures used to help guide them to that care? Are they satisfied with the parties who are managing their care, whether health plan, employer, physician, hospital, or any combination thereof?

SHIFT 8: FROM BARRIER TO BENEFIT

In contrast to traditional management and demarketing techniques for reducing demand, the best approaches to improving health and consumption of services will deliver *benefits* to consumers, rather than impose access *barriers*. Reducing injury and disease is something virtually all consumers would like to see. Ensuring the right care at the right time in the right place must mean "right" from the consumer's perspective, not simply that of providers and payers.

Effective health improvement, promotion, fitness, and wellness programs should enhance the quality of life for consumers, delivering benefits such as greater energy, optimism, better appearance, and performance in sports and on the job. They should also add to the quantity of life consumers enjoy, with attendant benefits to their loved ones. Consumers, by avoiding service use, can avoid wasted time, out-of-pocket expense, and opportunity costs.

Through reformed patterns of actual use of services, consumers avoid the risks, inconvenience, pain, and discomfort of unnecessary and inappropriate care. They gain the benefits to health and quality of life that come from getting the right care in the right place from the right providers at the right time. They avoid out-of-pocket deductibles and copays for services they don't need. They save lost time from work and enjoyable pursuits. There are plenty of benefits available from improving health and demand to entice consumers to better behavior, rather than relying on imposing barriers.

Care seeking is likely to produce some gains to some consumers, even when it could have been avoided, replaced, or reformed. Such benefits will hamper efforts to avoid all demand that is avoidable, replace all that is replaceable, and reform all that is reformable. On the other hand, there is plenty of opportunity for most consumers to gain under most demand improvement initiatives and for other stakeholders to benefit as well (Fig 1–2).

HOW DEMAND IMPROVEMENT BENEFITS SPONSORS

The focus of this book's approach to improving demand is rightly on benefits to consumers, since their enthusiastic cooperation is essential to success. Nevertheless, the sponsors of health and demand improvement initiatives, whether employers, health plans, providers, or communities, benefit as well. They achieve many of the same benefits they have sought through traditional management efforts aimed at providers or demarketing barriers to consumers, with significant added value as well.

Employers

From better employee, dependent, and retiree health, employers gain increased morale and productivity and reduced turnover and absenteeism, all of which help

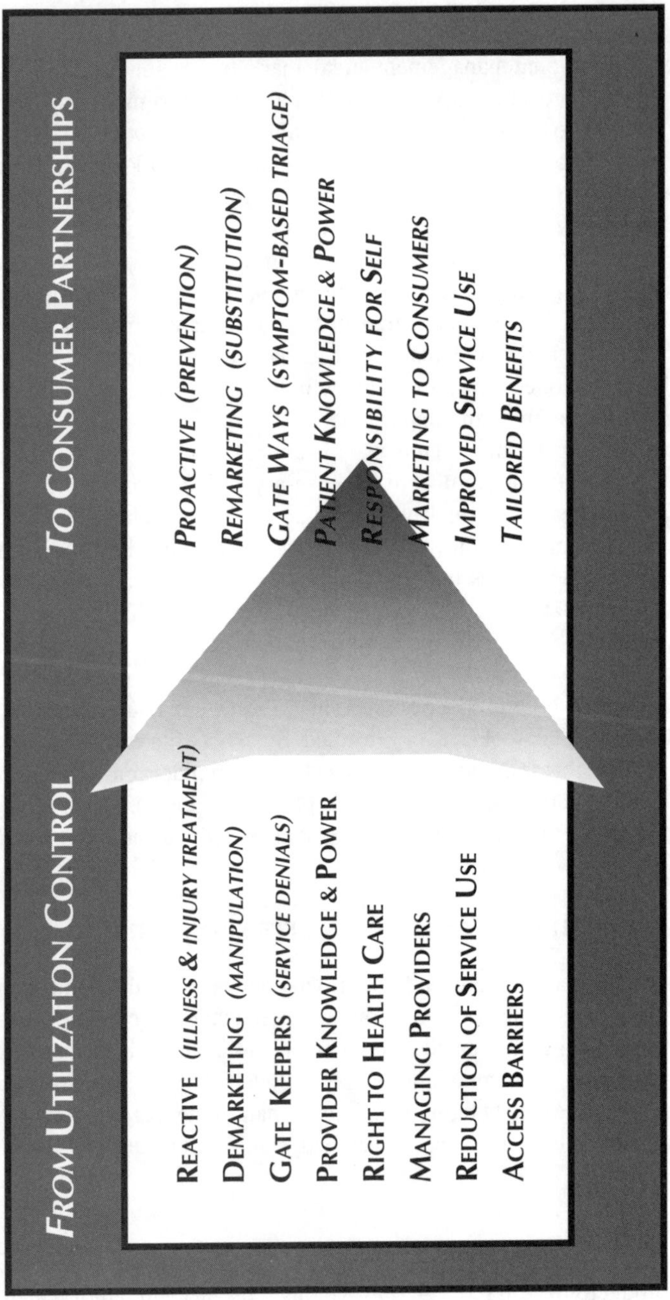

Figure 1–2 Paradigm Shift

FROM UTILIZATION CONTROL

TO CONSUMER PARTNERSHIPS

REACTIVE *(ILLNESS & INJURY TREATMENT)*

DEMARKETING *(MANIPULATION)*

GATE KEEPERS *(SERVICE DENIALS)*

PROVIDER KNOWLEDGE & POWER

RIGHT TO HEALTH CARE

MANAGING PROVIDERS

REDUCTION OF SERVICE USE

ACCESS BARRIERS

PROACTIVE *(PREVENTION)*

REMARKETING *(SUBSTITUTION)*

GATE WAYS *(SYMPTOM-BASED TRIAGE)*

PATIENT KNOWLEDGE & POWER

RESPONSIBILITY FOR SELF

MARKETING TO CONSUMERS

IMPROVED SERVICE USE

TAILORED BENEFITS

to reduce operating costs and improve profits. From demand and expenditures avoided through health promotion and worker safety they also can gain lower health insurance and workers' compensation costs to the extent that their insurance rates are affected by their own experience. Improved quality of demand for care of unavoidable problems also typically reduces disability and absenteeism costs and reinforces employee morale.

Health Plans

Health plans can expect higher levels of member satisfaction as consumers gain better health and quality of life. This will help with performance reporting, such as for National Commission for Quality Assurance (NCQA) accreditation and Health Plan for Employer Data and Information Set (HEDIS) quality indicators. It will promote member retention and stimulate word-of-mouth "advertising" with positive results on enrollment and market share.

The NCQA/HEDIS performance measures are largely dependent on consumer cooperation. Plans can only achieve high levels of immunization if consumers go to where shots are provided. They can only achieve high levels of prenatal care initiated in the first trimester when pregnant women promptly seek such care. Plans may pass on expectations of such performance to providers but can only succeed with the help of consumers.[16]

Avoided utilization means lower costs for plans, giving them competitive advantages over plans that do not optimize demand or are less successful at it. Improved use of care for unavoidable problems reduces plans' legal risks as well as potentially adding to cost savings, competitive position, market share, and profits.

Providers

Providers stand to gain patient satisfaction, retention, loyalty, and word-of-mouth effects as well. More satisfied patients are less likely to sue and can provide leverage for providers wishing to achieve, maintain, or improve the terms of managed care contracts. Provider performance on NCQA/HEDIS measures can be optimized only with consumer help.

Provider performance for health plan credentialing or public reporting will be enhanced by improved cooperation of consumers in prevention of disease and injury, as well as management of chronic conditions. When sharing risks under capitation payment systems, providers gain from avoided and improved utilization the same financial benefits as do employers and health plans.

Communities

Communities gain from demand improvement success, whether or not they are actively involved in efforts. They gain from improved citizen quality of life and clinical outcome improvements, as well as from reduction in expenditures. They save the social costs of poor health and misdirected demand and stand to save when health and demand can be improved among population segments that are paid for by government insurance programs. Communitywide gains among the uninsured and under-insured also benefit employers, health plans, and providers by reducing expenditures that produce cost-shifting to those sponsors.

REFERENCES

1. D. Powell, "Control Health Care Costs by Controlling Demand," *Human Resource Professional* 8, no. 2 (1995):19–22.

2. J. Fries, et al., "Reducing Health Care Costs by Reducing the Need and Demand for Medical Services," *New England Journal of Medicine* 329, no. 3 (1993):321–325.

3. D. Sobel, "Self-Care, Values Lead to Healthy Communities," *Health Progress* 75, no. 6 (1994): 70–72, 79.

4. "Wasted Health Care Dollars," *Consumer Reports* 57, no. 7 (1992):435–448.

5. T. Hancock, "Seeing the Vision, Defining Your Role," *Healthcare Forum Journal* 36, no. 3 (1993):30–35.

6. P. Kotler and R. Clarke, *Marketing for Health Care Organizations* (Englewood Cliffs, NJ: Prentice-Hall, 1987), 16.

7. J. Fries, "Reducing Need and Demand," *Healthcare Forum Journal* 36, no. 5 (1993):18–23.

8. G. Kindra and D.W. Taylor, "Demarketing Inappropriate Health Care Consumption," *Journal of Health Care Marketing* 15, no. 2 (1995):10–14.

9. R.S. MacStravic, "The Demise of an HMO—A Marketing Perspective," *Journal of Health Care Marketing* 2, no. 4 (1982):9–16.

10. "The Tricky Business of Keeping Doctors Quiet," *Managed Care Competitive Network* 5, no. 3 (1997):4.

11. S. MacStravic, "Remarketing, Yes, Remarketing Health Care," *Journal of Health Care Marketing* 15, no. 4 (1995):57–58.

12. E. Speedling and G. Rosenberg, "Patient Well-Being: A Responsibility for Hospital Managers," *Health Care Management Review* 11, no. 3 (1986):9–19.

13. P. Sommers and M. Thompson, "The Best Malpractice Insurance of Them All: Customer Satisfaction," *Health Marketing Quarterly* 1, no. 1 (1983):83–91.

14. S. MacStravic, "Marketing or Management: Which Way the Future?" *Journal of Health Care Marketing* 16, no. 2 (1996):10–13.

15. "Physician Triage Practice Reduces LOS, Saves HMO Dollars," *Healthcare Demand Management* 2, no. 6 (1996):88–90.

16. "From Eye Examinations to Vaccines, Here's What Medicare HEDIS Will Require Next Year," *Public Sector Contracting Report* 2, no. 10 (1996):150–151.

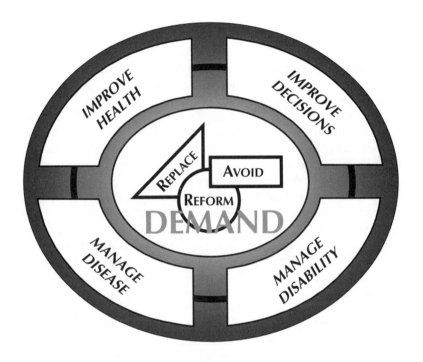

Chapter 2

THE FOUR DOMAINS OF DEMAND IMPROVEMENT

With the definition and contrasts made to other approaches for controlling utilization from Chapter 1, we now move to describing the basic domains of demand improvement. Efforts to improve consumer health and demand behaviors fall into four distinct, though related, categories of initiatives, each with a slightly different purpose:

1. Health improvement—Reducing morbidity and need for care
2. Decision improvement—Making better-informed care choices

21

3. Disease (self)-management—Improving process and outcomes through consumer management of acute and chronic conditions
4. Disability management—Doing all three in the workers' compensation/disability context

HEALTH IMPROVEMENT

This first of the four demand improvement domains is commonly referred to as health risk reduction, or health hazard management. We use the term health improvement here to emphasize the positive purpose of improving consumer health, though the results are similar. Health improvement aims at avoiding the need for health care in the first place by reducing preventable and avoidable disease and injury as much as possible. This, if successful, would significantly reduce the demand for illness-related and injury-related health services, leaving only unavoidable morbidity and the demand caused thereby.

Health improvement includes health risk reduction and health promotion as well as both primary and secondary prevention (tertiary prevention will be discussed under disease management). It includes health and fitness promotion and wellness programs aimed at encouraging "positive health" in addition to efforts intended to reduce the incidence and prevalence of specific morbidity. While the role and importance of providers in health improvement are fully acknowledged, the emphasis in this discussion, as throughout the book, will be on the behavior of consumers.

Health improvement reflects a desire to "move upstream" in managing care consumption by looking for opportunities to avoid the conditions that necessitate or at least stimulate demand at the source. Where efforts in controlling care *delivery* begin once consumers seek care, improving *demand* begins earlier to prevent the conditions that prompt demand, addressing need as well.[1]

Health improvement has four basic components: health promotion, risk reduction, prevention, and early detection. Each may be found described in other ways, but the basic ideas are consistent. Each plays a separate but significant role in the effort aimed at avoiding the need for health care in the first place. Where the other domains are more focused in terms of the consumers targeted for attention or the timing of interventions, health improvement generally aims at entire populations throughout their lives.

Wellness, Fitness, and Health Promotion

Programs variously referred to as wellness, health promotion, or fitness are important components of health improvement. Though each may be defined differently, all share an emphasis on protecting or improving some aspect of physical, social, emotional, and spiritual well-being throughout the population and on making consumers as resistant as possible to disease and injury.

Physical health or fitness is usually addressed through some combination of exercise and diet. While the emphasis of health promotion, wellness, and fitness programs is on improving health in a positive direction rather than preventing specific disease or injury, the success of such programs is usually *measured* in terms of reduced risk or lower incidence of morbidity and mortality. Since there is no overall "thermometer" or summary measure for positive health, lower risk or incidence of morbidity and mortality can be used for estimating value in planning and evaluating health improvement initiatives. (See Chapters 16 and 20 for further discussion of planning and evaluation.)

Health Risk Reduction

Related to wellness, fitness, and health promotion are health risk or health hazard programs. These aim first to identify, then to reduce the risks reflected in unhealthy behaviors. Health risk assessments or appraisals (HRAs), for example, are typically surveys of populations aimed at discovering patterns of self-reported behavior that represent low or high risk of disease or injury. They usually include questions on common hazardous behaviors, such as smoking, excessive alcohol use, and lack of physical activity that are associated with higher incidence of disease. Risk of injury is addressed by including questions about use of seat belts and motorcycle or bicycle helmets, drinking and driving, and participation in dangerous sports or hobbies, such as bungie jumping or sky diving.

In addition to behaviors, HRAs may ask consumers about their weight, body fat, cholesterol levels, blood pressure, and any chronic conditions they might have. While such self-reporting may be unreliable and inaccurate, it can provide a basis for early detection. By including questions on health status measures, HRAs can help identify the extent of a population's awareness of specific health conditions as a prelude to clinical verification or awareness promotion.

Perceived stress is often included, together, perhaps, with questions on, for example, how people cope with stress, degree of social involvement, availability of support groups. Spiritual health may be addressed through questions on one's orientation toward life, religion, and sense of self-worth and self-efficacy. Emotional health might be addressed with questions on, for example, one's sense of connectedness with others, optimism or pessimism, depression, and energy levels. Functional status is measured through questions on activities of daily life and ability to perform them independently. A wide variety of instruments are available to gauge perceived health status, such as the SF-36 and SF-12 questionnaires and Perceived Functional Status surveys.[2]

Data on health risks may be obtained through self-reporting by consumers in a survey, though such data may be unreliable if consumers report what they think surveyors want to hear, what they think they *ought* to be doing or feeling, or even what they *intend* to do rather than actual behavior and perceptions. Where there are financial incentives for low-risk behavior, consumers may exaggerate or underreport specific behaviors to qualify for the incentives. Moreover, only in rare instances will all consumers targeted for risk assessment complete and return questionnaires, so information is often incomplete, even where it is accurate.

On the other hand, since biases and the effects of financial incentives are likely to be constant over time, changes in self-reported health risk behaviors are probably good indicators of trends. Even if the levels of risk may be understated, the extent of changes in risk may be accurately estimated based on HRAs. Where more accurate measures are required, clinical testing may be used.

Ideally both self-reporting and clinical testing will be used, since each provides something the other cannot. Only surveys or interviews of consumers can identify most risky behaviors, though tests can detect unreported smoking and drug use. Only tests can detect, for example, high blood pressure, cholesterol, and human immunodeficiency virus (HIV), though home-testing devices are available. Combining both approaches, however, may seriously reduce the numbers of consumers whose risks are fully identified, since their participation in both surveys and testing is required.

Health risk assessments typically produce overall scores that attempt to reflect a summary measure of a consumer's health risk status. This measure may be stated in terms of expected years of life remaining, with riskier consumers having fewer years remaining for their age than their healthier counterparts or in terms of one's health risk age compared to chronological age. It may simply be a numerical score based on the number of risky behaviors or clinical risk measures identified.

Sponsors may be just as interested in consumers' risk of using health services and costing health insurance expenditures as in their health risks. In some cases health risk can be stated in terms of higher- or lower-than-average risk of dollar costs in, for example, health insurance claims, absenteeism, or disability. Specific consumers may be identified as having a past history-based use ratio of 2.50, for example, meaning that they use 2.5 times the average amount of service expenditures. (See Chapter 21 for further discussion.)

These summary measures can be useful in assessing the overall risk for a defined population or in gauging changes in risk for individuals. Only specific, individual behaviors and test results can truly be "managed," however. Even if employers, health plans, or individual consumers set goals and objectives in terms of risk score reduction, they must focus on specific behaviors and measures to achieve and monitor changes. One can vow to reduce an overall risk score by 10%, for example, but each person must make a specific behavior change to achieve such an improvement.

Primary Prevention

"True" prevention means preventing the incidence of disease or injury in the first place. This is defined as primary prevention. For diseases, prevention can often be achieved through modifying lifestyle behaviors (e.g., abstinence or use of condoms to prevent acquired immune deficiency syndrome [AIDS], avoiding or quitting smoking to prevent lung cancer). Using seat belts, safe driving, and generally careful behavior can prevent or at least reduce injury.

Often, however, prevention requires the cooperation of providers. Immunizations against a host of common childhood diseases and for tetanus, flu, and even pneumonia are recommended for specified populations at risk. Though providers must deliver the immunizations, consumers need to play their role as well, coming in for the shots and, in many cases, demanding immunizations to remind providers. Studies have shown far-less-than-perfect awareness on the part of physicians as to the importance of immunizations and nothing close to perfect performance in giving them to patients.[3] Health plans and employers can improve prevention by reminding providers and consumers and by offering convenient (e.g., shopping mall or worksite) opportunities and even incentives for getting needed immunizations.

Prevention through immunization creates costs to the system and so should be provided and consumed only where it makes sense. Not everyone needs to get a flu shot every autumn, for example; only those whose age or condition puts them at more than average risk should be immunized. Pneumonia vaccinations are only recommended for those at significant risk. It is a challenge shared by both consumers and providers to know who is at sufficient risk to warrant the effort by both. Chapter 10 will discuss the strategic issues related to choosing where to focus specific demand improvement efforts, including prevention.

Early Detection and Intervention

Though defined as secondary prevention, early detection and intervention are not aimed at preventing the incidence of disease or injury but at detecting morbidity at a stage when it can be more effectively and efficiently addressed. It "prevents" the consequences of delayed detection and treatment, rather than the original morbidity itself. Both early and accurate detection are emphasized in this component, since inaccurate detection can lead to unnecessary and inappropriate demand (false positives) or can delay intervention until too late (false negatives).

In some cases early detection relies chiefly on consumers. Breast self-examination by women and testicle self-examination by men are examples. Watching for early signs of cancer and prompt response to symptoms are ways that consumers can promote early diagnosis and treatment. By encouraging consumers to respond immediately to the kinds of chest pain that suggest a heart attack, for example, payers, providers, and public health agencies may reduce damage to the heart and the amounts of care and expense needed.

With the growth of home testing kits and devices, consumers can detect a variety of conditions before routine medical care might. Hypertension can be detected with a home sphygmomanometer, high cholesterol with a home test kit, and pregnancy with a home detection kit. Even AIDS/HIV can be detected through a home blood test kit, though clinical labs must process the blood sample. Concerned consumers can use these tests to promote earlier intervention by providers, if only to confirm or disconfirm the results. Payers and providers may find it cost-effective to provide or pay for such devices for high-risk individuals.

For most conditions, however, providers and clinical tests are required. Hypertension, high cholesterol, diabetes, and similar chronic conditions are more commonly detected through provider testing, even if home testing devices are available. Asthma, ulcers, congestive heart failure, depression, and similar clinical conditions can only be confirmed by physicians, even if strongly suspected by consumers. Other conditions, such as glaucoma, most cancers, and most infections can only be detected at a presymptomatic stage by trained professionals.

Both consumers and providers share an interest in the earliest possible detection of conditions where early detection makes a significant difference to outcomes and to the course and costs of treatment. At the same time, early detection that depends on providers adds to the costs of health care. In most cases screening everyone for every condition where early detection is beneficial would be impractical and uneconomical. The key is to identify who is *sufficiently* at risk due to lifestyle, age, family history, occupation, or other factors to make early detection worth attempting, for both providers and consumers.[4]

Specific suggestions on how to plan and implement effective health improvement initiatives, together with examples of successful efforts, are discussed in detail in Chapter 21.

DECISION IMPROVEMENT

Like health improvement, decision improvement can be aimed at every consumer in the population of interest. It applies only at specific moments in time, however, based on when particular important decisions are being made. It includes five basic types of decisions:

1. health plan selection,
2. provider selection,
3. urgent treatment choice,
4. elective treatment selection, and
5. end-of-life planning.

Health Plan Selection

Employers can be quite interested in the choices that employees and retirees make regarding health insurance plans. In some cases they may prefer that employees obtain insurance through their employed spouses, for example, and offer cafeteria plan alternatives to encourage *deselection* of their own insurance plans. This removes the deselecting employee and dependents from the employer's risk group entirely, saving potentially large amounts of expenditures. It may not change health care demand patterns, but it eliminates the necessity of one employer paying for whatever demand occurs.

More often, where there is a choice, the employer has a preference as to which plan the employee chooses. As employer purchasing coalitions emerge, or if medical spending accounts become national policy, consumers may see their options multiply from the one choice offered by their employers to three, five, eight, or more choices. The federal government is demonstrating a preference for Medicare beneficiaries to select HMO coverage, which should automatically save the government 5% of costs, since it only pays the HMOs 95% of prevailing local costs. Both federal and state governments are pushing Medicaid beneficiaries into HMOs, though often those beneficiaries have no other choice.

While steering employees and other beneficiaries into preferred health plans is chiefly aimed at reducing the sponsors' health insurance expenditures, it may, to some extent, be influenced by prospects of other benefits as well. Employers may come to prefer a health plan that adds value, such as healthier employees, lower absenteeism, higher productivity, and related cost savings over and above health insurance claim costs. Both governments and employers may come to prefer health plans whose providers deliver higher clinical quality and better outcomes, thereby reducing the risk that sponsors will be entangled in malpractice litigation or scandal. They should also be interested in health plans that maintain high levels of member satisfaction and retention.

Consumers are equally interested in health plan choice. They may insist that their employers offer more or different choices. They may request specific indicators of the clinical and service quality offered by health plans' networks of providers, indicators of success on HEDIS performance measures, member services, and claims processing performance. Increasingly, employers are empowering their employees to choose among health plans by offering more choices and by supplying more information on plan performance.

Provider Selection

Within the context of health plans, employers and plans themselves are interested in the provider selections made by consumers. Many insurers offer centers of excellence options, for example, in which consumers are urged to choose selected providers of high-cost treatment, such as open heart surgery or organ transplant, often in distant cities. Such providers are selected by payers based on some combination of proven quality and low price. The challenge is to get consumers to choose the select few over providers with whom they may be more familiar and for whom they have an established preference.

For managed care plans and wherever primary care physicians are paid on a capitation basis, the consumer's selection is a key event. Health plans are challenged to offer consumers enough choices to promote reasonable proximity and consumer acceptance. For consumers with a strong attachment to their personal physician, offering the option of keeping that physician may be what determines whether or not the consumer will choose that health plan.

For some plans, consumer choice of physician may be guided by preferred provider status (i.e., where the plan will pay a higher percentage of charges if the consumer goes to a preferred provider). A similar arrangement may apply to the hospital chosen and to ancillary service providers, such as physical therapists or home health care agencies. Self-insured employers or health plans may steer employees toward preferred providers because they offer lower unit prices or because they better manage overall costs of care or deliver higher clinical and service quality.

Steering consumers to a selected set of providers involves some legal risk for both health plans and employers if providers prove to deliver questionable quality. To control their risks, many payers are increasing the number of options available to consumers and are supplying them with more information on provider performance. Consumers who have more to do with selecting providers tend to be more satisfied with those providers.

Offering choices of "alternative" or "complementary" providers is a growing tendency as part of improving the marketing success and cost control of managed care. Many consumers have developed strong ties to chiropractors, acupuncturists, herbalists, naturopaths, and homeopaths, making them unwilling to switch to managed care if it means giving up or not getting coverage for use of such providers. By the same token, plans have frequently found that alternative providers treat patients at less cost.

Urgent Treatment Choice

One of the easiest and quickest ways to manage demand for health services is to intervene in choices consumers make when they feel the need for immediate medical attention. Consumer perceptions of what constitutes a "medical emergency" are often totally different from what professionals think; they may be outrageous at times. An ambulance may roll up to the door of a hospital emergency department carrying a patient with a sprained thumb! Countless patients show up at a hospital in the middle of the night complaining of problems they have had for days, even weeks.

Whether we define such cases as unnecessary or inappropriate, the point is, such demand is often replaceable. Capitated providers, plans, and employers sponsor or offer a variety of triage and self-care counseling services by phone, available 24 hours a day. They give away self-care books and pamphlets and provide self-care instruction and training so that consumers can and will treat a large portion of their routine medical problems on their own, without seeking professional help.

It is estimated that consumers diagnose and treat 80% to 90% of their own health problems at home, with no professional contact. Consumers are the true "primary providers." The challenge is to motivate and enable their self-treatments to be appropriately chosen and effectively carried out. *Giving* the right care in the right place at the right time is just as important as *getting* it.

The key in such situations is to accurately and quickly assess the seriousness of the symptoms experienced by consumers. On their own, self-care guides ask questions that help the consumer determine if a true emergency exists, or if self-care, a routine appointment, or a wait-and-see approach would make sense. Callers to phone triage services challenge triage nurses to make the same determinations, without claiming to make a diagnosis over the phone or talking callers out of getting care they should have.

Counseling services are aimed not simply at diverting consumers from using a level of care they do not need or seeking it earlier than they have to; they also promote early detection and intervention for truly urgent and emergent conditions where callers might be reluctant to seek care. Callers may be experiencing chest pain, for example, and fear the embarrassment of rushing to emergency care only to find out it is simple heartburn. They may be convinced that it cannot be serious but want the reassurance of a professional confirming their conclusion. In such cases triage nurses can prompt callers to get immediate care and will even call 911 on their behalf.

Triage programs can serve as gateways to care rather than gatekeepers. They can authorize immediate care at a hospital emergency department or urgent care center, for example. They can make a direct referral to a specialist, bypassing the primary physician who would normally have to make such a referral. They can even make an appointment for the caller to see a specialist or one with the caller's primary care physician where appropriate. In this way they become a consumer benefit rather than a bureaucratic nuisance.

Phone triage and self-care guides seem to work. Virtually every published report of their effects has demonstrated significant savings for both payers and providers, and as of this writing, there appears to have been only one instance of a successful lawsuit for bad advice. One safeguard for phone triage programs is that they are, in most cases, *doubly* voluntary: consumers do not have to call them before seeking care and do not have to follow the advice they get. At the same time, most such programs have achieved high levels of consumer participation, similarly high proportions of callers following the advice they get, and positive effects on both consumer satisfaction and member retention. (Specific examples will be discussed in Chapter 5.)

Elective Treatment Choices

In addition to phone counseling and self-care guides to help consumers make decisions about urgent care needs, a variety of information, education, and counseling services are available to help consumers make choices among elective treatment options. By definition, this involves situations where there are treatment options to choose among and where consumers have the time to make a considered decision.

Where phone triage services are based on a simple, single technology, namely, the phone, perhaps supplemented by a self-care guide, elective treatment decisions can be assisted by a wide variety of information technologies and multiple sources of information rather than one or two. They typically begin with the physician, who makes the initial diagnosis, or perhaps the specialist, who confirms it, and the personal, one-on-one counseling that occurs in that context.

To supplement this counseling, both to save physician time and to greatly increase the consumer's access to information, many other sources and technologies are available. Nurses and educators on the physician's staff may be brought in to help. Printed literature from medical associations and organizations such as the American Cancer Society and American Heart Association can be used. Resource centers such as those offered through Planetree program hospitals can provide consumers with entire libraries of information. Time-Life offered a set of videos recommended by former Surgeon General C. Everett Koop on specific conditions and treatments, though these failed to excite much interest.[5]

Beyond the printed word, many hospitals offer hundreds of audiotapes that can be accessed by phone covering specific conditions and treatment options. Videotapes and interactive video or computer systems can cover specific conditions and treatment options in depth, including comments from patients who have chosen different options. Consumers with access to the Internet can seek information from others faced with the same choice, over and above whatever information is given them by providers and payers.

In most cases promoting consumer involvement in making such decisions is prompted by experience showing that consumers tend to be more conservative than providers and more likely to choose medical over surgical alternatives and watchful waiting over aggressive intervention.[6] Not only are these choices less costly to payers, they also can reduce risks of nosocomial infections from hospital stays where outpatient options are chosen and adverse outcomes or complications from treatment where watchful waiting is preferred.

Even if this were not the case, there is value in consumer participation. In addition to the fact that consumers who are involved in choosing therapies tend to be more satisfied with the result, some of the technologies used to inform consumers can also test their understanding of their options, thereby "proving" informed consent was given and reducing risk of malpractice litigation.[7]

End-of-Life Planning

It is an unfortunate but unavoidable reality that consumer choices have to be made and that these choices make a major difference in the use of services and costs of care at the end of life. Such choices may also apply at the beginning of life for seriously compromised newborns, though options are severely circumscribed by government legislation and regulations under the Americans with Disabilities Act. For people who are terminally ill or who wish to spend their final days at home, special arrangements must be made to avoid unwanted and futile medical interventions.

Payers may promote end-of-life planning because of the money it saves. Studies have shown that patients who die with advance directives in place spend considerably fewer health care dollars than those without such directives.[8] Other studies have also shown that even with directives in place, there is often poor adherence by providers due to miscommunications, objections by relatives, fear of litigation, or other problems.[9]

Consumers can employ end-of-life planning so as to minimize the pain and indignities that may accompany an unplanned passing. Surely patients and their families should have the final say at such a time. Unfortunately the "default position" of providers tends to be to do everything possible, whether or not significant benefit is likely. Consumers must take an active, assertive role to be sure their wishes are followed.

Specific suggestions on how to plan and implement effective decision improvement programs, together with examples of successful efforts, are discussed in detail in Chapter 22.

DISEASE MANAGEMENT

This now familiar term, disease management, should probably be changed to "condition" management since it covers injuries as well as diseases and includes pregnancy, which is neither. To distinguish it from the wide range of programs through which *providers* manage conditions (e.g., case management, outcomes management), we should also probably call it "disease *self*-management," since we are talking about what consumers (i.e., patients and family/friend caregivers) do rather than what providers do. We use the term disease management because it is the familiar and accepted term.

In contrast to both health improvement and decision improvement, which can apply to any and all members of a population, disease management (sometimes referred to as disease state management) applies only to those segments of a population who (1) have a chronic condition, (2) are dealing with an acute illness or injury, (3) have a mental/behavioral health problem, or (4) are pregnant (clearly not a disease but managed in a similar fashion).

Its purpose is to empower consumers (who, by definition, qualify as "patients," since they are under a provider's care) or their caregivers to participate actively and effectively in managing their own or a loved one's condition. The challenges of disease management are somewhat different for acute versus chronic conditions and are unique for behavioral health problems and for pregnancy.

Acute Conditions

The challenges of influencing consumer behavior throughout an episode of acute illness or injury overlap with those of decision management up to the point where treatment begins. Sponsors want consumers to obtain the right care at the right place and time to ensure they are diagnosed and treated at a point where optimum efficiency and effectiveness are possible. Once diagnosed, with treatment determined, the acute disease challenge is to promote consumer contributions through their role in treatment, recovery, and rehabilitation processes. (We recommend the use of the terms "contribute" and "cooperate" rather than "comply" as a better way to approach this challenge, something consumers can be proud of. Who wants to be known for being "compliant"?)

Left to their own devices, consumers may not contribute. They may not get their prescriptions filled, thereby never initiating intended therapy. They may take their medications improperly: too much or too little at a time, at the wrong times, irregularly, incompletely. They may fail to initiate changes in behavior (e.g., bed rest, diet changes, activity modifications) or end them too soon. They may engage in activities or take other medications, food, or drinks that are contraindicated while they are taking medications for a specific condition.

While achieving patient contributions is most commonly a challenge once patients are discharged from care, it applies to periods of hospitalization as well. Increasingly the clinical paths and patient care plans that providers are using to make inpatient care more effective and efficient specify a role for the patient and often for family or other caregivers as well. Enthusiastic and effective cooperation in consumer roles can make a big difference to the success and cost of treatment. In hospital cooperative care units, contributions by patients and caregivers to the care process have reduced costs by 30% or more.[10]

For some conditions, tuberculosis (TB) being one of the best illustrations, patient cooperation in taking prescribed medications can be a long, complicated process, and the costs of noncooperation can be astronomical. Prescription drug treatment for TB takes a full year. Irregular and/or too quickly terminated taking of medications makes the condition resistant to conventional, inexpensive treatment and can raise the costs of treatment by $100,000 per case in addition to making the TB patient a risk to others.[11]

For many self-limiting acute conditions, failure to cooperate in treatment and lifestyle regimens may have little impact; it may even cost less if some treatments and medications are avoided. If correct diagnoses and treatment decisions are made by providers, however, the costs of noncooperation can be significant. The length of recovery may be extended, more serious conditions may arise, dramatic increases in expenditures may be needed to make up for failing to do it right the first time. The challenge is to make realizing the full potential of consumer contributions not simply a "power trip" in which providers insist on controlling their patients or patients insist on resisting, but a meaningful partnership in which providers and patients cooperate in achieving the best possible results.

Chronic Conditions

The most common applications of disease management are for chronic conditions. These have included AIDS, arthritis, asthma, congestive heart failure (CHF), chronic fatigue syndrome (CFS), chronic obstructive pulmonary disease (COPD), depression, diabetes, headache, hypertension, ischemic heart disease, low back pain, osteoporosis, ulcers, and many more. What they share in common is that the role of patients as well as their caregivers can make an enormous difference to the costs of treating consumers with such conditions—and the costs of this treatment can constitute the largest single reason for annual health expenditures for employers, health plans, and consumers.

Disease management applied to chronic conditions has produced savings in annual expenditures for individuals with particular chronic conditions of up to 80% or 90%.[12] It can have dramatic impact on total costs of care in a relatively short time, as patients and caregivers tend to be motivated to participate and often need only be trained and supported in playing their roles. Some may be of the old school, expecting providers to do everything, or may be fatalistic about their ability to make a difference and therefore poor candidates for active partnership. But most seem to be enthusiastic about the idea. (See Chapter 23 for some examples.)

Providers have not been uniformly enthusiastic either; some apparently feel that patients are ill suited or ill prepared to play a significant role or that providers should be the ones who manage disease. Once having experienced the difference that effective disease management can make to their patients' need for and consumption of care and to after-hours demands on their time, providers may become enthusiasts as well.

Behavioral Health

It is a well-established, though perhaps unfortunate, reality that behavioral or mental health problems have been treated as fundamentally separate from physical conditions. Health insurance coverage has long been more restricted for behavioral health care, perhaps because diagnosis and cure are determined cognitively and subjectively rather than via objective laboratory parameters.

There is growing recognition of both the medical/physical aspects of behavioral health problems and the impact that mental problems such as depression have on the demand for somatic medical care. These are pushing the inclusion of behavioral health in demand improvement efforts, even though it still lags behind physical health in medical insurance coverage. Because behavioral health necessarily focuses on consumer behavior, it clearly belongs among the disease management challenges covered in this book.

Pregnancy

The management of patient (and partner) behavior around an episode of pregnancy may seem inappropriate in the category of disease management, since pregnancy is by no means a disease. This discussion is included here because the challenges and the differences that a well-managed pregnancy makes are similar to those already described relative to acute, chronic, and behavioral health conditions. The techniques used to realize the potential for consumer contributions to better pregnancy outcomes are also essentially similar.

In one sense, engaging pregnant women and their partners as effective participants in managing pregnancy is one of the most promising areas for making a difference in health care expenditures, as well as in the health of society. Maternity is far and away the most common reason for hospitalization and accounts for a sizable proportion of all health care expenditures. One case of poor pregnancy management, reflected in the birth of an extremely premature baby, can cost hundreds of thousands, even millions of dollars, in treatment, compared to a few thousand for the normal delivery of a healthy infant.

Complicating the management of pregnancy are the large and growing risks of babies born with fetal alcohol or fetal drug syndrome. Both conditions are the direct result of pregnant women abusing their bodies and that of their babies in utero through the use of alcohol and drugs. Add to this the risks and costs associated with babies born with HIV and AIDS and the behavior of pregnant women can make billions of dollars of difference in the costs of care and uncountable difference to the quality of life for their babies and to the welfare of society.

In many ways the consumer role during pregnancy is similar to that of acute disease self-management; it includes self-monitoring and self-assessment for early detection of problems, keeping a pattern of physician or midwife appointments, taking prescribed treatment (e.g., vitamins), making changes in diet and activities, and avoiding contraindicated substances. Caregivers can play a significant role in supporting and reminding pregnant women of specific things to do and avoid, though it is the mother who bears by far the greater burden. (If everyone were sentenced to endure what most pregnant women experience during pregnancy and were required to control their behavior to the full extent expected of them, there would likely be lawsuits, media blitzes, and strident demands for reform legislation.)

Specific suggestions on how to plan and implement effective disease management programs, together with examples of successful efforts, are discussed in detail in Chapter 23.

DISABILITY MANAGEMENT

The term "disability management" is one already familiar to employers and workers' compensation insurance carriers. In this context we do not refer to "disability" in the normal sense of a permanent limitation, restriction, or disadvantage, but only in the narrow, insurance-dictated sense of a condition for which employers are liable to pay workers' compensation and short-term disability (STD) and long-term disability (LTD) benefits (i.e., employment-connected injuries or diseases). Improving consumer demand in this domain applies to disability benefits as well as medical care associated with such injuries and diseases. (For consumers who are disabled in the normal sense of the word and are not covered under workers' compensation, efforts to improve their quality of life, medical care, and utilization fall under the category disease management, even though in many cases an injury or genetic condition may be involved, rather than any "disease.")

This fourth demand improvement domain is actually a composite of the first three. It includes efforts to promote worker health and fitness plus reduce risk of occupational disease and injury, as does health improvement. It has a special emphasis on selecting providers and treatment options and on steering workers to the best time, place, and type of care, essentially decision improvement. It includes programs aimed at managing acute and chronic conditions attributable to the workplace, on achieving partnerships in efforts aimed at more effective, efficient, and timely cure or rehabilitation and return to work (i.e., disease management).

What puts this component in a category by itself is that it applies only to employed workers and to health plans and providers engaged in occupational health efforts under workers' compensation insurance. Though restricted to workers, it also has the potential added value of promoting employee morale and productivity, while reducing absenteeism and disability costs. Because workers' compensation and disability insurance have a history of fraud and abuse worse than that of conventional health insurance, disability management includes a number of issues related to union/management conflicts, litigation, and legislation that do not apply to the previous three domains.

Disability management, in addition to the other domains, represents an opportunity for dramatic improvements in health care demand and expenditures by consumers. Use of health care under workers' compensation amounts to 10% to 11% of all health expenditures, and the cost of workers' compensation insurance has increased at a rate far in excess of the increase in health insurance expenditures over the past two decades.[13] Moreover, employer attempts to restrict and reduce their workers' compensation liability have often led to shifting the burden to taxpayers.

Safety and Prevention

Like demand improvement in general, disability management includes an emphasis on the prevention of worker injury and occupational illness. By preventing morbidity, both the financial consequences and labor/management hassles in dealing with them can be avoided. Prevention efforts may include improving the work environment; ergonomic analysis and design of workplaces, furniture, and tools; equipment, policies, and procedures to promote safety; training in proper lifting, use of equipment, and safe driving; and safety clothing and protective devices.

Provider and Treatment Choice

Choice of providers has become a particular "cause" for employers after years of scandals regarding unscrupulous providers or those too receptive to employees trying to "game the system." Frequently employers have turned to preferred provider networks or a group of exclusive providers to prevent fraud and abuse. On the other hand, by creating a situation in which providers are more dependent on employer than patient goodwill, they have invited criticism and counterreform measures.

There have been numerous examples of effective management of episodes of injury/illness and treatment, resulting in dramatic savings for employers and improvements in the quality of life for employees. It would be unfortunate if disability management became permanently embroiled in labor-management conflict rather than a way to promote benefit to both.

Specific suggestions for planning and implementing effective disability management programs, together with examples of successful efforts, will be discussed in detail in Chapter 24.

Table 2–1 Goals of Demand Improvement

	IMPROVE HEALTH	IMPROVE DECISIONS	MANAGE DISEASE	MANAGE DISABILITY
AVOID DEMAND	• Health Promotion • Prevention • Risk Reduction		• Lifestyle Changes • Reduce chronic condition cases • Prenatal care	• Occupational safety • Ergonomics
REPLACE DEMAND		• Self-care • Urgent Treatment Choice	• Self-Management • Co-op Care	• Self-care in condition management
REFORM DEMAND	• Early Detection & Intervention	• Plan choice • Provider choice • Elective procedures • Urgent treatment • End of life	• Case Management	• Provider choice • Condition management

CONCLUSION

Each of the four demand improvement domains and their various components contribute significantly to the overall challenge of controlling health care utilization and expenditures through improving consumer health and demand behaviors. All four can save money for governments, taxpayers, employers, health plans, and providers through avoiding, replacing, or reforming demand (Table 2–1).

All four, if so planned and implemented, can deliver added value to employers through better worker morale and productivity, lower absenteeism, and reduced turnover. They can benefit payers and providers through promoting consumer premium and out-of-pocket payment reductions, enhanced quality of life, and thereby satisfaction and loyalty. Each also promises significant added value to consumers and to society as a whole in the form of better health, better control over health choices, and better outcomes of care.

REFERENCES

1. J. Fries, et al., "Reducing Health Care Costs by Reducing the Need and Demand for Medical Services," *New England Journal of Medicine* 329, no. 3 (1993):321–325.
2. F. Wolinsky and T. Stump, "A Measurement Model of the Medical Outcomes Study 36-Item Short-Form Health Survey in a Clinical Sample of Disadvantaged, Older, Black and White Men and Women," *Medical Care* 34, no. 6 (1996):537–548.
3. "Outliers—Kooped Off," *Modern Healthcare,* 3 February 1997, 76.
4. K. Griffin, "The Life Savers: 8 Medical Tests You Shouldn't Ignore," *Health* 10, no. 3 (1996):107–112.
5. "Outliers."
6. F. Fateman, "Multimedia Shared Decision Making Systems," in *The Next Generation of Health Promotion* (Boston, MA: Institute for International Research).
7. "Interactive Video May Change the Face of Medicine," *Marketing to Doctors* 5, no. 11 (1992):7.
8. W. Weeks, et al. "Advance Directives and the Cost of Terminal Hospitalization," *Archives of Internal Medicine* 154 (1994):2077–2083.
9. G. Kolata, "Living Wills Few, Frequently Ignored," *Denver Post,* 12 April, 1997, 12A.
10. J. Friedman, "Good Sam Pushes Program To Bring 'Partner' to Hospital," *The Business Journal,* 7 October, 1985, 6.
11. "Rx Compliance: Moving Beyond the Tip of the Iceberg," *1994 Planning Guide: Talk about Prescriptions* (Washington, DC: National Council on Patient Information and Education, 1994), 1–3.
12. L. Muir, "Disease Management," *Hospital & Health Networks,* 5 June, 1997, 24–30.
13. S. Akabas and L. Gates, *Planning for Disability Management* (Scottsdale, AZ: American Compensation Association, 1995), 2.

Demand Improvement Strategy Vendors

Andersen Consulting Health Services
  Practice
Pittsburgh, PA
  —*Healthcare informatics
    infrastructure*

Ashby • Montrose & Co.
Denver, CO
  —*Health, disease, decision and
    demand management; strategic
    planning*

Applied HealthCare Informatics,
  division of United HealthCare
Minneapolis, MN

Corporate Health Designs
Seattle, WA

Decision Support Technology
Wellesley, MA

Health Decision, International
Golden, CO

Health Enhancement Research
  Organization (HERO)
Birmingham, AL
  —*Predicting impact of interventions*

Health Management Associates
New Bern, NC

Health Management Corp.
Richmond, VA
  —*Planning and evaluation*

Healthcare Forum
San Francisco, CA
  —*Computer simulation
    "community builder" for
    planning community
    interventions*

Healthlink America
Indianapolis, IN

InforMedical
Bouder, CO
  —*Shared decision making, patient
    training technology*

Innovation Associates
Waltham, MA
  —*Computer simulation
    "microworld learning
    experience" for planning*

Johnson & Johnson Health Care
Systems, Health Management
Division
Piscataway, NJ
 —*Health risk appraisals, interest
 surveys, claims analysis, human
 resources cost analysis*

Lynch Consulting, Ltd.
Denver, CO
 —*Vision, strategy, program
 evaluation, predicting utilization,
 segmentation*

Medical Information Systems, Inc.
Lexington, MA
 — *"Wellcast ROI" predicting
 impact of interventions*

MediRisk, Inc.
Atlanta, GA
 —*Predicting Health Costs*

MedStat Group
Ann Arbor, MI
 —*Software, Information Systems,
 Consulting*

Mosby Health Services
St. Louis, MO

Riedel Associates
Conifer, CO
 —*Planning, positioning, marketing,
 promotion*

Strategic Marketing Gorup
Marblehead, MA

Summex Corp.
Indianapolis, IN
 —*Claims Analysis, Interest Surveys
 for Planning*

Total Health Management, Division of
Adventist Health Systems Sunbelt,
Inc.
Orlando, FL
 —*Health Risk, Claims Analysis for
 Planning, Evaluation*

Value Health Sciences, Inc.
Santa Monica, CA
 —*Research, Analytic and
 Consulting Services*

Chapter 3

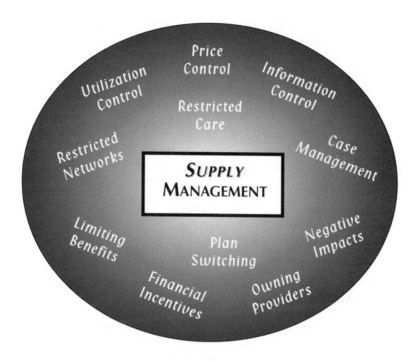

Price
Control

Utilization
Control

Information
Control

Restricted
Care

Restricted
Networks

Case
Management

**SUPPLY
MANAGEMENT**

Limiting
Benefits

Plan
Switching

Negative
Impacts

Financial
Incentives

Owning
Providers

PAST EFFORTS IN
UTILIZATION MANAGEMENT

In this chapter we will discuss supply management, or provider-focused utilization, controls used by employers, health plans, and governments. Such efforts have focused on restricting resources available for care, payment for care, and choices for providers in directing care of their patients. We will also discuss efforts by payers that have affected both providers and consumers through limiting choices of insurance plans, restricting what is covered in benefit packages, and denying information about or coverage for expensive treatments.

Payers have tried to influence provider decisions and care of patients through financial incentives and by restricting the flow of information to consumers. Some have taken on direct control of providers by owning and operating their own practices, while others have developed partnerships with provider organizations. Controls on the provision of care have had many positive results but have also created a significant backlash from providers as well as consumers and from media and politicians.

Until recently the most popular approaches to controlling utilization and expenditures for health services have been primarily aimed at the supply side, focusing on the provision of care rather than its consumption. There is no doubt that these approaches have had some success, though some notable failures as well. In this chapter we will cite the various supply, or provider-behavior, management techniques that have been tried and their successes and failures, and we will argue for the necessity of including consumption-focused, or consumer-behavior, improvement approaches as well.

RESOURCE CONTROL

The idea of controlling the supply of resources to control the use of those resources has been around for centuries. It was employed during the Depression to reduce the number of physicians being turned out by medical schools, thereby keeping meager patient revenues for those physicians who were already in practice. It was used in the Hill-Burton legislation to increase the availability of hospital facilities in rural areas, thereby enabling utilization to come closer to need.

Starting in the 1960s, Certificate-of-Need (CoN) laws were passed and implemented to control what was coming to be perceived as an excess of urban hospital capacity and wasteful duplication of expensive technology. That experiment, using resource controls to reduce utilization and expenditures, was largely a failure or, at best, a limited success. Most states have repealed their CoN laws, having discovered that they tended to delay rather than prevent capital expenditures and added enormous administrative and legal costs to the system.

CoN laws often created perverse incentives, counter to the intention of reformers. Knowing that a limited number of approvals would be forthcoming for any new technology (e.g., magnetic resonance imaging [MRI] or positron emission tomography [PET] scanner, laser surgery), providers submitted CoN applications as soon as they feared they might be left out rather than waiting to be sure there really was a need for the technology. Thereafter, providers would vigorously defend that need, thereby convincing themselves, if no one else. Moreover CoN laws promoted competition among hospitals to see who would "win" CoN approval rather than cooperation that might have been best for the community.

In the past, and where such laws persist, payers, especially large employers, have worked to influence specific capital spending plans by hospitals. In Toledo,

Ohio, the local Business Coalition on Health Care was able to get the state to overturn approval for a $23 million hospital expansion. In Arizona, businesses went even further, demanding that hospitals cap their rate increases as well as control their capital expenditures. Business coalitions in Iowa have opposed hospital replacement as well as expansion projects.[1]

In the absence of such laws, businesses have attempted to apply direct influence on hospital capital decisions. Businesses in Milwaukee, Wisconsin, challenged hospital construction projects. Houston (Texas) business leaders called on their colleagues who served as trustees in area hospitals to reconsider capital expenditure plans.[2] The Miami Valley (Ohio) business coalition opposed hospital bed additions in its area, while the Birmingham (Alabama) coalition influenced the denial of five hospital expansion projects in its jurisdiction.[3]

In recent years payers have moved toward promoting cooperation among hospitals rather than limiting resources. In Detroit, Michigan, for example, General Motors and the United Auto Workers (UAW) are promoting the cooperative development of technologies, combining high-cost programs such as open-heart surgery. In Flint, Michigan, where auto-industry employers account for 80% of local physician and hospital income, they make a formidable partnership.[4]

Despite such efforts, the "medical arms race" continues. Concerns over malpractice litigation force providers to have the latest technologies available, even where they offer only marginal improvement in quality with enormous multiplication of costs.[5] Hospitals and physicians have bought into the argument that they must each be full-service providers to capture managed care contracts.[6]

As the medical arms race continued and utilization of health care began to decline, the idea of controlling resources reemerged. The Pew Commission has called for closing 50% of all hospitals and 20% of medical schools by the year 2005, as well as reducing the number of nurses and pharmacists. Such reductions are argued to be necessary to revitalize the health professions and meet the health care challenges of the 21st century.[7]

PRICE CONTROLS BY PAYERS

In addition to putting pressure on resources, payers have sought to directly reduce what they pay to providers to cut their expenditures. This has be done simply through encouraging or forcing providers to cut their prices. It can be achieved through changing the methods used to calculate or negotiate payments. Finally, it can involve reviewing individual claims and prices for services already rendered.

The Pacific Business Group on Health saved over 9% through collective purchasing clout,[8] while the Minnesota Business Coalition negotiated limits on annual increases: 4.9% in 1996 and no greater than 6% in either 1997 or 1998.[9] Aetna's combination with United Healthcare is expected to give it irresistible clout in demanding provider price reductions.[10]

The Boeing Co. was able to force Wichita hospitals to reduce their prices toward levels that prevailed in the Seattle (Washington) market. Blue Cross in California started a "price war" by sending out a request for proposal (RFP) to hospitals statewide, inviting them to try to be among the low bidders selected for a limited network providing care for a new HMO.[11] With excess hospital capacity and a surplus of physicians, providers are finding themselves under pressure to cut prices just to maintain existing volumes.

When not pressuring providers to cut prices, payers are pushing for changes in the way prices and payments are calculated. They are looking to bundled pricing, combining hospital and physician charges with discounts from both.[12] Employers are moving to per case and per capita payment plans rather than discounted fee-for-service.[13] Insurers are negotiating procedure-specific fees with providers.[14] Not all providers, however, are accepting changes in payment systems without a fight. Physicians in one case filed a lawsuit contesting Aetna's attempt to force them to switch from fee-for-service to capitation payment.[15]

Once prices have been settled, payers look at individual claims for opportunities to save money. They may systematically review all claims for consistency, looking for examples of improbable services, such as delivery room charges for a male patient.[16] Determining which are charges for services not covered under the health plan saved employers 10.7% in one case.[17] Employees are frequently asked to help in such efforts, checking to be sure they actually received all the services that providers billed for.

Payer efforts to control resources and prices were aimed entirely at providers and have had some success. By and large, they did not affect consumers to any significant degree. They also have had only limited effect on providers and on health care utilization and expenditures. To supplement such efforts, payers have also sought to control the way providers deliver care to consumers and to limit what services consumers use. While some of these attempts have had the desired impact, more often they have had negative, often disastrous, side-effects, as we will describe.

RESTRICTING PROVIDER NETWORKS

Rather than pressure all providers they do business with to reduce prices, payers have moved to selecting a limited network of providers based on their quality and prices. Centers of Excellence programs are examples of payers narrowing their networks to a few high-volume, high-quality, low-cost providers for the highest-cost category of procedures, such as organ transplant and open-heart surgery.[18] When primary physicians accept capitation risk, they typically restrict the network of specialists and hospitals to whom they refer.

Essentially the entire panoply of three-letter acronyms for managed care—for example, preferred provider organization (PPO), exclusive provider organization (EPO), point of service (POS), HMO, and integrated delivery network (IDN)—involve restricted numbers of physicians or hospitals delivering care under insurance plans. While these devices are also ways to restrict consumer choice, they aim to reduce payer costs by inducing the select providers to bid low prices to be selected and negotiate or to accept dictated low prices thereafter to retain the business. The plans then use the financial disincentive of lower or no payment to nonselected providers to ensure that consumers use only the low-price providers selected.

While most employers[19] and unions[20] have accepted, even promoted, health plans that restrict provider selection, some are concerned about the potential negative impact such restriction might have on employee relations or the legal risk they might incur should they steer employees to negligent providers.[21] Though we know of no cases of an employee successfully suing an employer as a party to medical negligence, there is always the possibility.

Many employers have decided to engage in direct contracting with providers rather than deal with health plan "middlemen." In some cases this appears to reflect employer concern that plans are making too much profit and not sharing the savings they achieve with the employer.[22] In other cases employers seem to feel they can do a better job of "buying right"[23] in selecting providers than insurers can.[24]

One employer, Signet Bank (Richmond, Virginia) contracted with HMOs for estimated hospital costs. It paid hospital bills as they came in, sharing with HMOs whatever savings or overruns in expenses occurred.[25] Other employers have gone directly to providers for discounted contracts as preferred or exclusive providers for their employees and dependents. Employers are beginning to exercise this option where they, individually or collectively, enjoy negotiating leverage and where direct provider contracting is permitted by law.

RESTRICTING PROVIDER NETWORKS

- ✗ CENTERS OF EXCELLENCE
- ✗ PPO, EPO, POS, HMO PLANS
- ✗ DIRECT CONTRACTING

Limiting provider networks has not been accepted gracefully by providers, particularly those who have been or fear they will be left out of such networks. Legislation has been introduced in over half the states, though passed in few, that would require health plans to include every provider willing to live with health plan rules and payment systems.[26] Such "any willing provider" laws would severely limit health plans' abilities to influence providers.

Limiting the selection of providers available to consumers has hampered the market success of HMOs, PPOs, and EPOs. In turn, this has resulted in the growing popularity of POS plans that open up provider selection, though imposing extra out-of-pocket costs on consumers who take advantage of the privilege.

RESTRICTING THE DELIVERY OF CARE

Directly controlling the delivery of care by some combination of up-front permission, concurrent reviews, and retrospective reviews has been what distinguishes traditional indemnity insurers, who simply pay providers for the services they render, from those who "manage" care. Even where they do not restrict provider choice, payers can restrict the types and amounts of care that providers are allowed to deliver or at least get paid for. Payer efforts in this regard have often been the bane of their existence, however, angering consumers, providers, media, and politicians alike.

In one study utilization review of hospital care was listed as one of the three best cost saving tactics by 34% of payers surveyed. Forty-four percent of respondents had introduced precertification of hospital admission, and 24% had introduced concurrent or retrospective review.[27] Another study reported that employers who used concurrent review had saved an average of 6.1% on their claims costs.[28]

Not long ago second surgical opinion programs were all the rage, with payers hoping that a significant amount of unnecessary or questionable surgery would be avoided. Experience seems to suggest that despite its initial popularity, the pro-

RESTRICTING DELIVERY OF CARE

✗ UTILIZATION REVIEW
✗ SECOND SURGICAL OPINION
✗ PRECERTIFICATION / GATEKEEPING
✗ RESTRICTING MATERNITY LENGTH OF STAY

grams did not work.[29] They often cost more in additional fees for the second opinion than they saved in reduced surgery costs.[30]

Precertification of ED care has been one of the thorniest devices used in controlling delivery, despite well-known consumer abuse of EDs for nonemergency situations. Charges have been made that unqualified health plan staff are making life-and-death decisions over the phone about what is an emergency and are frequently making poor decisions. Cases where patients have died after being turned away stimulate lawsuits and are sure to attract media attention.[31]

Critics have argued that consumers perceiving themselves to be in an emergency situation cannot be expected to calmly call the health plan and wait for permission; and in many cases, such as heart attack, they should not delay. Some HMOs have been charged with intentionally making access to permission difficult by not publishing the number to call or by using an answering machine or service to answer the calls, with consumers waiting until a staff person calls later to discuss the case. Legislation has been proposed at both state and national levels to prevent such abuses by HMOs.[32]

It can be argued that precertification measures are really attempts to change consumer, not provider behavior, by forcing a review of consumer need for care before they can get it. Certainly when consumers call an HMO seeking permission to go to the ED and are refused, they know that they will have trouble getting coverage for the visit should they make one. They may even be convinced by the refusal that they should seek some other option.

However, it is more common for consumers to simply go to the ED, since they feel the immediate need for care; they may even have tried calling for permission only to encounter an answering machine. Once they arrive at the ED it becomes the provider's concern whether the visit will be covered. The managed care health plan typically requires ED providers to seek permission before they treat enrollees. The ED may worry who will pay if the health plan does not. And federal law requires EDs to accept and evaluate every patient to at least determine if a true emergency exists. Thus the ED is required to treat the patient, though the health plan is not required to pay for it.

So, too, the providers in the ED may have a different perception about the patient's need for immediate care, even hospitalization, as compared to the health plan staff person on the phone. Medical ethics require that physicians deliver the care they feel patients need. Yet fearing that the hospital will be stuck with the bill after the health plan has refused authorization, or that it will be struck from the list of preferred providers for disregarding health plan judgment, can providers be effective advocates for their patients?

The gatekeeper system used by most managed care plans requires consumers to obtain permission from their primary physician before seeking care from specialists or hospitals. This is often supplemented by a requirement that the plan approve such care as well. While this has been justified as helping in coordination of care, it is often seen as onerous by consumers. Recent "open access" options offer consumers ways of self-referring to specialists (though not hospitals) without requiring gatekeeper approval.

Requiring payer permission for keeping patients in the hospital has been used to reduce lengths of stay in maternity. After one scandal, the state of New Jersey passed a law requiring insurers to pay for 48 hours following a normal delivery, 96 hours post-Caesarean.[33] Media treatment of "drive-through deliveries" represented one of the early examples of "managed care bashing."[34] Eventually public and media outcry led to the 1996 enactment of federal legislation mandating minimum lengths of stay throughout the United States.

Despite the outcry over maternity, attempts by plans to dictate the length of stays of patients were extended to surgery as well as maternity. Some plans have sought to require that appendectomies and even mastectomies be done on an outpatient basis, limiting post-surgery recovery to under 24 hours. This has given media and litigators a host of new opportunities for bashing HMOs.[35]

GUIDELINES AND CASE MANAGEMENT

By contrast, one of the more effective approaches to controlling the provision of health services has been case management. By assigning a nurse, discharge planner, or social worker to take responsibility for a patient's entire stay and post-discharge care, hospitals have been able to reduce lengths of stay where diagnosis-related group (DRG)/case payment or capitation make such reductions desirable. The key is to reduce stays without increasing readmissions because discharge occurred too early. Under capitation, providers are expanding the concept to total care management, addressing the management of a complete episode of care from primary physician office visit to specialist referral, hospital admission and discharge, or nursing home or home care referral.[36]

The use of clinical paths, clinical maps, and clinical guidelines to cover specific categories of patients has also become a popular device for controlling the provision of care. These employ predetermined, written outlines of what care should be provided, in what sequence, and by which providers, thus helping to coordinate and speed up the delivery of services to eliminate wasteful duplication of services and reduce lengths of stay.[37] The same approach can be used to control provision of care over an entire episode, before and after hospitalization.[38] Effective case management requires and depends upon the participation of patients or family caregivers as well as professionals.

It has been argued that controlling physicians' clinical management of patients is the *only* way to reduce costs of health care.[39] For controlling physicians, specifically, clinical profiles comparing each physician's performance to that of peers and to agreed-upon guidelines have been recommended. By stamping out variations in physician practice, significant savings have been achieved.[40] New computer software programs help physicians select the most cost-effective treatment options in particular cases, saving money as well as reducing the need for utilization management efforts by payers.[41] Getting physicians to use new computer technologies is not always easy, but it has great promise when it can be achieved.[42]

RESULTS OF LIMITING PROVISION OF CARE

There are both direct and indirect effects of limitations imposed on providers. To measure the direct effects, specific instances of requests for approval that were denied, together with estimates of the expenditures that would have resulted if approved, are counted. Indirect effects are more difficult to measure, since they reflect providers' awareness that permission will not be given, providers not requesting approval, and providers simply not providing the care in question. Both effects are included when comparisons are made of utilization and expenditures with versus without provider controls or before versus after the use of provider controls.

There have been and still are champions of provider controls who defend such controls as ways of regulating health care utilization and expenditures. A study by the Robert Wood Johnson Foundation concluded that utilization management saved $51 per insured person per year in avoided expense. It saved $60 per person in hospital utilization at the cost of only $9 per person in additional outpatient utilization.[43]

There are also critics. Utilization management sets up an adversarial relationship between the payer and both providers and consumers. It imposes significant costs on health plans as well as on providers who must do the paperwork and make the calls to get health plan approvals. It imposes a hardship on consumers, particularly in emergency situations. And there seems to be some doubt as to whether, on balance, it has actually saved money.[44]

Vickery has described the effects in one system of precertification on hospital admissions. Health plan staff originally denied 30% of requests for approval; the plan medical director reviewed these denials and cut them to 9%; then patients or their physicians appealed and the number finally denied dropped to 2% of requests.[45] In general, care provision management techniques such as precertification and utilization review are thought to reduce use of services by roughly 1% each.[46]

EMPLOYERS CHANGING HEALTH PLANS

One of the most popular tactics for employers looking to control utilization has been to change their insurance: from traditional unmanaged indemnity to managed indemnity (includes utilization management) or from managed indemnity to

PPO, EPO, HMO, and POS plans. In effect, employers are buying the ability of such plans to control utilization, prices, provider selection, and whatever else it takes to manage expenditures.[47]

Many employers moved carefully into managed care, following a progression of incremental steps. Others went right to an HMO and looked for lower cost HMOs to change to for further savings. Federal and state governments have signed contracts with HMOs for Medicare and Medicaid beneficiaries and are moving all or most Medicaid beneficiaries into HMOs, involuntarily if necessary. Medicare enrollment in HMOs, where involuntary movement is impossible, has been growing only slowly.[48]

In a study by Northwestern National Life Insurance Company, employers were found to have saved $354 per employee per year through shifting from indemnity to PPO coverage (and getting their employees to choose such a plan), compared to $103 via utilization review and $25 through case management. This worked out to represent a return on investment of $10.85 for each dollar spent in the PPO switch, $6.59:1 for utilization review and $5.85:1 for case management.[49] Whether such relative savings and return on investment (ROI) ratios would apply to anyone else considering alternative strategies is likely to depend on each situation, of course.

Recently employers who were concerned about HMOs limiting their employees' choice of providers have added a POS option, allowing employees to go outside the limited panel of selected providers but at additional out-of-pocket cost to employees, both in higher premiums and in higher copayments for using out-of-network providers.[50]

Changes in health plans have frequently been highly effective. Xerox Corp. saved $1000 per employee per year by switching from traditional fee-for-service indemnity plans to HMOs. A survey found that 35% of employers listed PPOs as among the three best cost savings tactics, another 29% listed POS plans. Hospitals have moved into managed care plans for their own employees, with significant savings resulting.[51]

LIMITING HEALTH PLAN BENEFITS

Benefit decisions can influence both consumer and provider behavior in health care utilization. When these decisions are used positively, payers can design benefit packages that facilitate coordination of services, case management, and a seamless continuum of care. When benefit decisions are used negatively, refusal of coverage for treatments that consumers want and that providers determine they should have can result in a horde of unpleasant consequences for payers.

In a longitudinal study of five years of utilization of mental health services by federal employees, significant reductions were found when benefits were reduced. Although the numbers of people using the benefit actually increased from 2.13%

to 2.76% of employees, the average number of visits per user dropped from 19 to 13, more than making up for the increased number of users.[52]

Recent "attacks by anecdote" on managed care have most frequently resulted from denial of coverage for expensive, but potentially lifesaving care.[53] Denial of coverage for a bone marrow transplant for a woman with breast cancer resulted in an $89 million judgment against one HMO. *Time* magazine featured a similar case in a cover story on "The Soul of an HMO."[54] Such publicity probably had some influence on Blue Cross/Blue Shield of Michigan's decision to change its policy to cover bone marrow transplants in such circumstances.[55]

Controlling benefits through the use of drug formularies has been a frequently employed tactic. By listing only lower cost drugs as included in coverage, health plans can shift physician prescribing behavior. However, a 1996 study funded by HMOs themselves found that enrollees in plans with the most severely restricted formularies used other medical services twice as often as did enrollees in plans with no such restrictions.[56]

The very fact that health plans can be accused of "rationing" needed health services puts them at an extreme public relations disadvantage.[57] And the weakening public image of managed care has prompted a number of strenuous and expensive efforts to recover from the anecdotal attacks to which it has been subjected. The American Association of Health Plans and, separately, six of the largest HMOs in the country launched national public relations campaigns to "burnish the industry's image" and to influence threatened legislative intervention.[58]

FINANCIAL INCENTIVES

To a great extent capitation of providers, either separately for each provider's set of services or in "global capitation" covering everything, provides financial incentives to providers in the direction of minimizing unnecessary and avoidable utilization. On a positive side, this can motivate providers to work diligently on promoting patients' health and steering them toward the right care in the right place at the right time. On the negative side, it can motivate them to err on the side of less care to keep as much of their capitation payments as possible. If fee-for-service worked to promote too much care, it must be at least suspected that capitation can promote too little.

Financial incentives have long been used by medical groups in paying their physician members. Bonuses may be paid for "productivity," or the amounts of care physicians deliver, under fee-for-service payment systems. Under capitation bonuses are more likely to be based on unspent capitation amounts and overall profitability of the group. Many include quality and patient satisfaction measures relative to individual physicians in addition to how well they control the volume of services delivered.[59]

In addition to the built-in incentives of capitation, providers have to worry about the threat of deselection from preferred or exclusive provider networks if they are too aggressive or generous in providing care or referring patients elsewhere. Even though deselection is relatively rare, it produces the same kinds of horror stories among providers as coverage denials and drive-through deliveries have among consumers. The maxim that perception is everything applies to the effects of this threat on providers.[60]

To add to the effects of this "stick," many HMOs have offered the "carrot" of financial rewards for controlling utilization. Physician patterns of referral may be the basis for salary increases, special bonuses, or sharing in the profits of the plan.[61] Such incentive systems have been referred to by critics as a health plan "abuse" threatening to deny patients needed care and have been the subject of media and legislative attention.[62] The federal government has created rules restricting the payment of bonuses or other financial incentives to physicians that might induce them to limit the care they provide to Medicare or Medicaid patients.[63]

This same federal government is by no means averse to financial incentives per se. The Health Care Financing Administration (HCFA) announced a bonus plan applicable to medical groups that are able to reduce Medicare expenditures to levels below what was projected for specific populations.[64] In effect this program would give physicians financial incentives similar to those that are embedded in capitation contracts but applicable to fee-for-service patients.

While health plans are usually the ones who determine how to pay providers, employers and purchasing coalitions who have direct contracts with providers can use financial incentives as well. Randall Foods (Houston, Texas) combines a risk-sharing contract with financial incentives for the providers with whom it contracts.[65]

INFORMATION CONTROLS

Perhaps the most egregious example of controlling providers has been the controls over information exerted by health plans through "gag rules." Information controls have restricted the flow of information to consumers about:

- exactly what is and is not covered by insurance benefits, leaving a lot of questions to be decided later by the health plan (e.g., as to what is "experimental" or the "community standard" for care)[66];
- what expensive tests, treatment procedures, or providers outside the health plan network might be better for the patient than those the plan is willing to pay for[67];
- what financial incentives or other business arrangements between the payer and provider might tend to promote underserving, restrict access, or otherwise interfere with providers' ability to be patient advocates[68]; and

- any concerns, criticisms, objections providers have about health plans and their policies and procedures or specific decisions they have made.[69]

While there seems to be a difference of opinion as to how widespread such limits on communication may be, allegations of gag rules have joined the list of "HMO bashing" opportunities for media, organized medicine, and politicians.[70] Regardless of how common a problem it is, the media respond to anecdotes that make good stories, and politicians seem more willing to respond to the media than to HMO denials.[71]

Exacerbating the story of the woman suffering from stage IV breast cancer who was denied coverage for a bone marrow transplant was the charge that her physicians were prevented by their arrangements with the health plan from even mentioning this treatment option.[72] This case produced both a barrage of negative publicity and a $10.2 million judgment against the plan.[73]

Federal rules were promulgated in 1996 to address financial incentives that might promote providers' restricting care or information delivered to consumers. The rules first restrict the paying of bonuses or any incentives beyond those inherent in capitation that might promote underserving. They go on to give Medicare and Medicaid beneficiaries the explicit right to demand information on financial arrangements between plans and providers and require that they be given such information.[74]

Vague contractual language prohibiting providers from "any communication which undermines the confidence"[75(p.9)] of consumers has been employed to eliminate criticism of plans by providers. Such language can be interpreted to include discussion of treatment options not covered and specialists not offered by the plan, as well as financial arrangements between providers and plans.

While most plans deny having any gag rules in their contract, some have taken steps to respond to the storm of criticism about them. US Healthcare, for example, announced that it would *encourage* its contracted physicians to openly discuss treatment options, even if not covered benefits, arguing that it never restricted such discussion but did not encourage it either.[76]

It has been argued that gag rules are both difficult to enforce and unnecessary.[77] It may be that providers at risk for patients' selection of expensive procedures will reduce information flow to patients in their own financial interests.[78] Or the fear of deselection by the plan may be enough to keep physicians in line without contractual language. In fact, the 1996 federal rules specifically prohibit any form of retaliation against providers for discussing treatment options or contract terms with patients.[79]

In addition to federal regulation, state legislation has been proposed to eliminate restrictions on information flow to patients. The American Medical Association's Council on Ethical and Judicial Affairs adopted a position that gag rules were "an unethical interference in the physician–patient relationship."[80(p.8)] California professional liability insurers drafted legislation prohibiting such rules, recognizing their potential impact on malpractice litigation, while both New Jersey and New York have considered legislative and regulatory remedies against information restrictions.[81]

For their part it is incumbent on health plans to eliminate vague language and subjective practices relative to what services are covered benefits. Given publicity over huge profits and executive salaries in some health plans, it is an easy charge to make that plan decisions in "fuzzy" circumstances are made to increase their profits rather than benefit consumers.[82] The National Institute for Health Care Management proposed that benefit plans explicitly describe the criteria and processes used to determine what is a covered benefit, including both quality and cost.[83]

"OWNING" PROVIDERS

Yet another tactic used by payers to control utilization is hiring their own physicians, purchasing and developing practices and hospitals. Employers have moved into offering their own medical clinics at the worksite. Deere & Co. does so in a joint venture with the Mayo Clinic. Gates Rubber Co. has operated its clinic for decades.[84]

Some HMOs have owned and operated their own hospitals for decades (e.g., Kaiser Permanente and Group Health of Puget Sound). Staff HMOs such as Kaiser and Group Health have for decades contracted with or salaried their own physicians. Aetna and Prudential have hired doctors to work in their clinics.[85] CIGNA has purchased the Lovelace Clinic in Albuquerque.[86]

It is difficult to say how much "owning" providers adds to payers' ability to manage the provision of health services. Concerns and legislation relative to the "corporate practice of medicine," together with professional ethics and personal values, will necessarily limit owners' control over physicians. The ownership of hospitals entails such built-in overhead that payers have to be extremely careful about such an investment, and some payers are divesting hospitals they already own.[87]

NEW PARTNERSHIP EFFORTS

A few payers are expanding their roles and relationships with providers. Some are working with providers to develop Integrated Health Systems that integrate finance and delivery.[88] Others have introduced payment schemes that reward providers for better quality, rather than focusing exclusively on price.[89] One employer donated money to the local hospital, but with strings attached based on the hospital's achieving quality improvement goals.[90]

Another works closely with hospitals on case management for individual, high-cost patients, looking to smooth discharge planning and the continuum of care in cooperation with physicians and hospital staff.[91] The Ford Motor Co uses data-based report cards on care rendered to its employees as guidance to area hospitals in their own quality improvement efforts.[92] Analysis of the nation's "best purchasers" concluded that among the six characteristics common to the most successful payers is an emphasis on a long-term cooperative relationship with providers rather than an adversarial or even arms-length relationship.[93]

The most effective payers seem to be those who get actively involved in "managing" or at least influencing the day-to-day operations of providers. They create a sense that all are in it together and work to support as well as demand and reward quality and performance improvements. As employers become more experienced and sophisticated as purchasers, they are expanding their roles and urging providers to move into health and wellness and other consumer-focused activities.[94]

CONCLUSION

In general it seems that efforts to manage the delivery of care by controlling provider behavior have produced a mixed bag of results. Some have achieved significant, even dramatic reductions in health care costs. On the other hand, many have produced lawsuits, scandals, media criticism, and legislative involvement that have threatened the ability of health plans to manage care. It may be time to reconsider many of the supply-side efforts to minimize the delivery of services as ineffective and too costly. At a minimum we recommend that payers and risk-sharing providers alike carefully consider the potential advantages of turning their attention to efforts aimed at improving consumer health and demand behavior.

REFERENCES

1. G. Richards, "Business Examines Hospitals," *Hospitals,* 1 January, 1986, 61–69.
2. K. Pallarito, "Shaping Hospitals' Capital Spending Decisions," *Modern Healthcare,* 16 April 1990, 33–48.
3. L. Gross, "Coalitions Adopt Aggressive Stance," *Modern Healthcare,* February 1983, 62–64.
4. S. Schear, "Detroit's New Model for Health Care," *Business & Health* 14, no. 2 (February 1996): 46–53.
5. R. Denker and J. Ogilvy, "The Iron Triangle and the Chrome Pentagon," *Healthcare Forum Journal* 36, no. 6 (November/December 1993):72–77.
6. "Cost Containment in Managed Care Limited by Market Competition," *AHA News* 29, no. 41 (October 11, 1993):3.

7. "National Commission Calls for Closing of 20% of Medical Schools, Drastic Reduction in New Doctors, Nurses and Pharmacists," *Health Care Strategic Management* 14, no. 2 (February 1996):17.

8. "Coalition Employers Save 9 Percent," *Business & Health* 14, no. 2 (February 1996):61.

9. "Coalition Wins Premium Hike Limits," *Business & Health* 14, no. 2 (February 1996):61.

10. D. Burda, "Aetna Deal Signals Provider," *Modern Healthcare,* 8 April 1996, 2, 3, 13.

11. S. Heimoff, "Will Tier-Pricing Prove a Sign of the Times? Fallout from the California Blue Maneuver," *Strategic Health Care Marketing* 13, no. 3 (March 1996):1–3.

12. F. Curtiss, "Managed Health Care: Managed Costs?" *Personnel Journal,* June 1989, 72–85.

13. D. Cave and L. Turner, "10 Facts about Point-of-Service Plans," *HR Magazine,* September 1991, 41–46.

14. T. Droste, "Employers and Insurers To Seek Preset Prices," *Hospitals,* 20 January 1989, 70.

15. K. Pallarito, "Lawsuit Challenges Aetna of N.Y. Capitation Contracts," *Modern Healthcare,* 8 January, 1996, 22, 23.

16. N. Bell, "From the Trenches: Strategies That Work," *Business & Health* 9, no. 5 (May 1991):19–25.

17. Burda, "Aetna Deal Signals Provider," 2, 3, 13.

18. L. Christensen, "Change of Hearts," *Business & Health* 9, no. 6 (June 1991):18–26.

19. M. Kahn, "Employers Must Join Providers in Making Sticky Access Decisions," *Managed Care Outlook* 4, no. 23 (November 22, 1991):7.

20. N. Bell, "Workers and Managers of the World, Unite!" *Business & Health* 9, no. 8 (August 1991): 27–33.

21. P. Taulbee, "Hershey Using PaHC4 Data To Pick Quality Hospitals and Physicians for Network," *Healthcare Competition Week,* 30 September 1991, 3.

22. J. Kajander and M. Samuels, "The Other Side of Group Purchasing: The Employer's Perspective," *Health Systems Review* 29, no. 2 (March/April 1996):14–18.

23. M. Traska, "Corporate Execs Can Make a Difference," *Business & Health* 8, no. 7 (July 1990):43, 44.

24. M. Traska, "Xerox Reports HMOs Saving $1K per Insured over Fee-for-Service," *Managed Care Outlook* 5, no. 13 (June 19, 1992):4.

25. Bell, "From the Trenches," 19–25.

26. G. Bilchik, "Under Scrutiny," *Hospitals & Health Networks,* 5 May 1996, 24–32.

27. N. Lowndes, "Spring 1991 Health Care Study," *Medical Benefits,* 15 September 1991, 7.

28. J. Burcke, "Employers Cut Healthcare Spending, But Few Use Most Successful Methods," *Modern Healthcare,* 1 May 1984, 56.

29. F. Ham, "Who Will Pay for Health Benefits? Management and Labor Face Off," *Business & Health* 7, no. 8 (August 1989):29–34.

30. R. Henkoff, "Yes, Companies Can Cut Health Costs," *Fortune,* 1 July 1991, 52–55.

31. G. Henry, "Emergency Care under Managed Care: A Fatal Distraction?" *Health Systems Review* 29, no. 2 (March/April 1996):55–62.

32. "ACEP Challenges AAHP To Do More with 'Patients First' Initiative," *Health Care Strategic Management* 15, no. 2 (February 1997):6, 7.

33. "Parents Describe Tragic Results of Maternity Policy," *AHA News* 31, no. 38 (1995):3.

34. J. Ziegler, "Drive-Through Delivery: Bargain or Blunder?" *Business & Health* 13, no. 9 (1995): 19–25.

35. "New Flak over Drive-Through Mastectomies," *Business & Health* 14, no. 12 (December 1996): 10.

36. "Hospital Blazes New Trail with Cross-Continuum Case Management Program," *Hospital Case Management* 4, no. 1 (January 1996):1–3.

37. "Algorithms Boost Clinical Pathways' Effectiveness," *QI/TQM* 5, no. 8 (August 1995):94–97.

38. "Changing Physician Behaviors Can Lead to Profits," *Hospital Managed Care Strategies* 3, no. 12 (December 1995):137–138.

39. "How To Get Physicians To Manage the Costs of Care," in *Alliance for Healthcare Strategy & Marketing Annual Meeting* (New Orleans, LA: 1996), 22–37.

40. "Use Outcomes To Stamp Out Treatment Variation," *Patient Satisfaction & Outcomes Management in Physician Practices* 1, no. 8 (December 1995):88–90.

41. J. Montague, et al., "How To Save Big Bucks," *Hospitals & Health Networks,* 5 March, 1996, 18–24.

42. B. Bunschoten, "Pushing Physicians To Give Data Entry a Spin," *Health Data Management* 4, no. 3 (March 1996):82–87.

43. "UR Produces Net Savings of $51 per Person Annually," *Managed Care Stats & Facts,* 23 December 1991, 2.

44. M. Manley, "The Paradox of Utilization Management," *Hospital Managed Care & Direct Contracting* 2, no. 4 (October 1992):1–3.

45. "The New Discipline of Demand Management," *Healthier Communities Direct.*

46. H. Harrington, et al., *Demand Management,* Discussion Paper sponsored by the National Health Management Foundation, Washington, DC, 1993.

47. R. Herzlinger, "How Companies Tackle Health Care Costs: Part II," *Harvard Business Review* 63, no. 5 (1985):108–120.

48. C. Grahl, "Elders at Risk," *Managed Healthcare* 7, no. 10 (1997):40–41.

49. "How To Save $482 per Worker per Year," *Business & Health* 11, no. 10 (1993):21.

50. Cave and Turner, "10 Facts," 41–46.

51. J. Johnsson, "Managing Care: It's No Easy Feat When a Hospital's Employees Become Its Patients," *Hospitals,* 20 March 1992, 42–46.

52. D. Padgett, et al., "The Effect of Insurance Benefit Changes on Use of Child and Adolescent Outpatient Mental Health Services," *Medical Care* 31, no. 2 (1993):96–110.

53. *Healthcare PR & Marketing News,* 21 March 1996, 5.

54. E. Larson, "The Soul of an HMO," *Time,* 22 January 1996, 44–52.

55. "Blue Cross & Blue Shield Changes Policy: Will Cover Bone Marrow Transplants for Advanced Breast Cancer," *State Health* 3, no. 3 (1996):10, 11.

56. "Drug Formularies May Raise Medical Costs, Study Says," *Modern Healthcare,* 25 March 1996, 52.

57. E. Friedman, "Too Much of a Bad Thing," *Healthcare Forum Journal* 39, no. 2 (1996):11–15.

58. "Use Outcomes to Stamp Out Treatment Variation," 88–90.

59. R. Clarke, "Perception Is Everything," *Journal of Health Care Marketing* 15, no. 3 (Fall 1995):32, 33.

60. S. Luxemberg, "Bonus Plans That Go beyond Productivity," *Medical Economics* 71, no. 24 (1994):21–26.

61. Manley, "The Paradox of Utilization Management," 1–3.

62. L. Kertesz, "HMOs Battling Horror Stories, Lawmakers," *Modern Healthcare,* 8 April 1996, 44, 45.

63. R. Pear, "Feds Target HMO Rewards for Limiting Services," *The Denver Post,* 27 March 1996, 4A.

64. "Do-It-Yourself Managed Care," *Profiles* 352 (March/April 1993):18–27.

65. E. Weissenstein, "HCFA To Unveil Medicare Bonus Program," *Modern Healthcare,* 26 February 1996, 70.

66. "Decisions Strike Fear in the Hearts of Plans, Providers," *Capitation Management Report* 3, no. 1 (1996):1–5.

67. C. Bell, "Providers Should Weigh Risks of Risk Assumption," *Modern Healthcare,* 29 January 1996, 34.

68. M. Jaklevic, "Disclosing Doc Incentives," *Modern Healthcare,* 6 January 1997, 21.

69. " 'Gag Clauses' Rarely in Contracts, Not Often Used To Dump Physicians," *Managed Care Week* 6, no. 7 (1996):1, 2.

70. L. Kertesz, "AMA Opposes HMO 'Gag Clauses,' " *Modern Healthcare,* 29 January 1996, 8.

71. L. Kertesz, "HMO Groups Plan Counterpunch to Media Criticism," *Modern Healthcare,* 11 December 1995, 60–62.

72. Larson, "The Soul of an HMO," 44–52.

73. "Blue Cross and Blue Shield Changes Policy," 10, 11.

74. R. Pear, "Feds Target HMO Rewards for Limiting Services," 4A.

75. "Gag Clauses Restricting What Doctors Tell Patients Will Be This Year's Biggest Battle in States, Expert Says," *State Health Watch* 3, no. 1 (1996):1, 9.

76. "Critic of 'Gag Rule' Applauds U.S. Healthcare's Decision To Encourage Doctors To Talk to Patients," *State Health Watch* 3, no. 2 (1996):11.

77. Larson, "The Soul of an HMO," 44–52.

78. Friedman, "Too Much of a Bad Thing," 11–15.

79. E. Weissenstein, "Congressmen Propose Law Barring HMO 'Gag Rules,' " *Modern Healthcare* 26, no. 10 (1996):52.

80. Kertesz, "AMA Opposes HMO 'Gag Clauses,' " 8.

81. Luxemberg, "Bonus Plans," 21–26.

82. J. Asplund, "California Doctors Rip HMOs on Spending, Profits," *AHA News,* 26 February 1996, 1.

83. L. Kertesz, "Group Urges Rewrite of Benefit Contracts," *Modern Healthcare,* 18 March 1996, 16.

84. D. Brailer and R.L. Van Horn, "Health and the Welfare of U.S. Business," *Harvard Business Review* 71, no. 2 (1993):125–132.

85. Burda, "Aetna Deal Signals Provider," 2, 3.

86. M. Matheny and B. Bader, "What Happens When a Payer Owns or Controls a Hospital?" *Health System Leader* 1, no. 6 (1994):4–13.

87. K. Lumsdon, "To Buy or Not To Buy, That Is the Question," *Hospitals & Health Networks* 20 (1996):24–32.

88. *Health Gain: Improving the Health of Communities through Integrated Health Care* (Minneapolis, MN: Allina Health System, 1994).

89. "Outcomes-Based Payment Prompts Better Quality, Lower Costs in Minnesota," *Healthcare Systems Strategy Report* 11, no. 17 (1994):11, 12.

90. C. Lindquist, "Tying Hospital Gifts to Cost Cutting Incentives," *Business & Health* 2, no. 6 (May 1985):27, 28.

91. P. LeBrun, "Payers Step Up Roles in Discharge Planning," *Hospitals,* 16 June 1985, 98, 102.

92. N. Carroll, "Ford Has Another Idea," *Business & Health* 8, no. 6 (June 1991):79–82.

93. "Six Characteristics Common to 'Best' Healthcare Purchasing Performers," *Competitive Healthcare Market Reporter* 1, no. 2 (1993):6, 7.

94. R. Zaldiver, "Size No Reflection of HMO Quality," *The Denver Post,* 28 March 1996, 21A, 26A.

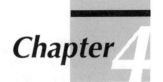

Chapter 4

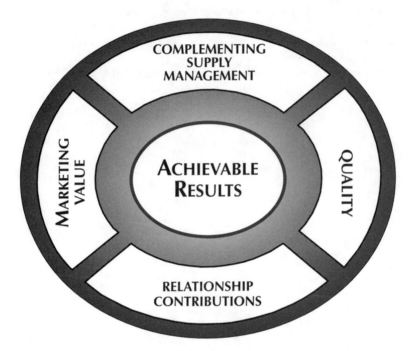

The diagram shows concentric ovals with "ACHIEVABLE RESULTS" at the center, surrounded by four domains: COMPLEMENTING SUPPLY MANAGEMENT (top), QUALITY (right), RELATIONSHIP CONTRIBUTIONS (bottom), and MARKETING VALUE (left).

WHY IMPROVE DEMAND ?

Having defined demand improvement and having described its four domains, and having discussed the limitations and dangers of controlling utilization from the supply side, it is time to discuss why it is advisable, if not essential, to improve demand. Arguments for improving consumer health and demand behaviors fall into these five categories:

1. It is a natural complement to controlling care supply or delivery.
2. It makes significant contributions to quality.

3. It makes significant contributions to marketing.
4. It adds value to key relationships.
5. It produces significant results.

COMPLEMENTING SUPPLY MANAGEMENT

Given the already described limitations and negative side effects of provider-focused efforts, turning to consumer behavior (i.e., their demands on health services) is simply recognizing the other side of the coin. It will be essential for health plans and capitated providers to manage consumer health and consumption of services in order to survive in a market unwilling to devote any more money to health care.[1]

Because supply-side efforts focused on providers or imposed barriers to consumer use of services, they failed to consider how to deliver benefits to consumers in order to engage them in demand improvement efforts. Consumers have been treated as enemies of cost controls and profits and as objects of the often draconian tactics described in Chapter 3. As a result, the contributions that consumers might make to controlling utilization have been overlooked rather than promoted.

Among the causes of utilization, morbidity is fundamental. If there were no illness or injury, there would be very little utilization. Yet supply-side efforts fail completely to address the need for care, focusing entirely on the quantity and quality of its provision. The limits of supply-side thinking are perhaps best illustrated by the case of medical providers from the United States looking at an outbreak of tetanus among newborns in India. Rather than building a neonatal intensive care unit to care for the newborns (estimated cost $400,000 per case), it was determined that by supplying midwives with a sterile kit of materials for cutting the umbilical cord, the epidemic was ended at a cost of roughly $.10 per baby.[2]

Providers tend to think in terms of the skills they have mastered and the technologies they are familiar with, and in some cases, the investments they have made. Self-referral has been frequently cited as a cause for overdelivery of care. Some multi-specialty physician practices put their individual specialties at risk when buying equipment. If the obstetricians order an ultrasound machine and fail to use it enough to generate the revenue needed to cover its costs, those obstetricians will have to cover the difference out of their own pockets.

By engaging consumers as counterweights to providers and consumer-focused thinking to balance provider-focused thinking, we have a chance to reduce the provider-generated variations in demand that have so long persisted among different communities.[3] Consumers at risk for the costs and side effects are unlikely to opt for questionable and clearly unnecessary procedures, once they are empowered to identify them.

Where capitation hasn't yet shifted provider thinking toward "less is better," consumer empowerment is another approach to countering the technological imperative that drives providers to perceive and define patient problems in terms of their own specialty and procedure capabilities.[4] Where supply-side efforts have aggressively attacked the quantity of utilization, consumer perspectives are needed to support provider concerns for quality.

As Goldsmith has described it, focusing on consumers, particularly on their health status and risks, is simply the third stage in the evolution of managed care once the potential of a provider focus has been exhausted.[5] Adding in a concern for and effective means to manage health risks and promote wellness is an essential component of managed care.[6]

O'Malley[7] enumerates seven elements that can and must be managed in managed care: (1) payments to providers, (2) provision of care by primary physicians, (3) referrals to specialists and hospitals by primary physicians, (4) delivery of care by the specialists and hospitals they refer to, and (5) profits of health plans on the supply side, plus (6) consumer lifestyles and (7) demand for services on the demand side. Focusing on consumers is at least two sevenths of the managed care challenge.

As Fries points out, both providers and consumers are responsible for excess demand.[8] So it makes sense to include consumers as partners in seeking the solution, rather than as simply parts of the problem. Consumers influence most of the factors in the chain of events that lead to utilization of health care, and certainly the early "upstream" factors of health behaviors, morbidity, response to symptoms and initiation of contact with providers.[9] To work on only the last few links in the "continuum of causality" is suboptimal at best.

It has frequently been argued that an essential requirement for a truly integrated health system is the alignment of incentives among all its members.[10] The problems and limitations of provider-focused efforts may have emerged because they have not aligned incentives so that consumers are included. Supply-side tactics for controlling utilization chiefly impose costs on consumers, rather than benefits. These include the out-of-pocket costs of deductibles and copayment for benefits denied and for obtaining care after precertification disapproval, or from out-of-network providers. They also include the costs of limited coverage, drug formularies, length of stay limits, and similar restrictions in terms of adverse quality of care impact.

As long as payers and providers treat consumers as objects to be controlled, rather than partners in achieving better health and utilization, the negative consequences of supply-side efforts are likely to continue, and managed care organizations will continue to take the heat for their more egregious acts.[11] Until consumers are engaged as active participants in managing their health and care consumption, efforts to control utilization will continue to be sub-optimal.

Consumers have a great deal to gain from demand improvement, and should be willing recruits into many kinds of initiatives. From health improvement they gain better health and quality of life and better outcomes when problems are caught and addressed early. From decision improvement they gain reassurance about the plans, providers, and procedures they choose; obtain immediate response when they can employ self-care; and avoid the hassles and out-of-pocket costs of innappropriate care. From disease management, they gain a reduction in chronic condition crises, better outcomes of care, and improved quality of life. From disability management they gain increased income and quality of work life. From demand improvement in general, they stand to gain reduced health insurance premiums, and a potential share in employer and government savings.

CONTRIBUTIONS TO QUALITY

Quality has long been thought of and treated as the exclusive domain of professionals. Indeed it is professionals who are held responsible for achieving and maintaining quality and are sued for quality failures. But as we continually redefine what we mean by health care quality and introduce new ways of measuring and reporting quality, the essential role of consumers is becoming clarified.

Consider the Health Plan Employer Data and Information Set measures promulgated by the National Council on Quality Assurance. While providers and health plans are to be held responsible for meeting HEDIS standards, they cannot possibly do so without the active cooperation of consumers. The following are just some examples:

- The proportion of pregnant women initiating prenatal care in the first trimester is one of the HEDIS quality indicators. How can providers meet HEDIS standards or do better than their competitors on this indicator unless pregnant women tell them about their pregnancy, come in for tests, and comply with the recommended pattern of prenatal visits? How can providers achieve reductions in adverse fetal outcomes, including low birthweight and infant mortality, unless mothers comply with prenatal regimens?
- The proportion of children who have received their full quota of immunizations is another quality indicator. How can plans and providers improve their performance on this measure unless parents bring their children to where immunizations will be provided?
- The proportion of members and patients who receive prescribed screening tests such as mammograms, Pap smears, prostate and colorectal cancer tests is another HEDIS quality indicator. If consumers don't make appointments and come in for tests, or send back specimens, what hope have plans and providers of meeting standards?
- How many diabetics have annual retinal eye exams and how many asthma patients are admitted to hospitals are indicators of the quality of care for patients with chronic conditions. What can providers do without diabetes pa-

tients coming in for the examination, and asthma patients managing their own condition so as to minimize acute crises?

It has been estimated that U.S. health care wastes at least $200 billion a year in overpriced, useless, even harmful treatments, and the bloated bureaucracy that attempts to control utilization.[12] While the focus of utilization control has been chiefly on eliminating avoidable expenditures, it clearly includes quality implications where harmful treatments can be avoided. Adding in the use of treatments from unqualified providers and "quacks," which are frequently not covered by insurance, hence not counted as health care costs, the consumption of harmful care has to be a major quality concern.

There are provider-focused efforts aimed at reducing harmful care but consumers are ultimately the only ones who can eliminate bad care by not using it. A well-informed and empowered consumer public can prevent the use of most harmful care through shared decision making and wise selection of providers. Poorly informed consumers, uncertain about the true motivations of payers and upright providers, are likely to be perfect targets for unscrupulous providers.

Consumer cooperation is essential to quality in a number of other ways. Obese patients challenge the skills of surgeons and represent high risks of poor outcomes. Similarly, overweight patients can make recovery from hip surgery problematic and increase adverse outcomes. Rehabilitation success after cardiac treatment depends on how well patients comply with diet and exercise regimens.[13]

For seniors, with their generally higher risk of disease and injury plus significantly higher levels of health care utilization, quality of care requires their active involvement. They may have to bring in and discuss multiple prescriptions (for example, with their pharmacist). Their participation in individual or group sessions on managing their chronic conditions in exercise and fitness programs is likely to be essential in achieving good health outcomes, maintaining their independence, and controlling their utilization.[14]

It is widely recognized that consumers are already the major primary provider of health care to themselves and their families, accounting for 80% of all the care needed in one example.[15] If payers and providers ignore the quality of consumer decisions regarding whether, when, and where to seek care, and how to care for their own problems, they cannot claim to be truly committed to, much less accomplished in, quality of care management.

Virtually every measure of quality being touted for public reporting for employer and consumer use in selecting plans and providers either depends partly upon or can be significantly affected by consumer behavior. By improving consumer health and care behaviors, plans and providers have a far better chance to meet quality standards and/or to beat their competition in terms of quality, thereby reducing their dependence on price-based competition alone.

MARKETING VALUE

Improving health and demand can add significant value and marketing advantage for providers and plans with respect to employer and union purchasers as well as consumer enrollees and patients. This contrasts sharply with controls on care delivery, which are uniformly onerous and unattractive to consumers as well as risky for purchasers.

The gatekeeper system is considered a nuisance, a barrier to getting needed care, and a barrier to HMO enrollment by large numbers of consumers. Recently HMOs themselves have recognized this fact and attempted to differentiate themselves from their competitors by offering alternatives. Qual-Med in Colorado has promoted its 24-hour phone triage system as a faster way to get a referral to a specialist when needed. The nurse-counselor can authorize such a referral and can even make the appointment over the phone rather than requiring the caller to go through an appointment with the primary physician gatekeeper.[16] United Healthcare offers "open-access" plans where consumers can refer themselves directly to specialists, counting on this provider selection freedom to attract consumers resistant to HMO enrollment.[17]

While surveys often show HMO enrollees to be as satisfied with their plan as indemnity and PPO enrollees, if not more so, one area where HMOs have not done well is on member satisfaction with the HMOs' "concern for their well-being." Given HMOs' public commitments to health maintenance, it does not look good when only 52% of those surveyed report themselves as "highly satisfied" on this dimension.[18] Investing more heavily and enthusiastically in promoting health and reducing health risks may be necessary if HMOs are to earn higher marks.

By actively promoting and achieving consumer health improvements, plans and providers alike figure to gain a competitive advantage over peers who give only lip service to health maintenance.[19] Members who feel their health has been protected or enhanced, their chronic conditions made more subject to their control, and their quality of life improved are more likely to remain enrolled.[20] All this adds to the potential for pricing advantages from reducing consumer need and avoidable consumption so as to reduce expenditures.

Both providers and health plans gain marketing adantages when they can, with consumers' help, improve their HEDIS performance scores. Employers and consumers are both likely to lean toward plans and providers that have the highest HEDIS scores, as those scores become better understood and more relied upon in making such choices. They also gain marketing advantages from happier, healthier consumer members and patients, through improved satisfaction levels, increased retention, and word-of-mouth advertising.

There are also significant potential marketing advantages relative to employers. By better controlling utilization through improving health and consumption behavior, plans can reduce the motivation for employers to shift costs to employees, promising better employee morale and less risk of labor unrest as a result. Any reduction in the more egregious provider-focused tactics in favor of consumer-focused effort is likely to reduce the risk of "HMO bashing" and ease the minds of employers contracting with or considering moving to an HMO.[21]

Demand improvement efforts have distinctly lower potential for media bashing than do supply-side control programs. This is not to say that they have no risk. Employers who steer employees to a notorious health plan, or to providers with poor track records, may find themselves lambasted in the media as well as in the courts. Plans, providers, or employers who engage in a "blame the victim" approach to consumers who fail to correct their bad health habits or comply with advice and regimens may find themselves tarred by the same brush as was used for provider control blunders.[22]

Still, employers can enjoy significant side effects from successful health improvement and consumption reform efforts by plans and providers. Improvements in productivity and morale as well as reductions in absenteeism and turnover have been frequently reported as results of wellness and fitness programs. (See Chapter 5 for specific examples.) The cost reductions that employers can enjoy as the result of successful consumer-focused efforts can help improve their profits and competitive position in world markets.[23]

Health plans that deliver such added value to employers can help overcome media exposures regarding their excessive profits and executive salaries. Otherwise, employers may shift to direct contracting, out of either a general dissatisfaction with HMOs or a perception that providers can do the job better without the "middle man."[24]

RELATIONSHIP CONTRIBUTIONS

A good relationship with consumers is first a foundation for successful demand improvement. Consumers who distrust or are skeptical about health plans, employers, or providers who try to alter their behavior are unlikely to respond positively. Past supply-focused efforts have greatly undermined consumer trust in every attempt to control their use of services. Fortunately, demand improvement efforts can strengthen the very relationships upon which their success depends. We will cite some of the ways in which demand improvement, through its four components, can help build and maintain good relationships among consumers and employers, health plans, and providers.

Health improvement enhances consumer quality of life and thereby consumer satisfaction and loyalty toward the employers, providers, and plans to whom they give the credit. Decision improvement not only helps consumers obtain the best responses to their care needs, it also reduces employer, provider, and plan litigation risks. Disease management enhances consumer quality of life, in addition to reducing provider utilization and payer costs. Disability management enhances worker morale and saves workers' compensation and disability costs for employers. As consumer health and demand improve, the population as a whole gains health and happiness and society gains lower health care expenditures with resulting new opportunities for investment in other areas of need.

Effective and successful demand improvement promises significant benefit to all who share in the causes and effects of health and utilization of health services. In turn these benefits stand to strengthen the relationships among all those involved and affected. And through stronger relationships, the effectiveness, efficiency, and success of demand improvement stand to increase.

As put forth by the National Health Council, patients (actually all consumers) have the following explicit "rights" in relations with payers and providers:

- to informed consent in treatment decisions, timely access to specialists, and protection of their privacy and information confidentiality,
- to concise, understandable information about their health plan benefits and about what is and is not covered,
- to knowledge of how coverage and benefit denial decisions are made and how they can be appealed,
- to thorough and understandable information about costs of coverage and health services,
- to a reasonable choice of providers and the information needed to make a good selection, and
- to full knowledge about what provider incentives or restrictions might affect practice patterns.

To balance these rights, the Council also promulgated this list of responsibilities for all capable consumers:

- to pursue healthy lifestyles,
- to become well informed about their health plans,
- to actively participate in health care decisions, and
- to cooperate fully in mutually determined courses of treatment.[25]

This combination of rights and responsibilities calls for a new relationship between payers/providers and consumers/patients. It addresses precisely those characteristics of interaction that are essential to improving consumer health and care behavior. Providing consumers with the information they need to appropriately select health plans, providers, and treatment options is exactly what decision improvement is about. Adopting healthy lifestyles is what health improvement promotes, while complying with *mutually determined* courses of action is the essence of disease management.

It is consumers' right and responsibility to create and sustain a working partnership with payers and providers, to be coinvestigators in examining problems, and to be coimplementers in carrying out their solutions. As plans and providers move away from their provider-control focus to consumer behavior improvement, they will necessarily have to acknowledge and promote the essential consumer role. As consumers enjoy the gains of improved health and consumption of services, they should more easily adopt and enjoy their rights and responsibilities in the partnership.

The idea of empowering consumers, through being motivated, enabled, and prompted toward better health and demand behavior, is not simply a political stance, nor just a pragmatic philosophy. It contributes directly to the achievement of health and demand improvement. The feeling of powerlessness, one of the most commonly cited social problems of our day, is directly related to the negative effects of workplace and personal life stress.

Powerless people, consumers who lack self-efficacy with respect to managing their own lives, have higher morbidity and mortality than the empowered.[26] Those suffering from "learned helplessness" cannot take full responsibility for their health and care behaviors. By empowering consumers, we can promote their active contribution not only to better management of utilization, but to their psychosocial and spiritual as well as physical health. In turn, empowered consumers will be able to carry out their responsibilities and enjoy their rights in managing their health and care consumption to their own benefit.

RESULTS ACHIEVABLE

Enlisting consumers in demand improvement as a complement to provider-focused efforts can make payers' utilization control efforts more successful. Shifting attention to consumer-focused demand improvement efforts may produce far more potitive impact on utilization than supply-side control efforts have ever delivered.

Consumer demands have frequently pressured providers toward overtreatment in the past, insisting on antibiotics for viral conditions, for example, or demanding additional tests out of fear of a more serious condition. Patients and family members concerned about pain and discomfort might insist on general anesthesia where a local would be better, on inpatient admission where an outpatient option would be superior, on Caesarean delivery versus normal delivery. Physicians have often felt forced to accede to such demands to maintain patient satisfaction and loyalty or protect against the possibility of litigation. Empowering consumers to reduce or reverse their demands for overtreatment will be essential to the full success of provider controls.[27]

Consumers are also needed as active partners to enable providers to achieve effective case and care management. To be able to discharge patients within per-case payment limits, for example, the patient or family members often have to be empowered to continue care at home. Patients might have to be kept in emergency departments unless they or someone at home can provide needed follow-up care

Table 4–1 Value of Demand Improvement Strategies for Different Constituents

CONSTITUENT ▶	BETTER HEALTH	BETTER UTILIZATION
CONSUMERS	✗ Enhance quality of life ✗ Avoid adverse health events ✗ Reduce lost work time & income	• Reduce out of pocket expense • Reduce premium costs
EMPLOYERS	✗ Improve productivity ✗ Improve morale & retention ✗ Reduce absenteeism	• Reduce absences for seeking care • Reduce health care use & expense • Reduce workers' compensation and disability costs
PROVIDERS	✗ Improve patient satisfaction and retention ✗ Reduce demand for services ✗ Promote patient volume / share ✗ Improve NCQA / HEDIS reviews	• Reduce malpractice risk • Reduce utilization expenses • Lower operating costs
HEALTH PLANS	✗ Improve member satisfaction and retention ✗ Improve NCQA/HEDIS reviews ✗ Promote member word of mouth advertising ✗ Increase market share	• Reduce legal risk • Lower capitation losses • Greater profits • Happier providers • Lower costs
COMMUNITY / SOCIETY	✗ Healthier communities	• Lower expenditures

and supervision. Parents of premature infants can significantly reduce their baby's stay in the hospital by learning to provide needed care in the home.[28]

In addition to improving the effects of supply-side control efforts, improving consumer health and demand can address the utilization problems mainly attributable to consumer behavior factors. It has been estimated that as much as 70% of morbidity and mortality is caused by lifestyle factors, which are not subject to supply control efforts.[29] As much as 40% of all utilization may be avoidable through improving consumer behavior.[30]

The $200 billion spent on overtreatment, overutilization, and attempts to control both would be significantly reduced if consumer health were significantly improved and consumer care decisions better informed.[31] The annual costs of high-risk/high-use Medicare beneficiaries has been calculated at 20 times as great as the costs for low-risk beneficiaries. As many as 25% of physician visits and 55% of ED visits may be avoidable.[32] Dramatic (50% to 75%) reductions in the use of and expenditures for care by asthma and diabetes patients have been achieved through empowering them to be effective self-managers.[33]

The potential for consumer-focused efforts to dramatically reduce annual health care expenditures for governments, employers, health plans, and capitated providers has been a major argument for champions of improving consumer health and care behaviors. At the same time uncertainty over the extent and probability of such reductions has been a major source of resistance to shifting away from supply-side measures. In the next chapter we will examine the evidence, considering what has already been achieved and what success might be confidently expected by sponsors who engage in health and demand improvement efforts.

Table 4–1 illustrates the extent to which consumers, employers, providers, health plans, specific communities, and society as a whole stand to benefit from successful demand improvement programs.

REFERENCES

1. J. Bensky and C. Reynolds, "Keeping Them Well," *Health Systems Review* 29, no. 2 (1996):20–24.
2. G. Annas, "Beyond the Military and Market Metaphors," *Healthcare Forum Journal* 39, no. 3 (1996):30–36.
3. T. Hudson, "Mirror, Mirror," *Hospitals & Health Networks,* 5 April 1996, 24–30.
4. M. Magee, "Information Empowerment of the Patient: The Next Payer/Provider Battlefield," *Journal of Outcomes Management* 2, no. 3 (1995):17–21.
5. J. Goldsmith, et al., "Managed Care Comes of Age," *Healthcare Forum Journal* 38, no. 5 (1995): 14–24.
6. B. Wolcott, "Demand Management: An Overview," *National Conference on Medical Management,* Chicago, IL, American College of Physician Executives, 5 May, 1995.

7. J. O'Malley, "Reducing Healthcare Costs with Demand Management," *The Alliance Bulletin,* August 1995, 3, 5.

8. J. Fries, "Reducing Need and Demand," *Healthcare Forum Journal* 36, no. 6 (1993):18–23.

9. J. Otis, *The Art and Science of Demand Management* (Oakton, MD: The Center for Corporate Health).

10. D. Coddington, et al., *Making Integrated Health Care Work* (Englewood, CO: Center for Research in Ambulatory Care Administration, 1996).

11. L. Kertesz, "Ruling in Kaiser Case Supports HMOs' Right To Withhold Care," *Modern Healthcare,* 26 September 1994, 30.

12. "Wasteful Health Care Dollars," *Consumer Reports,* July 1992, 435–448.

13. Bensky and Reynolds, "Keeping Them Well," 20–24.

14. "Demand Management Critical to Success in Senior Market," *Healthcare Demand Management* 2, no. 2 (1996):17–22.

15. M. Burke and J. Burke, "Managed Care Needs a Partner To Keep Its Promise," *Business & Health* 13, no. 10 (1995):72.

16. "Qual-Med To Introduce Fourth Generation Medical Management," *Health Care Strategic Management* 14, no. 4 (1996):15.

17. E. Narvaes, "HMO Expands Access," *The Denver Post,* 1 May 1996, 1C, 3C.

18. "All That Glitters," *Hospitals & Health Networks* 20 April 1996, 46–48.

19. J. Chutz, "How New Trends in DMS Can Help MCOs Gain Competitive Advantages," *Demand Management Services,* Dallas, TX, International Business Communications, Oct 19, 20, 1995.

20. D. Powell, "Use Demand-Side Management as a Cost Containment and Marketing Tool," *The Alliance Report,* March/April 1996, 1, 2, 5.

21. H. Meyer, "The Tide of Times," *Hospitals & Health Networks,* 20 April 1996, 34–40.

22. N. Wallerstein, "Powerlessness, Empowerment and Health," *American Journal of Health Promotion* 6, no. 3 (1992):197–205.

23. L. Chapman, "The Challenge of Managing the Demand for Health Care," *ACA Journal,* Winter 1994, 12–20.

24. "Beyond HMOs," *Hospitals & Health Networks,* 20 April 1996, 33–35.

25. "National Health Council Calls on Managed Care To Endorse Patients' Rights," *Health Care Strategic Management* 14, no. 2 (1996):17.

26. Wallerstein, "Powerlessness," 197–205.

27. M. Mihlbauer, "Controlling Consumer Demand: The Next Generation of Managed Care," *Medical Interface,* November 1992, 20–22.

28. R. Coile, "Integrating the Patient into Healthcare Systems," *Hospital Strategy Report* 5, no. 5 (1993):2.

29. Fries, "Reducing Need," 18–23.

30. Fries, "Reducing Need," 18–23.

31. "Wasteful Health Care Dollars," 435–448.

32. A. Kotin, "Using DMS To Manage Medicare and Medicaid Risk Contracts," *Demand Management Services,* Dallas, TX, International Business Communications 19, 20 October, 1995.

33. D. Vickery, "Toward Appropriate Use of Medical Care," *Healthcare Forum Journal* 39, no. 1 (1996):15–19.

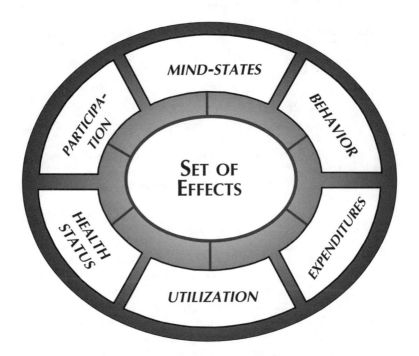

Chapter 5

**HOW WELL DOES DEMAND
MANAGEMENT WORK ?**

In previous chapters we have argued that improving consumer health and demand behaviors is an essential part of controlling utilization for both payers and providers at risk. While it is simple enough to identify the limitations and negative side effects of strategies aimed at managing provider behavior and tactics used thus far to restrict consumer access, it is quite another to demonstrate that improving consumer behavior will work better. The purpose of this chapter is to back up our arguments in favor of improving consumer health and demand behaviors with facts.

We will cite such facts in terms of a wide range of changes in consumer behavior, from involvement in health and demand behavior improvement activities to changes in their mind-state, behavior, health status, consumption of care, and reduced expenditures by payers and consumers as well as added value enjoyed by consumers, payers, providers, and society traceable to health and demand behavior improvements.

Since there is no national system for gathering all reports of success or failure in demand improvement, the examples we will cite are illustrations or examples, as opposed to scientific proof that it works. The reported examples range from weak, anecdotal discussions to rigorous controlled studies, but even the best involve selected populations rather than random samples, and their results could not be confidently extrapolated to all other populations.

While it would be tempting to argue that one or some approaches to specific demand improvement objectives are superior to all others, there is also no basis for supporting such an argument. Where controlled studies have been conducted, they compare some intervention to no intervention or, occasionally, a modest intervention to a more aggressive intervention of the same type. It would take an enormous investment in multiple, random-sample, controlled evaluations to find compelling evidence that some tactics always or usually work better than others. We can only present examples of the sort of evidence that is available, the sort of results that have been reported.

SET OF EFFECTS

Seven categories of effects measures can be used in demonstrating the worth of specific demand improvement initiatives:

1. Increased *participation* by consumers in specific programs/activities. This effect includes consumers' use of health services such as prevention, monitoring, and early detection aimed at reducing morbidity or subsequent use of acute health services.
2. Improvements in and reinforcement of consumer *mind-states*. This effect includes consumers' consciousness of and motivation to engage in improved behavior, their capability to adopt and persist in desired behavior (e.g., knowledge, awareness, beliefs, perceptions, attitudes, intentions, commitments, self-efficacy). Note that self-efficacy is a combination of competence and confidence. While competence can be partly demonstrated through knowledge and confidence, clearly mind-states, actual skill in performing an action can only be measured through how well it is carried out in practice (i.e., in behavior).
3. Improvements in and reinforcement of specific consumer health and self-care *behaviors*. This effect covers reductions in or elimination of dangerous

behavior; adoption, repetition, and continuation of desired behavior; and improvement in self-care and self-management skills performance.

4. Improvements in consumer *health and functional status*. This effect includes health maintenance or improvement and reductions in risk measures and morbidity.

5. Improvements in the appropriateness of health services *use*. This effect refers to the quantity or quality of demand for care.

6. Reductions in health care and related *expenditures* by consumers, employers, health plans, governments, at-risk providers, and society.

7. *Added value* derived from improved behavior or health status. This effect includes productivity/efficiency in the workplace, psychosocial/spiritual health gains for consumers, increased satisfaction, loyalty/retention, and market advantages for employers, health plans, and providers.

Often the measures in this set of effects occur in chronological order and reflect a natural or logical sequence of causation. As a result of participation in a class, using a self-care guide, or interacting with a video or computer information system, consumers experience mind-state effects. Because of these mind-state effects, behavior changes do (or do not) occur. Because of behavior changes, health status is affected. As a result of health status changes, different patterns of health service use occur, and as a result of these, different patterns of health service expenditures result.

Value-adding effects, however, are separate from and parallel to the six sequential effect measures ending in desired reductions in expenditures. They may include mind-state changes (e.g., worker morale, perceived quality of life, or health plan member or patient satisfaction), behavior changes (e.g., productivity, absenteeism, social involvement), quality of life (e.g., greater energy, longevity), health plan cost reductions (e.g., due to lower turnover), and employer cost reductions (e.g., due to less turnover, increased productivity). They are important when and because they add value that may make a difference in planning decisions regarding whether to undertake an initiative or in evaluation judgments on whether or not initiatives have produced positive results.

These "effects" do not always occur in order. Attitudes often change after and as a result of behavior change, as behaviorists tell us. Some mind-state changes may be needed to promote participation (e.g., persuading consumers to come to classes or to request a self-care guide). Changes in behavior can produce as well as be produced by mind-state changes, as when a successful experience with self-care increases consumer confidence in its future use. The order is not essential; each effect measure offers a basis for planning and evaluating initiatives in whatever order each occurs.

Each of these seven effect measures may be the specific objective of a given initiative, may be used as an interim tracking measure, or may be a basis for estimating the value of initiatives aimed at outcomes that are difficult to measure or that occur too far off in the future. Each has its own advantages and disadvantages as a basis for evaluation, depending on how well each reflects the outcomes of efforts and how well each can be translated into some measure or estimate of value.

In general the early-stage outcomes (e.g., participation, mind-states, health behavior) are easier and less expensive to measure, and are detectable earlier than later-stage outcomes (e.g., health status, utilization, expenditures, value-added effects). Unfortunately they are also more difficult to place a value upon, since all are means to an end rather than ends in themselves. From health status on, placing a value on effects is far easier, though not always in dollar terms.

In most cases it is wise to use one or more of the early-stage measures to track results early and to look for ways to improve impact even though assigning value is difficult. Waiting for later-stage effects and paying no attention to participation, mind-states, and behavior can delay the making of midcourse corrections. At the same time, tracking one or more of the later-stage effects is essential to determining and demonstrating the value of initiatives, so a combination of measures is advisable.

Without the ability to at least estimate dollar value, it is impossible to judge the financial return on investment of specific efforts. It may then be impossible to decide whether to continue a given initiative, to expand it, or to reduce it. It will also complicate decisions regarding how to share the costs of such initiatives among whatever payer/provider sponsors are involved or regarding how to share rewards among sponsors and consumers.

Each of the seven effect measures applies, to some extent, to each of the four demand improvement domains. In practice, what tends to be set as an objective and used for tracking is slightly different, however, for each of the four. We will discuss the seven effects in the context of each of the four domains. Where possible we will cite specific evidence of effects; where none were found, we will describe evidence to look for. (Note: The set of effects is a useful tool in planning, implementing, and monitoring demand improvement initiatives, in addition to its use in evaluating such initiatives. It will be discussed and used repeatedly in later chapters devoted to these applications.)

HEALTH IMPROVEMENT

In one sense health improvement represents the greatest challenge in evaluation because it focuses "upstream" on the factors that influence the need for health services and only indirectly affect demand. The occurrence of disease and injury, or at least symptoms thereof, are the initial drivers of health care consumption.[1] If we could eliminate or significantly reduce morbidity, we would significantly reduce utilization and expenditures, as well as improve quality of life, reducing absenteeism and probably worker productivity as well. Direct measures of the impact of particular health improvement initiatives have included the following:

1. *Increased participation.* Sponsors who have examined health improvement efforts have used every one of the seven effects in their evaluations, including participation. Aetna tracked the numbers of employees participating in "brown-bag-lunch discussions.[2] Secure Horizons health plan counted the number of senior enrollees attending wellness seminars.[3] Quaker Oats measured the number of employees completing Health Risk Assessments.[4] Coors achieved 97% employee participation in a blood pressure check.[5]

    Champion International got 82% of its employees immunized.[6] General Electric attracted more spouses (57%) than employees (54%) to participate in its wellness program.[7] Group Health of Puget Sound increased participation in its smoking cessation program from 125 to 2,000 enrollees in two years.[8] Westinghouse achieved 97% to 100% participation levels in its worksite exercise program.[9]

2. *Mind-states.* Aetna included self-efficacy ratings in its measures of wellness program effects.[10] Secure Horizons gauged participants' satisfaction with education content and their increased awareness of healthier lifestyle choices.[11] Healthtrac includes self-efficacy/control in tracking success of its stress management program[12]; AT&T tracks perceived stress reduction.[13] The National Heart, Lung and Blood Institute found a steady increase in public awareness of the dangers of hypertension resulting from 20 years of social communications efforts.[14]

    Ontario Hydro detected a heightened sense of employee awareness about health and fitness after its health risk assessment (HRA) survey.[15] Westinghouse found improved employee "mood scores" resulting from its exercise program.[16] A Canadian public education effort was evaluated in terms of public awareness and recall of specific health messages.[17] School efforts in promoting "Sun Safety" were judged by improved knowledge and understanding of skin cancer risks and avoidance measures.[18]

3. *Behavior.* Since health improvement focuses on changing consumer health/risk behaviors, it is understandable that heavy emphasis be placed on tracking changes in behavior. Aetna measured the number of employees shifted from the "sedentary" to "active" category through its education/persuasion efforts.[19] Secure Horizons found that only modest numbers of seniors increased their exercise activities.[20] Baker-Hughes reduced smoking prevalence from 34.7% to 29.1% of its employees.[21] A study comparing over 7,000 employees in a wellness program to an equal number of controls found the numbers of high-risk employees dropped by 14% among program participants.[22]

    The Health Project reported on five different payers (i.e., Blue Shield of California, Johnson & Johnson, Tenneco, Travelers Insurance, and Ventura County, California) who achieved significant improvements in health risk behaviors such as smoking, dietary fat, lack of exercise, and seat belt use.[23]

AT&T found 90% of its wellness program participants reported at least one positive change in lifestyle behavior over five years.[24] Stanford's Community Health Education program reduced smoking levels and promoted physician interventions in their patients' health behaviors.[25] A television promotion increased the numbers of people using a designated driver by 10%.[26]

4. *Health status.* Changes in health behaviors are supposed to result in measurable effects on health or risk status. Aetna, for example, found decreases in body fat percentage and cholesterol levels.[27] Blue Shield of California reduced back pain by 17.5% through an exercise program, while 68% of Coors' employee participants in a nutrition/exercise program achieved weight goals. Ventura County achieved reductions in blood pressure and blood glucose levels, though Tenneco found no decrease in injury rates for exercisers versus nonexercisers, perhaps because exercise can cause injury.[28]

AT&T's health promotion failed to reduce blood pressure, weight, or cholesterol levels, though it did improve high-density lipoprotein (HDL) levels.[29] On the other hand, the DANA Corp (Bristol, Virginia) reduced the number of its employees with high cholesterol by 12.5% and found 47% of employees had lower blood pressure.[30]

Screening or early detection of disease will not necessarily reduce expenditures, though it can extend life expectancy and improve quality of life. Pap smears are credited with reducing cervical cancer mortality by 50% in the past 50 years; mammograms along with clinical breast exams can cut breast cancer mortality by one third; bone density scans can identify risks and lead to prevention of osteoporosis.[31]

5. *Health service use.* Changes in health risk behavior and health status should produce differences in health service use. Aetna found its wellness program reduced physician and ED visits as well as hospital admissions.[32] Indian Industries (Evansville, Indiana) was able to reduce its hospital bed day rate from 399 to 221 patient days per thousand in just two years.[33] CIGNA reduced physician visits by 18.4% through the Healthtrac program,[34] while Mayo Clinic reduced pneumonia and influenza admissions by 48% to 57% through its immunization program.[35]

Utilization does not always decline through health improvement initiatives. In some cases HRAs can raise consumer sensitivity to their health, promoting additional physician visits. Health screenings may find a number of false positives or simply detect a number of problems that would not have shown up until later. Consumer attitudes toward medical efficacy and lack of social support can promote utilization even when health risks and morbidity decline.[36] A Canadian program of weekend health educational workshops, for example, found participants increased their use of physician visits, diagnostic services, and mental health counseling as compared to nonparticipants.[37]

To measure the *quality* of health care use, in addition to its quantity, it is necessary to include qualitative measures and to examine the effects of utilization on other effect measures. Changes in use patterns should ideally improve consumer health status, for example, or at least not harm health. The quality of utilization should be reflected in value-adding effects such as consumer quality of life, employer measures of morale and productivity or return to work, and provider measures such as professional satisfaction. In turn such measures add value to health plans through improved marketing success.

6. *Health care expenditures.* Looking at expenditures makes sense for all consumer health behavior improvement efforts, since it provides a direct dollar-for-dollar comparison to the costs of initiatives. In the course of investigating results reported for health improvement efforts, we identified over 50 articles and reports reflecting over 300 case histories of impact on health care expenses. In some cases employers and health plans looked at the annual increase in expenditures. Montana Power saw its rate increases go from 17% to 18% per year to only 12% to 13%.[38] Dominion Resources (Richmond, Virginia) kept its annual increases below 10% through its wellness program.[39] Healthtrac reported employers without wellness programs experienced annual rate increases twice as high as those with programs.[40]

In a review of worksite health promotion programs where health care costs were among the outcomes measured, 80% of such programs were rated as having "encouraging" results, with 13% "mixed" and only 7% "discouraging."[41] Storage Tech (Boulder, Colorado) reported no increase in its annual expense compared to average increases of 14.2% nationally, while Coors held its increase to 5.5%.[42] The City of Birmingham (Alabama) kept its annual expenditures the same for five years![43]

Other sponsors judge their success by comparing their expenditures to their peers. L.L. Bean reported its costs at $2,123 per employee per year, compared to a national average of roughly $4,000.[44] Providence General Medical Center (Everett, Washington) had annual claims costs 33.6% less than the other hospitals in its system.[45]

Many sponsors have reported absolute reductions in expenditures. Aetna estimated its savings at $1.6 million in combined reductions for health care utilization.[46] Steelcase (Grand Rapids, Michigan) estimated it saved $2,000 per employee over three years,[47] reducing medical claims from an average of $1,155 per employee to $537.[48] Quaker Oats claimed savings of $1.4 million per year.[49] One review of 200 cases found that eight of them reported savings of 20% or more in their first year.[50]

Sunbelt Manufacturing (Monroe, Louisiana) reported a reduction in its costs per employee from $2,600 to $1,000 per year over a five-year period.[51] A wellness program at a continuing care retirement community enabled its owners to reduce their required reserves for future nursing home costs from $16 million to $3 million.[52] The Bank of America saw costs for participants go down $164 per employee, while nonparticipants' costs went up $15.[53]

Expense reductions without considering the cost of achieving them can greatly overstate the benefits of wellness and other health improvement programs. The better evaluations report both, often translating them into return on investment ratios to show how many dollars were saved for each dollar spent. One review of 48 studies found that all studies that measured ROI found it positive, ranging from 1.9 to 6.0, which would be excellent returns for any investor.[54]

The federal Centers for Disease Control and Prevention (CDC) reported that worksite wellness programs normally generate ROI ratios of from 2:1 to 3:1.[55] Chapman reported ratios of 2.15 to 5.64 across 30 case studies (with the more rigorous studies tending to report the more positive results) in one review[56] and an average ROI of 5.94 in another review of 25 studies.[57] Among winners of the C. Everett Koop National Health Awards—payers who have been identified as having the best wellness programs—annual savings of 15% to 25% are common, though ROI ratios were not reported.[58]

Sponsors have reported savings for specific focused programs rather than wellness in general, or for wellness combined with counseling (decision improvement), and for programs focusing on chronic conditions (disease management). Union Pacific, for example, estimated savings of $56 per employee per year just from lowering blood pressure and cholesterol.[59] Coile estimates that quitting smoking saves $100,000 per lifetime in health and related expense.[60] Tenneco found that male exercisers cost $561 in medical claims compared to $1,003 for nonexercisers; among females, the difference was even greater: $639 versus $1,535.[61]

Medical Information Systems found that focusing on a small number of high-risk employees generated a savings ratio of 2.59 over four years.[62] Champion International reported $1,260,000 savings from heart risk reduction, compared to $240,000 for stroke.[63] Mayo Clinic estimated that pneumonia and flu vaccines saved $117 per person per year and would save $200 for seniors only.[64] An analysis of chicken pox vaccination estimated that it would save only $80 million a year in health care expense at a cost of $88 million, but that other expense, for example, for lost parent workdays, would mean additional savings of $384 million.[65]

A mammography promotion program at Zeneca Company (Wilmington, Delaware) determined that the early detection of breast cancer had saved it $250,000 over five years compared to the costs of later detection.[66] By targeting high-risk employees for its fitness program, General Electric Aircraft Engine Co. was able to reduce its medical expenditures per employee from $1,044 to $757, while costs for nonparticipants increased from $773 to $941.[67]

Although the vast majority of wellness/prevention/promotion programs report positive results (i.e., savings in health care expenditures), there are some exceptions. Chapman found that while careful evaluation showed "very strong support" for high-risk interventions and "strong support" for blood pressure reduction and exercise promotion, support was only "moderate" for smoking cessation and stress management and was "weak" for cholesterol, nutrition, and weight management programs.[68]

In a five-year tracking of Blue Cross employees, costs for participants in a wellness program were higher in every year except the first.[69] An analysis of early detection programs indicated that screening of the general population is rarely cost-effective. Programs should focus on those whose age, sex, family history, or behavior patterns make them high risks for the conditions being screened for.[70] In a survey of wellness professionals around the country, 2.2% of respondents reported their expenditures had increased, 14.1% were unchanged, 21.7% decreased, and 62% said it was too soon to tell what impact their wellness programs had.[71]

Some evaluation results need to be reviewed carefully. Decreases in the rate of annual increases in expenditures may be common to all payers, reflecting variations in health care inflation patterns rather than success of programs. Decreases in expenditures could reflect chance (e.g., not having a million-dollar case) or the effects of other factors. Having comparison groups (experimental design) that are well matched can reinforce positive findings, as can tracking program impact along the entire sequence of effects, which will tend to strengthen attribution of dollar savings to specific efforts.

7. *Added value.* Added value can be used to add to positive evaluation or, in some cases, may make the difference between a conclusion of failure or success. Where such effects can be translated directly into dollar savings, they can easily be added to health care expenditure reductions to augment the dollar value of results. Where these effects are not translatable, they can at least provide a basis for reconsidering a conclusion.

It is common for worksite wellness and fitness programs to include estimates of impact on absenteeism and productivity, for example. Both can be translated into dollar impact. Fitness programs have been shown to help in reducing worker injuries and workers' compensation costs. Aetna included all such dollar savings in its calculation of $1.6 million in savings.[72] Highsmith found its employees more energetic and self-reliant with greater fitness, but did not attempt to place a dollar value on this value-adding effect.[73]

In a survey of those who reported positive impacts from wellness programs, 91% indicated improved morale, 50% increased productivity, and 47.5% reduced absenteeism.[74] Dupont decreased worker absenteeism by 47.5% and Canada Life reduced turnover by 32.4%.[75] In a more general correlation, companies with healthier employees were found to have higher profits,[76] though more profitable companies may simply be able to afford more health-related programs for their employees.

Among winners of the Koop Awards, employers generally report improvements in productivity, absenteeism, turnover, and morale, in addition to health care expense reductions.[77] Other side effects that have been suggested include quality and quantity of life, employee loyalty and commitment, and job satisfaction.[78] Improved ability to balance the demands of home and work life has also been reported.[79]

DECISION IMPROVEMENT

1. *Participation.* For decision improvement programs, early success can be measured in terms of attendance at education programs or support groups relative to specific decisions. Training programs in cardiopulmonary resuscitation (CPR), caregiving, and self-care can track attendance and completion of training as early indicators of success. Requesting and using self-care guides, information services, and printed and visual materials are additional "participation" measures.[80]

2. *Mind-states.* Ratings of self-efficacy are probably the earliest indication of decision management impact. One program reported an 88% increase in participants' self-rated efficacy in handling childhood fever.[81] Satisfaction with involvement in efforts to improve decision-making capability is another useful mind-state measure. A study of self-care guide users found 61% reporting it improved their preparation for physician visits, 63% felt it helped their family's health, 47% said it helped them decide whether and when to see a physician, and 97% rated the guide as easy to understand.[82]

3. *Behavior.* Decision improvement aims at changing how people use health services, so about the only measures of behavior other than use of services that make sense in its evaluation are indications of using self-care instead. While most evaluations simply look at reductions in service use, one study found that 60% of callers to a phone triage service took care of the problem that prompted their call at home by themselves. It was estimated that without triage, only 10% would have done so.[83]

4. *Health status.* Since the aim of decision improvement initiatives is to improve the choices that consumers make, health status affects are typically not the focus of evaluation. In most cases changes in the decisions made are

checked to be sure they had no *adverse* impact on health status rather than looking for positive effects. Phone triage and treatment choice counseling services are followed up to be sure that patients steered to self-care or a less resource-intensive, lower-cost form of care are not worse off. Health plan and provider choices can be judged by differences in HEDIS health status measures that result.

5. *Health service use.* Health service use is precisely where decision improvement is supposed to see its impact felt. Since most sponsors of triage, counseling, education, and training programs intended to empower consumers to make better decisions are hoping for reductions in health care use, that is typically where they look for impact. Triage programs routinely report significant drops in use of ED or physician visits; one vendor of such a program claims 15% to 25% reductions in both.[84]

A review of self-care and triage programs in combination found reductions in physician office visits in the range of 15% to17% overall, or 22% to 35% in minor symptom visits.[85] Kaiser reported a 17% reduction in ambulatory care visits, with a drop of 35% in childhood fever visits.[86] An Air Force program reduced physician visits by 16% and ED visits by 28%.[87] Blue Shield reduced physician visits by 15%, minor problem visits by 34.6%.[88]

Decision counseling programs show reductions as well: 20% to 33% reductions in surgeries, for example.[89] A patient advocate nurse program helped achieve a reduction in hospital days.[90] At RCA, a nurse counselor helped reduce hospital bed-day use rates by 20%.[91] Interactive videos on benign prostate hyperplasia cut rates of surgery for that condition by 40%.[92]

While champions of decision improvement programs would insist that changes in utilization represent equally good care at lower costs, there seem to be few examples of triage counseling programs that aim specifically at improving the quality of use patterns. One exception may be the variety of social and commercial communications efforts aimed at getting people with chest pain to seek care earlier. Qual-Med HMO also claims that its outreach triage and phone counseling program encourages members to get the care they need when they need it rather than delay.[93]

6. *Health care expenditures.* With reductions in use will come reductions in expenditures, in most cases. Aetna reported its self-care program saved an average of $325 per person per year, while Union Pacific reported savings of $45.[94] One analyst estimated the normal savings from triage programs at $5 to $7 per member per month.[95] Another reported savings of 7% to 17% over two years.[96] An HMO executive claims that the HMO's self-care book alone saves $250 per member per year.[97]

A nurse counseling program reduced RCA's expenses by $53 (3.8%) per employee in the group who were used to judge the program, where costs increased by \$109 (6.0%) per employee in the control group.[98] Parker-Hennifan (Cleveland, Ohio) cut its cost increase to 8.3% compared to the national average of 15%, thanks partly to a nurse counseling service. Patients who had planned their end-of-life experience through advance directives (ADs) spent \$30,478 for their last hospitalization, compared to \$95,305 for those without ADs.[99]

Since triage and decision counseling programs cost sponsors money, the ROI from such programs is a major consideration. The CalPers system for California State employees determined a \$3:1 ROI ratio for its self-care program, while Bank of America retirees produced a \$6:1 ratio. An added advantage was that these savings occurred in the first year of the program.[100] Union Pacific reported an ROI ratio of \$2.77,[101] whereas RCA calculated a ratio of \$4:1.

Self-care books alone were reported to generate ROI ratios of \$2.50 to \$3.50.[102] In one of the few studies to compare different self-care approaches, the Wisconsin Education Association found that supplying employees with a self-care book alone produced an ROI ratio of \$2.40:1, where the same book combined with nurse counseling achieved a ratio of \$4.75:1, even with higher costs.[103]

7. *Value added.* We found no published studies of value-adding effects of decision improvement programs. If promoted correctly, however, they should be advantageous in attracting and retaining health plan enrollees given the advantages they offer to consumers. If the savings from such programs were shared with consumers, the effects could even be greater. By the same token, employers should be able to use results to promote employee recruitment and retention for the same reasons.

Consumers who call triage phone lines and gain confidence that they can handle the "emergency" problem themselves obtain the benefits of immediate treatment compared to travel, long waits, and copays that are likely to be part of the costs of going to an ED or urgent care source. They may also gain a sense of control over their own or family health, greater independence, and a sense of accomplishment.

DISEASE MANAGEMENT

1. *Participation.* Where sponsors employ education and training classes and seminars, or lend out written and visual materials, or offer libraries and information lines to consumers and caregivers concerned about chronic conditions, they can use participation measures to track early response. Patient Education Media, Inc, operating under the Time-Life Medical trade name, which markets a series of 30 videos on as many conditions, can track sales of those videos as a participation measure.[104]

2. *Mind-states.* While sponsors of disease management programs aim primarily for reductions in acute episodes and use of emergency care, there are a few who have tracked mind-state changes as well. The Arthritis Patient Self-Management Program offered by Eidetics, Inc (Watertown, Massachusetts) gauges participant perceptions of their sense of control over their condition, satisfaction with their health, and overall attitudes.[105] CareWise, Inc, formerly the Employee Managed Care Corp, (Bellevue, Washington) tracks participants' perceptions of self-efficacy and their ability to manage their own condition.[106]

3. *Behavior.* Desirable behaviors in disease management include making whatever temporary or permanent lifestyle changes are indicated by patients' conditions. Eliminating smoking, alcohol, and drugs while pregnant; reducing salt intake if suffering from congestive heart failure or high blood pressure; and avoiding allergy-exacerbating conditions are a few examples. The CareWise program tracks what positive changes in lifestyle its participants make.[107]

For acute conditions the key behavior is often complying with medications. One study reports that generally half of all patients fail to take medications as directed, with compliance ranging from a low of 24% for patients with cardiac arrhythmia to 82% for patients taking immunosuppressants. Though the costs of noncompliance vary as well, low-cost interventions such as reminders by drug companies, pharmacists, and physicians have proven effective at costs in the under $1.00 per month range.[108]

4. *Health status.* Effective disease management should be reflected first in disease patterns, at least for acute conditions and pregnancy. Most published studies seem to focus on pregnancy, noting the dramatic differences in adverse fetal outcomes that apply to those who manage their pregnancy well versus poorly. The CIGNA Healthy Babies program, for example, reported 95% of participants had full-term babies versus only 83% of nonparticipants.[109] Among its participants, 60% had normal, uncomplicated deliveries versus 40% of nonparticipants.[110] By focusing on high-risk mothers, the PreNatal Plus program was able to reduce the incidence of premature births from 3.4% to 2.7%.[111]

Health status improvements in acute conditions might be measured in terms of time for recovery and return to work or normal activity. Compliance with medication or lifestyle changes are process measures that should lead to better outcomes. For chronic conditions, functional status measures such as mobility, activities of daily living, and pain will work for many patients.[112]

5. *Health service use.* Disease management is often touted as offering significant and early reductions in health care utilization. An analysis of HMO efforts and results in disease management reported that 74% of the HMOs reduced ED visits, 73.7% cut hospital admissions, 48.8% lessened specialist

visits, 34.4% cut back on diagnostic tests, 33.3% reduced home health visits, 28.2% cut primary physician visits, and 25.5% made a dent in prescription drug use.[113] How much of a difference that makes in any given population depends on how many have chronic conditions, of course, but chronic disease patients often use five to ten times as much care as healthy ones, so a reduction in use by this high-use population should make a big difference.

Self-management by asthma patients has reduced ED visits up to 79% and hospital admissions by as much as 86%.[114] The PrimeCare asthma management program produced a reduction from 36% having an ED visit with 12% admitted to 11% having a visit and 4% admitted, roughly a two thirds reduction in utilization.[115]

For pregnancies, prenatal care in one case reduced use of neonatal intensive care unit (NICU) days by one week on average.[116] Participants in a prenatal care education program had a 19% Caesarean section rate, where nonparticipants had a 28% rate.[117] A Baby Benefit program reduced the use of NICU days per thousand births from 248 for nonparticipants to 184 for participants.[118]

Acute care, preadmission education and patient participation helped to reduce heart surgery average length of stay (ALOS) by 19%, and by training patients for their role in surgery, Kaiser was able to reduce overall surgical ALOS by 1.5 days (12%) per case.[119] Through phone monitoring of patients, a Veterans Administration (VA) medical clinic was able to reduce medication use by 14%, physician visits by 19%, hospital days by 28%, and intensive care unit (ICU) days by 41%.[120]

6. *Health care expenditures.* Disease management programs have had significant impact on total employee, enrollee, and community expenditures for health care, particularly among populations with high proportions of chronic conditions. One analyst estimated that it would save $2 to $3 per member per month across an entire population if as few as 5% had chronic conditions.[121] Increasing compliance with hypertension medication saved $82 per patient for established patients, $125 for new patients.[122]

Lovelace Health System (Albuquerque, New Mexico) was able to reduce ambulatory visits, hospital admissions, and ALOS for pediatric asthma patients enough to reduce expenses from $4,102 to $2,797 per patient.[123] The National Jewish Center for Immunology and Respiratory Medicine (Denver, Colorado) estimates reduction by two thirds in lifetime costs for treating asthma patients, though amounts vary for pediatric, adolescent, and adult patients.[124] PrimeCare (Wisconsin) saved $867,000 through its asthma management program, at a cost of $32,000, for an ROI ratio of $27:1.[125] Employee Assistance Programs for employees with behavioral health problems have been found to produce ROI ratios of from $5:1 to $7:1.[126]

Prenatal care has been a major source of reported savings in health care expenditures and one that pays off quickly, limited only by the normal gestation period. It has been estimated that prenatal care and compliance can save $3 per member per month across the entire enrolled population, depending on numbers of pregnant women in the population.[127] CIGNA found costs per delivery for participants in its Healthy Babies program were $5,141 versus $14,116 for nonparticipants.[128] Blue Cross/Blue Shield of New Hampshire saved $7,000 per participant in its high-risk mother program, for a total savings of $3.5 million.[129]

For individual, high-risk pregnant women, the combination of care and compliance can mean the difference between having an extremely premature (25 to 26 week gestation) baby, with costs in the quarter to half million dollar range, and having a normal, healthy baby with costs of a few thousand dollars. Ventura County, California had two low-birth-weight babies in the year before it initiated its prenatal program, costing $700,000, with none since the program went into effect.[130]

7. *Value added.* The greatest value-adding effects of effective disease management programs are found in the attitudes and quality of life of patients. In addition, they frequently save consumers significant out-of-pocket costs by reducing their use of services that have copayment requirements.[131] They can influence consumer decisions on plan selection and reenrollment, thereby affecting health plan market share,[132] though, as described in Chapter 23, this may prove problematic for the health plan.

Consumers should always gain a sense of control and greater independence as a result of the knowledge and skills they gain in managing their own conditions. They should gain reassurance, lessened anxiety, greater sense of security about such conditions, and, perhaps, increased self-worth as "experts" in their own conditions. They may find an enhanced sense of belonging through socializing in person at classes or support groups, for example, or via Internet chat rooms and similar technologies.

Often behavioral health interventions are judged by their impact on worker morale, productivity, and absenteeism, in addition to health care utilization and expenditures. Prenatal and parenting programs typically reduce the time women spend on maternity leave and produce additional savings to employers, in addition to health expenditure reductions.[133]

DISABILITY MANAGEMENT

1. *Participation.* Early indications of success for disability management efforts may be found in numbers of participants in safety education and training programs and in requests for safety information or equipment. Attendance at semi-

nars or lunchtime discussions of safety problems and workers' compensation costs may indicate to what extent employees take ownership of the problem.

2. *Mind-states.* Beyond attendance at programs, employees can be surveyed to learn if any changes in knowledge, attitudes, or intentions have been achieved. Are employees satisfied with the programs they attended? Do they consider workers' compensation expenditures and lost time from work problems they share with the employer or entitlements they would be loathe to give up?

3. *Behavior.* Specific behaviors of interest may be the numbers of employees wearing safety equipment, using safe lifting techniques, and following safety rules and guidelines, generally. Monitoring such behaviors may be essential to understanding changes in injury incidence and severity, as well the earliest indicators that efforts have had real impact.

   Creative Windows (Elkhart, Indiana) changed employee behaviors so as to reduce repetitive stress injuries (also called cumulative trauma disorders). By rotating assignments and redesigning tools and equipment to fit women, it was able to significantly reduce the risk of such injuries.[134]

4. *Health status.* Since employers are likely to have established counts of injuries that require days lost from work or medical treatment, monitoring health status effects should be relatively simple. Champion International saw its safety "incidents" drop from 689 in the year before its disability management back injury prevention program to 91, then 82 in the next two years.[135] Hon Industries cut on-the-job injuries by 67% and Shoney's by 30% through fitness promotion.[136] A small employer cut its lost-time accidents from 13 a year to 12 to 8, then averaged under 2.[137]

   The *Fresno* (California) *Bee* newspaper reduced its annual carpal tunnel injury claims from 24 to 13 in just one year of effort at a time when such injuries are increasing 20% per year nationwide.[138] Proportions of employees returning to work within projected recovery times or proportions able to return to their previous jobs can also be used as success measures.

5. *Health service use.* All the above examples represent probable reductions in health service use. In some cases employers may measure such use directly, looking for changes in which providers are selected, how many treatments employees have, and how long they stay in the hospital. They may benchmark their own experience against industry norms or best performers in terms of utilization for comparable injuries.

   Aetna Life & Casualty contacts their own injured employees to guide them in provider selection and includes work-hardening programs if they will be helpful in speeding up the employee's return to work. Its case managers help with transportation and use ergonomic specialists to make changes in the employee's work space if needed to accommodate any lasting disability or limitations.[139]

6. *Health care expenditures.* Successful disability management programs are most frequently reported in terms of the cost savings they produced for employers. Champion International found costs for participants in its back injury prevention program to be 30% lower than for nonparticipants.[140] Towers Perrin found that disability costs per case averaged $23,733 among employers with "good" disability management programs versus $43,300 for the rest.[141]

One injury/back pain prevention program saved an estimated $200 per employee per year.[142] Another saved $450 per employee one year with savings of $600 predicted for the next.[143] The Mannas Company reduced its disability costs by 90% through the simple expedient of making each manager accountable for such costs in the budget.[144] A small employer reduced its workers' compensation claims by $250,000 at a cost of $12,000, producing an ROI of over $20:1.[145]

Portland (Maine) Glass Company reduced its workers compensation costs by 65% through a five-year effort involving changing corporate culture, safety incentives, and case management.[146] Aetna reduced disability costs 16%, medical expenses by 27%, and income replacement by 5% over seven quarters.[147] Creative Windows reduced insurance costs from $600 per family to $260, while the *Fresno Bee* reduced its costs from $250,000 a year to $6,000.[148]

By managing disability cases itself and opting out of the state workers' compensation insurance program, permissable in Texas, the Design Resources Group (Dallas) was able to reduce its premiums from $250,000 to $83,000; Long John Silver's restaurant chain cut its claims costs from $2.6 million to $340,000 in two years.[149]

7. *Added value.* Disability management programs have the potential for producing all the value-adding effects of the other three domains in terms of employees and families (e.g., improved morale, quality of work life, productivity, retention, absenteeism). Absenteeism that results from disability days is directly reflected in employer costs and so would be included in expenditure savings.

By decreasing disability days per injury and helping workers return to work, Aetna has enjoyed significant improvements in productivity.[150] By temporarily assigning recovering workers to lighter tasks, the Portland Glass Company achieved similar gains.[151] Companies that have introduced work and process redesign to reduce injuries often find increased productivity results as well.[152]

The psychological and social benefits that employees may gain from disability management efforts include perceived control and autonomy relative to their own worksite health, enhanced security versus fear of disability, and sense of accomplishment. All the benefits available in the other demand improvement categories are available here.

CONCLUSION

It is clear from the hundreds of cases reviewed that the four domains of health and demand improvement initiatives hold tremendous promise as cost savings approaches for payers and providers, as well as quality-of-life improvement opportunities for consumers. Compared to supply-focused controls and consumer barrier alternatives, they promise far greater savings for the future, far fewer negative side effects on consumers and providers, and less risk of public and political backlash to sponsors.

The findings cited here cannot be construed as promises of what payers or providers will achieve in their own situations. Differences in who sponsors specific initiatives, characteristics of the consumer population and their relationship with sponsors, and how well strategies are chosen and tactics are implemented will create wide variation in results. The results achieved by others should at least be seen as benchmarks representing what can be achieved and as indicators of the potential that demand improvement holds.

Sponsors of particular demand improvement initiatives should pay special attention to the consumer benefit effects of their efforts. Virtually every such initiative should benefit consumers; that is what makes improving health and demand so much safer than controlling utilization from the supply side. It is also what should make it easier for sponsors to attract consumers to enthusiastically accept and participate in such initiatives. The more attention is given to such benefits up front, in planning and implementing initiatives, the better luck sponsors should have in achieving desired behavior changes and the value they hope to gain from them.

We have provided only a sampling of the effects achieved by sponsors in this chapter. Additional results are reported in Chapters 21 through 24 in discussions of each of the four demand improvement domains.

REFERENCES

1. D. Vickery, "Toward Appropriate Use of Medical Care," *Healthcare Forum Journal* 39, no. 1 (1996):15–19.

2. "Aetna Measures Success of Aenhance®," *Employee Health & Fitness* 17, no. 1 (1995):4, 5.

3. E. Alberti and J. Sutton, "Improving Outcomes Reporting in a Senior Wellness Program," in *Clinical Practice Improvement,* eds. S. Horn and D. Hoplevin (Washington, DC: Faulkner & Gray, 1994), 237–246.

4. E. Brown, "How Cost-Effective Are Wellness Programs?" *Managed Healthcare* 5, no. 1 (1995): 40–42.

5. J. Fries, "Health Risk Change with a Low-Cost Individualized Health Promotion Program," *American Journal of Health Promotion* 6, no. 5 (1992):364–371.

6. J. Fries, *The Health Project Methodology for Evaluating Effectiveness of Worksite Programs by the Program Selection Task Force* (Palo Alto, CA: Stanford University Press, 1994).

7. F. Cerne, "Local Alliance Calms Tempers and Tackles Health Costs," *Hospitals & Health Networks,* 20 November 1993, 54.

8. J. Montague et al., "How To Save Big Bucks," *Hospitals & Health Networks,* March 1996, 18–24.

9. S. Pronk, et al., "Impact of a Daily 10-Minute Strength and Flexibility Program in a Manufacturing Plant," *American Journal of Health Promotion* 9, no. 3 (1995):175–178.

10. "Aetna's Program Keeps Employees Out of the Hospital, Slashes Medical Costs," *Employee Health & Fitness* 17, no. 1 (1995):1.

11. Alberti and Sutton, "Improving Outcomes Reporting," 237–246.

12. *Healthtrac Case Study: Major Company in Financial Services Industry* (Palo Alto, CA: Healthtrac, Inc.).

13. M. Holt, et al., "Health Impacts of AT&T's Total Life Concept (TLC) Program after Five Years," *American Journal of Health Promotion* 9, no. 6 (1995):421–425.

14. "Long-Term Campaigns Show PR's Value: Multi-Year Efforts Document Rise in Awareness, Media Coverage," *Health PR & Marketing News* 5, no. 3 (1996):7.

15. A. Peck, "All Is Wellness," *Managed Healthcare News* 3, no. 8 (1993):22–24.

16. Pronk et al., "Impact," 175–178.

17. "Tracking Canada's Health Promotion Campaigns," *Health Promotion,* Winter 1988/1989, 22–26.

18. L. Loescher, et al., "Public Education Projects in Skin Cancer," *Cancer* Supplement 75, no. 2 (1995):651–656.

19. "Aetna Measures Success," 4, 5.

20. Alberti and Sutton, "Improving Outcomes Reporting," 237–246.

21. N. Bell, "From the Trenches: Strategies That Work," *Business & Health* 9, no. 5 (1991):19–25.

22. R. Bertera, "Behavior Risk Factors and Illness Day Changes with Workplace Health Promotion," *American Journal of Health Promotion* 7, no. 5 (1993):365–373.

23. Fries, *The Health Project Methodology.*

24. Holt, et al., "Health Impacts," 421–425.

25. P. Terry, et al., "Does Health Education Work?" *The Bulletin* 37, no. 2 (1993):95–109.

26. "TV Promotes Designated Drivers," *Medical Self Care* 54 (1990):13.

27. "Aetna's Program," 1.

28. Fries, *The Health Project Methodology.*

29. Holt, et al., "Health Impacts," 421–425.

30. C. Petersen, "Wellness Pays Off at This Firm," *Managed Healthcare* 6, no. 3 (1996):36.

31. K. Griffin, "The LifeSavers: 8 Medical Tests You Shouldn't Ignore," *Health* 10, no. 3 (1996): 107–112.

32. "Aetna Measures Success," 4, 5.

33. M. Battagliola, "One Company on the Wellness Frontier," in *The State of Health Care in America* (Montvale, NJ: Business & Health, 1995), 18.

34. Fries, *The Health Project Methodology.*

35. "Mayo Clinic Develops Disease Management Strategy To Handle Capitation," *Healthcare Leadership Review* 14, no. 7 (1995):9, 10.

36. W. Lynch, et al., "Predicting the Demand for Healthcare," *Healthcare Forum Journal* 39, no. 1 (1996):20–24.

37. M. Cousins and I. McDowell, "Use of Medical Care after a Community-Based Health Promotion Program," *American Journal of Health Promotion* 10, no. 1 (1995):47–54.

38. M. Battagliola, M. "Making Employees Better Health Care Consumers," *Business & Health* 10, no. 6 (1992):22–28.

39. K. Davis, "Now the Good News on Health Care," *Wall Street Journal,* 20 September 1993, A14.

40. M. Bricklin, "The Power of Proactive Prevention," *Prevention,* February 1994, 45, 46.

41. C. Heaney and R. Goetzel, "A Review of Health-Related Outcomes of Multi-Component Worksite Health Promotion Programs," *American Journal of Health Promotion* 11, no. 4 (1997): 290–308.

42. K. Smith, "Companies Find Savings in Wellness," *Rocky Mountain News,* 23 January 1994, 93A, 102A.

43. K. Pelletier, K. "A Review and Analysis of the Health and Cost-Effective Outcome Studies of Comprehensive Health Promotion and Disease Prevention Programs at the Worksite: 1991–1993 Update," *American Journal of Health Promotion* 8, no. 1 (1993):50–62.

44. C. Beadle, "Announcement of the 1994 C. Edward Koop Awards for Outstanding Health Care Programs," *American Journal of Health Promotion* 9, no. 2 (1994):104–106.

45. "Databases Provide Strong Basis for Demonstrating Wellness Payoffs," *St. Anthony's Managing Community Health and Wellness* 2, no. 4 (1995):7.

46. "Aetna's Program," 1.

47. Beadle, "Announcement," 104–106.

48. "For the Record," *Modern Healthcare,* 17 January 1994, 16.

49. E. Brown, "How Cost-Effective Are Wellness Programs?" *Managed Healthcare* 5, no. 1 (1995): 40–42.

50. "Can Prevention Lower Health Costs by Reducing Demand?" *Hospitals & Health Networks,* 5 February 1994, 10.

51. F. Cerne, "Dollars and Sense: Creating Incentives To Effectively Manage Change," *Hospitals & Health Networks,* 5 April 1994, 28–30.

52. M. Crowley, "Living Longer and Better Than Expected," *Health Progress* 73, no. 10 (1992):38–41.

53. J. Fries, et al., "Two-Year Results of a Randomized Controlled Trial of a Health Promotion Program in a Retiree Population: The Bank of America Study," *American Journal of Health Promotion* 7, no. 5 (1993):455–462.

54. K. Pelletier, "Healthy People, Healthy Worksites," *Healthcare Forum Journal* 36, no. 6 (1993): 34–39.

55. Bricklin, "The Power of Proactive Prevention," 45, 46.

56. L. Chapman, *Proof Positive: Analysis of the Cost-Effectiveness of Worksite Wellness,* 3d ed. (Seattle, WA: Summex Corp, 1996).

57. L. Chapman, "Meta-Analysis of Studies on the Cost-Effectiveness of Worksite Health Promotion Programs," The Art and Science of Health Promotion Conference (Orlando, FL: March 7–11 1995, American Journal of Health Promotion).

58. C. Petersen, "Wellness Program Promotion Continues at Top Speed," *Managed Healthcare* 3, no. 12 (1993):27.

59. Beadle, "Announcement," 104–106.

60. R. Coile, "Integrating the Patient into Healthcare Systems," *Hospital Strategy Report* 5, no. 5 (1993):2.

61. Fries, *The Health Project Methodology.*

62. J. Harris, "Forecasting: A Legitimate Health Promotion Business Tool," *Health Promotion Practitioner* 4, no. 12 (1995):4.

63. Beadle, "Announcement," 104–106.

64. "Mayo Clinic Develops Disease Management Strategy," 9, 10.

65. L. Scott, "Looking beyond Cost," *Modern Healthcare,* 28 February 1994, 36–40.

66. J. Wechsler, "Employers Offer Breast Cancer Screening for Employees," *Managed Healthcare,* November 1993, 50.

67. "The Wellness Wave," *Profiles in Hospital Marketing* 55 (1993):22–27.

68. Chapman, *Proof Positive.*

69. J. Sciacca, et al., "The Impact of Participation in Health Promotion on Medical Costs," *American Journal of Health Promotion* 7, no. 5 (1993):374–383, 395.

70. A. Stanaland and B. Gelb, "Can Prevention Be Marketed Profitably?" *Journal of Health Care Marketing* 15, no. 4 (Winter 1995):59–63.

71. "Impact of Wellness Felt in Worksites Nationwide," *Wellness Program Management Advisor* 1, no. 1 (1996):1–3.

72. "Aetna Measures Success," 4, 5.

73. D. Fenn, "Healthy Workers Cost Less," *INC.,* May 1995, 137.

74. "Impact of Wellness," 1–3.

75. Peck, "All Is Wellness," 22–24.

76. Brown, "How Cost-Effective," 40–42.

77. Beadle, "Announcement," 104–106.

78. S. McBride, "Prevention: Good Medicine, Good Business," *Managed Healthcare* 4, no. 11 (1994):26, 27.

79. "Aetna's Program," 1.

80. "Quantifying the Impact of Your Demand Management Programs," *Healthcare Demand Management* 2, no. 1 (1996):10–12.

81. Coile, "Integrating the Patient," 2.

82. "Quantifying the Impact," 10–12.

83. "Phone-Based Triage System Brings Bottom-Line Benefits to Pediatric Hospitals, Physicians," *Healthcare Demand Management* 1, no. 1 (1995):9–11.

84. R. Anderson and D. Smith, "Investment in Prevention Is a New Idea in Our 'Pay-Me-Later' Society," *AHA News* 28, no. 20 (1992):6.

85. Brown, "How Cost-Effective," 40–42.

86. Coile, "Integrating the Patient," 2.

87. J. Fries and D. Vickery, *Strategic Approach to Demand Management* (Golden, CO: Healthtrac/ Health Decisions, Inc.).

88. Fries, *The Health Project Methodology.*

89. Anderson and Smith, "Investment in Prevention," 6.

90. Battagliola, "One Company," 18.

91. P. O'Donnell, "Managing Health Costs under a Fee-for-Service Plan," *Business & Health* 5, no. 5 (1987):38–40.

92. Peck, "All Is Wellness," 22–24.

93. D. Algeo, "Doctor Forecasts Triage Prelude to Medical Golden Age," *Denver Post,* 16 March 1996, 1D–2D.

94. Beadle, "Announcement," 104–106.

95. Anderson and Smith, "Investment in Prevention," 6.

96. Brown, "How Cost-Effective," 40–42.

97. E. Sipf, "Employee Education Cools Fevered Health Care Expenses," *Denver Business Journal,* 9 July 1990, 9.

98. O'Donnell, "Managing Health Costs," 38–40.

99. W. Weeks, "Advance Directives and the Cost of Terminal Hospitalization," *Archives of Internal Medicine* 154 (1994):2077–2083.

100. J. Fries, "Health Care Demand Management," *Medical Interface,* March 1994, 55–58.

101. M. Goldstein, "Emerging Data Show Programs Are Effective," *Modern Healthcare,* 21 August 1995, 144–146.

102. S. Siegelman, "Health Plan Options: Inquiring Employees Want To Know," *Business & Health* 9, no. 1 (1991):14–22.

103. "Insurer Gets Cost Savings from Demand Management," *Accountability News for Health Care Managers* 2, no. 8 (1995):2, 3.

104. "Outliers—Kooped Off," *Modern Healthcare,* 3 February 1997, 76.

105. R. Davis and J. Hay, *Arthritis Patient Self Management Program Outcomes Analysis* (Watertown, MA: Eidetics, Inc., 1994).

106. Promotional brochure. Bellevue, WA: Employee Managed Care Corporation.

107. Promotional brochure.

108. J. Mandelker, "Monitoring Drug Compliance Can Reduce Total Medical Plan Costs," *Business & Health* 11, no. 6 (1993):26–35.

109. J. Burns, "The Need for More Rigor When Measuring and Reporting Results," *Business & Health* 13, no. 1 (1995):8.

110. Goldstein, "Emerging Data," 144–146.

111. Montague, et al., "How To Save Big Bucks," 18–24.

112. Davis and Hay, *Arthritis Patient.*

113. "HMOs Aggressively Developing Disease Management Programs: Cost Reductions Reported," *Healthcare Demand & Disease Management* 3, no. 6 (1997):94–96.

114. Bricklin, "The Power of Proactive Prevention," 45, 46.

115. Montague, et al., "How To Save Big Bucks," 18–24.

116. Montague, et al., "How To Save Big Bucks," 18–24.

117. J. Packer-Tursman, "A Growing Priority," *Managed Healthcare News* 2, no. 9 (1993): 57, 58.

118. "With Program Evaluation, Don't Close Barn Door after the Horse Is Out," *Employee Health & Fitness* 17, no. 11 (1995):121–126.

119. M. Buser, "Pre-Established Care Guides Patients to Recovery," *California Hospitals* 7, no. 4 (1993):10–12.

120. J. Wasson, et al., "Telephone Care as a Substitute for Routine Clinic Follow-Up," *JAMA* 267, no. 13 (1992):1788–1793.

121. Anderson and Smith, "Investment in Prevention," 6.

122. Mandelker, "Monitoring Drug Compliance," 26–35.

123. J. Byrnes, *Using Real World Technology To Measure Outcomes* (San Francisco: Congress on Health Outcomes and Accountability, 1995).

124. "Asthma Program Slashes Hospitalization Costs," *Disease State Management* 1, no. 3 (1995):331–333.

125. Montague, et al., "How To Save Big Bucks," 18–24.

126. "When 'Warm Fuzzies' Don't Work: Use Hard Facts To Prove Your Value," *Wellness Program Management Advisor* 1, no. 3 (1996):4, 5.

127. Anderson and Smith, "Investment in Prevention," 6.

128. Burns, "The Need for More Rigor," 8.

129. "Concord, N.H.," *Modern Healthcare,* 23 November 1992, 26.

130. Fries, *The Health Project Methodology.*

131. Montague, et al., "How To Save Big Bucks," 18–24.

132. Promotional brochure.

133. E. Zicklin, "Prenatal Teamwork Fosters an Employer/Employee Partnership," *Business & Health* 10, no. 4 (1992):36–40.

134. B. Dimmitt, "Repetitive Stress Injuries: Relieving Pain at the Bottom Line," *Business & Health* 13, no. 5 (1995):21–24.

135. Beadle, "Announcement," 104–106.

136. L. Driscoll, "Compensating for Workers' Comp Costs," *Business Week,* 3 February 1992, 72.

137. "Making Safety Pay," *Profiles in Hospital Marketing,* January/February 1993, 2–5.

138. Dimmitt, "Repetitive Stress Injuries," 21–24.

139. "Aetna Finds Success with In-House Integrated Disability Program," *St. Anthony's Managing Community Health and Wellness* 2, no. 7 (1996):5.

140. Beadle, "Announcement," 104–106.

141. I. Bremer, "A Workplace Armageddon," *Corporate Finance,* March/April 1993, 18, 19.

142. Fries, *The Health Project Methodology.*

143. G. Leavenworth, "Big Savings for Small Companies," *Business & Health* 13, no. 1 (1995):38–42.

144. Driscoll, "Compensating," 72.

145. "Making Safety Pay," 2–5.

146. "Safety Programs Pay Off," *INC.,* May 1996, 114.

147. "Aetna Finds Success," 5.

148. Dimmitt, "Repetitive Stress Injuries," 21–24.

149. G. Leavenworth, "What If You Opted Out of Workers' Comp?" *Business & Health* 13, no. 8 (1995):23–28.

150. "Aetna Finds Success," 5.

151. "Safety Programs Pay Off," 114.

152. Dimmitt, "Repetitive Stress Injuries," 21–24.

PART II

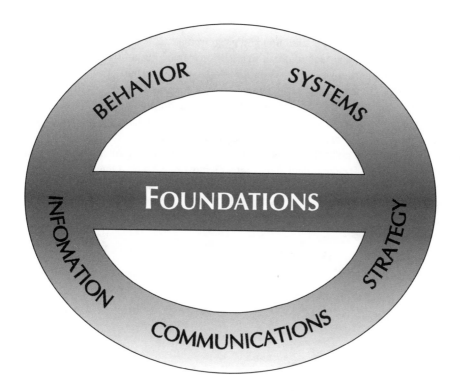

Part II supplies information on the basic foundations for demand improvement. It is intended to be of value to readers who are interested in the intellectual and practical tools available to support both strategic thinking and tactical interventions relative to consumer health and demand behaviors. These foundations should be of particular interest to those with strategic responsibilities, though readers with programmatic responsibilities should find them helpful as well.

Chapter 6 discusses the wide array of theoretical models available to aid in understanding, predicting, and/or influencing consumer health and care-seeking behaviors. It introduces the authors' own model, which emphasizes the options available for changing behavior. Chapter 7 provides both warnings and advice relative to the limits of simple cause-and-effect models and suggests ways to extend the vision and thinking of strategists and planners relative to improving demand. Readers already familiar with these behavior models and systems thinking may skim these chapters to see how we suggest employing both in specific challenges.

Chapter 8 describes the kinds of information foundations necessary for sponsors to carry out strategic planning and programmatic efforts. Chapter 9 examines the communications technologies available for reaching and empowering consumers, with particular emphasis on new and evolving technologies. These chapters are recommended to both strategic and programmatic readers, either for immediate challenges they are facing or for reference purposes.

Chapter 10 describes the strategic foundations for determining whether and how to invest in demand improvement. It covers the wide range of options available to the many potential sponsors of demand improvement interventions. It addresses the key strategic decisions sponsors must make and suggests criteria and concerns relative to those decisions. It also offers a list of vendors of strategic services potential sponsors might consider in addition to relying on their internal capabilities. We believe every reader should at least review this chapter.

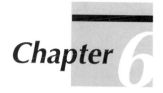

Chapter 6

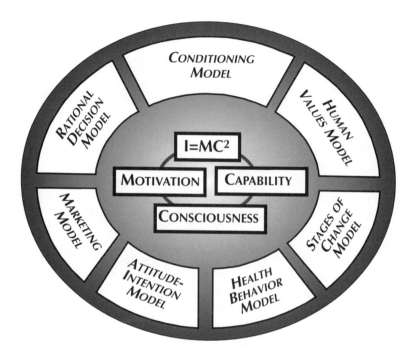

CONDITIONING MODEL

RATIONAL DECISION MODEL

HUMAN VALUES MODEL

I=MC²

MOTIVATION   CAPABILITY

CONSCIOUSNESS

MARKETING MODEL

STAGES OF CHANGE MODEL

ATTITUDE-INTENTION MODEL

HEALTH BEHAVIOR MODEL

BEHAVIORAL FOUNDATIONS

Since the focus of demand improvement is on improving consumer health and demand behaviors, we believe it is helpful to include some discussion of what is known about the causes of human behavior and ways to change it. In this chapter we will briefly describe and discuss the variety of models that have historically been used to understand, predict, and influence human behavior. We have adopted an eclectic approach, borrowing from what we feel are the best points of many models, to develop our own model, combining motivation, capability, and consciousness as the three most effective foundations for improving consumer health and demand behavior.

Readers already fully conversant or simply not interested in the behavioral foundations for managing consumer health and demand behaviors may wish to skip the first part of this chapter and move directly to the discussion of our composite model.

Understanding, predicting, and influencing human behavior have been the aims of a wide variety of sciences and pseudosciences, from psychology, sociology, anthropology, and social psychology to hypnotism, marketing, politics, and counseling. We take a pragmatic approach to these foundations for improving consumer health and demand behaviors; we are interested in whatever works, regardless of discipline.

Some disciplines seek mainly to *understand* behavior, perhaps to *predict* it. Many are truly "academic" in the sense that they are meant to delight the mind without necessarily changing anything. Others are intent upon *influencing* behavior, with political, commercial, or altruistic motives, perhaps, but with the conscious intention of changing how people act. We fall into this latter group, and we incorporate insights from any and all disciplines that will help us.

There have been serious efforts to understand and describe human motivation going back at least as far as Plato and Aristotle. Those acknowledged as history's greatest minds have addressed the problem.[1] We have looked for insights from all of them, for ideas on the best "leverage points" that offer significant opportunities to intervene so as to improve consumer health and demand behaviors. In the process we examined the complex, dynamic system of factors affecting behavior to find some places where specific initiatives can best promote and reinforce positive behaviors or extinguish negative.[2]

In the wide variety of disciplines concerned with understanding, predicting, and influencing human behavior, there are many theories about what makes us behave as we do, each discipline having many theories.[3] We will review a selection of these theories or models of behavior under seven categories:

1. rational decision models,
2. conditioning models,
3. human value/need models,
4. marketing models,
5. attitude/intention models,
6. health behavior models, and
7. stages of change model.

Following this review we will describe our own pragmatic model based on all seven categories, one that we feel can help sponsors of behavior improvement initiatives understand and select the best strategies and tactics for specific challenges.

RATIONAL DECISION-MAKING MODELS

Many analysts of human behavior have stressed the rational, intellectual bases for action, where we deliberately *decide* how to act. Such models assume that motivation to act already exists, that we merely have to choose how to act. One of the most common models is the problem-solving approach, as postulated by Dewey. We recognize some problem, search for alternative solutions, evaluate the alternatives, select and implement one, then evaluate the results.[4] This approach is frequently recommended for formal planning in organizations.

As we experience the consequences of our "solution" in one experience, we add the information to the process of identifying and evaluating alternative solutions for the next problem.[5] A key factor in such models is the set of solutions we call to mind and consider. The "evoked set" includes those options we are aware of and could list as possible solutions to our problem. The "consideration set" is a subset of those we are aware of that we consider the most viable choices. Typically the number we actually consider ranges from one to three.

A second major consideration in the rational decision-making model is risk. Not only are we looking for the best way to solve the problem; we are also looking to avoid the risks involved in making the wrong decision. The risks involved include (1) *financial* (we may waste or lose money); (2) *physical* (we may suffer bodily harm); (3) *performance* (our choice may not solve the problem); (4) *psychological* (we may feel foolish for making a bad choice); (5) *social* (we may lose the respect of others because of a bad choice); and (6) *temporal* (we may lose the time devoted to implementing the wrong choice and having to try again).[6]

If we are interested in influencing decisions made through such a model, we can address any of its content. We can attempt to alter (or reinforce) the way the problem is defined, the list of options considered, the types and perceived probability of consequences, and risks examined. We can take advantage of the "agenda-setting effect" by stressing information we want consumers to consider when making their decision. We can employ the "halo effect" by linking options to related factors we know consumers consider in a positive or negative light.[7]

CONDITIONING MODELS

The term "conditioning" harks back to Pavlov's work in training dogs to salivate to the sound of a bell by linking the noise to giving them food. Conditioning may be of the "respondent" type when consequences are applied *after* a given behavior, so as to reinforce it, or of the "operant" type when consequences are promised or threatened *before* a behavior in order to promote or reduce its being adopted. The model is often described as the "ABC" model: anticipation, behavior, consequences.[9] This model focuses on motivating people to behave in a fashion preselected by others, whereas the rational model assumes people are already motivated to act and will choose in their own fashion.

The conditioning approach may apply vicariously when people see others engage in a given behavior and experience the consequences thereof. This may occur in reality, observing the events as they happen, or by reading about it or seeing it on television, in a videotape, for example.[10] In psychology, it is called "behavior learning theory," learning from experience what happens if specific behaviors are adopted and learning to guide future behavior accordingly.[11] In management it is referred to as the "greatest management principle"—what gets rewarded, gets repeated.[12]

To employ rewards and punishments to influence behavior, it is essential first to understand what people consider to be positive and negative consequences. Because people value things differently, we cannot assume that the same consequences will work the same way for everybody. We must also recognize that the probability of consequences, in addition to what they are, affects their impact. If we see a given consequence as a direct and sure result of a given behavior, it will have more impact than an indirect and uncertain consequence.

Rewards must be viewed as equitable to be most effective. They must represent a fair "return" for the trouble involved or "switching costs" of changing behavior. They must also be seen as fairly distributed; each person converted must get roughly the same reward, and people already behaving "properly" should not see all rewards going only to those who convert. While conditioning models focus on motivating people, they cannot afford to ignore capability. It makes no sense to motivate people to do something if their own incapacity or external conditions make doing it impossible.[13]

Both positive and negative consequences can influence behavior, though positive are generally thought to have more lasting and predictable effect. The promise or threat of a consequence can "unfreeze" a current behavior pattern and promote a change, while the delivery of that consequence can "refreeze" the new behavior.[14] Both extrinsic rewards, given by others, and intrinsic rewards, inherent in the behavior itself, can influence behavior, though it has been argued that intrinsic have more lasting effect.[15]

Some consequences act as "dissatisfiers"—they are able to dissuade people from a given behavior but not attract them to another. Others act as "satisfiers"— they are able to attract people to new behaviors and reinforce them in new patterns.[16] The key is to understand how particular individuals value specific consequences, how they impact each person.

HUMAN VALUE/NEED MODELS

To understand the effect or meaning of consequences, it is essential to understand human needs and values (i.e., what motivates them). Most people are familiar with the work of Maslow, for example, who portrayed five basic human needs in a hierarchy, beginning with physical/survival requirements, then safety/security, belonging/acceptance, self-esteem, and finally self-actualization.[17] He later added the need for understanding and aesthetic appreciation and downplayed the hierarchical order.[18]

Later Rokeach identified 18 "instrumental" values, basically traits that are culturally or personally admired and aspired to, such as honesty and fairness. In addition, he listed 18 "terminal" values, much like Maslow's "needs," including peace and brotherhood, safety, and respect.[19] Kahle and Kennedy offered a "List of Values" that added fun and enjoyment to the motivations that apply and described the distribution of value priorities among consumers.[20]

Homer and Kahle added people's desire for choices, for freedom, and for power over their own lives as an important value and described how values lead to attitudes, then attitudes to behavior.[21] Klein noted that values can affect behavior in terms of what we see as an uncomfortable situation we wish to get away from or as a desired situation we aspire to.[22] Frankl described how the ultimate power we enjoy is how we deal with and interpret what happens to us and added the need to find meaning in life to the values that motivate us. Frankl also championed the need to take responsibility for our own lives, arguing that responsibility is the necessary companion to liberty.[23]

Burnett and Lumsford argued that guilt is an important motivator, defined as the sense of having violated our own or family/cultural/society's norms. While people vary widely in their susceptibility to feeling of guilt and the motivating force it has in their lives, they are likely to try to avoid feeling guilty in the first place or to seek ways to make amends for transgressions.[24] Van Fleet listed 14 "motivators" that can be used to influence others, including pride, financial success, being best at something, and the opportunity for creative expression.[25]

It is clear that a wide variety of needs/values may motivate people at any given time. By understanding what drives people toward or away from given behaviors, we can at least hope to influence their behaviors. Knowing even their "attribution," the rationale they employ to explain their behavior, may be useful in addition to identifying the "real" reasons. Appreciating how situational factors can influence which values apply may also be necessary.[26]

MARKETING MODELS

Marketing attempts to motivate consumer behavior are based on the notion of an exchange of values.[27] We offer and deliver something of value to others in exchange for their doing something of value for us, a reciprocal arrangement.[28] In the simplest example, companies offer consumers food or gasoline or lawn care in return for their money. At a different level, they "sell the sizzle, not the steak," offering psychological or social benefits, such as social confidence via deodorant or mouthwash, promised romance via perfume or aftershave. These benefits are offered in addition to or instead of physical benefits.

Some claim that marketers can "create" demand by developing new ways to deal with basic needs or desires. Where we wish to attract consumers to unfamiliar products or services, we can offer free samples or trials. To convert the masses to a new behavior, we would employ mass marketing and advertising; to convert individuals, we use personal selling.[29]

Marketing suggests that we recognize differences among consumers, clustering them into segments rather than treating them as a homogeneous group.[30] Segments may be based on demographic differences (e.g., age, sex, residence, income, education, ethnic group—what is collected in census information). They may also be determined by psychographic factors (e.g., perceptions, attitudes, beliefs, values—what takes a special kind of survey to identify). In demand improvement efforts, behavioral segments are important (e.g., high versus low users of services, smokers, exercisers, seatbelt wearers) in identifying who are the best targets for specific attentions. (See Chapter 21 discussion of health risk assessment.)

Marketers also note that we can be influenced by what we perceive as the symbolic meaning of behavior, what a given behavior tells us and others about ourselves.[31] If we define ourselves as rebels, we may deliberately resist complying with what parents or authorities want us to do. By the same token, if others tell us we have certain traits, we may strive to "live up to our billing" and be receptive to changing or continuing behavior through the "Pygmalion effect."[32]

Marketers employ the "marketing mix" to influence consumers, noting that the benefits of behavior ("product" factors) and of barriers and facilitators ("place" factors), as well as negative consequences and costs ("price" factors), can make a difference. Sponsors would have to be sure that a given behavior "offer" represents a desirable and easily accessible balance between benefit and costs (value for the price) and a more desirable and accessible balance than competing behavior options.[33]

The fourth component of the marketing mix is "promotion," or telling people about the offer in order to make them want to accept it. While media advertising is most frequently associated with marketing as the foremost means of communication, word-of-mouth comments by satisfied (and dissatisfied) customers is recognized as equally important.[34] Marketers want to be able to offer a "better mousetrap," create an offer people "can't" resist, in order to entice consumers their way.[35] But marketers do not expect consumers to beat a path to the door without effective communications about it.

In marketing communications it is usually expected that consumers will pass through a series of stages before being converted. This hierarchy of effects[36] is sometimes described as AIDA (awareness, interest, decision, and action). Another description uses KAIB (knowledge, attitude, intention, and behavior). Both recognize a combination of rational, factual factors (awareness, knowledge) and emotional, judgmental factors (interest, attitude). Each assumes that a conscious choice precedes action (decision, intention).

It is widely recognized that the order in which the stages are followed is not always "logical." People may start with a feeling or a judgment and "back up" to rationalize their conclusion with facts. They may try a behavior without passing through knowledge, attitude, or intention and have the experience of the behavior or its consequences construct their knowledge and attitudes and determine their future intentions. Any one of these stages may prove to be a key leverage point in inducing changes in behavior.

While marketing models focus primarily on motivating customers, they recognize that internal and external "place" factors may affect the ability or convenience of customers to buy and that "promotion" is useful in raising customer consciousness in the first place or in reinforcing it periodically to attract and retain customers. It also emphasizes the value of establishing and maintaining customer loyalty, trust, and receptivity to future marketing efforts.

ATTITUDE/INTENTION MODELS

There are a wide variety of models that attempt to explain and offer opportunities for changing behavior in terms of attitudes and intentions. One of the most basic addresses "expectancy value." It includes attention to consumer attitudes toward a given behavior based on its expected outcomes, their probability, and the value placed on them.[38] It then adds consumers' perceptions of what others prefer or expect them to do, social norms, and how sensitive consumers are to external expectations or pressure. The combination determines consumer intentions, which, in turn, lead to behavior.[39]

In contrast to preceding models, which focus on the individual and on ways to directly influence individual behavior, this model recognizes the social nature of most behavior, its susceptibility to direct social influence (peer pressure), and indirect influence based on what individuals perceive others expect and prefer them to do. It deals primarily with motivation, though it recognizes the importance of the individual's perceptions of capability of behaving in a particular way, as well as the desire to do so. The model recognizes that not only the *nature* of consumer perceptions and expectations but their *strength* affects intentions toward specific behaviors.

While this model has been found to do well in predicting the behavior of populations, it has sometimes done poorly in regard to the behavior of individuals.[40] When expressed as social learning theory, this model includes the learned, symbolic meaning of behavior and the perceived behavior of others as important factors. It recognizes that people must be conscious of the specific behavior they are expected to adopt and must know precisely what it is in order to comply with social expectations.[41]

The importance of social factors is also addressed in terms of social support for specific behavior.[42] This can mean social norms and peer pressure but also includes the likelihood that others will offer assistance. Will family members help by reminding people of what, when, and how to perform a given behavior? Will they pitch in if a consumer cannot do it alone? The intentions and attentions of others affect the behavior of individuals.

People have been found to have different attitude/intention "styles," or normal approaches, to choosing which behaviors to adopt. These are similar to market segments, preferring analytical, methodical, spontaneous, or crafted ways of deciding what to do.[43] Each segment would have to be approached somewhat differently for the best mix of efficiency and effectiveness in behavior improvement initiatives.

Another of the models in this general category is the theory of planned behavior. It recognizes that perceptions of how one's individual behavior affects others can be important determinants of how we act. Concerns for the environment, for the general welfare, and for the perceptions that one's behavior will make a difference one way or the other have been shown to be significant factors in individual behavior.[44]

An equally important factor in these attitude/intention models is what is called "self-efficacy." This combines actual capability to perform a given behavior with self-perceived competence or confidence in performance. Even for people perfectly capable of performing a behavior, lack of confidence may keep them from ever doing so. Conversely some may have misplaced confidence and insist on engaging in behavior they are not competent at. If you are looking for someone to perform CPR on a heart attack victim, you want someone with both competence and confidence.[45]

Just as marketing models recognize that knowledge and attitude may succeed rather than precede behavior, so do attitude/intention models. The term "cognitive dissonance" refers to the well-documented tendency of people to make their attitudes and behavior consistent. In some cases this means that their behavior is determined by their attitudes, while in others it means the reverse.[46] For sponsors this means that if consumers can be enticed to engage in a desired behavior, their attitudes are likely to change accordingly, helping to promote repetition and continuation of that behavior.

HEALTH BEHAVIOR MODELS

There are a host of models that were developed, tested, and employed specifically in the promotion of consumer health behaviors.[47] The health belief model addresses what people who are well do to stay well.[48] This behavior is a function of perceived susceptibility to illness or injury, perceived effectiveness of steps to reduce risk, and cues reminding people exactly what to do.[49] This model is particularly applicable to health improvement; to prevention, wellness, and promotion; and to the safety and preventive aspects of disability management.

The health seeking model addresses what people who consider themselves to be sick do about it.[50] It includes checking with others for advice, trying self-care, identifying and examining treatment options, selecting and using treatment, adopting the "sick role" (e.g., staying away from work, reducing or modifying activity, asking for help), and evaluating results of treatment. This model is particularly applicable to decision improvement and disease management.

Health behavior models often look to tension or anxiety as motivators for behavior.[51] If well people are not concerned enough about their health or do not see themselves at risk, they may be unreceptive to attempts to attract them to wellness or prevention activities, screening tests, or risk reduction. If they are not worried about symptoms or worry too much about insignificant aches and pains, they may delay seeking needed care or seek it unnecessarily or inappropriately.

When the motivation for action is great (e.g., intense pain or anxiety or a strong commitment to health), the stimulus or initiating factor for action may not be much. A comment by a coworker that one does not look too well may prompt an immediate call to the physician. When motivation is low, however, the stimulation may have to be quite intense or may need to be repeated frequently by many others before action occurs.[52]

Related to self-efficacy, as described in the attitude/behavior models, is the notion of "locus of control." People who perceive external factors as the primary determinants of health (i.e., factors beyond their control, such as "fate," the environment, heredity, or the acts of others) are likely to be unreceptive to appeals for them to modify their own behavior. Those with a more internal locus are more likely to accept responsibility and be open to change.[53] Perceptions of self-efficacy with respect to health behaviors, combined with motivation and self-responsibility, are likely to be good predictors of which consumers will be receptive to specific initiatives.[54]

These models are often summarized in terms of predisposing, enabling, and reinforcing factors affecting health behaviors.[55] Predisposing factors include consumer characteristics such as self-efficacy, attitudes, and beliefs that motivate or make people more receptive to changing behavior. Enabling factors are those that make the behavior easier to adopt, repeat, or continue, such as guidebooks, reminders, checklists, or written instructions. Reinforcing factors cover rewards, support, peer recognition, and whatever makes repetition and continuation more likely.

STAGES OF CHANGE MODEL

The stages of change model was developed from analysis of how people changed their own behavior. It has been used by its developers primarily as a basis for counseling individuals as they attempt to make changes in their own lives. Since it focuses on how people change, however, it has equally valuable applications for sponsors interested in achieving behavior changes across a population. We feel it is easily the most useful of the models thus far discussed.

There are six stages of change in this model, suggesting a progression from thinking to action: (1) precontemplation, (2) contemplation, (3) preparation, (4) action, (5) maintenance, and (6) termination.[56] At the precontemplation stage people are not even thinking about changing; they are complacent about whatever behavior others may think of as problematic and are not really open to advice or programmatic efforts aimed at getting them to change. They require the proverbial knock on the side of the head to awaken their consciousness to at least thinking about changing their behavior.

At the contemplation stage they are thinking about changing but have not yet made a definite decision or have not committed themselves to change. They are receptive to additional information and may be willing to participate in educational programs about the behavior in question. It may take some time and significant effort, however, before they actually develop a commitment to change and actually do so.

In the preparation stage they have made the decision and have promised themselves, perhaps have "signed a contract" with others and have made public their intention. They have set a date to adopt the new behavior to either quit the old or start the new. They are ready but have not yet started. Something may prevent them, still, so the commitment or intention may never be translated into action.

At the action stage people have begun the new behavior; they have stopped smoking, have started exercising, have begun using the blood glucose monitor for their diabetes, have started wearing a seat belt, or are using safety equipment at work. Where the behavior in question is a one-time effort, such as turning down the thermostat on their water heater, they have done it. For behavior that must be repeated or continued, they may still lapse, skipping some, most, or all occasions when they should be persevering in the behavior.

In the maintenance stage, they have turned the desired behavior into a habit, repeating or continuing it on a regular basis, with no more than an occasional lapse. They are not discouraged by lapses, simply making up for it the next time. If they overreact to lapses, they may revert to the contemplation, preparation, or action stages (not precontemplation) and require new attention to get them back to action and maintenance.

At termination they do not terminate the behavior. Rather the behavior has become so ingrained a habit that they would not even consider returning to their old ways. (We would call this stage "permanence.") They and sponsors can forget about it; no further attention on their part or intervention by others is needed. They are truly converted and for good. Sponsors can terminate their efforts as long as converts remain in this stage. Only time will tell how many are truly in this stage, however, and sponsors may have to intervene again at some point in the future. Moreover, some desired behaviors are to be repeated so infrequently that they are likely to require at least a reminder versus no attention.

This model has applications in sponsor planning, learning the status of consumers targeted for attention so as to pick the most promising targets or to design different approaches to people at different stages. Different tactics tend to work better for people at different stages in the change process. (See Chapter 17.) Individuals should be counseled differently in their self-change efforts depending on where they are along the six stages (see Table 6–1).

The stages of change model has been tested on a wide variety of "problem" or health risk behaviors, from smoking and drug use to delinquency, unsafe sex, and poor diet. It has also been used to examine moving women toward greater use of mammography screening. The proportions of people found at different stages of change varies with each behavior. Mostly precontemplation and contemplation stages are found among smokers, for example; many more people are in preparation and action stages relative to diet and nutrition, but there is frequent lapsing rather than maintenance of improved behavior.[57]

The probability of the success of interventions is largely determined by what stage people are in when approached and the extent to which interventions are geared to the right stage. Among smokers, for example, only 10% of those in the precontemplation stage were found to have quit after a program of interventions over 18 months. By contrast, 15% of those who began from the contemplation stage and 24% of those in the preparation stage had quit over the same period.[58]

For those in the precontemplation stage, consciousness raising through external sources and self-reevaluation have proven helpful in moving people to contemplation. Once in contemplation people may respond well to emotional arousals, such as learning of the death of a friend from a behavior-related condition or the offer of rewards. In preparation, the making of a public commitment or the signing of a "contract," even if legally unenforceable, can help move people to action. Once in the action stage, the individual's own efforts to find a substitute for an undesired action (counterconditioning) and efforts by others to remove reminders and reduce opportunities for negative behavior (environmental control) are more effective. The support of others (helping relationships) is particularly valuable in the maintenance stage.[59]

Because this model focuses specifically on encouraging and enabling individuals to change their behavior and has been tested successfully with a number of health risk behaviors, we consider it potentially the most useful of those discussed. Because it focuses primarily on individual motivation, however, we feel that efforts aimed at improving consumer capability and at reinforcing as well as raising consciousness deserve attention as well.

Table 6–1 Tailored Interventions for Prochaska's Stages of Change

STAGE OF CHANGE ▼	TAILORED INTERVENTIONS	OBJECTIVE OF INTERVENTION
1, 2	CONSCIOUSNESS RAISING *SPONSORS: EDUCATION, SOCIAL ADVERTISING*	*AWARENESS OF ISSUE & POTENTIAL VALUE / HARM VALUE OF CHANGE*
2, 3	EMOTIONAL AROUSAL *SPONSORS: PUBLICITY*	*ENGAGE EMOTIONS PERSONALIZE RISK / VALUE*
1, 2, 3, 4	SOCIAL LIBERATION *SPONSOR: ADVOCACY, SOCIAL MARKETING*	*EXTERNAL FACILITATORS NONSMOKING AREAS, LOW FAT FOOD IN RESTAURANTS*
4, 5	HELPING RELATIONSHIPS *SPONSOR: PROVIDE / FACILITATE SUPPORT GROUPS*	*ENLISTING OTHERS: FRIENDS, FAMILY, COUNSELING, SUPPORT GROUPS*
2, 3	SELF-REVELATION *SPONSOR: COUNSELING, GROUP DISCUSSIONS*	*RECONSIDERATION OF ISSUE IN LIGHT OF PERSONAL VALUES, SELF PERCEPTION / EXPECTATIONS; EVALUATE PROS & CONS*
4, 5	ENVIRONMENTAL CONTROL *SPONSOR: POSITIVE PROMPTS WHILE REDUCING NEGATIVE PROMPTS*	*REMOVE CAPABILITY, MAKE LESS CONVENIENT, REMINDERS*
4, 5	INCENTIVES *SPONSOR: REWARD, RECOGNITION & DISINCENTIVES*	*INCENTIVE / MARKETING: SELF & GROUP PRAISE*
4, 5	COUNTERING *SPONSOR: EDUCATION, GROUP DECISION SUPPORT*	*IDENTIFYING WAYS TO AVOID TEMPTATION, SUBSTITUTE BEHAVIORS*
3, 4, 5	COMMITMENT *SPONSOR: NEGOTIATION, GROUP SUPPORT*	*MAKING PERSONAL THE PUBLIC PROMISE TO CHANGE*

(SEE FIGURE 7–1)

COMPOSITE MODEL EQUALS BEHAVIOR IMPROVEMENT

Numerous attempts have been made to validate particular models that explain or enable us to predict or influence human behavior. It turns out that most models seem to work at least some of the time; no one model consistently performs best in all applications. One study asked health behavior change professionals about what factors were the best predictors of three behavior changes: (1) smoking cessation, (2) exercise, and (3) weight loss. They rated the best predictors as intention to change first, self-efficacy second, social support third, with time availability, peer pressure, convenience, beliefs about susceptibility to harm, amount of change required, and knowledge/beliefs about the consequences of changing roughly tied for fourth.[60]

Since this was a study of what professionals perceived, rather than what actually worked, it is an opinion poll rather than a scientific comparison of models. No study we could find compares all the models described in this chapter to each other with respect to all the health and demand behaviors of interest; indeed, no such study seems feasible. On the other hand, we believe that the basic ideas of all these models can be synthesized into a composite model for practical application.

The composite model we will use to describe and discuss consumer behavior improvement initiatives is called the behavior improvement model and is summarized as $I = MC^2$; Improvement = Motivation × Capability × Consciousness. All three factors in the MC^2 have been addressed in previous discussions of the various models, though not necessarily using the same terms.

Motivation has been the primary focus of almost all the models, as the instigator of rational decisions; the basis for conditioning; and a major focus in marketing, human values, attitude/intention and health behavior models and in driving people along the stages of change. Capability or self-efficacy is recognized as a separate and important factor in conditioning, marketing, attitude/intention, and health behavior models and is a major focus in stages of change. Consciousness is addressed primarily in the marketing, attitude/intention, health behavior, and stages of change models.

Our behavior improvement model focuses explicitly on *changing* behavior rather than on understanding or predicting it, though understanding and predicting have their own value in planning specific initiatives. First, the model suggests that sponsors considering a demand improvement challenge look to discovering why consumers are not already behaving in the manner desired, particularly since improved health and demand behaviors are beneficial to consumers themselves.

What *barriers* to optimum behavior are getting in the way? Are problem consumers not *conscious* of better behavior options or totally unaware of the disadvantages of their current behavior and advantages of improved behaviors? Are they not *motivated* or are they undermotivated to behave in ways sponsors would prefer? Are there problems of *capability*? Do consumers lack skills or resources needed to engage in the desired behavior? Are they motivated and capable of the better behavior but forget to engage in it? In other words, do they have low or no *consciousness* of the behavior at the critical time?

Identifying barriers as belonging to one or more of the three MC² categories can lead to consideration of directly related interventions. If the problem is lack of consciousness, then build and reinforce consciousness; if too little motivation, figure out how to motivate consumers; if it is a capability problem, make them capable, or perhaps make them confident in their current capabilities. By the same token, strengthening one factor may overcome a barrier in another.

Where motivation is lacking or low, working on capability may overcome that barrier where motivation cannot be directly enhanced. Creating new capability has motivational impact of its own; we tend to want to do what we are capable of, if only to prove or maintain our capability. Easing capability barriers (i.e., making it easier to engage in a behavior, by making it, for example, more convenient or reducing the resources required) can tip the balance where motivation was insufficient to instigate a more difficult behavior.

Similarly, heightening motivation can enable consumers to overcome capability barriers. When people are merely leaning toward a desired behavior, they may find modest capability barriers significant, while if they are wholeheartedly committed to a given behavior, they may figure their own ways around capability barriers. They may learn the necessary skill or acquire the needed resources on their own if they want to badly enough.

Where initial consciousness is the problem, for example, where consumers are in the precontemplation stage of change, introducing a new and significant motivation, such as a contest or peer pressure, may be sufficient to stimulate contemplation. Where remembering is the problem, a high enough motivation may stimulate consumers enough to develop their own mnemonic device. Alternatively, making the desired behavior easier to perform may reduce consumer tendencies to forget.

Although identifying the barriers to desired behavior as belonging to one of the three MC² categories does not automatically determine which factor to address, it will help sponsors to at least avoid some unpromising initiatives. Where capability barriers are serious, it is likely to prove more efficient to address them directly rather than hope to supermotivate consumers, particularly if they have high motivation levels already. Where motivation is the barrier, enhancing capability will only help if it is low to begin with. Where consciousness is the barrier, awakening or reinforcing it is likely to be helpful.

Though motivation and capability may seem to be internal characteristics of consumers, they have external components as well. Similarly, while efforts to increase consciousness are most often generated externally, there are internal counterparts. The composite model includes both internal and external means of influencing motivation, capability, and consciousness to promote improvements in consumer health and demand behaviors.

MOTIVATION

Internal

Internal sources of motivation include basic instincts and values, perceived problems and aspirations, tensions, and anxiety. Perceived benefits of current or proposed behavior, as compared to the costs of either, the extent to which a given behavior is seen as protecting or enhancing dearly held values, the intrinsic worth and symbolic meaning of the behavior itself, and the probability of enjoying benefits as compared to the risks of suffering costs—all these are internal motivators.

To change or reinforce internal motivation, it is doubtful if basic values can be altered. By educating and persuading consumers it may be possible to get them to revise their estimate of the relative benefit/cost of specific behavior, however, or the probability of either applying to them. In some cases the behavior may be made more intrinsically rewarding or enjoyable, such as by including social activities. Consumers may be led to think more about the positive and negative consequences of specific behavior or to visualize themselves engaging in a desired behavior and enjoying its intrinsic consequences.

External

External (i.e., extrinsic) motivation comes primarily from two sources. External rewards and punishments, or conditioning efforts, clearly apply. So do expressions of what others want us to do; family, cultural, and social norms; peer influence; and example. While consumer sensitivity to extrinsic rewards and external influence is an internal factor, the rewards themselves and the application of social influence are external and can be enhanced by sponsors so as to improve behavior.

External rewards are perhaps the simplest to manage, though they impose costs on sponsors. (Specific examples are offered in Chapter 14.) Social influence is a little more complicated to employ in specific cases, though advocacy efforts (i.e., asking, educating, and persuading others to influence family members, co-workers, fellow citizens, and lawmakers) is common practice in a number of social improvement efforts. (Examples are offered in Chapter 13.)

CAPABILITY

Internal

Internal capability reflects the extent to which consumers have the knowledge and skills required to engage in a given behavior. In some cases physical limitations and disabilities may interfere with performance, though frequently special arrangements can be made to enable disadvantaged consumers to convert to the desired behavior. Where motivation has been stimulated or already is high, capability may still be a barrier to improvement.

Internal capabilities are addressed primarily through education and training, information, and social communications efforts. Capability may be included in marketing and negotiation tactics as "part of the package" where consumers indicate it is a problem. Promoting self-efficacy, either actual competence or confidence in one's ability or both, can be accomplished through a wide variety of one-to-one and mass counseling and communications activities. (See Part III for discussion of specific alternatives.)

External

External capability factors include whatever circumstances in the environment make adoption, repetition, and continuation of a desired behavior or cessation of an undesired behavior easy versus difficult for consumers. Making the "right" behavior more accessible, such as through worksite fitness or screening programs, or the "wrong" behavior more inaccessible, such as by eliminating cigarette vending machines, are familiar examples.

Improving the prevalence and effectiveness of managing chronic conditions may be achieved through making home glucose monitoring and lung function testing more convenient. Back safety may be facilitated by providing special back supports or new equipment. Making information on treatment options available via phone services, interactive video, and television may promote better informed consumer decisions just by making information more accessible.

CONSCIOUSNESS

Consciousness may have to be raised merely to get consumers to think about improving their behavior. Initial awareness may have to be stimulated in order to make consumers receptive to motivation and capability enhancement efforts. And even for fully motivated and capable consumers, consciousness may have to be reinforced occasionally to remind them of behaviors that have yet to become fully ingrained habits.

Internal

Awareness of the desirability and possibility of improving a behavior and knowing exactly what to do and when and where to do it are internal factors but are usually dependent on external consciousness raising and reinforcement. There are some examples of internal consciousness promotion, however. Perceptions of specific symptoms, coupled with knowledge or ignorance of their meaning, prompt most contacts with the health care system. Remembering when it is time for an annual physical, routine screening, or immunization may be enough to prompt action. Looking at oneself in the mirror, at the scale, or noticing how out of breath we are after climbing a flight of stairs may be sufficient to stimulate interest in behavior improvement.

People can arrange their own internal consciousness-reinforcing cues. They can place notes on the calendar or program their computer to remind them of appointments or prompt a daily exercise session, prenatal visit, or educational seminar. Conditioning oneself to have a mammogram on one's birthday or placing a piece of safety equipment where one cannot miss it are other examples of self-generated reminders.

External

Prompting from external sources is the most common form of consciousness raising. Social advocacy, public service announcements, posters, and billboards may be used to awaken the public about the value of desired behavior. Bulletin boards, newsletters, and memos may remind workers of onsite screening programs, fitness events, and immunizations, for example. Calls from physician office staff are commonly used to remind patients of annual checkups, prenatal visits, follow-up appointments, and other desired contacts.

Prompting is often the most undervalued and underused approach to stimulating behavior change or, more often, its maintenance. Even highly motivated, fully capable people may simply forget to take their medication, get a checkup, engage in exercise, or perform some routine behavior that easily slips one's mind. Reminders from family and friends can include the motivational impact of peer pressure. Most prompting is inexpensive and is likely to be cost-effective (see Table 6–2).

We see the $I = MC^2$ model as intersecting with the stages of change model. Stages of change describe the state of mind or behavior of consumers relative to particular behaviors. Motivation, capability, and consciousness are the three factors that can be selected for attention in order to move people from one stage to the next. Information on where consumers are along the stages of change and on which of the MC^2 factors represent barriers to behavior improvement should provide a sound basis for planning and implementing interventions (see Table 6–3).

Table 6–2 Behavior Improvement Model for Changing Health & Demand Behaviors

	FACTORS TO BE INFLUENCED	POSSIBLE SPONSOR INITIATIVES
MOTIVATION	*INTERNAL:* PERSONAL FEELINGS & VALUES; PERCEIVED PROBLEMS & ASPIRATIONS; EXPECTED OUTCOMES	• *FOCUS COMMUNICATIONS ON PERSONAL VALUES* • *ENSURE IMPROVED BEHAVIOR DELIVERS DESIRED RESULTS* • *PROVIDE AWARENESS / ENJOYMENT OF OUTCOMES*
	EXTERNAL: REWARDS & PUNISHMENTS; COMMUNITY NORMS, INFLUENCE	• *PROVIDE REWARDS, RECOGNITION, INCENTIVES* • *PROVIDE FAMILY & COMMUNITY SUPPORT FOR IMPROVED BEHAVIOR*
CAPABILITY	*INTERNAL:* ACTUAL KNOWLEDGE & SKILL; PERCEIVED KNOWLEDGE & SKILL; PHYSICAL & MENTAL LIMITATIONS	• *PROVIDE EDUCATION, TRAINING* • *ENABLE CONSUMERS TO PRACTICE SKILLS* • *ADAPT TO CONSUMER LIMITATIONS*
	EXTERNAL: ACCESS TO FACILITIES & SERVICES; ACCESS TO SELF-MANAGEMENT TOOLS	• *MULTIPLY ACCESS POINTS, COVER AS BENEFITS* • *MAKE MORE AVAILABLE, ELIMINATE BARRIERS*
CONSCIOUSNESS	*INTERNAL:* KNOWING WHAT, WHERE, & WHEN TO ADOPT BEHAVIORS; REMEMBERING AT RIGHT TIME & PLACE	• *PROVIDE WRITTEN MATERIALS, GUIDES, SUGGESTIONS* • *FACILITATE SELF-PROMPTING BY CALENDAR, COMPUTER*
	EXTERNAL: GENERAL KNOWLEDGE OF DESIRED BEHAVIOR; REMINDERS OF BEHAVIOR	• *MASS MEDIA REMINDERS* • *PERSONALIZED REMINDERS*

Table 6–3 I = MC² & the Stages of Change

I=MC² & THE STAGES OF CHANGE	PROCHASKA'S STAGES OF CHANGE					
	1	*2*	*3*	*4*	*5*	*6*
	PRE-CONTEMPLATION	CONTEMPLATION	PREPARATION	ACTION	MAINTENANCE	TERMINATION (PERMANENCE)
MOTIVATION CAPABILITY CONSCIOUSNESS	POSSIBLE AWAKEN	EMPHASIZE ASSESS EXCITE	EMPHASIZE ASSESS EXCITE	USEFUL EMPHASIZE REINFORCE	USEFUL EMPHASIZE REMIND	REMIND*

* While Prochaska defines the termination stage as requiring no intervention, we feel that for some infrequently repeated behaviors, e.g., those required at one, five, ten years, or longer intervals, reminders may still be needed.

Any combination of internal and external efforts focused on any combination of motivation, capability, and consciousness may prove to be what is needed or what works best in initiating or reinforcing behavior changes by consumers. Sponsors should attempt first to identify the current state of each factor in the population of interest. They should then select the best tactics available to stimulate and maintain desired behavior changes.

(Recommendations for making strategic decisions are covered in Chapter 10. Part IV is devoted to the discussion of how to make tactical choices for specific behavior improvement initiatives.)

REFERENCES

1. S. Klein, *Motivation: Biosocial Approaches* (New York, NY: McGraw-Hill, 1982).

2. D. Kauffman, *Systems1: An Introduction to Systems Thinking* (Boston, MA: Future Systems, Inc., 1990).

3. K. Wallston, "Theoretically Based Strategies for Health Behavior Change," in *Health Promotion in the Workplace,* 2d ed., eds. M. O'Donnell and J. Harris (Albany, NY: Delmar, 1994), 185–203.

4. N. Barnes, "What Dewey Didn't Tell Us: A Closer Look at Our Basic Assumptions in Marketing Health Services," *Journal of Health Care Marketing* 5, no. 4 (Fall 1985):59–61.

5. C. Surprenant and R. Dholakia, "The Product/Service Decision Process," in *Add Value to Your Service,* ed. C. Surprenant (Chicago, IL: American Marketing Association, 1987), 193–196.

6. L. Turley and R. LeBlanc, "An Exploratory Investigation of Consumer Decision Making in the Service Sector," *Journal of Services Marketing* 7, no. 4 (1993):11–18.

7. S. Burton, "The Framing of Purchase for Services," *Journal of Services Marketing* 4, no. 4 (1990):55–67.

8. W. Qualls, "Toward Understanding the Dynamics of Household Decision Conflict Behavior," *Advances in Consumer Research* 15 (1988):442–448.

9. B. Bergiel and C. Trosclair, "Instrumental Learning: Its Application to Consumer Satisfaction," *Journal of Consumer Marketing* 2, no. 4 (1985):23.

10. W. Nord and P. Paul, "A Behavior Modification Perspective on Marketing," *Journal of Marketing* 44, no. 1 (1980):36–47.

11. M. Rothschild and W. Gaidis, "Behavioral Learning Theory: Its Relevance to Marketing and Promotion," *Journal of Marketing* 45, no. 2 (1981):70–77.

12. M. LeBoeuf, *The Greatest Management Principle in the World* (New York, NY: Berkley Books, 1985).

13. D. Smith, *Motivating People* (Hauppauge, NY: Barron's, 1991).

14. E. Dichter, *Motivating Human Behavior* (New York, NY: McGraw-Hill, 1971).

15. A. Kohn, "Why Incentive Plans Cannot Work," *Harvard Business Review* 71, no. 5 (1993):54–63.

16. F. Herzberg, "One More Time: How Do You Motivate Employees?" in *Harvard Business Review Business Classics* (Boston, MA: Harvard Business School, 1991).

17. A. Maslow, *Motivation and Personality* (New York, NY: Harper & Row, 1954).

18. A. Maslow, *Motivation and Personality* 2d ed. (New York, NY: Harper & Row, 1970).

19. M. Rokeach, *Understanding Human Values* (New York: Free Press, 1979).

20. L. Kahle and P. Kennedy, "Using the List of Values To Understand Consumers," *Journal of Services Marketing* 2, no. 4 (1988):49–56.

21. P. Homer and L. Kahle, "A Structural Equation Test of the Value-Attitude-Behavior Hierarchy," *Journal of Personality-Social Psychology* 54, no. 4 (1988):638–648.

22. Klein, *Motivation.*

23. V. Frankl, *Man's Search for Meaning* (Boston, MA: Beacon Press, 1959).

24. M. Burnett and D. Lumsford, "Conceptualizing Guilt in the Decision-Making Process," *Journal of Consumer Marketing* 11, no. 3 (1994):33–43.

25. J. Van Fleet, *Conversational Power: The Key to Success with People* (Englewood Cliffs, NJ: Prentice-Hall, 1984).

26. L. Kahle, *Attitudes and Social Adaptation* (Oxford, England: Pergamon Press, 1984).

27. P. Kotler and R. Clarke, *Marketing for Health Care Organizations* (Englewood Cliffs, NJ: Prentice-Hall, 1987), 5.

28. L. Adams, "Inequity in Social Exchange," in *Advances in Experimental Social Psychology.* Vol. 2, ed. L. Berkowitz (New York, NY: Academic Press, 1965), 267–299.

29. R. Ott, *Creating Demand* (Homewood, IL: Business One-Irwin, 1992).

30. M. Greenberg and S. McDonald, "Successful Needs/Benefits Segmentation: A User's Guide," *Journal of Consumer Marketing* 6, no. 3 (1989):29–36.

31. T. Reynolds and J. Gutman, "Advertising Is Image Management," *Journal of Advertising Research* 24, no. 1 (1984):27–36.

32. F. Lewis and L. Daltroy, "How Causal Explanations Influence Health Behavior: Attribution Theory," in *Health Behavior and Health Education,* eds. K. Glanz et al. (San Francisco, CA: Jossey-Bass, 1990), 92–114.

33. S. Cook, "Foreword," in *The Quest for Loyalty,* ed. F. Reichheld (Boston, MA: Harvard Business School, 1996), xi–xiv.

34. B. Gelb and M. Johnson, "Word-of-Mouth Communication: Causes and Consequences," *Journal of Health Care Marketing* 15, no. 3 (1995):54–57.

35. G. Nastas, "A Customer Approach to Improving Financial Services Marketing," *Journal of Professional Services Marketing* 1, no. 3 (1986):49–58.

36. J. Mowen, "Beyond Consumer Decision Making," *Journal of Consumer Marketing* 5, no. 1 (1988):15–25.

37. R. Zajonc, "Feeling and Thinking: Preferences Need No Inferences," *American Psychologist* 35 (1980):151–175.

38. M. Fishbein and I. Ajzen, *Belief, Attitude, Intention and Behavior: An Introduction to Theory and Research* (Reading, MA: Addison-Wesley, 1975).

39. I. Ajzen and M. Fishbein, *Understanding Attitudes and Predicting Social Behavior* (Englewood Cliffs, NJ: Prentice-Hall, 1980), 42–52.

40. M. Ryan and E. Bonfield, "Fishbein's Intention Model: A Test of External and Pragmatic Validity," *Journal of Marketing* 44, no. 2 (1980):82–90.

41. C. Perry, et al., "How Individuals, Environments and Health Behavior Interact: Social Learning Theory," in *Health Behavior and Health Education,* ed. K. Glanz et al. (San Francisco, CA: Jossey-Bass, 1990), 161–186.

42. A. Smith, "Patient Participation in Changing Behaviors," *Home Health Nurse* 13, no. 2 (1995): 45–49.

43. K. Kolbe, *The Conative Connection: Uncovering the Link between Who You Are and How You Perform* (Reading, MA: Addison-Wesley, 1990).

44. S. Taylor and P. Todd, "Understanding Household Garbage Reduction Behavior," *Journal of Public Policy & Marketing* 14, no. 2 (1995):192–204.

45. Perry, et al., "How Individuals Environments and Health Behavior Interact," 161–186.

46. R. Jayanti, "Preventive Maintenance," *Marketing Health Services* 17, no. 1 (1997):36–44.

47. L. Festinger, *A Theory of Cognitive Dissonance* (Evanston, IL: Row Peterson, 1957).

48. J. Dearing, "Social Marketing and Diffusion-Based Strategies for Communicating with Unique Populations," *Journal of Health Communications* 1, no. 4 (1996):343–363.

49. I. Rosenstock, "The Health Belief Model and Preventive Behavior," *Health Education Monographs* 2 (1974):354–386.

50. U. Igun, "Stages in Health Seeking: A Descriptive Model," *Social Science in Medicine* 13A (1979):445–451.

51. R. Oliver, "Testing Competing Models of Consumer Decision Making in the Preventive Health Care Market," *Advances in Consumer Research* 5 (1978):277–282.

52. L. Wortzel, "The Behavior of the Health Care Consumer: A Selective Review," *Advances in Consumer Research* 3 (1976):295–301.

53. S. Gould, "Health Consciousness and Health Behavior," *American Journal of Preventive Medicine* 6, no. 4 (1990):228–237.

54. H. Becker, et al., "Self-Rated Abilities for Health Practices: A Health Self-Efficacy Measure," *Health Values* 17, no. 5 (1993):42–51.

55. R. Thompson, et al., "Primary and Secondary Prevention Services in Clinical Practice," *JAMA* 273, no. 14 (1995):1130–1135.

56. J. Prochaska, et al., *Changing for Good* (New York, NY: Avon Books, 1994).

57. J. Prochaska, et al., "Stages of Change and Decisional Balance for 12 Problem Behaviors," *Health Psychology* 13, no. 1 (1994):39–46.

58. J. Prochaska, et al., "In Search of How People Change: Applications to Addictive Behaviors," *American Psychologist* 47, no. 9 (1992):1102–1114.

59. Prochaska, et al., "In Search of," 1102–1114.

60. M.B. Love, et al., "Normative Beliefs of Health Behavior Professionals Regarding the Psychosocial and Environmental Factors That Influence Health Behavior Change Related to Smoking Cessation, Regular Exercise, and Weight Loss," *American Journal of Health Promotion* 10, no. 5 (1996):371–379.

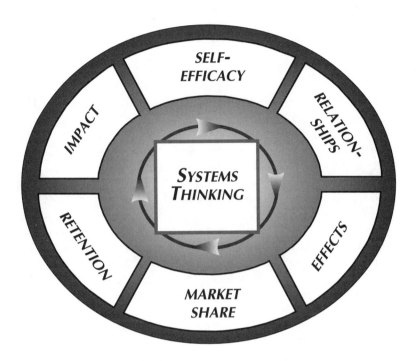

Chapter 7

SELF-
EFFICACY

RELATION-
SHIPS

IMPACT

SYSTEMS
THINKING

RETENTION

EFFECTS

MARKET
SHARE

SYSTEMS FOUNDATIONS

Two of the three foundations for demand improvement, set of effects and stages of change, are basically linear models. Consumers are thought to proceed in an orderly fashion along the set of effects, from participation to mind-state changes to behavior changes, which cause health status changes responsible for health care utilization and expenditure changes on one hand and value-adding effects on the other. They move from precontemplation to contemplation to preparation to action to maintenance and, finally, end up in the termination stage.

Not all movement is from left to right across the effects or stages. Consumers may require mind-state changes before they are likely to participate in some programs or may change their behavior because of changes in their health status. They tend to lapse backward among the stages of change, reverting to recontemplation or repreparation after lapsing from action or maintenance. These are natural exceptions to the "normal" order, however, rather than a different model.

IMPACT MYOPIA

A common risk in thinking about demand improvement challenges and initiatives is "impact myopia," a tendency to look for and at only the nearest, most immediate effects of possible interventions. The set of effects challenges sponsors to look beyond whichever effect(s) they focus on initially to the rest of the set, especially to possible added-value impact. Improving employee fitness can improve productivity and morale and reduce absenteeism and turnover, for example. These effects, in turn, should reduce, for example, the employer's costs and improve profits or market share, etc.[1]

In examining the costs of existing unhealthy behavior, it is often necessary to look past immediate effects. Smoking by pregnant mothers, for example, affects the health of their babies and tends to adversely affect the health and conduct of children throughout their lives. Second-hand smoke affects the health of non-smokers, adding to lung infections, asthma, and cancer costs. Smoking adds to risk of fires and the damage to life, health, and property that results. No assessment of the costs of smoking or value of quitting would be complete without consideration of such *extended* effects.[2]

Sponsors would be wise to at least try looking beyond even these extended effects to how the rest of the "system" might be affected. Improving employee morale and retention can both lead to improved customer satisfaction if, as is widely believed, happier employees deliver better customer service, and if retaining the same employees to interact with customers tends to strengthen loyal relationships. It may not be necessary or even helpful to place dollar figures on these extended effects, but recognizing their potential for adding still more value may enable sponsors to devise ways of including them in evaluation, thereby enabling them to monitor and report the added value they deliver. And by measuring and reporting the added value they deliver to others, sponsors can strengthen their relationships with other stakeholders and thereby gain themselves.

Clearly there is a limit to how far sponsors should look in space and time for extended effects. Tracking such effects can cost money as well as time and effort and may soon run into diminished returns. If other stakeholders fail to appreciate and attribute the extended effects to sponsors' efforts, the impact on relationships will be negligible. On the other hand, by tracking and reporting such extended benefits, sponsors can heighten stakeholders' perceptions of them and their likelihood of crediting the sponsor for them.

The prudent approach would be to look for any and all extended effects that sponsors think would be appreciated by stakeholders. By tracking and reporting these effects, then checking on stakeholder appreciation and attribution of them after reporting, sponsors can find out whether or not they are having positive impact on important stakeholder relationships. If not they can be dropped from tracking and reporting efforts. If so, sponsors may look for even further extended effects until they reach the point where stakeholders no longer appreciate or attribute them.

CIRCULAR EFFECTS

In addition to linear sequences with some lapses (repetition of steps) or exceptional reversals of the "normal" order and to extensions of effects in time and space, there are sequences of effects that are circular, where changes in one parameter of the model can bring about changes in both earlier and later parameters. While the normal and simple approach to thinking about and discussing causes and effects is linear, reality is often complex and nonlinear.

The complexities of interventions and their impacts have been recognized and described by a variety of authors, from Forrester's "systems dynamics" at the Massachusetts Institute of Technology in the 1960s[3] to Senge's "systems thinking" in 1990.[4] We believe these complex, nonlinear models are applicable and of special interest in regard to improving consumer health and demand behaviors.

The essence of systems dynamics (Forrester) or systems thinking (Senge) is "looping," the tendency of events to affect each other in a circular fashion. There are two types of loops or circles: balancing and reinforcing. In a balancing loop or system, changes in one factor or element of the system affect other elements in ways that end up tending to return the system to the status it enjoyed before the changes began.

One of the classic examples of a balancing system is the working of a thermostat. The temperature in the space governed by the thermostat changes. That change triggers changes in the mechanism of the thermostat, resulting in signals to the heating or air-conditioning unit to turn on. The effects of the heating or cooling unit operation are felt by the thermostat and result in a second signal to the unit to turn off once the preset temperature has been restored. The entire system is geared to recognize when the temperature is "wrong" and to return it to the "right" status.

The majority of systems are of this type; otherwise we would see too much uncontrolled change. A reinforcing system is rarer but more interesting and challenging. In a reinforcing system, once one factor changes in a given direction, it tends to promote continuing change in the system in the same direction rather than a return to the status quo. If the reinforcing system begins to change in a negative (i.e., unfavorable) direction, we call it a "vicious cycle." If it changes in a positive, favorable direction, it is a "virtuous cycle."

Examples of complex, looping systems in health care have been discussed for over 20 years.[5] If a hospital sees its quality of care go down, for example, this will reduce its attraction to physicians; as a result, the physicians will refer and admit fewer patients; revenues and profits will decline; the hospital will respond by reducing expenditures and cutting staff and investment in technology; as a result, quality will decline still further and the hospital will enter a vicious cycle of decline.

The complex dynamics involved challenge administrators to resist the obvious response of cutting expenses and instead to invest in quality improvement so as to reverse the direction of change entirely. Once this is done quality improves; attraction to physicians increases; admissions increase; revenue and profits increase; and this makes it easier to invest in further quality improvements to keep the virtuous cycle going (Fig 7–1).

When confronted with balancing systems, we can, at best, hope to improve the speed and efficiency of returning to the status quo. Otherwise such systems will be frustrating since they resist any permanent change, positive or negative. When confronted with reinforcing systems, the challenge is first to recognize that they are reinforcing systems, then to determine where we can intervene and how so as to get the system going in a favorable direction or to reverse its movement if it has already started going in an unfavorable direction.

Figure 7–1 Vicious or Virtuous Cycle?

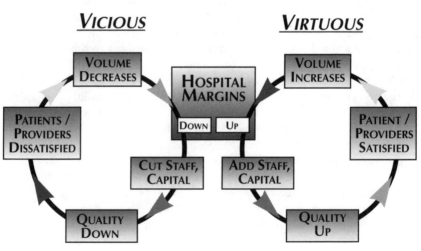

THE DYNAMICS OF SELF-EFFICACY

One of the most important factors in improving consumer health and demand behaviors is the combination of ability and confidence called self-efficacy,[6] or capability in the $I = MC^2$ model. Where consumers have the motivation but lack the capability (e.g., knowledge, skill, physical capability) to behave in a desired fashion, appealing to them to do so will have little effect. Even if they have the capability but have no confidence in their ability (i.e., do not believe that they have it), the results are likely to be the same: minimal or no response. If they have no real capability, but have misplaced confidence enough to try behaving in the desired fashion, consumers may respond but will be frustrated or obtain the wrong results and will lose confidence, making them unresponsive the next time.

By contrast, if they have both the necessary ability and justified confidence in that ability, and improve their behavior accordingly—*and* enjoy the positive results that have been mentioned in Chapter 5 (e.g., better health, quality of life, more immediate relief from anxiety or discomfort)—they will find that the experience reinforces their likelihood of repeating the desired behavior. This effect has been noted in training patients with arthritis in self-care, for example.[7]

Sponsors of demand improvement efforts can take advantage of this reinforcing effect. By intervening through a program to promote self-efficacy, perhaps a training and practice program, sponsors can increase the likelihood that consumers will engage in an exercise program (health improvement) or employ self-care appropriately (decision improvement). Once consumers experience the positive effects such behaviors have on them personally, they are both more motivated to repeat the behavior and more confident in their self-efficacy and so tend to repeat the behaviors more frequently, enjoying the positive effects even more (Fig 7–2).

Sponsors could also intervene by encouraging and reminding consumers to try the desired behavior, counting on the experience of doing so to reinforce consumer self-efficacy, increasing the frequency of the desired behavior and experiencing the positive consequences of increased motivation and self-efficacy, for example.

Within any reinforcing system, sponsors may have only one or multiple "leverage points" where they can intervene effectively.[8] The stages of change model requires intervention focused on the stage individuals are in at the time. The $I = MC^2$ model challenges sponsors to influence, build, or reinforce whichever of the factors is missing or weak.

RELATIONSHIP DYNAMICS

Consumers' relationship with sponsors is another key factor in demand improvement. If consumers distrust the employer, health plan, or provider who sponsors a given initiative, they are unlikely to respond in the desired fashion. If they trust that the sponsor truly has their best interests in mind and that the change in

Figure 7–2 Consumer Self-Efficacy

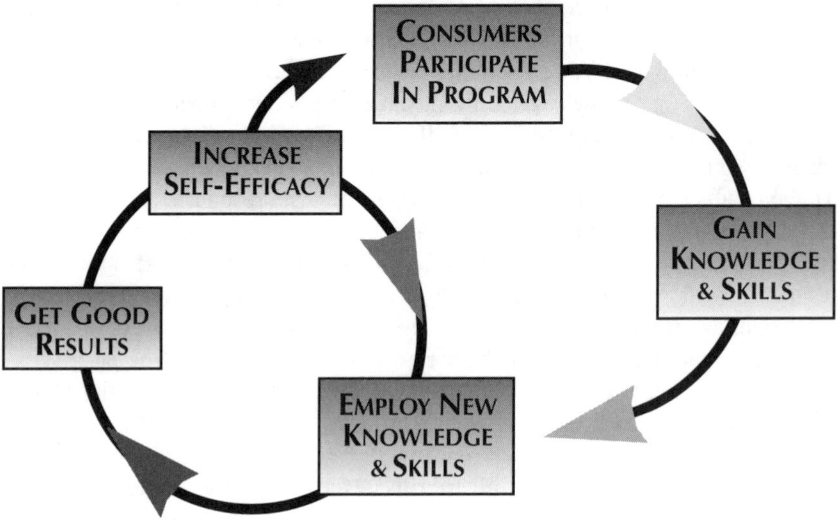

behavior will truly benefit them, not just the sponsor, then the desired response is more probable.

Once they make the desired response, they will presumably enjoy the positive benefits that naturally follow. This will tend to make them trust the sponsor more, making them more receptive to subsequent initiatives. Their response to these initiatives will, in turn, produce still further benefits to them and reinforce their confidence in sponsors, making them, for example, more receptive, responsive. Once consumer attitudes toward sponsors start moving in a positive direction, both the effectiveness and efficiency of future initiatives should improve.

By the same token, if a sponsor starts off on the wrong foot, attempting to improve consumers' behavior through oppressive means or deceptive information, trust will be eroded. Consumers will be unresponsive to sponsor appeals and will not change their behavior, not experience the positive consequences, perceiving such appeals as attempts to manipulate or coerce them, further undermining their trust and making even more unresponsive.

The size of the investment may also be a critical factor. If sponsors underfund particular initiatives, they may both doom the initiative to failure and make targeted consumers less receptive to subsequent efforts, even if those are adequately funded (Fig 7–3).

Figure 7–3 Consumer-Sponsor Relationship Dynamics Affecting Behavior Change

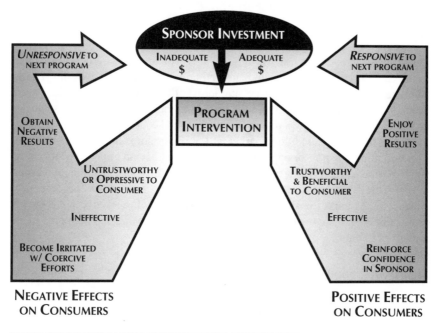

RETENTION DYNAMICS

One of the more serious barriers to sponsors' investment in demand improvement is high turnover among consumers. If employees change jobs frequently, if health plan members change plans at a rate of 25% each year, or if patients change provider allegiance at the drop of a hat, consumers may not be around long enough for changes in their behavior to benefit sponsors. Many health improvement initiatives take more than a year to affect consumer health, use of services, and expenditures. Many decision improvement and disease and disability management efforts tend to increase their effects over time, so high turnover among consumers may prevent initiatives from yielding a satisfactory return on investment.

Yet demand improvement initiatives, where they produce clear and significant benefit to consumers, will tend to promote retention. Effects on employee morale have already been cited among the effects of health improvement and disability management initiatives in Chapter 5. Higher member and patient satisfaction, loyalty, and retention are value-adding effects for health plans and providers. As demand improvement initiatives promote greater retention, they both improve the payoff to sponsors and add to their savings and profits, making them better able as well as more willing to invest further[9] (Fig 7–4).

DYNAMICS OF MARKET SHARE

Demand improvement has still further impact on sponsors. Where it saves on health care expenditures for health plans and providers and on both health and disability insurance costs for employers, it improves their market position. Employers, health plans, and providers can use the savings to reduce prices or increase quality and make themselves more attractive in the client and consumer markets.

In turn, added success in the market will bring in more clients and consumers. This will multiply sponsor opportunities to achieve demand improvement savings and to promote greater efficiency in specific efforts through economies and synergies of scale. This will, in turn, improve their savings and further enable them to enhance their market position and market share. It will also give them greater profits that will make them better able to afford to invest in demand improvement initiatives in the first place (Fig 7–5).

Figure 7–4 Sponsor's Benefit: Consumer Satisfaction

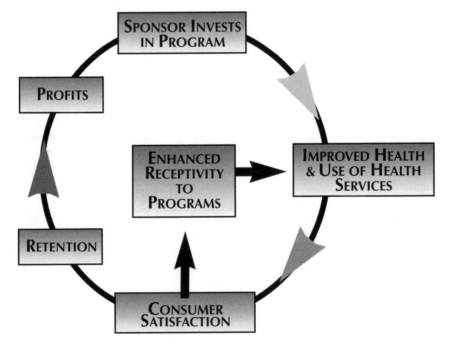

Figure 7–5 Sponsor's Benefit: Competitive Edge

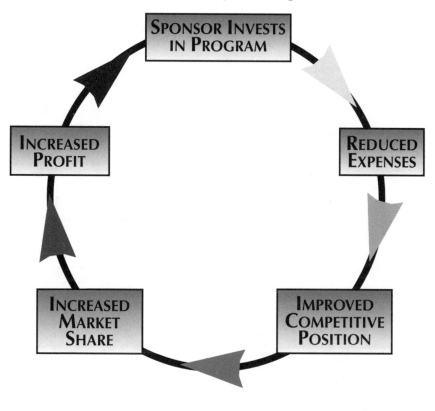

SET OF EFFECTS DYNAMICS

In Chapter 5 we discussed the set of effects of the four categories of demand improvement initiatives in a linear order. In reality these effects are capable of forming reinforcing loops. For example, changes in mind-states may have to be achieved before participation in a class or group effort or before reading of a self-care manual occurs. So mind-state changes may precede participation, in addition to resulting from it (Fig 7–6).

Similarly, the diverse value-added effects listed at the end of the linear description of the set of effects do not all come from reductions in expenditures, the immediately preceding effect. Added value also comes from improved health status (e.g., morale and productivity of workers). It can come from reforms in service use, as when well-chosen care speeds up return to work and thereby worker pro-

Figure 7–6 Set of Effects: Complex Dynamics

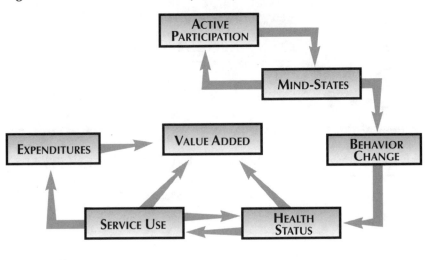

ductivity. Improvements in service use can improve health status, just as changes in behavior do.

Yet another loop relates to the set of effects on consumers. As they move from participation to improved health knowledge and mind-states, to improved behavior and health status, to better utilization and expenditure savings for themselves, and to quality of life and other value-adding effects resulting from their progress through the set, they should become more receptive to further opportunities for participation, for example, and to changing other health and demand behaviors. This will increase their likelihood of having further positive experiences, reinforcing their receptivity to still further opportunities (Fig 7–7).

For sponsors the added effects in the set include the retention and attraction effects that consumer and client satisfaction and investment of savings can have on market success and financial performance. These, in turn, make further investment in demand improvement initiatives both more possible and more rewarding. Thus the set of effects loops to make possible, for example, further participation, mind-state, and behavior improvements as well as improvements in sponsor market success, as previously depicted in Fig 7–5.

In most cases the existence of the reinforcing systems we have described has not been demonstrated. Because it is easier to think in linear terms, sponsors and scientists alike have planned and evaluated demand improvement initiatives chiefly in linear fashion. Where no one has looked for reinforcing effects, they

Figure 7–7 Set of Effects: A Complex Consumer Dynamic Loop

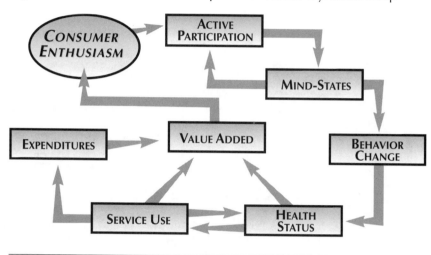

have not been found and reported. The challenge is to look for them, in both planning and evaluation of specific initiatives.

It is a relatively simple matter to at least agree in conjecture as to what looping dynamics might apply in a given situation. The examples described in this chapter offer a number of possibilities, though there are probably many more. We recommend that sponsors include the possibility of effects on consumer self-efficacy, receptivity to future initiatives, loyalty, and retention, for example, in planning and evaluating each initiative. In addition, it would be wise to include market effects, financial performance, and similar value-adding effects.

As we warned in our discussion of the set of effects, the farther the set is followed, the greater the difficulty of attribution. Many factors other than demand improvement efforts may be influencing consumer satisfaction, trust of sponsors, retention, and related effects. Even more factors are likely to be at work relative to market position and financial performance. Each sponsor can at least come closer to a reasoned judgment about whether particular initiatives have particular effects by planning for them and including them in evaluation deliberately, as opposed to speculating about them after the fact.

Where sponsors determine that a systems dynamics reinforcing loop is present, they should give special attention to ensuring that the direction of change produces a "virtuous" rather than "vicious" cycle (i.e., moves the parts of the system in a positive rather than negative direction). Each of the loops described in this chapter merits attention in that regard.

REFERENCES

1. J. Burns, "Better Benefits Foster Increased Productivity," *Managed Healthcare* 7, no. 8 (1997): 58.
2. B. Coleman, "Parent Smoking Kills 6,200 Kids," *Denver Post,* 15 July 1997, 3A.
3. J. Forrester, *Industrial Dynamics* (Cambridge, MA: MIT Press, 1961).
4. P. Senge, *The Fifth Discipline* (New York, NY: Doubleday, 1990).
5. N. Stearns, et al., "Systems Intervention: New Help for Hospitals," *Health Care Management Review* 1, no. 4 (1976):9–18.
6. C. Perry, et al., "How Individuals, Environments and Health Behavior Interact," in *Health Behavior and Health Education,* eds. K. Glanz, et al. (San Francisco, CA: Jossey-Bass, 1990), 161–186.
7. K. Lorig and H. Holman, "Arthritis Self-Management Studies: A Twelve Year Review," *Health Education Quarterly* (in press).
8. D. Kauffman, *Systems I: An Introduction to Systems Thinking* (Minneapolis, MN: Future Systems, Inc., 1990).
9. F. Reichheld, *The Loyalty Effect: The Hidden Force behind Growth, Profits, and Lasting Value* (Cambridge, MA: Harvard University Press, 1996).

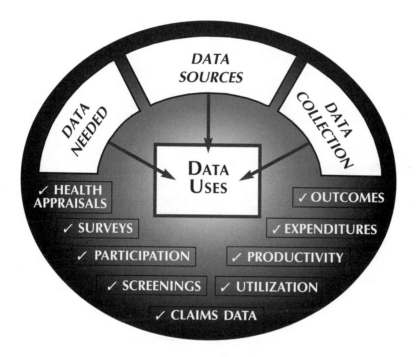

Chapter 8

DATA
SOURCES

DATA
NEEDED

DATA
COLLECTION

DATA
USES

✓ HEALTH APPRAISALS

✓ OUTCOMES

✓ SURVEYS

✓ EXPENDITURES

✓ PARTICIPATION

✓ PRODUCTIVITY

✓ SCREENINGS ✓ UTILIZATION

✓ CLAIMS DATA

INFORMATION FOUNDATIONS

To plan, implement, and evaluate the most effective and efficient strategies and tactics, it is essential to have the right information. In planning, information promotes better decisions in targeting the right consumers and most promising behavior changes to go for. In implementation, information helps keep initiatives focused and permits midcourse corrections to promote achieving desired outcomes. In evaluation, information enables sponsors to find out and place a value upon what changes occur in what success measures, determine which effects can be attributed to their efforts, and learn how to do better next time.

In this chapter we will discuss the types of information that can deliver value in particular initiatives, where and how such information can be found or generated, and how to use it. We will begin with a discussion of basic demographic information about the population of interest. We will then describe information based on the seven set of effects categories described in Chapter 5, together with $I = MC^2$ and stages of change information that can be used in selecting consumer targets, setting objectives for, and evaluating results of specific initiatives.

DEMOGRAPHICS

The first category of fundamental information relates to the demographics characteristics of the population of interest. Such information precedes the set of effects but can be instrumental in understanding and analyzing the data directly pertinent to planning and evaluating initiatives.

Demographic data include the basic facts about populations of interest, the kinds of data normally collected in the decennial census: for example, age, gender, ethnic group, education, occupation, income, place of residence, and family members. Information on ethnic group can help anticipate some health problems, such as higher incidence of diabetes among Hispanic populations and higher blood pressure among African Americans. The number of childbearing-aged women in the population will suggest the need for family planning or prenatal care services.[1]

Education levels will help in planning educational efforts, and language spoken will indicate whether information, surveys, and educational efforts should be translated into languages other than English. Income levels will give some indication as to the potential impact of cost or transportation problems as deterrents to participation in particular efforts. Family size and ages of family members will point out likely patterns of problems or the need for childcare to permit family participation.

For community populations, census data should provide most demographic information of interest. For health plan enrollees and employee, dependent, and retiree populations, insurance or personnel records should do the same. In special cases, surveys may be needed to supplement already existing data. Suggestions for conducting surveys will be offered later in this chapter.

SET OF EFFECTS INFORMATION

Participation

Where initiatives are to be focused on promoting participation in health-protecting or health-promoting activities, it is essential to have baseline data on who is already participating in what (see Table 8–1). Who is already engaging in sponsored wellness activities, attending educational seminars, getting scheduled immunizations or screening tests, or using self-care guides? Who is already attending or has attended

Table 8–1 Consumer Data Required for Program Planning

SET OF EFFECTS	DATA NEEDED	PROGRAM USE
ACTIVE PARTICIPATION	X WHO IS PARTICIPATING X IN WHAT PROGRAMS	• TO IDENTIFY POPULATIONS FOR SPECIFIC INTERVENTIONS • TO SET OBJECTIVES FOR PARTICIPATION
MIND-SET CHANGES	X PREFERENCES FOR SPECIFIC TYPES OF PLANS X PREFERENCES FOR SOURCES OF INFORMATION X EXPECTATIONS FOR DESIRED BENEFITS X PERCEIVED BARRIERS X AREAS OF RECEPTIVITY	• TO SET GOALS FOR PROGRAM INTERVENTIONS • TO IDENTIFY APPROPRIATE MODELS FOR CONTENT DELIVERY • TO DETERMINE WHETHER CONSUMER WILL ACCESS APPROPRIATE SERVICES • TO REDUCE PERCEPTION OF INAPPROPRIATELY DENIED CARE • TO ENHANCE RECEPTIVITY TO SPONSORED PROGRAMS
HEALTH BEHAVIORS	X HEALTH RISK BEHAVIORS X SELF-HELP SKILLS X RESOURCES ACCESSED	• TO PREDICT UTILIZATION • TO TARGET NEEDED SELF-EFFICACY SKILLS & SET OBJECTIVES • TO UTILIZE RIGHT LEVEL OF SERVICE AT RIGHT TIME
HEALTH STATUS	X PERSONAL FAMILY HEALTH HISTORIES X GENETIC RISK FACTORS X DETERMINATION OF CURRENT SYMPTOMS, DISABILITIES & PROBLEMS	• TO IDENTIFY KNOWN HEALTH RISK FACTORS & TARGETS • TO MEASURE AND MONITOR TARGETED EFFORTS • TO MODIFY BEHAVIORS • TO IMPROVE HEALTH STATUS
SERVICES USED	X QUALITY OF UTILIZATION X QUANTITY OF UTILIZATION X MEASURED AGAINST DESIRABLE UTILIZATION	• TO IDENTIFY PROBLEMS & TARGETS • TO SET GOALS FOR OPTIMUM UTILIZATION • TO TARGET IMPROVEMENT OPPORTUNITIES
RESOURCE COSTS & EXPENDITURES	X RESOURCES CONSUMED X EXPENDITURE LEVELS	• TO MEASURE $$ SPENT AGAINST $$ SAVED • TO MEASURE ATTITUDES TO PRICE & DISCOUNT INCENTIVES
VALUE ADDED & BENEFITS DERIVED	X BASELINE INFO ON HEALTH & ATTITUDES X ENROLLMENTS & DISENROLLMENTS X PROFIT PERFORMANCE	• TO MEASURE CHANGE IN HEALTH & QUALITY OF LIFE • TO SUPPORT STRATEGIC PLANNING • TO MANAGE MARKETING FUNCTIONS & PROFITABILITY

education and training programs on the use of blood-sugar monitors and peak flow meters as part of managing their chronic conditions? Who has been educated in using safety goggles, seat belts, or other safety equipment or procedures on the job?

Such baseline information is useful first in evaluating past efforts. Finding out how many of the people who were educated, trained, or screened have changed their behavior appropriately offers insights into the effectiveness of past efforts, in addition to supplying data on the extent of the current challenge. Knowing how many have participated or are participating in programs sponsored by other interested parties can help determine whether additional sponsors and programs are advisable.

Having baseline data on current and past participation is also essential in setting goals and evaluating efforts. There is no point in setting a goal of getting 50% of all children in a population immunized if 60% have already been immunized. The level of current use of a self-care guide can also suggest how difficult or easy it might be to achieve some desired participation goal. Goals should not be arbitrary but should be based on what is realistic as well as desirable for a population. Evaluation should note how much participation has changed rather than simply what level has been achieved.

Information on participants can also help identify those consumers who may serve as models for their peers, who may be enlisted as word-of-mouth ambassadors in promoting the same or similar programs to their peers. Past participants can also help as advisors on how to improve programs to make them more attractive or satisfying, though insights from participants should always be supplemented with ideas from nonparticipants on why they have not participated.

Information on participation and participants may be obtained from the programs in which they were involved, from the sponsor's past records, or from those of other partners. In the absence of reliable records, populations of interest can be surveyed on their past and current participation. Given poor memories, added to the tendency of some to report what they feel they should have done or what surveyors want to hear, actual records are normally the preferred source.

Mind-States

The existing mind-states of the population of interest is second in importance only to their current behavior patterns. Identifying their state of readiness in terms of the three mind-state stages of change (i.e., precontemplation, contemplation, or preparation) is critical to selecting which consumers to go after and what types of interventions to employ. Determining their present status regarding motivation, capability, and consciousness is vital to understanding why they are not already evidencing desired behaviors and to formulating tactics to move them from one stage of change to the next.

Current states of knowledge, beliefs, perceptions, and attitudes may form the basis for setting goals, designing programs, and evaluating results of initiatives. In community planning, citizen concerns and worries about health, perceived needs and problems, and preferences for community action often form the basis for planned interventions.[2] For enrolled and employee populations, levels of interest in learning about wellness and health promotion or in participating in fitness and self-care can suggest their receptivity to new initiatives.[3]

Employee preferences regarding benefits or types of health plans and the importance they place on choice of providers or on coverage for specific services may well determine their potential for being steered in a direction desired by employers or unions and can help in designing benefit packages as well as screening health plans. Senior attitudes toward prescription benefits, aversion to deductibles and copayments, or desires for provider choice can guide health plan efforts in designing Medicare HMOs and promoting enrollment.

Identifying consumers' preferred sources of information and their preferred providers for specific health promotion, prevention, education, counseling, and support services will help sponsors decide who is best suited to implement specific programs. Determining their attitudes toward self-care versus dependence on professionals, self-responsibility versus external locus of control, and their perceived competence and confidence (self-efficacy) will give sponsors a good idea as to the challenge they face in promoting self-care and chronic condition management.[4]

In designing initiatives, and particularly in developing ways to promote them, knowing what benefits consumers are interested in can make all the difference. Are they hoping for wellness programs to make them feel better, look better, perform better, live longer, or enjoy life more? Do they see fitness activities as reducing stress, enhancing productivity, improving their job performance and security, reducing their risk of disease and injury, or improving their recovery therefrom?[5]

What motivational status are consumers in? Do they see no value in the desired behavior or misperceive the benefits of their present behavior? Do they believe their present behavior is admired by their peers or are they rebelling against what others expect of them? Are they ignorant of the risks of their current behavior, or do they feel immune to far-off threats? Why do they not want to improve?

What motivational barriers do consumers perceive to participation in activities under consideration or already offered or to adopting and persisting in a desired pattern of behavior? What do they see as workplace, sociocultural, and family norms relative to specific behaviors? What do they perceive their reference groups are doing in terms of health and demand behaviors? Given the effect of social norms and models, it is helpful to know what consumers think others are doing and thinking, in addition to what they themselves have in their minds.[6]

What internal/personal or external/environmental barriers do they perceive to their capability? Are they conversant with self-care and chronic condition or disability self-management but lacking in confidence in their own skills? Are opportunities for exercise inconvenient because of time or place factors? Do they lack funds to secure early detection screening, or is the safety equipment clumsy for them to use?

Are they even conscious of a better behavior and of the risks of their present behavior compared to the benefits of a better alternative? Do they want to do better but frequently forget to take their pills or floss their teeth? Do other activities submerge their intent to exercise so that it slips their mind most of the time? Do they recall if they are due for a routine physical or prostate check?

Since the purpose of most reform initiatives is to change consumer behavior, identifying where they are in the stages of change is especially useful. Sponsors may choose to focus exclusively on those at the preparation stage, for example, knowing they are more likely to change behavior, or design separate programs for those at different mental stages.[7]

Discovering what specific activities consumers are receptive to, what education and training programs they say they would attend, and what wellness and fitness activities they would engage in can be critical in making program decisions. Even where their preferences may be for programs of unproved or doubtful efficacy (e.g., weight loss), it may prove important in building and sustaining relationships for sponsors to heed their requests.[8]

Identifying patterns of mind-states is also the basis for psychographic segmentation—grouping consumers based on attitudes, preferences, wishes that make subsets of the population similar to each other and different from other subsets. Consumers with low levels of self-efficacy, for example, may require more and different forms of attention as compared to those with fairly high levels. Trying to meet the needs of both with the same program could leave the former frustrated and the latter bored, where separate programs could achieve desired results with both.

Discovering the present mind-states for populations of interest will almost always require some form of survey or group discussions, perhaps both. Health plans and many providers are likely to be familiar with survey research and focus group techniques; employers and other providers can secure outside help from market and public opinion research firms. Within integrated systems, virtual or actual, partners can share the costs of outside services since all will share the benefits of better information.

Health Behaviors

The list of behaviors that might be of interest to sponsors is probably endless. Commonly behaviors of interest include exercise/fitness activities; diet/nutrition habits; smoking; alcohol and drug use; safety in work, home, driving, sun, and sexual activity; sleep patterns; social activity; and support groups. In addition, sponsors may seek to identify current levels and patterns of self-care—for example, when used, how often, for what problems, and with what results. Identifying chronic condition self-management activities and skills may also be of interest.

At the community level, determining first aid, CPR, and similar self-help skill levels can also be important to estimating the level of assets and needs among populations of interest. Finding out how many people use alternative care providers, from chiropractors to *curanderas*, and for what conditions may disclose problems or potential solutions unknown heretofore. In general, learning what people do when confronted with specific symptoms can indicate what kinds of interventions are needed and possible.

For identifying patterns of health-risk behaviors, health-risk appraisals are especially suited. (See Chapter 21.) These same surveys can also be used to identify health-related interests and concerns and perceived health and functional status. They have the advantage of being able to summarize patterns of behaviors in terms of a health-risk or life-expectancy score, which can both indicate the overall risk for a population and stimulate individuals with poor scores to make changes.[9] (See Table 8–2.)

Survey results may be supplemented with sponsor records, such as measured worksite fitness participation, observations on safety equipment use, and records on seat belt use in accidents. In most cases, however, overall information on a population can only be gathered through questionnaires or interviews. This means relying on what consumers report about their own behavior, with all the limitations that entails. There are means to promote more accurate disclosure of behaviors that consumers may be unwilling to discuss (to be discussed later in this chapter). There are also clinical tests that can be used to check on or supplement reports on some behaviors, such as smoking and drug use.

Determining where members of a population are along the three behavioral stages of change is as valuable as knowing whether or not they are engaging in a desired behavior. Those just initiating a behavior change (the action stage) may benefit from recognition and reward programs or from social support programs, for example. Those who have been engaged in a desired behavior for some time but are subject to frequent lapses (maintenance stage) may benefit from reminders or monitoring and reporting of their success (e.g., weight loss or blood pressure measurement). Those truly habituated to the desired behavior (the permanence or "for good" stage) may be removed from the list of those requiring anything more than occasional prompting so that efforts can be focused elsewhere.

(While those at this last stage of the stages of change theoretically require no attention, there are some behaviors that occur so infrequently that a reminder is likely to be needed even for those thoroughly motivated and able to repeat them. Annual or biennial mammography screening, pneumonia vaccination every five years or tetanus every ten are examples of infrequent behaviors that are more likely to be correctly repeated with the help of reminders.)

A key issue in all attempts to determine health behavior patterns in a population is whether the information is needed and will be used at the population or individual level. Where only population data are needed (i.e., knowledge of the patterns that prevail throughout an employee, enrollee, or community population of interest), samples will suffice rather than information on everyone, and individual anonymity can be guaranteed. This greatly facilitates the task and can enhance the accuracy of the behaviors reported.

Table 8–2 Examples of Available Tools for Data Gathering

DATA SOURCE ▼	REPRESENTATIVE TOOLS
CONSUMER	✗ HEALTH RISK APPRAISALS ✗ SURVEYS ✗ CONFIDENTIAL REPORTING
ANY SPONSOR	✗ PROGRAMS OFFERED ✗ PARTICIPATION DATA ✗ AGGREGATE CLINICAL SCREENINGS
PHYSICIAN	✗ INDIVIDUAL CHECK-UPS ✗ CLINICAL SCREENINGS
HEALTH PLAN	✗ HEALTH CARE UTILIZATION DATA ✗ CLAIMS DATA ✗ EXPENDITURE DATA
HOSPITALS	✗ ED VISITS, ADMISSIONS ✗ LENGTH OF STAY
EMPLOYERS	✗ WORKERS' COMPENSATION / DISABILITY COMPENSATION RECORDS ✗ PRODUCTIVITY, ABSENTEEISM DATA
PUBLIC AGENCIES	✗ IMMUNIZATION STATISTICS ✗ HEDIS COMPARATIVE DATA

For health risks (health improvement) to be most effectively addressed, however, it is necessary to know precisely which individuals practice what behaviors. Only with such information can customized reports and corrective action plans be generated for individuals.[10] This means potential embarrassment and even fears about job or insurance security for consumers and therefore high likelihood of low participation or organized resistance.[11]

For decision improvement efforts, knowing who has received self-care materials; who has accessed information on plan, provider, and procedure choices; and who has asked for advance directive forms is essential. In disease management knowing who has been taught or trained for self-management of chronic conditions, who has accessed sponsor information or support group assistance, and who has obtained prescribed prenatal or behavioral health treatment is necessary for evaluation. In disability management being able to determine which individuals have had which interventions and how they have behaved subsequently is as vital as knowing what injury rates, utilization, and expenditure levels are true for the employee population as a whole.

If only population-based data are available, sponsors can determine what changes have occurred in any of the set of effects measures. Unfortunately they will not be able to say whether changes are attributable to their efforts. What if adverse fetal outcome rates go down overall, but not among the women participating in prenatal interventions? What if heart disease problems decline, but not among those who quit smoking? Only by tracking the changes across the set of effects *by individuals* can sponsors determine whether they have achieved results as opposed to mere chance developments.

Whenever information on individuals is necessary, threats to privacy and confidentiality of sensitive information arise. One way to reduce such threats is to rely on personal physicians as the only persons who will have access to individual information on health status and behaviors. It is hoped that most consumers would accept their personal physician being privy to the most intimate details of their lives if they trust their physicians and feel the information will be used in their best interests.

For consumers who lack such trust, arrangements can be made so that only consumers themselves will know what status and behaviors pertain to them. Confidential identification codes can be assigned to individuals so that individual information may be processed, reports and corrective recommendations generated, and changes recorded over time, with only the individual able to examine the information knowing to whom it pertains. Such systems will be unwieldy and more expensive to employ and are likely to require the services of an outside firm. But these systems may be the only way some consumers will accept the risk.

Perhaps the best approach is to obtain individual consumer approval for the types of information to be collected, stored, analyzed, and reported and for the people who will have access to such information. Since the goals of demand improvement include the improvement of consumer health and quality of life, there is at least a hope that consumers will consider strictly limited loss of privacy a worthwhile price to pay.

Health Status

Basic personal and family health histories are essential to effective improvement of health and demand. Past diseases and injuries as well as prior hospitalizations and procedures are typical items in medical histories. Physicians at risk for the health and demand of specific populations are likely to have their own ideas of what specific items should be included in histories. Consumers may have the same kinds of trust or objections to physicians knowing some specifics in their past.

Health status measures should include all the risk factors that are best, or in some cases only, identified through clinical measures: for example, blood pressure, blood sugar, cholesterol and HDL/LDL levels, body mass index, HIV/AIDS, cardiac irregularities, and lung function. Here, too, physicians responsible for the population of interest will have their own ideas as to what measures should be routinely used for which consumers.

Current symptoms, disabilities, or problems may also be identified in clinical assessments of health status or may be reported by consumers as part of health appraisals. The numbers, types, and frequency of medications being taken for what conditions should also be included. Perceived health and functional status is equally important. Perceived health status, for example, has been found to be one of the best predictors of impending mortality.[12] Functional status will identify consumers who may need special support or customized interventions because of difficulties with daily life activities.

Health status measures such as perceived health and functional status can only be obtained via survey, such as the SF-36 form in common use.[13] Other health status measures may also be obtained through asking consumers, since many will know their last blood pressure, cholesterol, blood sugar, or HIV/AIDS status. Such reports need not be relied upon, but they can indicate consumer awareness of their health status and willingness to discuss it. Confidentiality of such information may have to be guaranteed in the same manner as health behavior data.

Health status measures can be obtained through mass screenings as well as individual checkups. Screenings can be both more efficient and can reach more people, particularly where they are conducted at the worksite, in malls, or at other easily accessible locations. Multiple opportunities and arrangements may be needed to obtain both upfront and monitoring measures of health status for particular populations, so no one method ought to be relied upon.

Health utilization and claims data can supplement both clinical tests and self-reported conditions. Past claims data may be more reliable than consumer memory and may reflect conditions not screened for and procedures not reported to current personal physicians. The unfortunate insurance practice of "underwriting" so as to exclude people with preexisting conditions from coverage or of dramatically increasing their health insurance costs makes full disclosure by consumers less popular and sharing of claims information among insurers more common.

For community health status, screening fairs and self-reporting may be relied upon more than for enrollee and employee populations. Mortality data and reportable morbidity such as medical treatment misadventure and communicable disease will be available from public health agencies. Crime statistics, domestic violence, education, joblessness, income, and similar measures may also be used as indicators of community health in the largest sense.[14]

Health Services Utilization

Current utilization data are likely to be used as the basis for identifying problems and setting goals by sponsors. Specific patterns, as opposed to overall levels of utilization, can also be useful in selecting consumer targets for attention and selecting strategic focus. By comparing both to prevailing risk-adjusted averages or benchmarks reflecting best practices, sponsors can determine where their greatest problems and opportunities are.

In most cases a branching logic applied to overall utilization data will aid in selecting problems and opportunities. If overall hospitalization levels are high, discovering which medical categories and diagnosis groups appear high should lead to identifying intervention potential. High levels of Caesarean section deliveries in maternity, or coronary artery bypass graft (CABG) surgery for heart disease, or lumbar surgery for back problems, for example, will enable more effective targeting than is possible through overall levels alone. Sponsors will still have to decide whether consumers are the best focus for intervention as opposed to providers, of course.

Because specific types of utilization are substitutable, both the quality and quantity of utilization need to be addressed. An unusually high level of ambulatory surgery may not be a problem but a sign of effective reductions in inpatient surgery. High levels of primary physician visits may reflect more use of preventive and promotion services or less reliance on specialists rather than a problem situation. Early detection may cause a one-time surge in utilization that is highly desirable.

Analysts of utilization data should employ some kind of template indicating what types and amounts of desirable utilization should be found, in addition to indicators of inappropriate or unnecessary use. Immunization, screening, and proper symptom response should be looked for and identified as a problem when missing. Avoidable utilization (i.e., the use of services that is deemed appropriate and necessary given the symptoms that prompted it but where the symptoms could have been prevented) should be a particular focus.

Similarly, data reflecting utilization that was delayed past the point where the most cost-effective interventions are possible should be avidly sought. Arrival at the emergency department hours after the onset of heart attack symptoms or diagnosis of breast cancer at stages III or IV should be investigated as serious problems in consumer behavior. Identifying and addressing the reasons for such suboptimal use of services can at least help others.

In most cases health service utilization information will be obtained through provider and payer records. Consumers may be surveyed to learn of their recalled utilization patterns where such records are not available, as with new employees, enrollees, or a community population. Recall of physician and outpatient use may not be reliable beyond a few months, or hospitalizations beyond a year or two, but where there is no other choice, consumer reporting is probably better than not knowing.

For utilization of services not covered by insurance, particularly for alternative providers, self-reporting by consumers may be the only source of information available. Insurers may not care about such information, though high levels of use of noncovered providers may warn of or explain disenrollment. Employers and providers should be interested, though perhaps for different reasons. It might turn out that some alternative providers prove more cost-effective in treating some conditions—chiropractors for low back pain, for example[15]—in which case employers may rethink their benefit plans. Providers should ideally know all of the treatments their patients are getting if ever they are truly to coordinate the full continuum of care. Those at risk may find that referring some patients to alternative providers is in their own financial interests as well as better for their patients.

Health Care Expenditures

Actual expenditures for health care, by employers and insurers and by providers at risk, are likely to be the major focus of sponsors' planning and evaluation activities. While other problem and outcome measures may be accorded some value in their own right, chances are the dollar effects will always at least be included. Dollars saved have that attractive property of being easily comparable to dollars spent in promoting health or improving consumption of services. Identifying out-of-pocket expenditures by consumers can help in selecting and motivating targets for attention.

In most cases payer and provider records will contain most of the expenditure information of interest. Exceptions arise relative to consumer out-of-pocket expenditures. Where deductible levels are not reached, consumers may not have reported their expenditures to payers, for example. Providers may have data on collected copayments, but payers may be in the dark about them. For uncovered services, including the use of alternative providers not included in the network, only the consumer may know about levels of expenditures.

Surveying consumers, in addition to analyzing claims data and provider financial records, can help sponsors learn something of consumer attitudes toward prices and value. Where consumers are unaware of and do not share in the discounts offered by providers to payers, for example, they may blame providers for outrageous prices, thus undermining their trust and confidence in their providers. Surveys may reveal that consumers have delayed or avoided using services they should have sought because of financial barriers.

Added-Value Effects

What were described as value-adding effects in discussing the worth of health and consumption behavior reforms need not be treated as accidents or unexpected outcomes in planning or evaluation. In fact, unless front-end data are collected on parameters that may be positively or negatively affected by demand improvement efforts, there may be no way of detecting value-adding effects.

While data on past absenteeism levels, turnover, and productivity may be available in the employer's records, information on morale, commitment, job satisfaction, attitudes toward management, and similar psychological parameters will not be available unless they have been measured before an intervention is undertaken. Similarly, unless payers have both tracked and learned reasons for enrollment and disenrollment, they may be unable to discover whether changes were due to health-promoting efforts or variations in job turnover, changing residence, and similar "nonvoluntary" reasons for disenrollment or new enrollments.

Identifying baseline levels of such added-value parameters can also be helpful in designing and justifying particular interventions. Programs that promise significant value-adding effects, such as fitness activities' impact on safety and productivity, may be seen as more valuable even though their direct return in health care expenditures may be less than competing investment options. In some cases the prospect or discovery of valuable "side effects" may make the difference between choosing a program or not or continuing versus terminating it. Unless the full scope of value-adding parameters is measured at baseline and tracked during and after implementation of an intervention, sponsors may be unaware of these effects or forced to guess about them.

CONDUCTING SURVEYS

In many of the information categories, a survey is recommended or required to collect the necessary data. While this is not a book on conducting surveys, we will suggest some important considerations and offer some simple suggestions for making surveys work.

Sample versus Population

As discussed under health behavior information, there are times when the entire population should be surveyed. At other times, however, a sample may be all that is necessary. To identify the major interests of an enrolled, employee, or community population, for example, or to determine their level of concern over a specific problem, a representative sample will do as well and, in some cases, better than a survey of the entire population.

There is a respected maxim in research: it is better to get responses from 100% of a good sample than from a self-selected set of respondents from the entire population. In most cases a representative sample of 400 to 1,600 people can give a more accurate picture of the pattern of facts and perceptions in a large population than will a self-selected group of many thousands more if not truly representative. The problem in a self-selected sample arises from two significant factors about which surveyors are likely to be ignorant: what caused the people who did respond to do so, and what caused the people who did not respond to not do so.

Even if a sample is huge, say 10,000 people in a population of 1,000,000, if it is self-selected, surveyors have to wonder whether, by how much, and in what ways the 10,000 who answer a survey differ from the 990,000 who did not. It could be they felt more strongly about the issues addressed, or enjoy participating in surveys, or do almost anything they are asked. The point is, they differ in at least one dimension from nonrespondents: they responded. Surveyors have to wonder if they differ in other important ways as well.

By contrast, the uncertainty involved in a representative sample is at least controlled. Statistics tell us that if a random sample of 400 people breaks down into 50% in favor and 50% opposed to some idea, the chances are 95 out of 100 that the "true" proportion in the entire population from which the sample was drawn, even if that population was in the billions, is no more than 5% different from the sample either way.

If the challenge is to discover how many (what proportion) in the population exercise at least 30 minutes at a time at least three days a week, we can ask a sample of 400 and be 95% sure that whatever the sample results are, the proportion in the population is within plus or minus 5% of the sample proportion. If we need to be more precise, a sample of 1,600 will tell us within plus or minus 2.5%. If we can live with less precision, a sample of only 100 will tell us within plus or minus 10%. Even a sample of 25 will be within plus or minus 20% of the true figure 95% of the time.

If what we are interested in is something other than a proportion, such as the average weight, body mass, blood pressure, or cholesterol level of the population, the calculation of the sample size required to obtain a desired precision is a little more complicated, but the desired precision can be achieved with some sample in almost all cases. Any standard statistics text or qualified statistician can explain the process.

Promoting Response

Whether a sample is used or the entire population is to be surveyed, it is helpful to have as high a response rate among those surveyed as possible. For populations, anyone who fails to complete a health risk appraisal, for example, is simply an unknown for risk reduction purposes. For samples, nonrespondents introduce the same potential for self-selection bias as with a population.

To promote high levels of completion of surveys, there are a number of suggestions that have been used by surveyors over the years and found effective:

- Make the experience enjoyable if possible. Make it a social event for a sample in the workplace, at a senior center, or wherever members of the population or sample of interest congregate.
- Make it rewarding if possible. Sending a small incentive with the survey, such as a dollar bill, has significantly increased response rates; promising an incentive such as a free self-care guide or a chance in a lottery for a big prize such as a vacation trip can work equally well.
- Make responding as easy as possible. Include a self-addressed stamped return envelope and use simple language, large print for seniors, and check marks or fill-ins for scanning (include a pencil). If possible, offer multiple channels for returning the survey or even completing it (e.g., by phone or mail, drop points in the cafeteria, return mail).
- Describe exactly how the survey will be used and particularly how it will benefit the respondents and those they represent (e.g., indicate that not only their opinions/concerns, but those of people like them will be unreported or underrepresented if they do not respond, and describe the difference it will make if they do).
- Address confidentiality/privacy issues directly. If a sample survey is being taken, it should be anonymous, with no way individual respondents could be identified; if the entire population is being surveyed, describe how privacy and confidentiality will be protected.
- Indicate when and how they will hear about the results of the survey (e.g., indicate whether they will get a copy of individual results or see a report).
- Convince them that their input will make a difference, that the organization or individuals sponsoring the survey are committed to addressing what they learn through it and reporting what they do to address specific input.
- Prepare respondents beforehand with a phone call or letter telling them about the survey and why they should participate. At work, supervisors are likely to be the best at this; in the community, peer volunteers can provide the preparation.

- Supply prompts after the survey goes out—for example, phone calls, personal reminders, or postcards—to remind the forgetful.
- After the survey, thank all respondents, report results, and describe actions taken so that they will be enthusiastic about participating the next time.

INFORMATION SYSTEMS

For sponsors who have long-term relationships with and risk responsibility for a consumer population, extensive information systems are needed to maintain and offer effective access to the types of information described. Planning, monitoring, and evaluation efforts will be more effective and efficient if the requisite information is readily at hand. Implementation of reminder systems requires that information be available on who is to be prompted for what behavior and how best to reach such people.

For risk-sharing partners, special issues arise regarding which among them shall own and operate the information system and how access and use of the information will be controlled. However committed they are to the partnership, employers, health plans, physicians, and hospitals may wish to maintain their own information system so as to protect against the effects of dissolution of any particular partnership. Moreover, each may be concerned about a different population, since employees may choose from among multiple plans, plan members may come from multiple employers, and patients may come from multiple plans and employers.

A shared information system to which all interested parties have access (with controls on privacy and confidentiality) and which all such parties "own" as long as they have a legitimate interest in the data may be a way to avoid wasteful duplication and expense for information. Each of the risk-sharing partners will have to decide whether the benefits and risks of shared systems represent the best alternative.

HOW TO USE THE INFORMATION

Information on any of the seven measures in the set of effects can be used first to select specific consumers as targets for attention. This may involve selecting nonparticipants as opposed to current or past participants, for example, those especially receptive to change (stages of change), those most motivated and capable, or those at highest risk. Programs may be designed exclusively for one segment, or separate programs may be designed for different segments, where this will improve the effectiveness or efficiency of efforts.

Information may be used to set priorities across different consumer groups or behavior patterns, though an investment sufficient to cover multiple initiatives may be preferred to a toe-in-the-water, incremental approach. (See Chapter 10.) With baseline information, goals can be set for long-term outcomes and objectives for the first program year. The value of achieving each objective can become the basis for justifying budget allocations, while the value of overall goals serve in arguing for strategic resource allocations.

Specific tactics and levels of effort can be tailored to segments or adjusted to specific findings. Where motivation and capability relative to a desired behavior are high, for example, initiatives can be lower key, perhaps simple reminders or support. Where motivation is low, incentives, facilitators, and other higher level and higher cost tactics may be needed. (See Part III.) People already engaged in a desired behavior (action and maintenance stages) but somewhat irregular in adherence should need far less in the way of reminders, incentives, and support than do those for whom even initiating the behavior represents a drastic change and significant switching costs (precontemplation and contemplation stages).

Perhaps the best use of information is in customizing recommendations, plans, and tactics to individuals, wherever the information is specific to individuals and customization is cost-effective. A "continuous behavior improvement" plan for each targeted consumer can personalize the approach taken to the unique perceptions and values of the individual. It can also provide a personal improvement monitoring system that tracks not only changes in behavior but improvements in health status, quality of life, and other values of primary interest to the consumer.

Finally, the same information used in planning and implementing programs should provide the basis for evaluation of results.[16] The state of a given measure at baseline serves as the comparison for tracking progress and outcomes over time. As sponsors learn more about how measures early on in the set of effects are linked to changes in utilization, health care expenditures, and valuable side effects, they can get early indications of how successful specific initiatives promise to be.

INFORMATION EXAMPLES

There have been hundreds of studies, published and unpublished, offering information of value in early consideration of where to intervene in reforming health and demand behavior. We offer a sample here as indications of the extent of specific problems and their impact on health care and related expenses.

Dangerous Behaviors

- Smoking is frequently cited as one of the most serious health risks. It has been accused of being the true cause of 400,000 deaths a year.[17] One account claims it is responsible for $22 billion a year in medical costs alone.[18] Another gives it credit for $65 billion in total costs to society,[19] while yet another claims it is responsible for 18% of all preventable health care expenditures.[20]

  Among specific populations at risk, smoking has been linked to 19% higher costs for seniors in one study[21] or $312 in added costs per year in another.[22] At Control Data Corporation, smokers were found to have 25%

more hospital days than nonsmokers[23]; at Dupont, they added $960 to annual costs per smoker.[24] Claims costs per smoker have been reported as 18% higher than for nonsmokers,[25] as 31% higher[26] and 52% higher,[27] with hospitalization and absenteeism 50% higher[28] and lifetime health costs one-third higher despite shorter lifetimes.[29] Smoking has been reported to add $28.50 per month to health care costs.[30]

- Alcohol and drug abuse have also been frequently cited as significant risks, cited in one analysis as the highest-impact factors in $87 billion of preventable health expenditures,[31] with alcohol the cause of 100,000 deaths a year and drugs 20,000.[32] Alcohol was blamed for $13.5 billion in medical claims alone[33] and for $4.2 billion, 20% of all Medicaid claims.[34]

  Between 9% and 39% of seniors using ED care have been found to have alcohol problems.[35] Alcohol abuse has been found to increase claims costs by 83% and drug abuse by 80%,[36] with an additional $389 per year in added costs attributable to alcohol abuse in another study.[37] When alcohol *use* as opposed to *abuse* was analyzed, however, it was found to be associated with lower health care use in one case[38] and 10% lower claims costs in another.[39]

- Lack of exercise has been blamed for costs being 8% higher,[40] and as much as 82% higher than they need to be.[41] It accounted for $130 added expense per employee per year in one study[42] and has been estimated to be responsible for 11.4% of preventable expenditures.[43] Men who followed good exercise habits were noted to have annual insurance costs 44% lower than their sedentary counterparts; with women, the costs were 58% lower.[44]

- Poor diet and nutrition have been linked to 41% higher annual health care costs,[45] adding $32 per person per month in another study[46] and $1.4 billion per year in a third.[47] Poor coping with stress is blamed for 40% of all preventable costs,[48] increasing costs by 13% in one study[49] and 53% in another.[50] Failure to use seat belts was tied to $272 added costs per year in one study[51] and 35% higher costs in another.[52] "Bad driving," which can include speeding and driving after drinking, is blamed for 25,000 deaths a year[53] and 10% higher costs.[54] Unsafe sex is claimed to be responsible for 1.6% of preventable expense.[55] Poor compliance with medications has been linked to 125,000 deaths a year, $8 billion in wasted health care expense plus $1.5 billion in lost productivity and 20 million lost work days.[56]

Expensive Conditions

The following are considered to be expensive conditions:

- Hypertension has been cited as the cause for claims costs being from as little as 7% higher than average[57] to as much as 54%[58] and 68%.[59] It was blamed for adding $373 per person in annual employee costs[60] and 11.7% of all preventable expenditures.[61] Among seniors, where it is far more common, high blood pressure has been linked to costs being 11% higher,[62] adding $527 per year per person.[63]

- High cholesterol has been blamed for costs being 30% higher,[64] adding $34 per person to monthly premiums[65] and $370 per year.[66] Among seniors it has been linked to 6% higher costs[67] and annual per person costs $117 higher.[68] Apparently it makes less of a difference to seniors. In at least one study, high cholesterol levels made no difference in utilization or expenditures.[69]
- Obesity, or an unhealthy weight level, has been blamed for expenditures 87% higher in one case,[70] for hospital costs being 143% higher in another,[71] for 37% higher claims, and for 22% more physician visits in a third.[72] It has been held responsible for $14.7 billion, or 17%, of all preventable costs.[73]
- Adverse fetal outcomes add dramatically to maternity costs. In contrast to normal, full-term babies who generated costs per baby averaging $11,209 in their first 18 months of life, normal premature babies generated $36,134 and extremely premature babies $89,426.[74] End-of-life (the final 18 months) costs represent 20% of lifetime health care costs, while 30% of all Medicare expenditures occur in the last year of life.[75]
- Chronic conditions add greatly to health care utilization and expense, particularly when not well managed by consumers and providers. Estimates are that $92 billion a year is spent on diabetes, for example; patients with diabetes are five times more likely to be hospitalized; diabetics make up 4.5% of the population but account for 15% of all expenditures.[76] Asthma has been found to account for up to 40% of avoidable hospitalizations in a Medicaid population.[77]

HEALTH-RISK COMBINATIONS

While each of the risk behaviors and conditions add significantly to health care utilization and expenditures, they can be even more devastating in combination. The combination of seven factors (e.g., smoking, obesity, lack of exercise, high blood pressure, high cholesterol, drinking, and lack of seat-belt use) added over $1000 in costs per employee for one employer.[78] If consumers had three of five risk factors (i.e., smoking, obesity, high blood pressure, high cholesterol, diabetes), their annual costs were twice those for no-risk consumers; if they had all five, costs were eight times higher.[79]

Among seniors, those who both smoked and had high blood pressure had costs $1,249 higher than for those who had neither risk factor; if they also had high cholesterol, costs were $1,757 higher.[80] Seniors with the same combination in another study had costs $1,000 per year higher.[81] Estimates indicate that up to 60% of all hospital days are preventable.[82] Half of all expenditures,[83] with estimates ranging from $68[84] to $87[85] billion a year are related to health risk factors and therefore avertable.

For employers, the combined costs of health insurance and worker disability have been estimated to represent 11% of total payroll and climbing.[86] If total costs, including amounts paid by employees, costs of sick child care and elder care, Medicare surcharges, Occupational Safety and Health Administration (OSHA) compliance, state taxes for Medicaid and indigent care, reserves for future retiree medical costs, higher life insurance premiums, and disability management costs were included, the figure would be much higher.[87]

LIMITATIONS OF INFORMATION

There are limits to how useful such information will be in developing reform strategies and tactics. Problems of definition make comparisons problematic and can be misleading. Unless uniform criteria for *high* blood pressure and cholesterol; *poor* diet, stress coping, driving, and exercise habits; "obesity"; and alcohol "abuse" are used, it is impossible to rely on published studies for suggestions as to the right problems to attack or goals to set. For example, alcohol *use* seems to reduce costs, while *abuse* increases expense, so the definition of terms can make all the difference.

Risk factors are commonly expressed in terms of the additional costs or use each "causes" per individual having the factor. But the number of people with a given factor can vary widely across populations; what may be a huge problem in one workforce may be virtually undetectable in another.

The impact of a risk factor can be exaggerated if it tends to be found in conjunction with other factors. Smoking and drinking often are found together, for example, so how can we tell how much of a difference each one makes by itself? Lack of exercise and poor diet are linked to obesity; stress is associated with a number of risk factors, including high blood pressure, smoking, and drinking, so which is the "cause" we ought to attack?

One finding related to risk factors is particularly worrying or promising, depending on one's perspective: their negative synergy. Having more than one risk factor is associated with higher costs and utilization than the sum of the effects of each would suggest. In a study of seniors, for example, smoking added $312 to annual costs, high blood pressure $527, and high cholesterol $117. People who had high blood pressure and smoked had costs higher by $1,249, whereas the sum of both factor's effects is only $839. If the same people also had high cholesterol, the combined effect was an additional $1,757 in costs versus only $956 as the sum of all three.[88]

Such findings and others that consistently show the same pattern[89] indicate that consumers with multiple risk factors represent the greatest potential payoff, if they can be "converted." On the other hand, such people may be insensitive to health concerns or leave everything to fate, thereby making them the most difficult to convert.

One assumption to be avoided in interpreting the risk information presented is that by changing specific risk behaviors, the amount of added cost each represents can automatically be saved. People with histories of high-risk behaviors will not necessarily revert to the utilization and cost patterns of those with lifelong healthy habits. There may be residual damage that will reduce the potential savings, or poor health habits may be correlated with poor utilization patterns.

Similarly, changes in health status measures may not immediately be followed by reductions in utilization or costs. Effects may take some time to be felt or may have caused physiological changes that continue to put an individual at risk. Reduction in cholesterol may not create reduction in plaque already occluding coronary arteries; high blood pressure may have already damaged organs. The only way to learn how much specific changes in health risks will impact health care use and costs is to see what happens in each case.

Perhaps the most significant limitation to information is that it takes time and resources to obtain it. Sponsors should consider the benefit for the cost of information, just as they do for any investment. Relying on the published experience of others or on an intuitive understanding of the population of interest will almost always prove cheaper and enable earlier action than the collection and analysis of information about that population. It also entails significant risk, since populations tend to be different from each other and to change over time, making extrapolation from past experience dangerous.

REFERENCES

1. J. Kurtenbach and T. Warmoth, "Strategic Planning Futurists Need To Be Capitation-Specific and Epidemiological," *Health Care Strategic Management* 13, no. 9 (1995):8–11.
2. Scovill, M. "Using Data in the Community Health Assessment Process," *Inside Preventive Care* 1, no. 12 (1996):1, 4, 5.
3. "Use of Survey Data in a Corporatewide Health Promotion Program: The Metlife Experience," *Statistical Bulletin* 73, no. 2 (1992):28–35.
4. C. Kraft and P. Goodell, "Identifying the Health Conscious Consumer," *Journal of Health Care Marketing* 13, no. 3 (Fall 1993).
5. R. Strauss and D. Yen, "How an Expert Corporate Fitness Program Might Be Designed," *Health Care Supervisor* 10, no. 3 (1992):40–55.
6. "Shaping a Healthy Culture," *Workplace Health,* May 1993, 1, 5.
7. "Adopt 'Stage Model' of Behavior Change To Improve Results of DM Programs," *Healthcare Demand Management* 2, no. 3 (1996):41–43.
8. C. Petersen, "Employers, Providers Are Partners in Health," *Managed Healthcare,* January 1995, 36–38.

9. "Assessment Programs Counsel Patients To Make Lifestyle Improvements," *Inside Preventive Care* 3, no. 1 (1997):1–4.

10. Strauss and Yen, "How an Expert," 40–55.

11. "Survey by Kaiser Raises Eyebrows," *The Denver Post,* 21 December 1995, 1A, 12A.

12. S. Pak and L. Pol, "Segmenting the Senior Health Care Market," *Health Marketing Quarterly* 13, no. 4 (1996):63–77.

13. F. Wolinsky and T. Stump, "A Measurement Model of the Medical Outcomes Study 36-Item Short Form Health Survey in a Clinical Sample of Disadvantaged, Older, Black and White Men and Women," *Medical Care* 34, no. 6 (1996):537–548.

14. Scovill, "Using Data," 1, 4, 5.

15. M. Konner, *Medicine at the Crossroads: The Crisis in Health Care* (New York, NY: Pantheon, 1993), 18.

16. G. Leavenworth, "Making Data Work for You," *Business & Health* 14, no. 2 (1996):33–40.

17. M. McGinnis and W. Foege, "Actual Causes of Death in the United States," *JAMA* 270, no. 1 (1993):2207–2212.

18. "Medical Costs of Bad Habits and Violence Is $43 Billion: AMA," *Medical Interface,* June 1993, 21.

19. R. Whitmer, "Why We Should Foster Health Promotion," *Business & Health* 11, no. 13 (1993):68, 74.

20. J. Lautzinger, et al., "Projecting the Impact of Health Promotion on Medical Costs," *Business & Health* 11, no. 4 (1993):40–44.

21. H. Schauffler, et al., "Risk for Cardiovascular Disease in the Elderly and Associated Medicare Costs," *American Journal of Preventive Medicine* 9, no. 3 (1993):146–154.

22. M. Minkler, "Critical Issues and Trends," *American Journal of Health Promotion* 8, no. 6 (1994):403–412.

23. K. Sandrick, "Controlling High-Risk Behavior Can Lower Health Costs," *AHA News* 23, no. 15 (1987):5.

24. D. Fenn,"Healthy Workers Cost Less," *INC.,* May 1995, 137.

25. "The Wellness Wave," *Profiles in Hospital Marketing* 55 (1993):22–27.

26. "Data on 6,000 Workers Dramatize Financial Toll of High-Risk Behaviors," *Employee Health & Fitness* 17, no. 7 (1995):73–76.

27. L. Yen, et al., "Associations between Health-Risk Appraisal Scores and Employee Medical Claims Costs in a Manufacturing Company," *American Journal of Health Promotion* 7, no. 7 (1991):504–511.

28. "The Wellness Wave," 22–27.

29. J. Fries, et al. "Reducing Health Care Costs by Reducing the Need and Demand for Medical Services," *New England Journal of Medicine* 329, no. 5 (1993):321–325.

30. C. Petersen, "Unhealthy Practices Exposed," *Managed Healthcare* 5, no. 7 (1995):8, 10.

31. Lautzinger, et al., "Projecting the Impact of Health Promotion," 40–44.

32. McGinnis and Foege, "Actual Causes of Death," 2207–2212.

33. "Medical Costs of Bad Habits," 21.

34. K. Pallarito, "20% of Medicaid's Hospital-Care Costs Traced to Substance Abuse," *Modern Healthcare,* 19 July 1993, 8.

35. W. Adams, "Alcohol Abuse in Elderly Emergency Department Patients," *Journal of the American Geriatrics Society* 40 (1992):1236–1240.

36. Yen, et al., "Associations," 504–511.

37. Fenn, "Healthy Workers," 137.

38. Sandrick, "Controlling High-Risk Behavior," 5.

39. "Data on 6,000 Workers," 73–76.

40. "Data on 6,000 Workers," 73–76.

41. Yen, et al., "Associations," 504–511.

42. Fenn, "Healthy Workers," 137.

43. Lautzinger, et al., "Projecting the Impact of Health Promotion," 40–44.

44. Strauss and Yen, "How an Expert," 40–55.

45. "Data on 6,000 Workers," 73–76.

46. Peterson, "Unhealthy Practices Exposed," 8, 10.

47. Lautzinger, et al., "Projecting the Impact of Health Promotion," 40–44.

48. Lautzinger, et al., "Projecting the Impact of Health Promotion," 40–44.

49. "Data on 6,000 Workers," 73–76.

50. Yen, et al., "Associations," 504–511.

51. Fenn, "Healthy Workers," 137.

52. Yen, et al., "Associations," 504–511.

53. McGinnis and Foege, "Actual Causes of Death," 2207–2212.

54. "Data on 6,000 Workers," 73–76.

55. Lautzinger, et al., "Projecting the Impact of Health Promotion," 40–44.

56. S. Neibart, "An Innovative Drug Compliance Program," *Medical Interface,* May 1992, 29–30.

57. "Data on 6,000 Workers," 73–76.

58. Yen, et al., "Associations," 504–511.

59. Sandrick, "Controlling High-Risk Behavior," 5.

60. Fenn, "Healthy Workers," 137.

61. Lautzinger, et al., "Projecting the Impact of Health Promotion," 40–44.

62. Schauffler, et al., "Risk for Cardiovascular Disease," 146–154.

63. Minkler, "Critical Issues and Trends," 403–412.

64. Yen, et al., "Associations," 504–511.

65. Peterson, "Unhealthy Practices Exposed," 8, 10.

66. Fenn, "Healthy Workers," 137.

67. Schauffler, et al., "Risk for Cardiovascular Disease," 146–154.

68. Minkler, "Critical Issues and Trends," 403–412.

69. "Data on 6,000 Workers," 73–76.

70. "Data on 6,000 Workers," 73–76.

71. "Health Risks and Their Impact on Medical Costs," *Health Promotion Practitioner* 4, no. 12 (1995):3.

72. "Healthy Habits Are Cost Effective," *Business & Health* 13, no. 2 (1995):14.

73. Lautzinger, et al., "Projecting the Impact of Health Promotion," 40–44.

74. M. Cameron, "Prenatal Care: A Small Investment Begets a Big Return," *Business & Health* 11, no. 6 (1993):50–53.

75. R. Coile, "Healthy Communities: Reducing Need (and Costs) by Promoting Health," *Hospital Strategy Report* 6, no. 4 (1994):1–7.

76. E. Meszaros, "Diabetes Management: Management by Patients," *Managed Healthcare* 5, no. 6 (Supplement DSM):12–14.

77. *Colorado Medicaid's Primary Physician Initiative and Ambulatory Care Sensitive Hospitalizations* (Denver, CO: Colorado Health Data Commission, August 1995).

78. Fenn, "Healthy Workers," 137.

79. J. Fries, "Reducing Need and Demand," *Healthcare Forum Journal* 36, no. 6 (1993):18–23.

80. Minkler, "Critical Issues and Trends," 403–412.

81. Schauffler, et al., "Risk for Cardiovascular Disease," 146–154.

82. D. Axene and R. Doyle, *Analysis of Medically Unnecessary Inpatient Services* (Seattle, WA: Milliman & Robertson, Inc., 1994).

83. N. Bell, "From the Trenches: Strategies That Work," *Business & Health* 9, no. 5 (1991):19–25.

84. "Continuum of Care," *Hospitals & Health Networks,* 5 August 1993, 21–22.

85. Lautzinger, et al., "Projecting the Impact of Health Promotion," 40–44.

86. "Average of $3995 Spent on Health Care," *Business & Health* 13, no. 1 (1995):16.

87. L. Chapman, "Examining Benefit- and Program-Related Health Costs," *Employee Health & Fitness* 16, no. 8 (1994):110–112.

88. Minkler, "Critical Issues and Trends," 403–412.

89. Fries, "Reducing Need and Demand," 18–23.

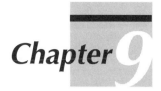
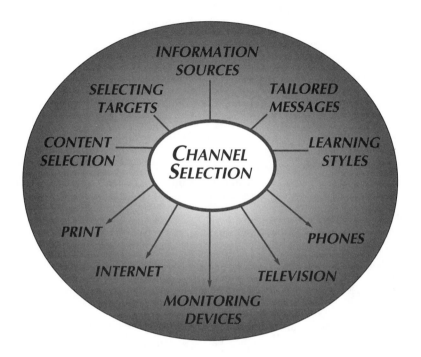

In Chapter 8 we described the information foundations for improving consumer health and demand, the types, sources, and uses of information in designing, monitoring, and evaluating specific interventions. In this chapter we will address the communications technologies available for implementing interventions, the use of communications to influence consumer behavior, and ways of getting information *to* consumers rather than about them.

Technology does not mean equipment and machines; it addresses whatever means or techniques are used to achieve a purpose. Handwriting and printing are communications technologies, as are speaking and signing. Body language, psychodrama, television and computers, phones, faxes and modems, radio, telegraph, landlines, and fiber-optics are all technologies. While modern and still-developing technologies open up all kinds of new possibilities for communicating information, they also greatly complicate the task of deciding which ones to use for specific interventions.

LEARNING STYLES

Information technologies can be categorized in a variety of ways. Based on the ways different people learn, we can describe technologies in terms of aural, visual, and experiential. Aural information is delivered through what people hear from radio to audiotapes and from the audio components of television, computers, and video. Visual information includes all forms of print media, graphics (including cartoons), videotapes, computers, and television. Experiential information comes through the experience of *doing* as opposed to seeing or hearing, and represents what hands-on skill training communicates.

For the average person, visual information is usually more powerful than aural, though the combination is more powerful, still. Experiential information is essential in conveying most skills, such as using blood glucose monitors or peak flow meters for diabetes and asthma, though many people may be able to learn their use through aural and visual information alone (e.g., instructions and diagrams) and gain self-efficacy through their own practice.

Discovering which learning styles are preferred by individuals can help make communications by providers to their patients more effective. For employers and health plans faced with communicating to diverse populations, a combination of approaches is likely to be more effective than relying on one only. Since each intervention is an opportunity to learn what works best with a specific population, choices of aural, visual, or experiential approaches should be tested to improve effectiveness over time.

COMMUNICATIONS TARGETING

There are also three categories of communications approaches based on how specific information will be to individual targeted consumers. At one extreme are mass communications technologies intended to reach all targeted consumers with the same information in the same form. This approach is usually the most efficient, since each piece of information is applied to everyone in the target population. It also tends to be the least effective, since it fails to deal with the diversity of people's interests, stage of readiness to change, language skills, and other factors affecting their receptivity to the information.

In the middle are technologies for communicating information that are differentiated for specific groups or segments of the population. These may be selected by sponsors based on their understanding of differential preferences within a population of interest, or past experience on what works best. They may also be selected by targeted consumers, choosing the technology which they prefer on an individual basis. Differentiated technologies tend to be considerably more effective than mass communications, though they are also significantly less efficient.

At the other extreme are customized information technologies, where each message is tailored to an individual as to content, approach (aural, visual, or experiential) or both. Customized content is most easily communicated on a one-to-one basis, but is often used in computer-generated health risk assessment reports and recommendations, for example (see Chapter 21). Customized information tends to be by far the most effective, though also the least efficient.

COMMUNICATIONS SOURCES

The communication of information can be carried out in four combinations of targets and sources. One combination is one-to-one counseling, where a physician, counselor, or educator conveys information to one consumer. This is easily the least efficient combination, though it is often the most effective. It easily permits customization and usually includes opportunities for consumers to ask questions, raise concerns, and assert their own values. As an interactive mode, it can add greatly to impact.

The one-to-many approach to communicating information is one we are all familiar with from school, political speeches, sales presentations, and similar experiences. The only limit to how many are in the audience is the level of interest in the population and the size of the physical or technological accommodations. This can be the most efficient technique for communicating, when large numbers of targets are addressed by one person.

The limitations of one-to-many communications tend to be in effectiveness. Because it involves a number of consumers in contact with the same source and communication, it is unlikely to best meet the expectations and needs of all. It cannot be customized. As numbers of targets increase, for efficiency, the opportunities for interaction diminish, so this mode is less effective for that reason as well.

The many-to-one mode is probably the least frequently used approach to communications, since it is the least efficient. It is most frequently used in peer influence situations, where family members, friends or coworkers communicate norms and expectations to individuals whose behavior is targeted for change. If the right set of peers is involved, this can be the most effective means of combining motivational, capability-enhancing, and prompting communications.

This approach can also be used in physician or other provider practices, where teams of nurses, educators, and other staff, for example, can share responsibilities for communications to and from individual patients. Each member of the team may perform those communications functions each is best suited for, thereby making communications more effective, though this is still likely to be inefficient compared to other approaches.

On the Internet, however, the technique of *pointcasting* makes it possible for sponsors to use a many-to-one approach to sending customized information to preselected individual Internet addresses. This technique was originally designed as a paid subscription service whereby consumers and businesses select from a menu of news clippings, stock updates, and similar timely information rather than wading through a wide variety of publications. Health care providers, health plans, and demand improvement vendors can use the same technology to send customized reminders and health or demand suggestions to selected consumers. (Consumers can use the same links to report condition self-monitoring measures such as weight and blood sugar, for example, as part of health risk reduction and disease management initiatives.)

The many-to-many mode of communication is also less common, though growing in popularity with the Internet. Support groups of consumers faced with the same treatment choices (decision improvement) or coping with the same condition (disease management) are examples of this mode. Members of the same class or training program can be encouraged to share insights and concerns (health improvement and disability management). In Internet applications, this type of communication is now possible on an international basis, with "chat groups" including providers as well as consumers.

Many-to-many communications links are almost always interactive dialogues rather than one-way "multilogues." Since interactive communications tend to be more effective, this mode combines the effectiveness strengths that come with many sources with the added power of interaction. It can be efficient as well where the number of interactions is great and volunteer support group participants are involved rather than paid professionals.

It is impossible to recommend one mode as always better than the rest, given the wide variety of consumers, behavior changes, situations, and economics potentially involved. On the other hand, experience with worksite health promotion suggests that one-to-one counseling is often necessary to achieve continuing lifestyle changes, and is more effective in any case. A review of 36 published cases found positive results in 80% of cases where individual counseling was included in the intervention versus 45% when absent[1] (Fig 9–1).

TACTICAL APPLICATIONS

Each of the communications technologies may be useful for any one of the tactics available to improve consumer behavior (Chapters 11 through 15). Com-

Figure 9–1 Communication Modes (Personal & Electronic)

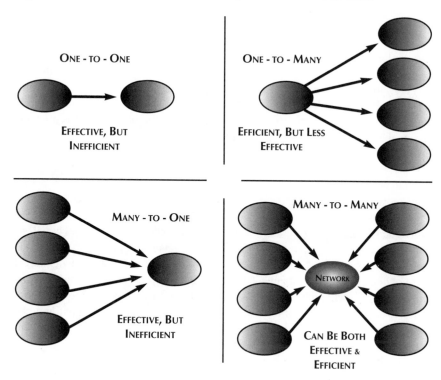

munications may remind consumers of behaviors they should adopt or avoid. A variety of information technologies may teach, train, persuade, or simply inform consumers to promote their self-efficacy. Social advocacy uses mass communications to reach large numbers of consumers.

For incentives and marketing tactics, communication is an essential, though insufficient component. In negotiation and empowerment, the tactic tends to dictate that one-to-one and interactive modes are used, though other modes are possible. The use of communications, in general, and of specific technologies will be greatly influenced by which tactics are chosen.

COMMUNICATIONS RELATIONSHIPS

One of the most critical dimensions of communications is the relationship between the sponsor and target of communication. In this context, the relationship applies strictly to the role each plays in the communications themselves. Each may play an active, passive, or interactive role.

In one category consumers are active and sponsors passive. This may be called "inbound" communications technologies, where sponsors make the information available and rely on consumers to actively access it. Common examples include phone access to medical information on audiotapes or computer access to prepared information on web sites via Internet.

A sponsor can use passive technologies to enable consumers to obtain information they are already interested in. Usually sponsors can track how many consumers call a phone center or "visit" an Internet web site, so they can determine which topics or information items are most popular. Normally they cannot track who is getting the information, however, and doing so may be seen as a violation of consumers' privacy.

Passive communications technologies rely on consumer interest and may not reach those that sponsors are most interested in reaching. Where sponsors do not even know who is accessing the information, they may find it impossible to judge whether it is having the desired effects. It is a useful and relatively inexpensive technique for making information available to interested consumers, nevertheless.

In another category sponsors are active and consumers passive. "Outbound" communications technologies include mass communications via all media, direct mail, phone, Internet, audiotapes and videotapes, books, pamphlets, and flyers, essentially any technique a sponsor chooses to use. In contrast to inbound, sponsors will know whom the information reaches (with some exceptions) and can control who gets what information. Because they control outbound communications, sponsors can determine when and where consumers get the information, as well as who, what, and how.

Outbound communications can be very ineffective, however, if consumers who get the information are not particularly interested or receptive, whereas inbound communications virtually guarantee only interested consumers get it. By carefully selecting who will be reached, and by using differentiated or customized approaches, sponsors can improve the effectiveness of outbound communications. Moreover, since they will know who received it, they can track the effects of specific communications far better than with inbound.

With increasing capabilities for customizing outbound communications, from direct mail to Internet, sponsors can tailor specific messages to the language spoken, learning style, interests, and stage of change and behavior change objective of individual consumers. Such messages can include requests for responses that can be made directly to automated systems that will record who responded how so as to enable constant monitoring and prompt evaluation of outbound communications efforts.

Interactive communications, where both sponsors and consumers actively participate, can enjoy the advantages of both inbound and outbound. If the communication is initiated by consumers, the sponsor can assume they are interested and probably receptive to the information. Through the interaction, the sponsor can learn who made the contact and thereby track effects and plan future contacts.

If the contact is initiated by the sponsor, and consumers indicate willingness to interact, the sponsor may assume at least some level of interest and receptivity among those who continue the interaction. Since the sponsor knows who was contacted, the information of who was versus was not interested can be recorded. Interaction makes it much easier to customize or at least differentiate the information that will be communicated to individual consumers, thereby promoting impact.

There are really two types of interactive communications: delayed and on-line, or real-time. If a consumer initiates a call and asks for information to be sent, or sends in a card or coupon requesting some information, that is interactive communication, though delayed. If a caller to a phone service leaves a voice-mail message, a user of e-mail leaves a message, or a visitor to a web site does so and the sponsor responds, that is interactive, though delayed. The sponsor can identify the caller for tracking and further communications, though the delay limits the exchange of information.

On-line interaction can occur in person, during visits to a provider, or interactions during a class. It can happen by phone, as when consumers call a phone triage or treatment counseling line, or sponsors call to carry out a health risk assessment or remind consumers of an upcoming screening or time for immunization. It can also take place via computer network if both parties are on line together. Since real-time interaction is one on one, it will tend to be inefficient, though it can also be highly effective.

The key to choosing which communications technologies to use is to start with the purpose, outcome objectives, and intended audiences rather than become enamored with a specific technology for its own sake. Each technique has its own strengths and limitations and is likely to do better for some purposes than for others. The numbers of consumers to be reached, their access via specific technologies, and their preferences for some over others should be as important as sponsor preferences.

Where relationships with consumers are important, and high response rates are desired, preference should probably lean toward customized and interactive techniques, geared to individual learning styles. Efficiency and effectiveness will often have to be traded off against each other. Just as a variety of messages delivered through multiple media tends to promote advertising effectiveness, so should sponsors think in terms of multiple technologies rather than rely on one.

NEW TECHNOLOGIES—EXAMPLES

It is always dangerous to discuss specific examples of new technologies in a book. Technology can change so fast as to make what we say obsolete or inaccurate by the time the book is published. Nevertheless, there are already many promising new examples of computer and interactive telecommunications technologies being applied to improving health and consumption behaviors that deserve mention.

The Internet

The number of people active on the Internet is relatively small but is doubling each year. According to one study, roughly 50% use the Internet for personal communications versus 35% business and 15% academic, and almost two thirds (64%) limit their contacts to under 50 sites, while 75% limit their visits to under 100.[2] The challenge to users is to find one's way through the enormous amounts of superficial and irrelevant information to find a few gems. The challenge to sponsors thinking of using this technology is to promote the right consumers having access to and competence in surfing the Internet.

Blue Cross/Blue Shield in Wisconsin offers a WorldWideWeb page as a general source of health information. Its HealthNet Connections program offers provider directories and treatment discussions as well as health and wellness information and advice.[3] Long Beach (California) Community Hospital and Medical Center allows patients to register on-line, reducing waiting time and promoting consumer preference when choosing a hospital. The neurology web site at Massachusetts General Hospital (Boston) enabled one patient to recognize his own symptoms as indicating a rare genetic disorder, download the information, and take it to a physician for confirmation of the diagnosis.[4]

The National Library of Medicine sponsors a Web page, "Internet Grateful Med," where visitors can find vast amounts of information on health and disease. Visitors have included a woman who found the probable cause of her series of miscarriages and was able to have a successful pregnancy and healthy baby as a result. Another recognized the symptoms of the rare "Harlequin Syndrome" and was able to get treatment.[5]

The CHESS program at the University of Wisconsin offered AIDS/HIV patients Internet access to faculty physicians and to each other and found that participants reported higher quality of life, understanding of their condition, and social support, as well as lower care consumption, with their hospital expenditures going down by $148 each, while costs for a control group without access went up $457, a difference of $605 apiece.[6]

The same CHESS program was made available to a group of 8 low-income women with breast cancer who had no computer skills. They described the system as easy to use and helpful, reported low-stress, and visited the system 886 times over 15 weeks, roughly 7 times a week each, averaging an hour at a time. While originally intended to give them access to physicians, it proved even more helpful by giving them access to each other as a computer support group.[7]

The Internet offers "chat rooms" that are perfect for support groups. Consumers who share a chronic condition, a choice of treatment, or life-threatening condition can log on and share problems, insights, and coping suggestions with each other, in addition to using the Net to learn more about their condition.[8] Consumers can use chat rooms to obtain information on treatments and specialists they might never otherwise hear about, though there is no "quality control" over the information and advice they might get.[9]

Group Health of Puget Sound (Seattle, Washington) offers Internet users opportunities to sign up for programs such as its Women's Forum, a Hot Topics home page information source, tracking how many visits it gets and what information gets downloaded to monitor its members' interests. Those who sign up for programs can be targeted for additional mailings or other contacts.[10]

The Internet can be used to gather information from consumers, as well. It is a growing basis for market research, where surveys can be conducted virtually overnight, if necessary, and computer conferences used like focus groups.[11] Consumers can use Internet links to do their own research through on-line research services, walk through decision maps to select from alternative treatments, and obtain information on plans and providers.[12]

There is great interest among consumers in getting health information. One analyst projected that the proportion of consumers reporting themselves as "concerned about their health" would increase to 50%, rising from only 5% in the 1960s, with a similar growth in the numbers actively doing something about their health. Interest among Internet users was already at 85%, with a surprisingly high interest level among seniors, who see the Internet as a new socializing opportunity.[13]

The issue of quality control will have to be addressed and resolved in order for the Internet to achieve its potential in improving the quality as well as quantity of information available to consumers. The wildest of rumors and idiosyncratic and anecdotal information are available on the Internet alongside rigorously tested and verified research. Unfortunately, there is little help for consumers trying to determine which is which.

The efforts underway by the Health Information Technology Institute, established by Mitretek systems (McLean, Virginia), should help. It has the involvement of organizations such as the American Medical and Nurses Associations and other health and consumer organizations in addressing the quality issue. While at this writing its efforts are just beginning, it appears to be at least a step in the right direction.

Other Computer Technologies

For consumers not on the Internet, there are still a variety of ways that computer technology can be used to improve their health and utilization behavior. Computerized health risk assessments, for example, can be offered in physician offices, worksites, or public health fairs to give instantaneous results.[14] Software programs can be purchased to give consumers ready access to information on CD-ROM.[15]

AIDS patients can be given or loaned home health workstations to connect with provider information systems.[16] Patients with a variety of conditions can report specific symptoms and biomarker tracking measures via computer to providers.[17] Packaged information can help consumers choose health plans and providers, make better decisions about their own health, manage their own chronic conditions, and remind themselves of, for example, scheduled screenings and physicians' appointments.[18]

Consumers do not even need their own computers to take advantage of the technology. They may use computers in their physician's office, worksite, or health plan clinic. Patients might use a smart card, for example, to record participation in a wellness/fitness program, enabling them to get an update on progress to date.[19] Hospitals have set up computer information access in mall kiosks, where registered nurse (RN) counselors, libraries of books and videos, and classrooms can supplement the new technologies.[20]

Workers can use a computer-based expert system provided by their employer to design a customized exercise program for themselves.[21] One program offers homeless drug addicts and street people a voice-mail system they can access by pay phone to send and receive messages. The sponsor uses it to remind them of screening checks and clinic appointments, while the consumers gain a way of reaching and being reached by friends.[22]

Another example of new computer technology at work where users do not need a computer is PregNet. Low-risk pregnant women call in via touch-tone phone, answering prerecorded questions by pressing the right buttons. The computer generates a customized letter for each caller based on the pattern of answers. It was found that not only were women perfectly comfortable interacting with a computer, they often gave more complete and honest information than was characteristic of personal interactions. The system promoted tighter monitoring of the women's conditions via weekly phone contacts, and reduced the average number of prenatal physician visits from 14 to 9 per low-risk pregnancy.[23]

Interactive TV

Beyond today's computer and modem links is the emerging potential for combined TV-computer technologies. Already there are cable-TV networks, such as America's Health Network, offering health information and home-shopping services for health-related products. Disney is working with Eli Lilly in Celebration City, Florida, to fiberoptically wire every home into a broadband digital network combining voice, video, and data capabilities. The system will offer e-mail, bulletin boards, software, a video library, videoconferencing, consumer access to their own computerized medical records, wellness/prevention reminders, and health promotion advice.[24]

Eventually computerized communications systems such as Disney and Eli Lilly are developing can link health plans, physicians, hospitals, pharmacists, and community health organizations to promote and track improvements in both the provision of services and their consumption, in addition to better health for the community. Pharmacists, for example, can use such systems to monitor patient compliance, identify the best generic equivalents for prescribed drugs, and check on any contraindications among prescriptions.[25]

AT&T is working on a comprehensive, interactive communications network that will include Health & Fitness Services linked to Mayo Clinic; First Aid and self-care information; an encyclopedia of health information; advice relevant to specific life stages and disease conditions; and fitness/exercise and medical consumerism information—all in the home.[26]

Personal health information systems are seen as the wave of the future.[27] Computer-TV systems can offer therapeutic learning programs, interactive information searches, self-help electronic communities, and similar capabilities that dramatically augment the potential of what we have accomplished thus far with our limited technologies.[28] Consumers will be able to use the screens of their TV to order up information, while providers will be able to follow up such information requests with personalized messages, standard and customized written, audio, and video materials.[29]

Home testing, measuring, and reporting of acute and chronic conditions are already available for inclusion in integrated health information networks. Comprehensive, interactive, seamlessly connected, user-friendly systems for shared decision making and consumer health empowerment are at least possible.[30] Whether the possibilities will be realized and have the promised benefits is yet to be seen.

CAVEATS

None of these new technologies is the panacea for communications problems and challenges. Quality control over the information and advice available on the Internet is only slowly emerging. Much of the information may come from quacks interested in promoting their own dubious services. Many sources may be misguided zealots who have the perfect answer that is simple, understandable, easily performable by the consumer, but wrong and potentially dangerous.[31]

Providers are quite concerned over the kinds of information that consumers might get via new technologies, and the effect that such information might have on the patient-physician relationship. Consumers are likely to find conflicting and confusing advice on the Internet, or may simply encounter too much information to handle.[32]

Perhaps the greatest challenge with respect to these new technologies is getting them to the people who can most benefit from them. Will market forces alone be sufficient to promote and finance the construction of a national information infrastructure adequate to reach every citizen? Will everyone be able to learn how to access and use the new technologies effectively and efficiently? Can we control or at least help consumers choose quality information and advice? Who will pay for all this?[33]

There is probably enough potential benefit to payers, health plans, and providers at risk to justify the investment in a universal health information infrastructure. The question is, will enough sponsors have confidence in the potential and be willing to work together to realize it? Will enough sponsors be willing and able to accept short-term financial and political risks to engage in the necessary long-term investment?

REFERENCES

1. C. Heaney and R. Goetzel, "A Review of Health-Related Outcomes of Multicomponent Worksite Health Promotion Programs," *American Journal of Health Promotion* 11, no. 4 (1997):290–308.

2. R.P. Heath, "Miles of Files," *Marketing Tools,* June 1996, 24–28.

3. "Payer Finds New Way To Reach Its Customers," *Health Data Management* 4, no. 3 (1996):68.

4. M.C. Jaklevic, "Internet Technology Moves to Patient-Care Front Lines," *Modern Healthcare,* 11 March 1996, 47–50.

5. A. Landers, "Medical Help on the Internet," *The Denver Post,* 9 July 1996, 4E.

6. D. Gustafson, et al., "The Use and Impact of a Computer-Based Support System for People Living with AIDS and HIV Infection," in *JAMIA Symposium Supplement* (American Medical Information Association, 1994) (unpaginated).

7. F. McTavish, et al., "CHESS: An Interactive Computer System for Women with Breast Cancer Piloted with an Under-Served Population," *JAMIA* 1994, 599–603.

8. L. Brakeman, "Get Interactive," *Managed Healthcare* 6, no. 5 (1996):79, 80.

9. D. Levy and M. Snyder, "In the Wired World, A Trove of Health Data," *USA Today,* 6 March 1996, D1, D2.

10. C.D. Shepherd and D. Fell, "Marketing on the Internet," *Journal of Health Care Marketing* 15, no. 4 (Winter 1995):12–15.

11. R. Iyer, "The Internet: A New Opportunity for Marketing Research Firms," *Quirk's Marketing Research Review* 10, no. 5 (1996):22, 30.

12. D. Weiss, "Using Information Technology To Improve Health Care Delivery," in *Demand Management ® for Health Care* (Chicago, IL: Strategic Research Institute, 1996) (unpaginated).

13. J. Flower, "On the Horizon: The Market Impact of Healthcare Technology," *Alliance for Healthcare Strategy & Marketing Annual Meeting,* New Orleans, LA, March 4, 1996.

14. G. Montrose, "Demand Management May Help Stem Costs," *Health Management Technology* February 1995.

15. M. Chamberlain, "Health Communication: Making the Most of the New Media Technologies— An International Overview," *Journal of Health Communication* 1, no. 1 (1996):43–50.

16. T. Ferguson, "Consumer Health Informatics," *Healthcare Forum Journal* 38, no. 1 (1995):28–32.

17. K. Kline, "Tapping into Home and Office PCs: Biomarker Tracking with Integrated Education Material," in *Multimedia Patient Education* (Phoenix, AZ: Institute for International Research, December 1, 2, 1994) (unpaginated).

18. C. Gieber, "The Future of Healthcare on the Internet," *Alliance for Healthcare Strategy & Marketing Annual Meeting,* New Orleans, LA, March 5, 1996, 63–71.

19. R. Cross and J. Smith, "The New Value Equation," *Marketing Tools,* June 1996, 20–23.

20. M.C. Jaklevic, "Hospitals Expand via Mall Centers," *Modern Healthcare,* 3 June 1996, 50, 51.

21. J. Evans, "Artificial Intelligence: The Latest in Wellness Technology," *The Alliance Report,* March/April 1996, 3, 7.

22. Ferguson, "Consumer Health Informatics," 28–32.

23. "Information Technology Helps Slash Maternity Costs," *Healthcare Demand Management* 1, no. 3 (1995):33–37.

24. "Disney's Latest Experiment: High-Tech Health Care," *Health Data Management* 4, no. 3 (1996): 8–10.

25. R. DuBosar, "Moving the Retail Medication Market—Electronically," *Managed Healthcare* 6, no. 5 (1996):S32–35.

26. Gieber, "The Future," 63–71.

27. M. McDonald and H. Blum, *Health in the Information Age* (Cambridge, MA: Environmental Science & Policy Institute, Harvard University, 1992).

28. Ferguson, "Consumer Health Informatics," 28–32.

29. "The Cutting Edge of Marketing Information," *Marketing Tools,* June 1996, 31–38.

30. L. Harris, "Differences That Make a Difference," in *Health and the New Media,* ed. L. Harris (Mahwah, NJ: Lawrence Erlbaum, 1995), 3–18.

31. P. Noonan, "Internet's Health Pipeline Not Immune to Quackery," *The Denver Post,* 11 March 1996, 1E, 4E.

32. Levy and Snyder, "In the Wired World," D1, D2.

33. F.D. Fisher, "But Will the New Health Media Be Forthcoming?" in *Health and the New Media,* ed. L. Harris (Mahwah, NJ: Lawrence Erlbaum, 1995), 209–227.

Chapter 10

STRATEGIC ISSUES

✓ *SPONSORSHIP*
✓ *OBJECTIVES*
✓ *TARGETS*
✓ *RESOURCES*
✓ *ROLES*

MEASURES FOR:

✗ *MONITORING*
✗ *EVALUATION*
✗ *GOAL SETTING*

MAKING DECISIONS

DEVELOPING A STRATEGIC FOUNDATION

WHAT IS A STRATEGY?

Traditionally strategy has addressed the big picture, "the war," in military terms, while tactics focus on the little picture, "the battle." In practice, strategy looks farther into the future and wider in space, considering a larger system of causes and effects, while tactics focus on the here and now and on specific, often single causes and effects. The distinction tends to be one of degree, rather than kind; strategy involves the bigger issues and addresses the bigger concerns.

Developing a strategy means making a series of decisions in a way that recognizes their interactions and interdependence. The set of strategic decisions once made will then guide specific tactical choices. In theory, strategy is *deliberate*, chosen at the beginning of a planning effort to guide later tactical decisions. As often as not, however, strategy is *emergent* (i.e., it is put together as a way of making sense out of tactical decisions already made and actions already taken). There seems to be no clear, scientific evidence that deliberate strategy works any better than emergent; either approach can work. The main value in having a strategy is to promote the recognition and consideration of the interrelatedness of decisions and actions.

Whether a deliberate or emergent approach to strategy is chosen, there are a number of decisions that will affect how specific health and demand improvement initiatives are designed and executed. When they are made to guide tactical choices, they serve a strategic purpose, whether made at the beginning or in the middle of an overall effort. It is these decisions and how to make them that will be discussed as "strategy" in this chapter. The tactics available to execute a strategy will be discussed in Part III.

STRATEGIC DECISIONS

The primary decisions that together make up a strategy for improving consumer demand are:

1. Should you engage in health and demand improvement?
2. Which and how many outcomes will be pursued?
3. Which consumers and types of behavior will be addressed?
4. Who will participate and play what roles in the overall effort?
5. What resources will be devoted to the effort?

We recommend that these decisions be addressed in the order presented, though circumstances may sometimes dictate otherwise. Clearly a decision is needed first about whether or not to engage in demand improvement, since a "no" answer makes the rest of the decisions moot. However, to make the first decision, sponsors must examine the prospects for improving outcomes that matter, so the first decision requires consideration of the second.

Once desired outcomes have been determined, the necessity of identifying the consumers and behaviors that most affect those outcomes logically follows. It is possible that the outcomes selected will immediately suggest partners who should be involved in the strategy and that what we have listed as step 4 will come before step 3. If so, the recommended order may be reversed for these two steps. We strongly recommend, however, that decisions on resources be left for last, rather than made earlier, where they will limit strategic thinking. (Note: Because strategic decisions are, by definition, highly interconnected and interdependent, each decision made should be considered a "draft" decision, recorded in pencil rather than etched in stone, ready for alteration if a subsequent decision so dictates.)

SHOULD A GIVEN SPONSOR DO IT?

While we feel that we have presented compelling arguments for engaging in demand improvement, generally the decision for specific payer and provider organizations is by no means automatic. For payers it is usually a fairly simple matter of determining whether they will gain enough in saved expenditures or value-adding performance effects and soon enough, to justify the investment. For providers more complex considerations are involved.

Payers

Both employers and health plans are directly at risk for the costs of health care and for other performance measures amenable to demand improvement interventions. They directly benefit from health care and workers' compensation/disability expenditure savings, unless they have passed on the risk to others, and even where the risk is passed on, they stand to benefit in subsequent years' price negotiations if they have succeeded in reducing expenditures. In addition to health care savings, they stand to gain from added-value effects such as employee or member retention and loyalty. Employers gain as well if productivity, turnover, absenteeism, and financial performance improve.

Changes in the health care environment may affect payers' motivation to engage in demand improvement. If health insurance reform results in the enactment of a community rating requirement, in contrast to the experience rating that now prevails, employers will lose many of the financial benefits they gain from their own initiatives. Similarly where employer coalitions have fostered wide health plan choices among their employees, similar to the 15 to 20 options available to employees in Minnesota,[1] any health and demand improvements they achieve among their own employees will disappear into the experience of the many plans that cover their employees, and only health plans and providers at risk will directly benefit.

Health plans must consider whether they will both succeed in improving demand and enjoy the fruits of their success. If governments and employers insist on following up a plan's expenditure savings by demanding corresponding premium reductions, plans may lose enthusiasm for continuing to work toward such savings. On the other hand, if plans are the only ones who benefit from demand improvement savings, why should governments, employers, and providers, even consumers have any enthusiasm for getting involved?

The most important strategic questions for payers are whether there are both significant values in and probability of succeeding. Are current employee or member health behavior patterns, health status measures, utilization patterns, and expenditure levels sufficiently worse than normal or "best practice" to suggest plenty of room for improvement, or are they already so good that little improvement seems possible? Are value-adding parameters such as productivity, absenteeism, retention, and market share as good as they're likely to get or below par? If less than perfect, can they be more effectively and efficiently enhanced through demand improvement initiatives than via some other approach?

Turnover of employees and members is also likely to be a major factor in determining the potential for demand improvement success. If turnover is extremely high, consumers may not remain long enough in a relationship to the sponsor to be amenable to behavior changes, and the consequences of such changes may not occur soon enough to have any real value to the sponsor.

Each potential sponsor will have to analyze its own unique situation to make the right strategic decision regarding the potential for and the probability and value of demand improvement success. Fortunately the same data needed to make that decision will provide essential insights into determining desired outcomes, identifying targets, and formulating behavior change goals for specific efforts.

Providers

For physicians, hospitals, and other providers, the question requires looking at a number of additional considerations and weighing possibly conflicting values. Mission commitments may drive providers to seek health status and demand improvements even where those will *not* produce positive financial returns. Not-for-profit providers may be motivated by a desire to protect their tax exempt status and aim for health status or utilization improvements that benefit the larger community though they produce a financial loss to the providers.

Turnover is a consideration for providers, as it is for payers. If patients have little loyalty to specific providers, changes in patient health status or demand may impact providers generally but not because some engage in conscious improvement initiatives while others do not. Since improving patients' health is a strong driver of loyalty to providers, demand improvement may be chosen as a way of improving loyalty, thereby changing the turnover situation. (The same possibility exists for payers.)

The most complicating consideration, however, is the conflicting impact of demand improvement on provider performance under capitation versus fee-for-service financing. Where the net effect of improved health status and demand in a targeted consumer population is reduced utilization of a provider's own services and most of the provider's revenue is derived from FFS arrangements, what financial sense does it make to deliberately *reduce* its volume and revenue where that is the expected result of demand improvement?

If capitation financing is the rule and providers share the same risk as employers and health plans, the issues are similar, but where FFS financing is dominant or significant, the net effects on providers will vary. There is no cut-off point in the mix of capitation and FFS population served, volume, or revenue where it will automatically be more financially advantageous to invest in demand improvement versus not. Each situation must be judged on its own, based on the full set of utilization and revenue effects expected, together with the impact on margin given cost reductions achievable with reduced volume.

Of course, providers operating under wholly or predominantly FFS payment systems may choose only those demand improvement initiatives that will improve their FFS performance. Hospitals may seek to enhance their market share, volume, and revenue by using health improvement or physician referral programs to enhance their reputations and increase consumer preference for their facility. Physicians may add to volume and revenue by increasing use of their early detection services, such as mammography.

Providers may save money by reducing avoidable or inappropriate demand. Hospitals may avoid capital investments and added operational expense by cutting back on inappropriate use of their overcrowded emergency departments, or unnecessary procedures in their overutilized surgery suites. Physicians may improve their financial performance by reducing avoidable and inappropriate use of poorly paid services or by poorly paying populations.

There are likely to be many opportunities for health and demand improvement initiatives that would improve consumer demand while enhancing provider performance under FFS financing. Providers need to consider the combination of effects of specific initiatives—on consumer health status, use of services, quality of life, patient loyalty, and retention—in comparison to specific changes in utilization of the provider's services, resulting revenue, and financial performance.

The provider decision may be further complicated by long-term marketing strategy. It may make no financial sense *now* to engage in demand improvement because the net financial effects would be negative. But might the provider gain significant marketing advantage by becoming and being known for delivering greater value to payers? Would payers shift enough contracts and covered lives to a provider known for high *demand* quality to make up for the loss in volume? Might they shift more contracts and covered lives to capitation because of provider success in improving demand, and thereby change the net financial effects of demand improvement? Or would payers simply pocket the added profit they gain from provider demand improvement success?

Here, too, the decision must be made on a case-by-case basis, with the added challenge of forecasting what market effects are likely. How will payers respond, and how will competitors react once they get wind of what's happening? Will the first provider who gambles on becoming a demand improvement champion win a permanent market advantage or merely enjoy a brief surge? How great a difference will it make, for how long? Forecasting the future in health care is anything but easy, and forecasting how both payers and competing providers will react to demand improvement initiatives and success is likely to be among the most difficult of tasks.

It is essential that providers at least consider the strategic marketing effects of a yes or no decision regarding demand improvement. Undoubtedly their competitors are at least thinking about the same decisions, and payers are thinking about the possibility of partnering with providers committed to or successful in demand improvement.

Complicating the decision for any potential sponsor is the impact of other sponsors' decisions. If most or major employer clients are actively engaged in demand improvement initiatives, should the health plan jump in as well? If plans and employers are heavily invested, does it make sense for providers to become involved? What will be the reactions of potential partners if any one employer, health plan, or provider makes a unilateral decision (Exhibit 10–1)?

Exhibit 10–1 Strategic Decisions: Should You Do It?

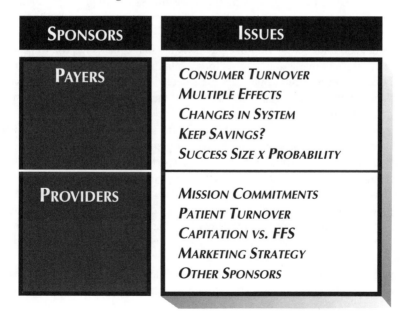

SPONSORS	ISSUES
PAYERS	CONSUMER TURNOVER MULTIPLE EFFECTS CHANGES IN SYSTEM KEEP SAVINGS? SUCCESS SIZE x PROBABILITY
PROVIDERS	MISSION COMMITMENTS PATIENT TURNOVER CAPITATION vs. FFS MARKETING STRATEGY OTHER SPONSORS

WHAT OUTCOMES SHOULD BE PURSUED?

Sponsors may look at any one or a combination of the four demand improvement domains for the best opportunities in improving health or decisions and managing disease or disability. Each may be selected for the particular outcomes it promises. Health improvement outcomes could include reductions in or earlier detection of morbidity, better quality of life, and lower expenditures for life-threatening conditions, for example. Decision improvement outcomes could include shifts in plan enrollment, provider choices, use of emergency services, high-cost procedures, or end-of-life care. Disease management outcomes might be reductions in acute episodes or use of emergency services. Disability management outcomes could be reduced injuries, lower expenditures, or earlier return to work.

Sponsors should recognize the interdependence of most such outcomes. Reducing morbidity should automatically reduce the use of acute and chronic care services, so where health and demand improvement outcomes are to be separately sought, sponsors need to estimate the overlap. For example, if improved health would reduce demand by 20% and better decisions would reduce it by 20%, the combined effect is likely to be less than the total of the two (e.g., if the efforts overlap completely, the net effect would be a 36% reduction rather than 40%, 80% × 80% = 64%, or the original demand would remain).

On the other hand, specific outcomes may have synergistic impact on other factors of interest. Improvements in employee fitness can improve productivity and reduce accidental injuries in addition to lowering conventional health insurance risks. Improvements in demand patterns can save health plan enrollees out-of-pocket costs and thereby improve their satisfaction, enhancing HEDIS performance ratings and marketing success for the plan as well as retention of current members. Where particular outcomes are selected to start the strategic thinking and planning process, sponsors should consider the applicable systems dynamics applying to the relationships among them.

The set of effects discussed in Chapter 5 offers seven categories of outcome parameters that might be chosen as the basis for strategic interventions. We recommend that improvements in the first three (participation, mind-state, and behavior) be treated as means to an end rather than ends in themselves. None of the three has clear, intrinsic value; each is valuable when and because it leads to a subsequent, valuable outcome. Sponsors would find it impossible to use improvements in any of these outcome measures as a basis for deciding how much to invest in demand improvement *except by estimating the impact of such improvements on subsequent parameters in the set.*

The first three effects are useful in planning specific tactical initiatives, particularly measures of consumer behavior, as will be discussed in decision 3, as well as in tactical planning in Chapter 16. They are also helpful in monitoring the early impact of such initiatives, but we feel the later measures in the set are better suited as strategic outcome measures. If a behavior change is chosen as the focus for strategy, for example, that choice can compromise the selection of tactics. (See Chapter 17.)

The last two measures in the set (health expenditures and value-added effects) might be selected as outcome parameters for strategic purposes. We see potential risk as well as value in such a choice, however. Sponsors who clearly and solely aim to reduce health care expenditures have already experienced the backlash from many of the supply-focused strategies they chose with that in mind. An exclusive focus on reducing expenditures as the aim of demand improvement strategies is equally risky.

Health plans that aim solely to reduce expenditures and thereby gain significant benefit in terms of shareholder value, profits, and executive salaries are likely to fare no better in public acceptance, media attention, and legislative assaults than they have in the past. Moreover, they are likely to find their risk-sharing partners unreceptive to the idea of helping them, particularly if there is no sharing of the resulting savings.

The greatest risk, however, is likely to be that sponsors concerned only with reducing expenditures will end up choosing demand improvement initiatives that turn out to have negative impact on equally valuable parameters, such as consumer health, quality of demand, customer satisfaction, and loyalty. It is far better to at least include, if not focus on, other outcomes of value.

Many of the value-added effects may seem suitable for strategic focus. Sponsors who start their strategic thinking with the intention of improving employee, member, or patient quality of life can hardly be criticized for such a focus. On the other hand, they may find that the most appropriate means to that end have nothing to do with and no impact on health care utilization, expenditures, or sponsor performance. They may produce value to consumers but none to themselves. While this is hardly reprehensible, it is likely to be impractical for all but the most altruistic of sponsors.

Strategy consciously, even exclusively, aimed at increasing employee, health plan member, or patient retention is unlikely to arouse the negative responses that a similar focus on reducing health expenditures would have. On the other hand, it is also unlikely to arouse enthusiasm among potential partners or among consumers, since only the sponsor benefits. Moreover, loyalty and retention will usually be enhanced because of improvements in consumer health and/or demand, so why not aim at these outcomes in the first place?

A similar caution applies to employers. Improvements in value-added parameters such as absenteeism, productivity, and financial performance may be the ultimately desired outcomes for employers. If these are the primary or exclusive focus for strategy, however, will other risk-sharing or community partners want to help? Will consumers (i.e., employees) commit themselves to achieving improvements that will benefit only the employer? Where such value-added gains for the employer are the direct result of improved employee health status and use of services, why not aim for these in the first place?

Sponsors can, of course, gain added value, themselves, by aiming for value-added effects of other risk-sharing partners. If a health plan aims for (and achieves) improved productivity, morale, and retention among the employees of its clients, it may gain increased client satisfaction and loyalty. The same applies to providers who achieve improved member retention among the plans with which it contracts. Following outcomes through systems dynamics to their full set of effects should help sponsors decide which to choose as the deliberate, public goals for their strategy.

In general, we believe that changes in health care expenditures and value-added measures are best reserved for *evaluation* of strategic efforts and specific initiatives. First, they are likely to be measurable much later than the other parameters in the set of effects. Second, choosing them as the explicit and exclusive purpose for demand improvement may create "political" problems among consumers targeted for attention and/or among other risk-sharing partners or the public, media, or government (see Exhibit 10–2).

The best outcomes to use as a focus for strategic efforts are those that have the best *total* effects—on the effectiveness and efficiency of planning and the actions that emerge from it and on public, risk-sharing partner, and consumer responses to the strategy itself and its resulting actions. We believe the types of outcomes best for strategic use according to these criteria are health status and use of services, with *quality* rather than *quantity* of utilization paramount.

By aiming first and foremost at improving consumer health status and the quality of consumer demand for health services, sponsors have the kind of outcomes that should anger no one and more probably elicit enthusiastic cooperation and support from a variety of potential partners, including consumers themselves. Moreover sponsors can confidently anticipate that health and demand improvement outcomes, once achieved, will end up producing significant expenditure savings and value-adding performance effects, without the negative fallout from choosing such outcomes as the explicit focus for strategy.

This is not to say that the outcomes stated as the primary focus for strategy should be "faked" for purposes of misleading the public, consumers, or potential partners in specific efforts. It is unlikely that the real motivation behind initiatives can be hidden for long, and "leaks" or even suspicions about the true purposes of effort, where they are different from publicly claimed reasons, will undermine the trust that is essential to long-term success in improving demand and in relationships with strategic partners.

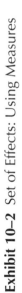

Exhibit 10–2 Set of Effects: Using Measures

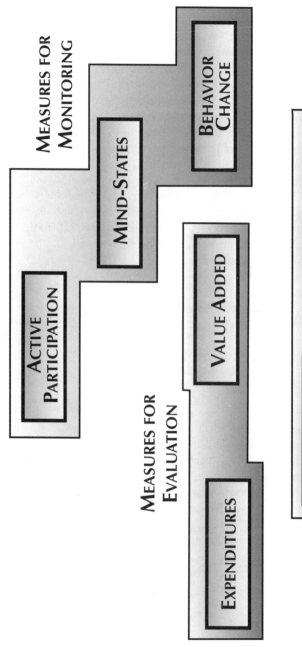

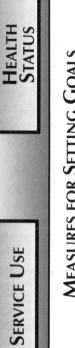

How Many Outcomes?

Which outcomes (i.e., measures) are selected for strategic focus will have great impact on subsequent decisions and on many other factors as well. A second critical choice in formulating the desired outcomes for specific efforts is how many to go after. The history of health and demand improvement initiatives thus far indicates that most sponsors start small, with only one outcome and one program. In most cases this is essential to gaining confidence in the idea and in the sponsor's, potential partners', or vendors' ability to deliver results. With success in initial ventures, sponsor confidence grows and additional efforts are undertaken.

There is nothing wrong with such an incremental, "toe-in-the-water" approach. Selecting the most promising outcomes, then planning and implementing efforts that pay off soon and significantly represents a sound, pragmatic approach. With significant experience in health and demand improvement behind us, however, there is ample reason to consider taking on multiple aims, with the intention of enjoying more and greater outcomes earlier than can be achieved through an incremental approach. (More on this subject under the Resources discussion.)

While most sponsors have begun by selecting a single or a few outcomes as goals for efforts, some more experienced organizations have broadened their scopes. Health Partners (Minnesota), for example, aimed for a variety of outcomes related primarily to health status, though with obvious demand implications: reduce heart disease events by 25%; increase proportion of children immunized from 75% to 95%; reduce infant/maternity complications by 30%; and increase the number of high-risk members screened for diabetes.[2]

Impact of Outcomes Selection

A frequently debated issue in selecting a strategic focus relates to consumer health versus demand. Should payers and providers look at promoting health and reducing morbidity, for example, expecting health improvements to produce reductions in demand and expenditures? Or should they wait till consumers initiate contact with the health care system before trying to modify their behavior, aiming to replace a significant portion of demand through self-care or reform it through improving the quality of demand?

It has been noted that differences in morbidity account for a far smaller portion (under 15%) of explained variations in health service use than do consumer demand attitudes—perceptions of need (roughly 40%) and preferences for treatment (roughly 40%)—so why focus on morbidity?[3] Unfortunately, the fact that *differences* in morbidity explain so small a portion of *variations* in health care use does *not* indicate that morbidity is a minor factor in generating consumption of services in the first place. It tells us merely that other factors have more to do with the differences in use patterns across populations.[4]

Sponsors are usually not interested in reducing variations in utilization patterns across populations but in reducing avoidable, replaceable, and inappropriate demand within a given population. Whether this can best be accomplished by reducing morbidity and the need for care in the first place or by rechanneling demand once need has arisen is a key strategic question whose answer is likely to be different for different populations.

Each sponsor should look at the specific population of interest. Does it have an unusual pattern of some diseases or injuries? How many of these are preventable or better treated if detected earlier? Or are morbidity patterns typical, even admirable, but demand for care includes a lot of inappropriate and unnecessary utilization? The particulars of each population will indicate whether health or demand or a combination of the two is the more promising focus for attention.

Even if the initial strategic focus is on improving the quality of demand, this may prove to be best accomplished by improving health in a given population, rather than by focusing on demand per se. For example, if claims data indicate that a large amount of avoidable demand is attributable to the incidence of respiratory flu in the population, sponsors may aim to reduce its incidence, through flu shots, perhaps. Conversely, they may aim, instead, for encouraging and enabling consumers to employ self-care once they experience flu symptoms rather than seek professional services. After prevention and replacement, sponsors might aim to persuade consumers not to insist on antibiotic treatment as a means of reforming demand.

It should be remembered that prevention may have less impact on consumer satisfaction and loyalty than it should. The problem with prevention is that it results in something not happening, and the absence of morbidity may not be noticed by consumers and therefore not felt as a benefit. Moreover, even if consumers notice the absence of morbidity, they may not attribute it to the sponsor's efforts, instead thinking it was luck, fate, or their own efforts that were responsible.

A key impact of the selection of the types of outcomes desired relates to whether they are best achieved through direct or indirect interventions. The distinction between the two is anything but clear, but it is significant. Direct outcomes are those that are most readily obtained through specific, easily identified changes in the behavior of consumers. Improving breast cancer mortality and reducing costs of its treatment by increasing the numbers of cases detected early is a good example. Reducing the incidence of communicable disease by increasing immunization or changing risky behaviors is another.

Indirect outcomes are those whose causes and means of intervention are more community-wide and social. Reducing violence and achieving specific reductions in gunshot, domestic violence, or child abuse cases are likely to require efforts to reduce poverty and hopelessness and promote cultural changes and other broad-brush initiatives with more remote connection to the outcomes stated. Where the health of populations is concerned, sponsors may well find that the most promising interventions require broad social action rather than their direct, personal effort.[5]

Perhaps the biggest strategic question sponsors face in regard to selecting a focus for their initiatives is how far "upstream" to look for intervention opportunities. Some have argued, for example, that we must first address the fundamental social causes of disease and injury—factors such as unemployment, race relations, crime, and a culture of violence—and work on community infrastructures, transportation, and education systems to promote better health.

Others have suggested that we need to change individual attitudes and cultures as a precondition for changing consumer behavior. We must promote self-responsibility and accountability for individual behavior first before we can achieve significant improvements in behavior. It has been suggested that we *mandate* healthy lifestyles, for example, requiring that consumers qualify for government or commercial insurance by cleaning up their health behaviors and getting appropriate immunizations and screening.[6] We should all be responsible for keeping up with required "body maintenance" to validate our "owner's warranty" for our own bodies.[7]

The outcomes themselves are neither direct nor indirect; it is the types of interventions required that fall into either or both categories. However, given the interdependence of means and ends in strategy, once certain outcomes have been chosen, certain types of interventions tend to follow. Sponsors should at least be open to considering whether social problems and solutions should be included, even highlighted in their health and demand improvement strategy. This will have much to do with their selection of partners for specific efforts (Decision 4). (See Exhibit 10–3.)

Setting Goals

The selection of outcomes determines the parameters or measures of health and demand on which sponsors will focus their strategic thinking. Setting a goal goes one step further by deciding in what direction the parameter will be changed and perhaps by how much and when as well. The *Healthy Communities 2000* report by the Surgeon General sets specific health parameters to be achieved nationwide by the year 2000, for example.[8]

Neither a specific achievement nor a time frame is essential for strategic purposes. Sponsors, in many cases, would be advised to select the direction that would reflect improvement in a parameter (usually self-evident), then go through the rest of the strategic decisions before settling on specific goals. The only thing they need to set a goal is a measure of where they are starting from and a clear indication of the direction they wish to go.

Sponsors may choose what improvements to aim for through any number of approaches. They may follow what is most popular in their industry or area or

Exhibit 10–3 Strategic Decisions: Which Outcomes?

RANGE OF POSSIBILITIES	TOOLS
• CHOOSE ONE AND MONITOR SUCCESS *OR* CHOOSE MULTIPLE, INTERLINKED GOALS • CHOOSE GOALS THAT GUIDE INTERNAL ACTION AND/OR FOCUS ON EXTERNAL STAKEHOLDERS • FOCUS ON HEALTH AND/OR DEMAND GOALS • FOCUS ON SOCIAL AND/OR CLINICAL GOALS	• *USE HEALTH CLAIMS ANALYSIS, HEALTH RISK ANALYSIS AND STAKEHOLDER INTEREST ANALYSIS TO ASSIST IN CHOICE* • *MAKE CHOICE BASED ON CONTRIBUTION OF PROGRAM TO ALL CONSTITUENCIES*

what has led to the greatest success by others. They may learn what other stakeholders, including consumers themselves, would most like to see achieved. They may hire consultants or conduct their own analyses to discover which are the most serious problems or most improvable measures.

All of these approaches offer value. The most popular and successful programs are likely to be easier to find support for, and the experiences of others may be good indicators of what will work. Unfortunately each situation and population is likely to be unique, and following the herd may also prove disastrous. Asking risk-sharing partners and consumers what goals they would like to achieve can increase the probability of their enthusiastic cooperation but may not result in the kinds of outcomes of greatest value to the sponsor.

Analysis of the sponsor's own population at risk to identify salient patterns of morbidity or health behavior that lie behind unusual patterns of demand and expenditure or performance problems is likely to provide a better, though slower basis for selection. Such analysis may well shift focus from a particular indicator of excessive demand to the specific health or disease condition most amenable to improvement—perhaps preventable communicable disease, acute episodes among patients with chronic conditions, or inappropriate use of emergency care for minor problems, for example.

We recommend a combination of health claims analysis, health risk analysis, and stakeholder interest analysis for setting goals in health and demand improvement. Each adds something worthwhile to the process, though the use of all three adds to the cost and time commitments of sponsors. Because the choice of which outcomes to pursue is so critical to the rest of the strategic planning process, and to the probability of achieving success effectively and efficiently, we feel it is worth the investment.

The results specified as the desired outcomes driving the planning and implementation of health and demand improvement initiatives should be selected in light of *all* the contributions they can make. The best choices can enhance the logic and effectiveness of planning, and the enlistment of enthusiastic participants and supporters. They can guard against the negative public relations impact of sponsors' initiatives seen as entirely self-serving and help ensure that everyone shares in the benefits achieved.

WHICH CONSUMERS AND BEHAVIORS?

Regardless of which goals are selected as the basis for developing strategy, the focus for intervention will at some point require specific changes in consumer health and/or demand behaviors in order to achieve the goals. Improving health status may require improving consumer health risk or employee safety behaviors or enlisting more consumers to participate in immunization or early detection programs. Improving demand may require their engaging in self-care, using triage and decision counseling services, and more closely monitoring and managing their occupational disabilities and chronic conditions.

There is a direct, but not automatic connection between outcomes and behavior. As sponsors choose which behaviors are the best to change in pursuing a selected outcome, they may have many options. Improved use of emergency care may be achieved by reducing risky behavior or by increasing self-care, for example. Improvements in cancer mortality may be achieved through improved lifestyles, earlier detection, or better choices of treatment and provider selection. Deciding which behaviors are most promising is often a difficult choice.

While changes in mind-states are often essential to achieving behavior change and behavior changes are essential to achieving health status, demand, expenditure, and organizational performance improvements, the basic focus for health and demand improvement is consumer behavior. By identifying the specific changes in (and continuations of) consumer behaviors required to achieve desired outcomes, sponsors lay the groundwork for identifying which consumers are to be targeted for attention and who should be enlisted in efforts to achieve the behavior changes.

To some extent the selection of desired outcomes may already dictate or at least limit selection of consumer behaviors. Improvements in health status, for example, typically presuppose changes in health risk behavior, safety, and prevention or early detection behavior. Improvements in demand per se lead to the selection of necessary changes in specific consumer decisions, or in how consumers manage acute or chronic conditions.

In most cases, however, the translation of outcomes into required behavior will not be automatic; there are likely to be multiple possibilities. An improvement in cardiac health status, for example, may be sought through reducing smoking behavior, increasing exercise, changing diet, or improving stress management and coping skills, or any combination of these. A desired reduction in use of emergency medical services may be sought through promoting safer driving, greater use of phone triage services, or better management of chronic conditions.

Translating goals into behavior changes should be based on two independent considerations: (1) which behavior changes will have the greatest impact on achieving the outcome goal; and (2) which behavior changes are most likely to be achieved earliest. The first consideration reflects the *contribution* that the behavior will make; the second reflects the *probability* of realizing that contribution. The combination of contribution and probability estimates indicates the potential *value* of any behavior change.

For example, if improvement in health status is the selected goal, sponsors may consider the relative promise of smoking cessation, childhood immunization, and fitness promotion as the three most likely behavior change categories available. Analysis of the numbers of smokers and their attitude toward quitting, of current levels of exercise and physical condition and attitudes toward fitness, of the incidence of communicable diseases among children, and related attitudes of parents (see stages of readiness discussion in Chapter 6), will suggest both the extent of the problems and the likelihood of solving each (Exhibit 10–4).

Deciding which and how many consumers to target for intervention can also be greatly influenced by, or greatly influence, choices of goals and categories of behavior. Sponsors of health improvement initiatives may aim at all consumers or may deliberately select those at highest risk. Programs or goals addressing changing demand behaviors or expenditures may aim for the highest users of health services or those on whose behalf the most money is spent.

Exhibit 10–4 Strategic Decisions: What Behavior?

CHALLENGES

DETERMINE SPECIFIC CONSUMER BEHAVIOR CHANGES TO ACHIEVE GOALS AND CHOOSE THOSE THAT:

- **WILL HAVE GREATEST IMPACT ON ACHIEVING GOAL**
- **WILL BE ACHIEVED EARLIEST & EASIEST**

It is a common convention, for example, to talk about the "20/80 rule" in health care—the 20% of consumers who account for 80% of utilization and expenditures. Studies suggest that, in fact, 10% of consumers account for 70% and that 5% account for 60% of health care expenditures, while 50% of consumers might be deliberately ignored because they account for only 3% of the burden.[9] One study indicated that 1% of Americans account for 30% of all expenditures![10]

Mathematically this means that there are a few people who use an enormous amount of our health resources. At an average annual expense per person of $4,000, for illustration, a 20/80 division means that the 20% in a 20/80 split account for an average of $16,000 apiece versus only $800 apiece for the other 80%. In a 10/70 situation, the 10% account for an average of $28,000 apiece versus $1,333 for everybody else. In a 5/60 pattern, the 5% account for an average of $48,000 apiece versus $1,684 for lower users. In a 1/30 pattern, those 1% account for an average of $120,000 apiece versus $2,828 for everyone else. In the four scenarios, high users cost between 20 and 40 times as much per person as the rest of the population.

Unfortunately membership in the high-user versus low-user group, however defined, is often not constant from year to year. Some are only in the high-user group due to a terminal condition and are not around the next year; others are cured of the reasons for their high use, and their high use cured them. Moreover, high users can often only be identified retrospectively, after their high use and expense show up in claims. At that point, it is likely to be too late to do anything about it.

The types of high users most appropriate as targets for intervention are those whose high usage patterns persist over time. Consumers with chronic conditions are good examples. People with diabetes average 3.5 times as much utilization and expense as the rest of the population, for example.[11] If diabetes cannot be successfully prevented, then early detection and effective management can dramatically reduce its burden on society and its sufferers. People who regularly use emergency departments for minor problems or who demand physician attention for colds and minor injuries more appropriate for self-care may also be selected for special attention.

People with asthma are also high users of medical care and expense. But the fact that this is true in general does not always make them good prospects for attention. When Georgia Blue Cross/Blue Shield looked for cost savings opportunities, it expected asthma to be high on the list. But analysis of actual claims data over two years revealed that patients with asthma comprised only 3% of its population at risk. Moreover, such patients were already being well managed by their physicians, so its initial expectations were wrong.[12]

High *risk* consumers, by contrast, are identified by the *probability* that they will generate high use and expense *in the future*.[13] They may be targeted for health promotion or prevention to reduce their risk levels or for self-care and chronic condition management once they develop symptoms. Unfortunately people at the highest risk may turn out to be the most difficult to reform, as was found in one survey of employees.[14]

Rather than focus on consumers who are the biggest problem, sponsors might identify those who are most amenable to behavior change. It makes sense, at a minimum, to identify who is interested in changing behavior and what specific benefits they might be looking for as consequences of behavior change. Consumers interested in fitness might hope for more energy, a better appearance, or just feeling good, for example. Knowing what specific motivating factors make people receptive to the idea of behavior change can help sponsors decide not only who to go after, but what kind of appeals to use in attracting them to participate in programs.

A promising approach would identify the consumer segments most receptive to changing behaviors, those already considering changes who see significant benefit and low switching costs in changing. Psychographic segmentation models employ surveys to identify clusters of consumers with similar attitudes, such as the "independently healthy," who are very much into sports and exercise, nutrition, and healthy lifestyles, and "naturalists," who rely on natural foods, alternative medicine, and macrobiotic diets, for example, to keep them well.[15] By analyzing the proportions of a given population that fall into specific segments, sponsors can estimate how many consumers would be good prospects for what initiatives.

The stages of change approach to selecting consumers for behavior change (Chapter 6) identifies where people are in the process of change, from not even thinking about it to active consideration, preparation, and implementation. The farther along people are in the process, the more successful efforts are likely to be. On the other hand, when the largest proportions of consumers are at the earliest stages, interventions may prove overly expensive and largely unsuccessful (more about how this model can be used for selecting tactics in Chapter 17).

The more promising prospects may be those whose motivation barriers appear to be easiest to overcome and who have no capability barriers. Perhaps those with minor capability problems but high motivation would be the best prospects. Those with high motivation and capability who need no more than some consciousness raising or reminding should be among the easiest consumers to convert. Good research into the MC^2 status of the population of interest will help identify the best prospects and thereby make interventions more efficient.

Of course, the best prospects, however identified, may promise the least return. They may already be low risk in terms of lifestyle and low users of health services. If they are among the 50%, 80%, 90%, or 95% who have lower need or demand for care, there may be little prospect of significant health improvement or expense reduction through reforming their behavior. If, as has been reported, 50% of the population account for 3% of health expense, then converting all of them to the best possible patterns of health and consumption behaviors can reduce total health expenditures by only 3% at maximum.

It is the combination of how much will be gained by converting consumers and how easily/efficiently they can be converted that indicates who are the consumers most suitable for intervention, not either of the factors alone. If the estimated value of a conversion goal can be expressed in dollars, and the ease of doing so in probability terms, then the dollar times probability amount for different targeting options would indicate where the greatest potential value lies.

At the strategic level, identification of the consumers and behaviors to be improved is based on the general set of outcomes desired. It sets the stage for subsequent tactical planning of specific initiatives. At the tactical planning level (see Chapter 16), sponsors may discover that their early estimates of what outcomes could be achieved at what costs were in error, and they may have to reconsider the feasibility or desirability of pursuing the selected consumer behavior changes. Thus all strategic decisions are of a "draft" nature not only relative to each other, but relative to subsequent tactical considerations (Exhibit 10–5).

WHO PARTICIPATES IN WHAT ROLES?

There are four classes of potential role players who may be considered as part of developing and implementing strategy. First are those within the sponsor organization—which departments and professions are likely to be most successful? Second are those who are part of whatever risk-sharing arrangement applies to the population of interest—the employer, health plan, and physicians plus hospitals or other organizations united in risk-sharing responsibility for the same population. Third are the health-related organizations in the community who might play a contributing role in efforts aimed specifically at the same risk population or at larger populations that include the risk group. Fourth are outside vendors of strategic services, including information development and analysis, planning and evaluation.

Exhibit 10–5 Strategic Decisions: Which Consumers?

CHALLENGES
• HIGH USERS *OR* LOW USERS
• HIGH-RISK CONSUMERS *OR* LOW-RISK CONSUMERS
• THOSE READY FOR CHANGE *OR* THOSE WHO NEED TO CHANGE

Internal Responsibility

However many stakeholders are involved in formulating strategy, someone needs to be specifically responsible and accountable for implementing the strategy and achieving the goals. The most important decision in this regard may be whether to assign responsibility and resources within the sponsor organization or turn to outside help. Other stakeholders or outside vendors may be better equipped to carry out specific initiatives. Once having assigned the job to an outside organization, it may prove irresistible to continue the outsourcing, since there are likely to be synergies or economies in having the same organization implement a growing strategy and investment.

If the decision is to develop and implement the strategy internally, there is still the question of where to assign responsibility. The human resources department or subsidiary units devoted to employee development and training or benefits administration may seem a likely choice for programs aimed at employees, for example, though they may have no competence or interest in improving health and demand behavior. The marketing or public relations staff might be an option if their abilities in influencing external attitudes and behavior can be translated into internal success. Health education professionals may be appropriate if they can expand their skills to encompass the full set of tactics available for improving behavior. (See Part III.)

There appears to be a trend toward employers assigning responsibility for a variety of demand improvement initiatives to employee assistance program (EAP) staff. Where these programs started by addressing employee stress and personal problems, they are frequently being asked to address overall wellness, managed care relationships, absenteeism, and disability problems as well. Some are conducting health and life issues education, sponsoring support groups and engaging in prevention efforts. While the majority of EAP programs use outside contractors, insiders are also selected in some cases.[16]

Just as motivation and capability are key in selecting consumer targets and designing tactical initiatives, so they are the appropriate basis for deciding where to assign responsibility for demand improvement efforts. Who is best equipped to carry out specific initiatives? Who has a relationship with consumer targets that will promote success? Who has incentives to do the best job? As additional initiatives are decided on, who is likely to be best at handling their diversity?

Risk-Sharing Partners

Given the large number of interested parties, it is no easy task to decide who should participate in any overall strategy. Obvious stakeholders include the employer or union that pays the costs and enjoys the benefits of improved health and demand behaviors, as well as value-adding performance improvements, plus any insurers, physicians, and hospitals at risk for the consequences of such behavior. Consumers themselves are clearly interested parties, and arguably belong on the list of risk-sharing partners in planning any overall effort.

The same criteria apply in deciding which are likely to be the best sponsors as were relevant to assigning internal resources and choosing between make and buy options. Which of possible partners has the best combination of motivation and capability? How long are partnerships likely to last compared to the time required to achieve desired outcomes? Who will gain in addition to the originating sponsor and how much? How will savings and other financial gains as well as costs for initiatives be shared?

Community Stakeholders

In addition to risk-sharing partners, there are many other organizations that might be willing and able to play a significant role. Government agencies, such as public health departments, are already involved in environmental health risks, immunization programs, communicable disease control, and delivering health care to the disadvantaged. Businesses and governments in Hawaii developed an effective partnership for statewide health management, for example.[17] The federal HCFA has promised greater involvement in promoting the health of Medicare beneficiaries and providing information so that both Medicare and Medicaid beneficiaries can make better health plan and provider choices.[18]

Community health and welfare organizations are potential partners, as well. Efforts to promote community health may be carried out in partnership with schools, senior centers, neighborhood health centers, churches, health clubs, essentially anyone who can help. The Danbury (Connecticut) Hospital partnered with local libraries to make health information more accessible to consumers.[19] Working with either government or community organizations will broaden the focus beyond the set of employees, health plan enrollees, or patients that payers and providers are most interested in, but might achieve specific results more effectively and efficiently.

Schools can be partners in efforts to promote exercise or better diets in the young. Universities may be interested in conducting research helpful in identifying the best consumer targets. Businesses may be helpful partners as well. Local restaurants and grocery stores may help in promoting lower fat diets. Packaged food companies may help by promoting their own healthier products, or drug companies their medications.

Vendors

The growing list of vendors offering demand improvement services includes a number who offer strategic assistance. Some focus on information systems and software to enable sponsors to carry out their own strategic analyses; others conduct analyses for sponsors. Most offer consulting services to help sponsors make strategic decisions and follow up with help in planning and evaluating specific initiatives and overall programs.

Some of the strategic services vendors also offer packaged initiatives in one or more of the demand improvement domains. Sponsors should be wary about choosing such vendors, who may have an understandable bias toward the domains in which they sell such initiatives. Selecting a vendor to plan and evaluate initiatives who will carry out such initiatives invites the risk of finding the appearance of success, even where there is little evidence for it.

If outside vendors are selected, they may be contracted to perform on a fee-for-service or risk-sharing basis. Fee for service is by far the most common basis for most outsourcing of services, though the method most preferred by health care buyers may be risk sharing. Sponsors should consider which type of payment offers the best set of incentives for vendors to perform well and deliver real value.

Increasingly vendors are accepting risks for results. For specific disease management programs, for example, 13 vendors were found that guaranteed savings to their clients. Many also took on risk for specific quality outcomes and satisfaction levels. As competition among vendors increases and each must constantly make the case for sponsors outsourcing programs versus running their own, such guarantees seem likely to become even more common.[20]

CHOOSING PARTNERS

An important question relates to who among the obvious stakeholders is willing to partner with which others. Small employers who may have little capability for engaging in reform initiatives on their own may find strength through employer alliances, for example.[21] Individual physician practices may find that by working with their peers, they can achieve the critical mass needed to initiate efficient efforts.

Hospitals may partner with their peers, including direct competitors, in initiatives that offer benefit to both parties, as well as improvements in community health. Three competing hospitals in Fort Wayne, Indiana, for example, collaborated on a video covering how best to use physicians, avoid unnecessary care, stay healthy, and plan for terminal illness.[22] Even health plans might find it expedient to work together on specific projects.

Working with stakeholders in other categories is equally possible. Hospitals and businesses are frequent partners. Bellin Hospital in Green Bay, Wisconsin, sponsors an employer-provider coalition aimed at improving health and reducing costs to the community.[23] Intermountain Health Care in Utah works with employers to promote better health and more informed use of health care.[24] BP Oil and Nestle/Stouffer partnered with University Hospital in Cleveland, Ohio, to reduce injuries and provide more accessible medical care on site.[25]

Health plans or physician groups can work with each other. Employers and integrated provider networks are partnering through direct contracting.[26] Hospitals and health plans can be logical partners under global capitation. Hospitals, employers, and health plans have a long-established partnership in Rochester, New York, promoting better access and lower costs in health care.[27] Additional examples of stakeholder cooperation in specific programs are offered in Chapter 19. It is a relatively simple matter to elevate such partnerships to the strategic level.

Enlisting other stakeholders in the planning effort automatically brings with it the risk that the outcomes chosen for emphasis, the behaviors for change, and consumers selected as targets will be different from what the original sponsor intended. This is another reason why strategies are written in pencil until they are complete. Sponsors must consider whether the added value available through the participation of other partners outweighs this risk.

Consumers targeted for attention and behaviors for change may not match the interests of sponsors and risk-sharing partners. In addition, a large group of diverse community organizations may have difficulty in deciding on a combined strategy, in obtaining the necessary resources to carry it out, or in achieving meaningful results. Political infighting may hamstring the most well-meaning of coalitions, and sponsors may end up waiting forlornly on the sidelines for anything to happen.

The key to deciding whether to partner with community organizations, and to selecting which are the best partners, is the identification of commonalities. Do community organizations share an interest in the same populations as sponsors—as each other? Does the population of interest lend itself to an integrated approach? The Rural Prevention Network in northeast Michigan allied hospital and health department, rural health centers, and local physicians in a wide-ranging effort to promote health and prevent disease[28] (Exhibit 10–6).

WHAT RESOURCES?

It is a common, though unfortunate, practice in many organizations to budget resources for new initiatives in advance before any strategic or tactical choices are made. This arises from conventional budgeting and financial management practice, though it is particularly problematic when related to health and demand im-

Exhibit 10–6 Strategic Decisions: Who Participates?

STAKEHOLDERS	CONSIDERATIONS
• EMPLOYERS / UNIONS WHO PAY COSTS • INSURERS / PROVIDERS AT RISK FOR CONSEQUENCES • CONSUMERS • GOVERNMENT AGENCIES • COMMUNITY HEALTH & WELFARE ORGANIZATIONS	• *WHO IS WILLING TO PARTNER WITH OTHERS* • *HOW TO KEEP OBJECTIVES ALIGNED* • *HOW TO ALLOCATE RESPONSIBILITY* • *WHO IS RESPONSIBLE FOR MANAGING (HUMAN RESOURCES AND/OR MARKETING)*

provement initiatives. In many cases the value of possible initiatives may be great enough, and the likelihood of realizing that value high enough, that sponsors may consider spending as much as they can afford on as many initiatives as they can implement rather than restrict themselves at the outset to a minimal or moderate investment.

The most common approach to embarking on a demand improvement strategy is to start small, with one program to test the water, then build up to more initiatives over time. The most common beginning for most sponsors is to find out about or be approached by a champion of one specific type of intervention. If it looks promising and can be fit into existing budgets, it is adopted. If successful, it may well be continued, and the sponsor may even look for another promising initiative.

Such an approach has the advantage of putting little at risk if the initial effort fails to deliver anticipated results. The people who propose the idea and those responsible for its implementation are at less personal risk if there is little at stake. Starting slow may allow sponsors to learn as they go in what may be unfamiliar territory. Countering all these perfectly valid reasons for an incremental approach is the fact that so many initiatives have track records involving dramatic returns on investment.

For illustration, let us say that a very careful, risk-averse sponsor picks one good enough initiative proposed by an internal champion or external vendor. That initiative can deliver an annual net savings or performance contribution of $50,000. If the sponsor continues the same program with the same results, it will end up with a total return of $250,000 over five years. (We recognize that specific initiatives may run into diminishing returns over a five-year period, but they are equally likely to have diminishing costs. Whether net returns will diminish or grow over time is for experience to determine—we have used a steady return for illustration only.)

Let us contrast that with a somewhat more ambitious sponsor who examines the situation strategically, looking for and identifying the most promising of all interventions, given the sponsor's unique population, claims patterns, consumer behavior patterns, attitudes, and readiness to change. Let us say that by selecting the best, rather than the first good-looking program to come along, the sponsor can obtain an annual return of $100,000, for illustration. The sponsor that implements and continues that one program, which returns an annual net savings of $100,000, will end up with total savings of $500,000 in five years, double the return compared to the sponsor who did not take a strategic approach.

However, imagine that another sponsor took an even more confident strategic approach, not only continuing its first investment but implementing and continuing a new initiative each year, based on careful analysis of which seemed most promising, increasing its total investment as each initiative proves itself. Let us suppose that each initiative produces an annual return of $100,000 in net savings and performance improvement.

For the first initiative, continued for the same five years as comparable sponsors, total savings will be $500,000. By adding a second initiative in the second year, this sponsor realizes an additional return of $400,000 for that one in the remaining four years of the period. The initiative begun in the third year contributes $300,000; the one from the fourth year, $200,000; and the last one, begun in the fifth year, contributes $100,000. The total return from all five initiatives over the five-year period is $1,500,000, six times as much as was achievable with one good enough initiative and three times as much as with one best initiative.

Imagine yet a fourth sponsor who is willing to commit to all five programs immediately, implements all five in the first year and continues all five for the same five years. Each produces a net return of $100,000 for all five years, so each contributes a return of $500,000 over the five-year comparison period. With five such programs all contributing for five years each, the sponsor realizes a total return of $2,500,000, fully ten times as much as was possible with one promising initiative, five times as much as with one best initiative, and $1,000,000 better than an incremental approach[29] (Exhibit 10–7).

Of course, there is likely to be a practical limit to how many programs can be implemented at one time, even if many promise significant net savings and ROI ratios. Staff resources may preclude anything but a one-at-a-time or incremental approach. Employees, members, and patients may have limited interest in or time to participate in multiple initiatives. Even if five or more programs could be funded, each promising significant return, sponsors may lack the energy and management time to implement them all.

On the other hand, many programs target different people (e.g., prenatal care engages only pregnant women, back injury prevention only those at risk because of lifting, diabetes and asthma management only consumers and families so af-

Exhibit 10–7 Strategic Decisions: What Resources?

SITUATION: 5 PROGRAMS, EACH PROMISE SAVINGS OF $100,000 PER YEAR	
INVESTMENT OPTIONS	**5-YEAR SAVINGS**
• ONE PROGRAM FOR FIVE YEARS • INITIATE 1 NEW PROGRAM PER YEAR / MAINTAIN OTHERS • INITIATE 5 PROGRAMS & MAINTAIN FOR 5 YEARS	• *$500,000* • *$1.5 MILLION* • *$2.5 MILLION?*

flicted). Many immunization efforts require only a brief participation; triage and decision counseling programs only apply at specific moments in time. The right set of behavior change targets and objectives may permit implementation of many initiatives at once without disrupting anyone's life unduly. Outside vendors can greatly expand the potential for implementing multiple programs. And the plan, employer, or provider who succeeds in many at once may gain a significant edge over more timid and gradualist competitors.

How Long To Invest?

About the only useful guidance that seems offerable regarding how long to continue investing resources in a given strategy or specific initiative is not to quit while it's still working. In many cases it may take some time before a strategy or program pays off. One employer found its strategy cost money the first year, broke even the second, and finally returned a net savings the third.[30] Another found its ROI ratio was only 1.84:1 in the first year of its multifaceted strategy, but 2.15:1 in the second year and 3.15:1 by the third.[31]

Some initiatives, by their very nature, will take time to deliver positive returns. An early detection program, for example, will tend to add a new group of consumers requiring treatment to those who were diagnosed in the normal course of events, doubling up on costs during the first year of implementation. Cholesterol and blood pressure reduction may take years, even decades, to make a difference in morbidity, utilization, and expenditures.

Once an initiative is paying off, however, it makes no sense to discontinue it as long as it is working. With annual ROI ratios averaging 2:1, 3:1, or more, and the common pattern of rising returns over time, it would cost a payer or provider money to discontinue an investment that pays off at 100%, 200%, or more per year. Even if it requires adding staff or borrowing money to initiate a strategy or keep it going, such returns on investment would make the gamble worthwhile.

HOW TO MAKE STRATEGIC DECISIONS

Perhaps the first consideration in making strategic decisions is who will make them. The general rule in such matters is to consider how important it is to choose the "right" strategy (whatever that may mean) versus achieve or maintain acceptance by and working relationships with key stakeholders. Normally some balance of the two is needed, if some involvement by other stakeholders is worth the trouble.

This is particularly true for the stakeholders most frequently ignored, consumers themselves. Their participation may help sponsors design a better program by introducing information and perspectives likely to be missing otherwise. It will also help promote consumer acceptance of the strategy and specific initiatives designed with their participation, by giving them a sense of personal ownership of the planned initiatives and desired results. Moreover, involving consumers will help promote their satisfaction with and loyalty to the employer, health plan, or provider sponsors, thereby promoting added performance value by itself.

Determining who will be involved is half the challenge in making strategic decisions. The other half deals with the process and criteria to be used in making specific decisions. The first and most important criterion has already been cited relative to selection of consumers to target for attention; the combination of payoff and probability. When applied to overall decisions about what to do, it works the same way: what promises the best mix of results and the greatest likelihood of achieving them?

Chapman has suggested that sponsors look at the combination of how common a problem is, how much it costs, and how variable it is across consumer populations.[32] The first two criteria address the seriousness of the problem, thereby the potential value of solving it. The third at least suggests the possibility of solving it—if others have kept the problem and its costs low, there must be a way for us to do so as well.

Choosing specifically on the basis of anticipated return makes good sense where dollar values can easily be assigned to results. However, the *amount* of the return should be given greater weight than the ROI ratio. One program may promise a 20:1 ROI ratio, for example, saving $20 for every dollar invested. If it can only take a $1,000 investment, however (i.e., if the initiative is focused on few people or modest changes), then the return will only be $20,000, or a net gain of $19,000.

Another initiative might have an expected ROI of only 2:1. If the sponsor can invest $100,000 in the program and realize $200,000 in savings, or a net gain of

$100,000, that is far better than a net gain of $19,000. A high ROI ratio may suggest that one initiative warrants greater confidence than another, implying that even a mediocre job of implementation is sure to deliver at least some net return. It does not tell us which initiative will do the most good, however, only which will do the most good for each person it applies to. If a given high-ratio initiative can only be applied to a few people, it cannot have the same amount of return as one that applies to everyone, or even a large number.

Sponsors may look to their peers for guidance in developing strategies. What have other employers, health plans, physicians, or hospitals done and how well did it work for them? Reports indicate that employers are the most active sponsors, with exercise/fitness, smoking cessation, stress management, substance abuse, back care, diet/nutrition, blood pressure, cholesterol, and weight management the most popular initiatives.[33]

A Marion Merrill Dow report suggests that by the year 2000 smoking cessation will be the most popular, with 79% of employers including it, followed by wellness (70%), mammography (68%), cholesterol (65%), blood pressure (62%), weight management (59%), prenatal care (58%), annual checkup (57%), prostate screening (55%), and Pap smear (51%). All initiatives addressed are increasing in popularity except for nutrition education, which fell from 27% to 13%.[34]

Health plans have not invested nearly as heavily in health or demand improvement, having devoted their attention primarily to controlling providers, as discussed in Chapter 3. On the other hand, HMO plans are likely to become more active in improving consumer health and demand, using their own devices or outside vendors.[35]

Hospitals have traditionally offered a wide variety of patient education and rehabilitation services. Many have invested in fitness centers, both as mission extensions and revenue generators, though they serendipitously fit with expense reduction efforts under capitation financing. Those following the Planetree Model have developed extensive libraries, resource centers, and information programs to empower patients and their families to be active and effective partners in both their inpatient care and overall disease management.[36]

Physicians are likely to vary widely in terms of what strategies they use for promoting patient health and appropriate use of services. Under capitation, many physicians have exchanged their answering services for full-fledged telephone information resources and triage and counseling programs, often with hospital help.[37] Where "cognitive" services, such as counseling patients in lifestyle improvement and risk reduction, are poorly paid under FFS, they can be rewarding investments under capitation.

There are many sources of help in advising potential sponsors on strategic issues. The American Institute for Preventive Medicine, for example, offers advice in the wellness, promotion, and prevention area. The US Public Health Service offers "Put Prevention into Practice" materials. The Healthcare Forum offers a wide range of materials on community health assessment and strategies for healthier communities. Local universities, particularly those with epidemiology faculty, plus local hospitals and governments may be sources of assistance. Vendors such as Johnson & Johnson, Health Decisions International, and Summex Corporation, as well as the Kaiser health plan, offer claims, interests, and health risk analyses to help sponsors identify the most promising opportunities. (See the end-of-chapter appendixes for listings of available resources for specific forms of assistance.)

Thanks to computer technology, we have the capability to examine far more data and address far more considerations in developing strategies. A computer-driven "expert system," for example, can enable sponsors to customize strategies and programs to their unique situations and values.[38] Other computer systems can simulate the effects of various interventions to suggest which ought to be included in a given strategy.[39]

In getting started it is usually wise to shoot for the "low-hanging fruit." Investing in initiatives that will produce a large, visible return in a short period may be necessary to securing ongoing support for the idea of improving demand or at least for focusing on consumers. Self-care programs have produced dramatic savings in their first year, for example.[40] Prenatal care has had similar results, though somewhat more delayed.[41]

Interventions that pay off quickly and consistently can help build confidence in the general idea of reforming consumer health and consumption behavior and in the four specific domains of demand improvement or their components. Sponsors may then be able to include initiatives that have a longer payoff period, once confidence in results has been achieved. It may be that only a brave few will consider implementing multiple initiatives from the outset, though this strategy may prove to be the best rewarded.

REFERENCES

1. D. Olmos, "Eyes on Minn. Health-Care Experiment," *The Denver Post,* 27 October 1996, 2A, 8A.

2. Olmos, "Eyes on Minn.," 2A, 8A.

3. D. Vickery, "Toward Appropriate Use of Medical Care," *Healthcare Forum Journal* 39, no. 1 (1996):15–19.

4. "New Approach Launched To Prevent Disease," *Health Care Strategic Management* 12, no. 5 (1994):4.

5. E. Friedman, "Redrawing the Line," *Healthcare Forum Journal* 39, no. 5 (1996):11–14.

6. R. Annis, "Mandated Care: Making Healthy Lifestyles Mandatory," *Wellness Program Management Advisor* 3, no. 10 (1994):8.

7. T. O'Neal, "Issuing a Service Warranty on the Human 'Engine,' " *AHA News* 31, no. 38 (1995):6.

8. "Toward Healthier Communities," *Hospitals & Health Networks*, 5 July 1994, 18.

9. S. McEachern, "Disease Management: They All 'Say' They're Doing It," *Health Care Strategic Management* 13, no. 6 (1995):1, 19–23.

10. "Study Shows 1% of Americans Use 30% of Health Expenditures," *Business & Health* 11, no. 12 (1993):10.

11. "New Approaches To Manage Diabetes," *Business & Health* 14, no. 1 (Supplement A 1996):1–30.

12. "Use This Tool To Identify Best DM Investments for Your Enrollee Population," *Healthcare Demand & Disease Management* 3, no. 6 (1997):89, 90.

13. "Comparing Costs by Health Risk," *Business & Health* 12, no. 3 (1994):12.

14. F. Kraft and P. Goodell, "Identifying the Health Conscious Consumer," *Journal of Health Care Marketing* 13, no. 3 (Fall 1993).

15. *Profiles of Attitudes toward Healthcare* (San Gabriel, CA: PATH Institute, 1996).

16. C. Petersen, "Employee-Assistance Programs Shaping 'Lean and Mean' Firms," *Managed Healthcare* 7, no. 8 (1997):6, 10, 62.

17. J. Lewin, "Prevention in Paradise," *Healthcare Forum Journal* 36, no. 6 (1993):22.

18. "HCFA Introduces Consumer Information Strategy To Improve Healthcare," *Healthcare Financial Management,* July 1994, 8.

19. "This Medical Library Is Not for Doctors Only," *Profiles in Healthcare Marketing* 46 (1992):48–50.

20. J. Burns, "DM Vendors Talk the Talk and Walk the Walk—And They Guarantee Their Results," *Managed Healthcare* 7, no. 8 (1997):18–21, 25.

21. F. Cerne, "Local Alliance Calms Tempers and Tackles Health Costs," *Hospitals & Health Networks,* 20 November 1993, 54.

22. "Team Teaching a Healthcare Lesson," *Profiles in Healthcare Marketing* 57 (1994):8–11.

23. A. Van den Akker, "A Foundation for Leadership in the New Era of Healthcare," in *Personal Health Management* (Rancho Cordova, CA: Access Health, 1995), 1–4.

24. D. Woodbury, "Intermountain Health Care Teams Up with Employer To Promote Prevention," *Inside Preventive Care* 1, no. 12 (1996):7.

25. E. Meszaros, "Cheaper by the Dozen, Cheaper on Site," *Managed Healthcare* 4, no. 11 (1994):24, 25.

26. E.P. Gee and A. Fine, *Dealing Direct: A Strategy for Business-Provider Relationships* (Chicago, IL: American Hospital Publishing, 1997).

27. K. Pallarito, "Rochester Health Plan Studied as Model for National Health Reform," *Modern Healthcare,* 4 May 1992, 28.

28. B. Pfeiffer, "Rural Prevention Network Involves the Community in Health Improvement," *Inside Preventive Care* 3, no. 4 (1997):1–3.

29. S. MacStravic, "Choosing Your Investment in Reforming Consumer Demand," *Health Care Strategic Management* 15, no. 1 (1997):16–19.

30. D. Wise, "Weighing the Value of Prevention," *Business & Health* 12, no. 4 (1994):94–96.

31. S. Blair, "Health Promotion as a Business Imperative," *1996 Healthier Communities Summit* (San Francisco, CA: The Healthcare Forum, April 23, 1996), 181–198.

32. L. Chapman, "Six Questions To Ask When Setting Demand Management Priorities," *Inside Preventive Care* 1, no. 6 (1995):7, 8.

33. "Health Promotion and Wellness Climbs Higher on the Strategic Agendas of Health Care Chief Executive Officers," *Strategy Letter* (Marblehead, MA: Strategy Development Group, January 1996), 3, 4.

34. "Current Usage and Five-Year Projected Prevalence of Corporate Preventive Health & Wellness Programs," *Medical Benefits,* 30 March 1995, 3.

35. S. McEachern, "Risk-Shared Outsourcing Will Soar as Build-or-Buy Solution," *Health Care Strategic Management* 14, no. 1 (1996):1, 20–23.

36. J. Cassidy, "Patient Participation," *Health Progress* 73, no. 10 (1992):42, 43, 57.

37. "An 'Advice Nurse' Serves Your Patients—and You," *The Physicians Advisory* 94, no. 12 (1994):3, 4.

38. D. Strauss and D. Yen, "How an Expert Corporate Fitness Program Might Be Designed," *Health Care Supervisor* 10, no. 3 (1992):40–55.

39. M. Sandberg, "An Apple a Day Keeps the Doctor Away . . . and Costs Down, Too," *Managed Healthcare* 4, no. 7 (1994):30–32.

40. J. Fries, et al., "Randomized Controlled Trial of Cost Reductions from a Health Education Program," *American Journal of Health Promotion* 8, no. 3 (1994):216–223.

41. B. Pfeiffer, "Los Angeles OB-Gyns Reduce Low-Birthweight Rate to 4.3%," *Inside Preventive Care* 3, no. 4 (1997):5.

PART III

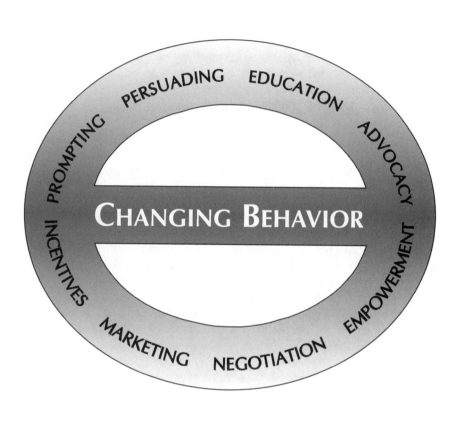

Improving consumer health and demand behaviors, whether promoting and reinforcing positive behavior or altering negative behavior, is invariably a complicated challenge. We have identified eight distinct approaches applicable to improving consumer health and demand behaviors:

1. Prompting
2. Persuading, or "Selling"
3. Educating
4. Social Advocacy
5. Rewarding/Punishing
6. Marketing
7. Negotiating/Contracting
8. Empowering

Each of these tactics addresses one or more of the $I = MC^2$ factors discussed in Chapter 6, motivation, capability, and consciousness, and may use an internal, external, or a combined approach to any of these factors. Each tactic varies in difficulty, cost, and effectiveness, though how well each is executed is as important as which is selected as the basic approach to achieving positive health or demand behavior change.

Of the eight, the first four involve a variety of ways of talking consumers into the desired behavior (i.e., communications tactics). These four will be discussed in Chapters 11 through 13. They can work where consumers are truly unaware of benefits they will gain by improving their behavior, need reminders, or perhaps need training in specific skills. In other words, they work in the simplest situations where relatively little has to be done to "convert" consumers to better behaviors. They may also serve to awaken consumers' consciousness in order to prepare them for more complex tactics and to remind converted consumers about something (e.g., details of what, when, and where they are already predisposed to do).

The final four tactics all involve going beyond communications by changing something about the experience or consequences of the behavior of interest, though each includes communication. They are recommended where communication alone will not work or has failed. All require knowing more about and working more closely with consumers than communications tactics alone and tend to cost more in time and resources. They will be discussed in Chapters 14 and 15.

The stages of change model, which so well describes the movement of people from progressive mind-states to progressive adherence to improved behavior, includes its own set of "techniques" applicable to particular stages. There are nine such techniques:

1. Consciousness raising: adding information about oneself and the problem to what one is aware of and thinks about relative to a given behavior;
2. Social liberation: advocating social actions that make the desired behavior easier to adopt and continue or offering more positive alternatives;
3. Emotional arousal: experiencing and expressing one's feelings about the behaviors at issue;
4. Self-reevaluation: clarifying the issues and values relative to a behavior;
5. Commitment: people committing themselves to action, to self-responsibility, and to self-efficacy relative to a given behavior;
6. Countering: finding better alternatives to a negative behavior;
7. Environment control: eliminating stimuli that tend to promote a negative behavior;
8. Rewards: giving oneself incentives to change behavior; and
9. Helping relationships: enlisting the help of others in supporting behavior change.[1]

Because these stages of change and techniques apply primarily to what people can do to change their own behavior or how therapists can help individuals achieve positive changes, they are not directly geared to most sponsors' efforts to change the behavior of populations. Moreover, because they have been used and tested primarily on negative, addictive behaviors (i.e., the health risk reduction component of health improvement), there are some adjustments needed to adapt them to other types of behavior.

In this part we will relate the stages of change and their techniques to the more general $I = MC^2$ model and suggest ways that sponsors can adapt self-change/therapeutic techniques to entire populations. We believe that the combined insights and experience embedded in these two models will offer the strongest available set of tactics for demand improvement.

The combination of inspiring (motivation), equipping (capability), and reminding (consciousness) people to adopt, change, or continue a given pattern of behavior may be seen as manipulative by some. Certainly there are unethical, misleading, and generally manipulative approaches that might be employed in the effort. Our position is that none of the tactics described in this part are manipulative per se. It is those sponsors employing the tactics, together with consumers who are the targets of such efforts, who will determine if they are manipulative or not.

Readers who function at the strategic level in deciding whether to engage in demand improvement in general or in any of its domains and components in particular are likely to find this part offering much more detail on these tactics than they are interested in learning. To them we recommend Chapter 17 on choosing tactics as suited to their needs. Those charged with the design or implementation of specific initiatives should find the level of detail, examples, and references in Chapters 11 through 15 more interesting and of practical use.

REFERENCE

1. J. Prochaska, J. Norcross and C. DiClemente *Changing for Good* (New York: Avon Books, 1994).

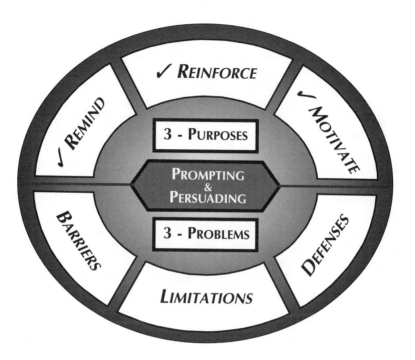

PROMPTING & PERSUADING

We have chosen to cover both prompting and persuading in this one chapter for three reasons. First, prompting belongs with almost all of the other tactics, particularly with persuading, as a complementary addition, wherever it is insufficient by itself. Second, prompting, by itself, is neither complicated nor challenging enough to describe and explain and thus would not fill a chapter on its own. Third, prompting in practice often includes some persuasive intent and effect due to the influence of the individuals and organizations doing the prompting.

203

PROMPTING

Prompting involves raising the consciousness or heightening the awareness of consumers relative to a specific behavior. This may be done at the beginning of a behavior improvement effort to awaken complacent individuals and populations to the possibility and desirability of changing behavior. In that sense it corresponds somewhat to the consciousness raising technique relative to stages of change. It is also used to reinforce and remind consumers already committed to or engaging in a desired behavior.

While its primary emphasis is on consciousness, prompting can have motivational impact through the effect of peer influence and authoritative or admired sources of the prompting. It can also add to capability by including information on when, where, and how to act that consumers were unaware of or needed a reminder to remember. In terms of the stages of change, prompting in the form of awakening consciousness applies at the beginning of the mental portion of the change process, where its reminder role applies during the time when improved behaviors are adopted, repeated, and continued.

The essence of reminding is to both specify the desired behavior and to prompt consumers to engage in it or avoid it as the case may be. In its various applications, prompting might be referred to as: (1) asking, (2) telling, (3) reminding, (4) nagging, or (5) demonstrating—whatever approach is effective for particular consumers targeted for attention.

These five words describe what is basically a single, basic approach: providing a cue or "prompt" to behavior to raise targeted consumers' consciousness about it. All involve simple communications, specifying or showing what positive behavior is to be adopted, repeated, or continued or what negative behavior is to be avoided, reduced, or ended. Each prompt can include information indicating when, where, and how the behavior is or is not to occur and should specify who is supposed to behave in the desired fashion. Prompting includes only basic reminders on how to do so, leaving education to provide more complex, capability building. It may also remind consumer targets of why they should engage in the behavior, though persuasion is used to convince them why in the first place.

Simple requests or orders will suffice in a wide variety of situations to bring about the desired behavior. When people are already motivated to behave in the indicated manner or to comply with an order/request—and when they are not hindered by incapacity or external barriers—the merest suggestion that they do something will suffice in most cases. The nonverbal cue of someone showing the way or the combination of telling and showing will often sway people to follow the leader.

As in all attempts to influence behavior, relationships with the targets of such efforts are key determinants of success. When trusting, friendly relationships are well established, a modest prompt, request, or suggestion will often suffice.

Where a relationship has not been established, some effort will often be needed by prompters to ingratiate themselves with targets before a request can be successful. Any standard text on sales will offer suggestions on how to create the requisite rapport.[1]

Clearly the vast majority of behaviors stimulated by external sources are prompted by simple requests: from spouses, parents, children; from bosses and coworkers; from customers and friends; even from absolute strangers. Where the requested action is simple enough, we tend to comply. When the request comes from a person in authority, we may feel compelled to do so.

For simple prompting to work, the behavior should be familiar, fairly simple to execute, and consistent with target values and attitudes. When reminders are used, they should address commitments targets have already made. For requests, prompts should be seen as involving behaviors that are commonly accepted and, ideally, strongly preferred among members of the target's peer group.

In many cases we intend or are committed to behave in a certain way—to brush our teeth, have a mammogram, get a checkup, monitor our blood sugar, wear a "hard hat." But if not reminded, we might simply forget to do so. If someone reminds us or if we arrange for a cue to prompt ourselves (e.g., note on the calendar, message on the computer) the cue will produce the right behavior with no further effort required.

In some cases a combination of external and internal cues are used to instigate action. The HealthPartners HMO in Minnesota uses staff personnel to call patients with congestive heart failure, asking them to check their weight. If the (disease management) patient detects a weight gain, that is an early sign of dangerous fluid retention, requiring immediate intervention. The external reminder causes the patient to look for the internal cue. This combination of prompts significantly reduced inpatient admissions for CHF patients and at very little cost.[2]

HealthPartners also uses its staff as "naggers" to remind high-risk danger management targets of the need to obtain preventive services. When reminders are repeated often enough, they can serve as an added motivating factor (i.e., anything to stop the incessant nagging). How many reminders and how frequently they will be perceived as nagging is, of course, a subjective judgment.

Some repetition may be essential. In a study of reminder letters aimed at prompting consumers to get a cholesterol screening test, half (50.2%) did not even remember receiving the letter, and 27.4% of the remainder could not recall what it was about.[3] For behaviors that are somewhat complex or unpleasant (the cholesterol screen requires going to a provider location and having blood drawn), many repetitions may be needed to induce a high response rate.

A key factor in determining the success of cues is the source of communication. We respond better to persons in authority (normally), to those we like or perceive to be like us. We are likely to respond better to attractive people with pleasant voices. We respond better when we get the same message from many people than when it is repeated many times by the same person.

The same logic applies when cues are physical—when demonstrating or modeling the desired behavior is involved. We will follow attractive people more readily and people we perceive as our peers. We will follow a crowd more often than a single individual. We will be guided more readily by people we know than by strangers.

Fellow workers can be helpful in prompting specific behaviors. The Northeast Georgia Medical Center in Gainesville uses employee volunteer "coaches" in each department to stimulate use of its wellness programs. This may involve no more than asking their peers: "Hey, are you going to the wellness brown bag lunch today?" Coaches are expected to model desired behaviors, attending classes and participating in "Heart Walks," for example, to reinforce their verbal cues.[4]

Trinity Medical Center in Rock Island, Illinois, encourages women to select their own "buddy" who will remind them to perform breast self-examinations on a monthly basis and offers preprinted reminders in the form of stickers to put on both prompter and promptee calendars.[5] Many hospitals use volunteers to call people, reminding them of health education programs they are registered for. Physicians and dentists routinely have their staff remind patients of upcoming appointments, sending postcards and similar prompts.

In the stages of change, helping relationships are suggested as ways to support change. While such relationships may focus on providing motivation and assistance to those aiming for behavior improvement, they may also include prompting. "Buddies" in a formal helping relationship can remind each other, or a sponsor's staff may help consumers by reminding them of the time for infrequently repeated behaviors, such as annual screenings or immunizations that are needed at multiyear intervals.

The timing of prompts can be critical. Where they are intended merely to jog the memory, sending them just prior to the desired behavior is usually best. Calls the night before an appointment or event are likely to be well received, though even the same morning or just before may work as well. Since consumers are likely to differ, trial and error may be needed to determine the best timing for specific people and behaviors.

Simple announcements, posters, e-mail messages, faxes, phone calls, memos, and any number or combination of devices may be used to communicate a prompt, in addition to personal contact. Barriers may arise due to illiteracy of targeted consumers or language differences. All consumers are likely to be suffering from "information overload" or communications "noise" from the thousands of messages they are exposed to daily. Whatever medium is chosen to deliver a prompt, the message must somehow get through the clutter.[6]

Asking someone to do something may seem a simple enough approach, but there are tricks of the trade that have been shown to increase the probability of the desired response. Since they are *tricks*, they always run the risk that targets will feel *tricked* when they are used. As in all tactical choices, decisions on what prompts to use and how to deliver them should be made with full consideration of their potential impact on relationships, with both the target consumers and other stakeholders.

One well-documented adjunct to simple requests is touching the other person. When done tastefully and with the right people, interpersonal touch has been shown to improve attitudes toward the requester and to promote compliance with the request.[7] Sales professionals have to learn how to "ask for the sale" in clever ways, such as asking when the customer wants the product rather than whether. Once familiar with the technique, customers may feel manipulated and resist the prompt, however.[8]

There may be a limit on how many times the same consumers will respond to requests from the same source. If the prompted behavior is seen as doing the requester a favor, then a sense of equity may require that favors be reciprocated before the behavior is repeated. If responding proves beneficial to the prompted consumer, willingness to respond again to the same prompter can be enhanced.

To use prompts effectively, behavior improvement sponsors must choose carefully which consumers to use it for, relative to which behaviors, and under what circumstances. They should be sure that target consumers are motivated to comply and have no barriers to compliance. Sources of prompts, their frequency and timing, and how they are delivered and worded are all factors in determining success.

As the simplest, typically least expensive, and easiest to implement quickly, the use of prompts should almost always be among the tactical options considered. Where a low proportion of responses is all that is needed, it may be wasteful to use any other approach. Group Health of Puget Sound (Washington), for example, has an "I'll Try Anything Once Club" whose members (employees, physicians, enrollees) agree only to be placed on a list of people to be asked for volunteer activities. Callers simply contact enough people on the list to get the number they need to help, even if the success rate for this simple prompt is low.

Where other tactics are necessary, prompts should almost always be included. There is no point persuading consumers to act in a certain way or in training them how, then not prompting them as to when and where to act. Reminders may be necessary for the most highly motivated and capable consumer, given the press of other obligations and activities. Knowing exactly what action is desired, where and when it is to occur, and being sure that one is among those who are supposed to engage in it are all essential to effective prompting (Exhibit 11–1).

PERSUADING, OR "SELLING"

Persuasion is a communication tactic focused on *motivating* targets to adopt, repeat, or persevere in a particular behavior by "talking them into it." It presupposes that capability is not a problem, neither internal or external, but that more

Exhibit 11–1 Prompting

DEFINITION	✗ A SPECIFIC COMMUNICATION TO REMIND CONSUMERS TO ENGAGE IN AND/OR AVOID CERTAIN BEHAVIOR
OBJECTIVE	✗ TO REINFORCE COMMITMENTS ALREADY MADE SO CONSUMER ENGAGES IN DESIRED BEHAVIOR
EXAMPLES OF TECHNIQUES	✗ REMINDERS TO PARTICIPATE IN PROGRAMS OR HAVE HEALTH STATUS CHECKED ✗ REMINDERS TO USE SAFETY EQUIPMENT ✗ POSTERS & OTHER PRINT MEDIA TO JOG MEMORY
SUGGESTIONS	✗ TARGET THOSE WHO ARE MOTIVATED TO BEHAVE IN INDICATED WAY AND/OR COMPLY WITH REQUEST ✗ TARGET THOSE NOT HINDERED BY INCAPACITY OR EXTERNAL BARRIERS ✗ TARGET AND PACKAGE CLEVERLY SO MESSAGE GETS THROUGH THE CLUTTER & IS NOT PERCEIVED AS NAGGING ✗ PROMPT FOR BEHAVIOR THAT IS FAMILIAR, SIMPLE & CONSISTENT WITH CONSUMER'S VALUES AND ATTITUDES

than a prompt to heighten consciousness is required to stimulate compliance. Persuasion may employ entirely factual, objective information, appealing to rational, intellectual criteria. It may also employ emotional content, instead of or in addition to factual.

There are limits to the power of factual persuasion in converting consumers to a new behavior. According to an article in *Health Commons Update,* "Information alone cannot be viewed as the single ingredient necessary to trigger individual behavior change."[9] Arguments and emotional appeals, peer pressure, and similar approaches may be required. At the same time, persuasive communications should not be thought of as limited to conversion efforts; it can be equally useful in reinforcing motivation and behavior among the already converted.[10]

Effective persuasion focuses on the fundamental values of target consumers. The cleverest arguments delivered by a charismatic spokesperson can fail utterly if they address the values of the sponsor rather than those of the target of the message. Persuasion works best when people come to believe that they (or someone important to them) will benefit from changing their behavior, and that their basic human values will be protected or enhanced.

In designing persuasive communications, behavior engineers should identify which values are "engaged" relative to a specific behavior. Why are consumers acting the "wrong" way now? What values are being protected or enhanced by their "wrong" behavior? What values will be protected or enhanced if they change that behavior? What are the switching costs involved in altering current behavior patterns?

Relationships are pivotal in persuasion as well as in simple prompting. Trust and rapport determine whether persuasive information will be believed and arguments given serious weight by audiences. Where consumers believe the persuader is truly committed to or at least cares about their welfare rather than the persuader's personal interests or hidden agendas, then "sales" are a lot easier to make.[11]

Ideally the aim of persuasion ought to be to help consumers make the best choices or at least choices that lead to high levels of consumer satisfaction.[12] This requires that persuasive facts and arguments address consumers' basic human values and show how they will be protected or enhanced through specific behaviors. The extent to which personal values are affected by the behavior in question must be sufficient to "unfreeze" consumers from their negative behaviors, "convert" them to the positive behavior, and "refreeze" them into repeating and continuing new habits.

Persuasion Research

In selecting consumers as targets for persuasion, deciding that a persuasion tactic will be used, and designing the specifics of communications, research is often worthwhile, if not essential. In any "conversion" effort, identifying consumers' stages of readiness is helpful.[13] Determining why they are not already behaving in the desired fashion is vital. Identifying their level of capability, perceived external barriers, and self-efficacy are equally necessary.

Identifying consumer differences in "persuasion style" can be helpful in selecting differentiated approaches to different consumer segments. Some respond best to "tellers," high in credibility, and to arguments based on logic and evidence. Others respond better to "compellers" in positions of authority who can hint at rewards and punishments and status and prestige and who emphasize the consequences of not complying. Still others are better approached by "fellers" who can tear down their objections and appeal to tradition and examples of others. "Wellers" rely on empathy and trust, shared experiences and feelings, promising support and appealing for cooperation. "Sellers" carefully identify their audiences' values, needs, and concerns, stressing how consumers benefit from complying, while "Gellers" articulate shared visions and common goals, idealistic arguments and altruistic motivations.[14]

Research can be useful in identifying the channels consumers prefer in receiving communications and in what mode they prefer information to be delivered (e.g., individual or group sessions, summaries or full details).[15] Finding out what personal sources of health information consumers prefer and believe will help in deciding whether physicians, hospitals, health plans, or employers are in the best position to affect consumer behavior. Research can identify target consumers' states of knowledge, beliefs, perceptions, and attitudes—what changes in which will be needed to alter their behavior and what values can be appealed to for which consumers?[16]

Who Can Persuade?

Among effective sources of persuasion are persons in authority, such as managers and supervisors, if the behaviors in question are related to their "legitimate," accepted jurisdictions. Informal leaders can often be more effective in the workplace. Physicians and nurses may have the highest credibility when persuasion focuses on health effects of particular behaviors. Hospital staff may be ideal sources for reaching inpatients or ED visitors. Employers have access advantages for their employees and may be best at using arguments based on the effects of behavior patterns on employee and company success and survival. Health plans may still enjoy trust and credibility and have the database for selecting high-risk targets.

Peers are often powerful sources of persuasion. Someone who has been through it can be the most credible source of persuasion on what happens if people do not adopt positive behaviors (e.g., don't wear seat belts, use safety equipment, take medications), or do engage in negative behaviors (use drugs, drink and drive, use tobacco). Family and friends, coworkers, and members of the same peer group communicate cultural as well as personal preferences for consumers' behavior. Spouses, as sources of persuasive arguments and example, have been cited as one of the reasons married people tend to be healthier.[17]

The source for persuasive communications should be as carefully selected as the content. Behavior engineers should be willing to look beyond their own skills to consider consumers' friends and family as well as outside experts and people in authority. In selecting full-time persuaders for staff positions in health plans, hospitals, practices, or worksites, it is best to choose people who are good at empathy and building rapport and who wish to have an impact on others (i.e., who have strong dominance drives).[18]

Who Can Be Persuaded?

The best targets for persuasion, or any other behavior engineering effort for that matter, are those who promise the best combination of payoff and probability (i.e., impact and ease of conversion). In many cases high-risk, high-user populations are chosen because their conversion to preferred patterns of behavior will make the greatest difference to demand quality and quantity and health care expenditures. In other cases highly health conscious and concerned populations are chosen because they are easiest to convert.

Problems arise when combining the two criteria for target selection because they may not be correlated. Highest risk populations may be intractable, and behavior change efforts are likely to run into diminishing returns as they convert the most convertible early and are left with the stubborn holdouts. High-interest targets may already be models of healthy lifestyle, disease self-management, and prudent use of services, hence promising few opportunities for conversion.[19]

Most importantly, persuasion should only be employed with consumers who are fully capable of converting to the desired behavior. Education, particularly including training and practice, is often required as a complement to persuasion so that capability and self-efficacy can be addressed simultaneously with motivation. Target consumers should also be at one of the susceptible stages of readiness (e.g., contemplation or preparation for conversion; action, including relapse; or maintenance for reinforcement), in addition to being capable, where persuasion is to be used.

When To Persuade

The timing of persuasion efforts can be an issue in some cases. When public media attention has been given to some health or health-related news event (e.g., when a famous person has just died of breast cancer or AIDS, that may represent a unique opportunity for persuasive communication on the subject). Choices of plans and providers have their own schedules—most often annually for commercial plans, monthly for Medicare.

Some individuals may be particularly susceptible to or resistant to conversion at specific times. Soon after being diagnosed with a chronic condition, though perhaps not immediately thereafter while in denial, patients may be most receptive to disease management efforts. Just after an acute episode of a chronic condition may be another opportune time. Soon after pregnancy begins is both a receptive time and the best point to begin prenatal care. Just after a friend or family member has contracted or died from a condition may be an opportune moment for persuasion on prevention or management.

Persuasion is often used in conjunction with other tactics. It can be employed to entice consumers to attend an educational program, for example, or to contact a health information phone line or web site. It is frequently used whenever rewards or punishments are to employed and when marketing efforts have improved the offer. Persuasion can be used in a two-stage effort, as when widely targeted communications are used to stimulate interest and inquiries, then respondents are given additional direct-contact sales attention to complete the conversion. In all such cases the timing of communication should be based on fit with the other tactic used.

How To Persuade

There are innumerable texts on persuasion and sales and a limited capacity to cover the subject as part of one chapter. There are some general guidelines that appear valuable, however, and likely to apply to most persuasion challenges. There are also some tricks of the trade worth considering, though with the same caveats as applied to prompts in terms of moral/ethical concerns and their effects on relationships.

Marketing has identified three separate bases for persuading customers: product, place, and price. (The fourth "P" of the marketing mix, promotion, is persuasive communication itself.) If we can persuade consumers that a new behavior offers a better mix of these three, better than they previously thought and better than their present behavior, then those consumers ought to convert to the new behavior.

"Product," in the context of health and demand behaviors, refers to all the positive consequences of adopting, repeating, or persevering in a given behavior. The benefits of a behavior change—in terms of protecting or enhancing basic human values, solving a problem, or achieving a goal—tend to be the most powerful basis for persuasion. The benefits of consumers' present behavior, as consumers perceive them, are often the most important sources of resistance to change, the basis for "switching costs" that may have to be overcome.

Benefits may come in the form of identifiable physical health gains: protection against disease and injury, greater energy, or improved functioning. They may include a variety of psychosocial advantages as well: greater security/reduced anxiety; sense of being welcomed into, accepted and respected by a group; self-esteem and a sense of accomplishment; sheer fun and enjoyment; a greater sense of autonomy or control over one's life; desirable learning and understanding—any of the fundamental values discussed in Chapter 6.

"Place" factors include everything that people perceive as making a given behavior easy or difficult to adopt, repeat, or continue. If they can be persuaded that suggested forms of exercise are easier than they thought, that an educational program is convenient for them to go to, that using a phone or computer information and triage service is easier than their original perception, then they may be more open to the new behaviors. The key is to deal with what makes consumers perceive something to be easy or difficult.

"Price" covers whatever negative impact on their values consumers perceive a given behavior to have. It can include pain and discomfort, embarrassment and indignity, or any damage to the kinds of psychosocial values that offer potential "product" benefits. Out-of-pocket financial costs are sometimes involved, but need not play a part; there are plenty of other costs potentially included. Whatever benefits accrue to consumers from their negative behavior, as consumers perceive them, are potential switching costs when they give it up.

Persuasion relies on convincing consumers that the mix of benefits, convenience, and costs of the desired behavior are more attractive than they thought, and more attractive than their current behavior. Effective communication may convince consumers that the mix itself is better, that they should have greater confidence in experiencing the benefits and convenience they want or in realizing benefits sooner. Guarantees, endorsements by respected authorities, and testimonials from their peers can all raise consumers' assurance that they will get what they want, where skepticism may have held them back previously.[20]

Advertising research has shown the persuasive power of demonstration, of modeling, as a vicarious learning experience. Stories in the newspapers, case histories, testimonials, and videotape "slices of life" that show people very like target consumers changing their behavior, obtaining the promised benefit, and experiencing convenience and minimal costs can be significantly more powerful than arguments or promises. Encouraging and enabling targets to contact others who have had and will brag about their positive experiences, using phone, mail, Internet, fax, or e-mail, can achieve high levels of conversion.

Tailor messages as much as possible—to individuals if feasible and cost-effective or at least to consumer segments where applicable.[21] Studies suggest, for example, that boys are more affected by appeals to status; girls to relationships. Men are more likely to downplay their doubts in personal interactions; women to understate their certainty. Ethnic minorities are likely to respond better to appeals tailored to their interests and in their language.[22]

Use a variety of communications channels rather than rely on one. Combine personal contact, phone, and mail. Use multiple sources rather than rely on one: physicians, peers, family, and friends. Use multiple arguments, not just one. Use multiple repetitions versus expecting one to do the trick. A repeated "drip-drip" approach at a low pressure level can wear down resistance.[23] A multiplicity of approaches will help increase the probability that the intended targets are reached by persuasive messages. Multiple messages also tend to have a synergistic effect greater than multiplication of the same single message, source, and medium.

In personal counseling, plan to spend 50% of the time (or more) listening rather than talking. Encourage targets to voice their objections and work them into the argument by overcoming them. An objection that targets do not have enough time (e.g., for regular exercise) can be addressed by asking them what they would do if they had the time, then what they can afford, or even what they would prefer to eliminate from their busy schedule.[24] Translate arguments into personal terms: "you will" . . . die of cancer, enjoy greater energy, reduce your dependence on others, for example, rather than "people have" or "studies show," for example.[25] Give targets a reason to act now, "ask for the sale" rather than assume they will act just because they appear to be persuaded.[26]

In impersonal communications, promise less than consumers will experience rather than more so that they will have a pleasant surprise and feel they made an excellent choice. Promising more and delivering less will make people regret, possibly reverse, their conversion and will eliminate trust in any future communications from the same source—even on the same subject.[27] Make messages honest and complete; include the downside as well as upside wherever there are both. A "two-sided" message pointing out some drawback to conversion will be believed more readily than one promising only positive results.[28]

Fear appeals can be effective in some circumstances. Since there are proven negative consequences to engaging in and continuing a wide variety of health and demand behaviors, pointing out such consequences is part of full disclosure and honest communications. However, the first response by many people to scare tactics is to deny their truth or applicability in order to reduce their own anxiety immediately. If fear appeals are used, they should be coupled with advice people can implement immediately to reduce the fear created: "come in"; "see your doctor"; "write for help," for example, or denial is likely to win out.[29]

Giving people a benefit in advance, such as doing them a service or sending a free gift, can create a "favor debt" that predisposes targets to comply with persuasive communication.[30] Try using the "Pygmalion effect" by communicating both high expectations for consumers' behavior and high confidence that they will live up to those expectations.[31] The "Avis effect" is similar, involving communicating to others, such as peers or the public, the same high expectations and confidence in the behavior of identified consumers. The "agenda-setting effect" works by stimulating people to think about criteria and concerns they might otherwise ignore, even if the information is not new.

Exhibit 11–2 Persuasion

DEFINITION	X MOTIVATING CONSUMERS TO ADOPT, REPEAT, OR PERSEVERE IN PARTICULAR BEHAVIOR THROUGH COMMUNICATIONS ALONE
OBJECTIVE	X TO HELP CONSUMERS MAKE BEST CHOICES, CHOICES THAT LEAD TO HIGH LEVELS OF PERSONAL SATISFACTION
EXAMPLES OF TECHNIQUES	X SPONSOR CONVINCES CONSUMER OF POSITIVE CONSEQUENCES OF CHANGING BEHAVIOR X SPONSOR ADVISES CONSUMER ON MAKING CHANGE EASY X SPONSOR SHOWS CONSUMER HOW COSTS OF OLD BEHAVIOR ARE HIGH
SUGGESTIONS	X TARGET THOSE WHO PROMISE BEST COMBINATION OF PAYOFF & PROBABILITY X TARGET THOSE WHO ARE HIGHLY HEALTH CONSCIOUS / CONCERNED X USE WHEN A PERSON IS IN CRISIS WHERE NEED IS GREATER THAN RELUCTANCE TO CHANGE X IDENTIFY CONSUMER'S LEVEL OF CAPABILITY, PERCEIVED EXTERNAL BARRIERS & SELF-EFFICACY

Make sure that persuasive messages include a full description of exactly who is to do exactly what, where, when, how often—exactly the same level of detail that would be used where a simple prompt is employed. If capability is an issue, or self-efficacy and confidence are factors, include descriptions, diagrams, or maps, for example, that will point out how consumers are to behave. While persuasion focuses on motivation, including information to remind and enable consumers will augment its effect, unless they feel their intelligence has been insulted.

To confirm that persuasion has had the desired effect, have people describe, in their own words, what they are going to do and how and why they are going to do it.[32] Getting them to voice their intentions aloud creates almost a "contract" effect and reinforces their commitment to the desired behavior. It takes advantage of "cognitive dissonance," since most people tend to try to make their actions consistent with their words. It also provides a test to be sure they know the behavior details regarding what, when, and where as well as how and why.

While many of these "tricks of the trade" have good track records in persuasion and sales, they may contravene ethical standards and moral principles of some health professionals. They may also risk damage to relationships with other stakeholders and with consumers themselves, who may feel tricked or otherwise manipulated. The safer alternative may well be to approach each behavior engineering challenge as a *shared problem to be jointly solved*. Get on the same side of the table with consumers and look for ways to achieve something together.[33]

To make this approach credible, as well as to create essential trust, identify what *you* expect to gain from the conversion, as well as what the consumers gain. In any capitation payment system, physicians, hospitals, health plans, and employers should gain financially from healthier consumer behavior, from improving the quality, and from reducing the cost of health service use. Making this financial gain clear up front will make a partnership approach more credible to consumers.

A true partnership approach in which behavior engineers communicate openly with consumers and develop ways to share gains will promote more lasting working relationships for future challenges. Shared goals, efforts, and accomplishments will strengthen the partnership and lead to positive expectations about future efforts. Open, honest communications will promote trust and openness by consumers. Sharing gains will make consumers truly feel that everyone is working together as members of the same team[34] (Exhibit 11–2).

REFERENCES

1. J. Carew, *You'll Never Get No for an Answer* (New York: Pocket Books, 1987).
2. R. Winslow, "An HMO Tries Talking Members into Healthy Habits," *Wall Street Journal,* 6 April 1994, B1, B6.

3. S. Ornstein, "Barriers to Adherence to Preventive Services Reminder Letters: The Patient's Perspective," *Journal of Family Practice* 36, no. 2 (1993):195–200.

4. "Hospital's 'Health Coaches' Spread the Word," *Employee Health & Fitness* 18, no. 1 (1996):10–11.

5. R. Weiss, "Market Response Systems: A Community Interface," *Health Progress* 75, no. 6 (1994):68–69.

6. L. Chapman, "Awareness Strategies," in *Health Promotion in the Workplace,* 2d ed., M. O'Donnell and J. Harris, eds. (Albany, NY: Delmar, 1994), 163–184.

7. J. Hornik, "Tactile Stimulation and Consumer Response," *Journal of Consumer Research,* December 1992, 449–458.

8. R. Cialdini, *Influence: Science and Practice,* 3d ed. (New York: Harper Collins, 1993).

9. E. Young, "Social Marketing: Where It Has Come From; Where It's Going," *Health Promotion* (1988):2–5, 26.

10. P. Sherlock, "The Irrationality of 'Rational' Business Buying," *Marketing Management* 1, no. 2 (1992):9–15.

11. J. Carew, *You'll Never Get No for an Answer.*

12. G. Moskoff, "Want Satisfied Customers? Get a New Attitude about Learning," *Marketing Executive Report* 3, no. 6 (1993):1, 12.

13. J. Prochaska, J. Norcross, and C. DiClemente, *Changing for Good* (New York: Avon Books, 1994).

14. E. Zuker, *The Seven Secrets of Influence* (New York: McGraw-Hill, 1991).

15. L. Meszaros, "Various Communications Forms Team Up To Deliver Knowledge," *Managed Healthcare* 6, no. 12 (1996):50–52.

16. P. Allessandra, P. Wexler, and R. Barrera, *Non-Manipulative Selling,* 2d ed. (New York: Prentice-Hall, 1987).

17. "The Wedding Bell Health Plan," *Health* 9, no. 4 (1994): 12–13.

18. "Selling Wellness to a Suspicious World," *Health Care Advertising Review,* March/April 1996, 1–8.

19. N. Jeffrey, "Wellness Plans Try To Target the Not-So-Well," *The Wall Street Journal,* 20 June 1996, B1, B6.

20. R. Dawson, *Secrets of Power Persuasion* (Englewood Cliffs, NJ: Prentice-Hall, 1995).

21. R. Hampson, "Death of a Truly Great Salesman," *Seattle Post-Intelligencer,* 25 November 1993, F4.

22. D. Tanner, "The Power of Talk: Who Gets Heard and Why," *Harvard Business Review* 73, no. 5 (1995):138–148.

23. "Drip Marketing—Or How To Cultivate High Potential Patients or Clients," *The Practice Builder* 12, no. 2 (1994):1–3.

24. "I Don't Have Time for Exercise," *Health Promotion Practitioner* 5, no. 3 (1996):3.

25. M. Oechsli, "How To Unleash the Power of the 'Pygmalion Effect,' " *Sales and Marketing Executive Report* (undated sample received May 1994), 6–7.

26. H. Fahner, "Getting Commitment from the Buyer," *Sales and Marketing Executive Report* (undated sample received May 1994), 4.

27. D. Caracciolo, "'Marketers Should Never Sell' Is a Myth To Be Avoided," *Marketing News,* 13 September 1993, 4.

28. R. Dawson, *Secrets of Power Persuasion.*

29. T. Backer, E. Rogers, and P. Sopory, *Designing Health Communication Campaigns: What Works?* (Newbury Park, CA: Sage, 1992), 30–32.

30. R. Dilenschneider, *Power and Influence: Mastering the Art of Persuasion* (New York: Prentice-Hall, 1990).

31. R. Miller, P. Brickman, and D. Bolen, "Attribution vs. Persuasion as a Means for Modifying Behavior," *Journal of Personality & Social Psychology* 31 (1975):430–441.

32. "Let Yourself Be Influential," *The Pryor Report* 7, no. 1A (1990):2.

33. G. Moskoff, "Want Satisfied Customers?" 1, 12.

34. J. Case, "Opening the Books," *Harvard Business Review* 75, no. 2 (1997):118–127.

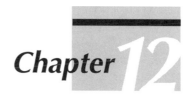

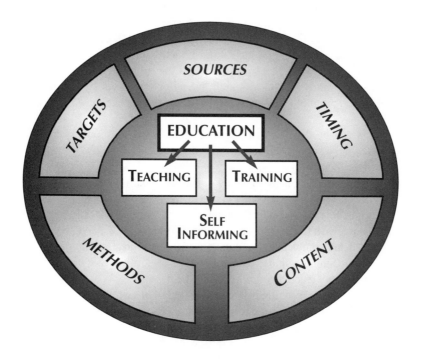

Chapter 12

EDUCATION

The American Academy of Family Practice defines patient education as "the process of influencing patient behavior, producing changes in knowledge, attitudes and skills required to maintain or improve health."[1(p1)] Among the four communications tactics used to improve consumer behavior, this chapter will define education as an alternative or complement to the persuasion tactics covered in the previous chapter. In the $I = MC^2$ context, education tactics are designed to improve consumer capability, giving them the knowledge, skills, and confidence (self-efficacy) they need to adopt and continue healthy behavior and appropriate demand for health services. Persuasion is aimed strictly at motivation and prompting at consciousness.

Education can also provide the basis for consciousness raising in the stages of change model by supplying additional information that will cause consumers to awaken to the possibility of changing behavior, moving them from the precontemplation to the contemplation stage. Education by a provider may be most effective in this regard, though also least efficient. Education by health plans and employers may be more efficient, though less effective in consciousness raising where members or employees question the motivation or expertise of these sponsors.

Education can be thought of in terms of three separate though related processes—teaching, training, and self-informing, as discussed below:

1. Teaching. Teaching is the enabling of people to learn (i.e., acquire knowledge and understanding) through the active intervention of individual teachers and programs. It is instigated by the sponsor with some specific objective in mind. To distinguish it from persuading, it consists of factual, objective, and hopefully balanced and complete information on subjects of interest, helping consumers learn something of value to them, in addition to whatever value it represents to the sponsors of teaching efforts (Exhibit 12–1).

2. Training. Where teaching is intended to impart knowledge, training is aimed at enabling consumers to acquire specific skills, in first aid, self-care, shared decision making, gauging blood-sugar (diabetes) or peak flow (asthma) levels, and using safety equipment or new procedures, for example. It may be initiated by consumers seeking out someone to help them learn a skill or by trainers seeking to impart a skill. At its core, training includes enabling consumers to become better learners and more assertive participants in making health decisions, improving their ability to add to the effectiveness and efficiency of health service encounters. The object is that they not only should acquire specific skills but also should gain full confidence in their use, so they will have no hesitancy in employing them at the appropriate time (Exhibit 12–2).

3. Information (self-informing). Complementing teaching and training, which involve the active intervention of educators and trainers, are information sources that consumers may access on their own.[2] In this definition the search for information is initiated by consumers, though it may be promoted by payers or providers. Such information may be accessed impersonally, through books and written materials, audiotapes and videotapes, interactive video and television systems, computers, or any variety of technological means. (See Chapter 9.) It may also be accessed personally through calls to

Exhibit 12–1 Teaching

DEFINITION	✗ SPONSOR-INITIATED COMMUNICATIONS ENABLING CONSUMERS TO ACQUIRE KNOWLEDGE & UNDERSTANDING
OBJECTIVE	✗ TO IMPROVE CONSUMER *CAPABILITY* BY ENABLING THEM TO GAIN KNOWLEDGE ABOUT HEALTH & DEMAND THAT THEY CAN AND WILL USE TO IMPROVE THEIR BEHAVIOR
EXAMPLES OF TECHNIQUES	✗ MEMOS, NEWSLETTERS, WRITTEN MATERIALS, PERSON-TO-PERSON & PERSON-TO-GROUP COUNSELING & PRESENTATIONS, AUDIOTAPE / VIDEOTAPES, INTERACTIVE VIDEO & TV
SUGGESTIONS	✗ INCLUDE WAYS OF ENHANCING CONSUMER CONFIDENCE & SELF-EFFICACY AS WELL AS KNOWLEDGE ✗ USE RESPECTED, TRUSTED, AUTHORITATIVE & CREDIBLE SOURCES, INCLUDING PEERS ✗ USE MULTIPLE FORMATS & VEHICLES, MULTIPLE SOURCES ✗ MAKE SURE INFORMATION IS ACCURATE & UP-TO-DATE. TEST KNOWLEDGE ACQUIRED TO EVALUATE TEACHING & PROMOTE SELF-EFFICACY

Exhibit 12–2 Training

DEFINITION	X SPONSOR-INITIATED BUILDING & REINFORCEMENT OF CONSUMER SKILLS
OBJECTIVE	X TO IMPROVE CONSUMER CAPABILITY BY ENABLING THEM TO GAIN SKILLS THAT THEY CAN & WILL USE TO IMPROVE THEIR HEALTH & DEMAND FOR HEALTH SERVICES
EXAMPLES OF TECHNIQUES	X SELF-TRAINING MANUALS & GUIDES, ONE-ON-ONE SESSIONS, GROUP SESSIONS, SIMULATIONS / VIRTUAL REALITY EXPERIENCES
SUGGESTIONS	X USE RESPECTED, TRUSTED EXPERTS & PEERS WHO CAN PERFORM SKILLS WELL THEMSELVES X OFFER MULTIPLE OPPORTUNITIES & VEHICLES X TEST SKILL PERFORMANCE TO EVALUATE TRAINING & PROMOTE SELF-EFFICACY X INCLUDE OPPORTUNITIES FOR SUPERVISED PERFORMANCE OF SKILLS

triage nurses, treatment counselors, support group members and others qualified to offer information of interest (Chapter 22; Exhibit 12–3).

The combination of teaching, training, and information aims first at enabling consumers to acquire knowledge and skills, get answers to questions, involve themselves in medical decision making, and otherwise become well-informed, competent, and confident partners with providers and other stakeholders in managing their own health affairs. Its second aim is to empower consumers to take responsibility for their own health and demand behaviors, reducing their dependence on providers and enabling them to ensure that their values are considered, if not dominant, in making personal health decisions.[3]

While these tactics are aimed principally at improving or reinforcing the ability of consumers to act, they have the added effect of boosting motivation as well. People with newly acquired knowledge and skills are likely to want to use them at the appropriate opportunity and sometimes even at inappropriate opportunities. Part of the challenge in promoting self-efficacy is to ensure that consumers have the ability to discern when they should use their capabilities and when to look elsewhere.

WHO CAN EDUCATE?

As was true for prompting and persuading, the sources of education can make a significant difference in whether they will be sought by consumers and what impact they will have. Authority, expertise, and credibility are as essential to education as they are to persuasion. Being taught or trained by someone who is enthusiastic about the knowledge and skills being covered and is committed to their being mastered by participants can make all the difference in the effectiveness of teaching and training efforts. Information offered by authoritative, credible, and respected sources, as perceived by consumers, is more likely to be sought and used.

Physicians and other health professionals have distinct advantages as educators. The personal physician can convey information in person and through handout materials, bulletin boards, libraries, and many other channels.[4] The American Academy of Family Practice has taken a strong position calling for family physicians to take a leadership role in health education.[5] Even as they shift to a partnership rather than authoritarian relationship with patients, providers are essential and significant players.

Unfortunately physicians are typically not trained in educating patients and may not see education as part of their role. They are also unlikely to be cost-effective, given their remuneration levels. On the other hand, they may find it worthwhile to seek training in patient education, including techniques such as group counseling, through which they can be more cost-effective.

Exhibit 12–3 Information

DEFINITION	✗ PROVIDER-INITIATED ACCESSING OF DATA, REPORTS & EXPERIENCES OF OTHERS
OBJECTIVE	✗ TO ENABLE CONSUMERS TO DISCOVER FACTS THAT WILL HELP THEM MAKE BETTER DECISIONS ABOUT HEALTH & DEMAND
EXAMPLES OF TECHNIQUES	✗ PHYSICIAN OFFICE BULLETIN BOARDS ✗ HOSPITAL LIBRARIES & RECORDS ✗ HEALTH PLAN INFORMATION SERVICES ✗ INTERNET ACCESS WEB SITES, CHAT ROOMS
SUGGESTIONS	✗ MAKE MULTIPLE AVENUES AVAILABLE FOR ACCESSING INFORMATION ✗ KEEP CURRENT THROUGH REGULAR UPDATING ✗ CREATE SUPPORT GROUPS FOR CONSUMERS WITH SIMILAR NEEDS ✗ ENLIST COMMUNITY INFORMATION ORGANIZATIONS TO HELP

Under fee-for-service payment systems, physicians have often found that playing an educator role was financially unrewarding, the kind of "intellectual service" that insurers refused to cover. Into the vacuum they left have stepped a number of proprietary vendors who have responded to the demands of health plans, employers, and consumers. It will be a challenge for physicians to reestablish a significant role.

Hospitals, their nurses, and educators have been valuable sources of information, teaching, and training for patients. Conventional and interactive television have been supplied in inpatient rooms.[6] Patient education programs, scheduled for patients before, during, and after episodes of treatment, have long been part of the hospital mission. Newsletters are commonly used by hospitals to convey information of interest to patients between episodes.[7] Flower Hospital in Sylvania, Ohio, offers Internet linkage for health information sources to patients, local residents, and businesses.[8]

Universities have begun to take on an active role in consumer health education. The University of Wisconsin, for example, operates a computerized health enhancement support system (CHESS) as part of a chronic pain management program.[9] It enables patients facing a wide variety of chronic conditions and life-threatening situations to obtain information from providers, peers, libraries, and self-help support groups. It is offered through HMOs and hospitals to improve consumers' emotional well-being, reduce health-risk behaviors, and improve the cost-effectiveness of health service use.[10]

Employers have an extensive, if not widespread history of educational efforts aimed at employees. Southwest Airlines, for example, has worked on conveying to employees the extent of health care costs by translating dollars of expenditure into the number of airline peanut packages and six-packs of beer "spent" per month.[11] Unions have been equally active: the Chicago Truck Drivers, Helpers and Warehouse Workers Union uses monthly meetings for employees and quarterly meetings of retirees and dependents to report on how their money is being spent as well as to promote wellness and health programs.[12]

Health plans are investing in the education of their members. Kaiser offers the HealthDesk software program to facilitate member access to information on such subjects as women's health, nutrition, stress, and heart problems.[13] US Healthcare provides its members an Internet World Wide Web site with menus offering information on prevention, self-care, chronic condition management and treatment options, with upwards of 3,000 "hits" a day from members.[14]

Group Health of Puget Sound offered its members a catalog of hundreds of free educational programs to excite their interests, with a 16% response rate.[15] It also offers health information via the Internet for members with computers.[16] Harvard Community Health Plan gives selected high-risk members a computer to facilitate access to triage, health-risk appraisals, monitoring, and chronic condition management information, as well as a vehicle for reminding the members of appointments and prompting them when it is time for immunizations, for example.[17]

WHO ARE THE BEST TARGETS?

Research is needed to identify the best consumers to target for particular teaching and training efforts, those segments most interested in which types of information. Ideally teaching and training efforts should be designed with at least a rough notion as to where the targets start from and what knowledge, beliefs, and skills they already possess. This will help make programs more effective and efficient, enabling consumers at different levels of interest, readiness to change, or existing knowledge to be approached separately, for example. It also provides the basis for evaluation of specific programs, looking for changes in knowledge, beliefs, skills, and confidence that have been achieved.

Like persuasion, education programs should be aimed, wherever possible, at individuals and segments who promise the greatest benefit if converted to the desired behavior and have the greatest probability of conversion. Family members should be included in efforts where their support and influence are likely to be felt. Programs should be customized to individuals and groups with particular needs or unusual access problems.

Workers are ideal targets for union and employer initiatives, for example. On-site programs can be both effective and efficient for larger employee groups. The growing ranks of "telecommuters" working at home can be accessed by the same computers that make the arrangement possible, with education, training, and prompting on "desk exercises" a natural opportunity.[18] Consumers with computers can be reached through a variety of health education software programs.[19] A modem means Internet possibilities can be included.

TIMING

The timing of programs aimed at teaching, training, and informing consumers can be a critical factor in their effectiveness and efficiency. The ideal timing is "just in time": when targets are both most receptive to/interested in the information and as close as possible to using it. Specific life events that create some type of personal crisis, such as the diagnosis of a new condition, may be optimal educational opportunities in terms of receptivity.[20] Timing to match that of the opportunity for use depends on the situation.

For example, timing of teaching, training, and information related to pregnancy is relatively simple, with nine months lead time. Preoperative and preadmission education is easy enough when elective procedures are involved, and it has been shown to have significant positive effects.[21] The best timing for information on managing chronic conditions may be soon after diagnosis or right after an acute episode.

Many health plans offer orientation sessions immediately after new members join. For member service information and advice on how to access health information, this may be good timing. For information on use of health services, however, few members may recall the information and advice they are given, unless their need for care arises soon thereafter. Most orientation efforts should be supplemented by access to as-needed information so that consumers can determine the timing for obtaining precisely the information they want when they want it.

HOW BEST TO EDUCATE

An essential task in designing and implementing successful education programs is making them sufficiently attractive and satisfying so that desired participation and impact can be achieved. A marketing approach based on product, place, and price factors should help in this challenge, just as in persuasion efforts. The difference is that in education, the marketing mix focuses on design of the teaching, training, or information program itself, in addition to communications about it.

The focus of all such programs should be on delivering added value to consumers, over and above what is necessary to achieving a behavior change objective.[22] Consumers should enter educational encounters with expectations of quality-of-life improvement and the enhancement or protection of their basic values. It should be as easy as possible for them to participate in programs and to access information, and there should be multiple opportunities for doing so rather than a "one-size-fits-all" approach. Costs of participation, in time, dollars spent, and risk to self-esteem, for example, should be minimized or at least commensurate with the value promised and delivered.

Programs need to be geared to individual interests and learning styles. Some people prefer hearing information, others prefer seeing and reading, while still others need to practice their learning in terms of guided behaviors. One health education publication suggests adjusting the approach used to the mix of participants in terms of:

- Scientific learners—respond to data, experiments, studies, and statistics;
- Inner-self learners—want personal growth and understanding;
- Anticipators—need to examine new ideas conceptually before accepting them;
- Validators—need to test ideas in practice, choose own approach;
- Accomplishers—want to solve a specific problem, achieve an objective;
- Role takers—visualize new selves or situations, strive to get there; and
- Emulators—model behavior after someone they admire, respect.[23]

To achieve the highest levels of participation in teaching/training programs or the highest use of information sources, design and implement the entire experience from the consumer's perspective. Plan every effort, from building initial awareness to consumers' calling for information or registration, to coming to a program location, room comfort, teaching and training experience, drills and simulations, learning checks, follow-up for feedback and reinforcement, to reporting opportunities to apply what was learned. For information services, manage initial awareness, the contact process, finding the desired information, validating it, and using it, with both user-instigated and provider-initiated feedback opportunities. Enlist volunteer consumers to make "dry runs" through the entire experience to identify and correct snags before inviting wide-scale participation.

Set explicit objectives for each encounter: specific knowledge, beliefs, skills, and confidence to be gained. Plan the experience to achieve those objectives and evaluate results to see how well they are achieved. Couple teaching and training with persuasion and prompts where needed to achieve the ultimate behavior change objectives and evaluate how well those are achieved as well.

Education in the form of announcements and displays may be used to promote participation in specific teaching or training programs and to attract users of information services. Persuasion techniques and prompting are likely to be helpful as well. Rather than rely completely on communications, incentives may be offered to consumers: reduced fees or free teaching and training, even "frequent flyer" bonuses for completing a course or participating in multiple courses may be used. To promote use of a triage or decision counseling information service, copayment levels may be reduced. (See Chapter 14 on incentives.)

CONTENT SUGGESTIONS

Teaching and training programs may work better for some targets if they begin by promoting self-esteem. One such approach asks participants to list or recite what they have learned since birth. Virtually everyone will be able to come up with an impressive list of knowledge and skills, from learning to walk, talk, read, and write to learning multiplication tables and local geography, for example. While none of the items on the list may be particularly impressive, the sheer length of the list should remind participants of their innate capability to learn.[24]

Make sure that the content of educational efforts reflects the values and perceptions of learners, rather than those of health professionals and sponsors. All too often, participants are turned off by obvious biases resulting from the training and socialization of professionals or special interests of payers or pharmaceutical vendors, for example.[25] If participants feel content is geared to promoting the sponsor's interests rather than those of the consumers, they are likely to treat the information content as so much advertising.

VERIFICATION

Include verification of learning in teaching and training programs. In teaching, ask participants to express what they have learned in their own words, both to verify the correctness of their learning and to reinforce their confidence in it.[26] In training, give participants the opportunity to demonstrate their skill wherever possible: using dummies for CPR, using exercise equipment on site, or showing their skills with blood sugar monitoring/insulin injection or peak flow measurement, for example.[27]

Formal assessments of learning may be used in decision counseling. Enabling consumers to check their own learning via interactive video and computer programs creates nonthreatening opportunities for them to monitor their own progress and see where they need additional help. Once they have "passed," demonstrating full and accurate understanding of the options, they can truly be said to have given "informed consent" to whatever they choose. This not only promotes better outcomes and patient satisfaction; it also reduces the risks of litigation against providers.[28]

For information services, verification can be attempted by making follow-up contacts to callers in phone access programs, to requesters of written information, and to Internet surfers. The information seekers can be asked if they located the information they sought and can be requested to summarize what they learned from the experience. This may provide opportunities to correct misinterpretations of information as well as evaluate the effects of specific programs.

METHODS

Just as multiple repetitions of prompts and persuasion from multiple sources makes these approaches more effective, so do they aid educational efforts. Especially where participants are not getting their education just in time, some repetition may be needed to keep their knowledge and skills at effective levels when the time comes to use them. Given the many different learning styles affecting consumers, having visual, audio, graphic, and experiential opportunities will help reach everyone. Getting the same basic information from multiple sources adds to its credibility and impact.

In a systematic study of educational efforts aimed at reducing heart disease risks among auto industry workers, the University of Michigan found that supplementing formal classes and in-plant media presentations with group discussions and one-on-one counseling, social support systems, and plant-wide "corporate culture" communications significantly increased participation in programs. Participation was up to eight or nine times higher where multiple channels of communication were used, and health risk reduction results were much greater.[29]

Health and demand-related education can be delivered in conjunction with other communications in order to increase efficiency. Physicians can send health messages and advice in greeting cards to patients. Employers can include, for example, health messages in other announcements, memos, and on bulletin boards.[30] Hospitals can include customized health information in their inpatient television programs.[31]

Using multiple sources can include the use of peers and "reformed" high-risk consumers as teachers and sources of information. Assigning "buddies" who have already mastered skills or who can remind targets of desired behaviors has proven effective. Employing a diversity of experiences, such as role playing, group sessions, and exercises, in addition to lecturing, has improved results of teaching programs.[32]

While we are just beginning to test the effectiveness and efficiency of new technologies, early results suggest that they are generally superior to older approaches. Interactive video and television technologies seem to work better for both children[33] and adults[34] than do their passive counterparts. Computer-based, multimedia training has proven more effective and efficient than using live trainers.[35] Consumers have indicated preference for computer-driven information access as compared to human counselors, considering their lower availability compared to 24-hour, easy access to computers.[36]

There are many home software programs already available to supplement information sources offered by payers and providers. The Home Medical Advisor Pro, Mayo Clinic's Family Health Book, and Medical House Call all offer information and advice on symptoms, treatments, and over-the-counter (OTC) medications.[37] CD-ROM software such as The Family Doctor, Complete Guide to Symptoms and Illnesses, and Personal Pediatrician and Family Pharmacist make enormous amounts of information readily available to computer-equipped homes.[38] This is expected to be among the fastest-growing opportunities for software and Internet information vendors.

It has been argued that computer-based education is sometimes better than that offered by physicians and professional educators. Computers can include drills, tests, and simulations that would stretch the skills and time available to professionals. Computer programs include the ongoing ability to check on learning in a way consumers find more acceptable than being quizzed by other persons. They allow consumers to access the information they want when they want it, rather than trying to fit into a physician's busy schedule.[39]

Enabling patients to surf the Internet for information can save time for physicians, though it also runs the risk that patients will discover information calling into question their physician's diagnosis or treatment.[40] Using e-mail permits educators to customize the content and timing of messages to individual consumers.[41] Communications sent via e-mail can await consumers' availability and interest and can be read at their leisure.[42] It can be used both ways, for consumers to request information and ask questions as well as to receive educational messages.[43]

By tracking contacts from consumers to information services, as well as registrations to teaching and training programs, payers and providers can build a database on who is interested and informed and has been taught and trained on what subjects. Such information can then be used to select who should be targeted for additional related educational efforts or who needs to be selected for special attention due to lack of response.

Additional technologies are available for educational purposes. The Starbright Pediatric Network offers a PC-based "virtual playground" for seriously ill, hospitalized children to connect with each other across distant hospitals, as well as to entertain themselves and reduce their pain, anxiety, and depression. The program has resulted in reductions on requests for pain medication as much as 50% in hospitals making it available.[44]

HMOs can enlist their members as "health partners" in the "Put Prevention into Practice" program, providing an on-line prevention news service customized to individual households and accessed either on home computers or employers' computer workstations. The system offers, for example, personal monitoring for diabetes, prompts for appointments, immunizations, and screening tests in addition to ongoing prevention education.[45]

SPRINT has rolled out the Public Information Exchange service, linking businesses, consumers, and sources/distributors of information such as federal government agencies, consumer organizations, public health and human service agencies, and libraries. Its subset Public Health Information, sponsored by the National Health Council (comprising over 40 of the largest voluntary health organizations, plus state and local governments, physician groups, and provider organizations), combines vast information resources available through the Internet and is capable of sending information on line, via fax, e-mail, or conventional mail services.[46]

Interactive video has been successfully used by physicians and payers for years in counseling patients on treatment options.[47] Interactive television has been employed in hospitals.[48] The Jones Education Network is developing a consumer health network, mirroring the growing number of specialty news networks, to make both news and feature information widely available to cable subscribers.[49] On-line Internet services are available describing the wide variety of information services, support groups, and self-help organizations accessible via the Internet.[50]

Not that everything is wonderful in cyberspace. Consumers may find locating the right source of information difficult, time consuming, and therefore expensive. They may encounter wildly conflicting suggestions and experiences among their peers, and some of the weirdest advice imaginable. With no quality control on access to the Internet, it is truly "caveat emptor" in ways that licensure and certification of providers has greatly reduced. Despite these limitations and frustrations, the Internet seems to be the fastest-growing and highest potential source of health education for consumers.[51]

Despite the vast array of education sources, vehicles for transmitting and accessing information, and the best techniques for increasing consumer knowledge and skills, it is clear that information alone is not a sufficient, though it may be a necessary, cause of meaningful and lasting consumer behavior change. The better we master the use of information, the closer we can come to reaching its full potential. But we cannot overcome its inherent limits; hence additional approaches will be discussed in the following chapters.

REFERENCES

1. *Patient Education: A Leadership Role for Family Physicians and the AAFP* (Kansas City, MO: American Academy of Family Practice, 1993), 1.

2. S. Davis and J. Botkin, "The Coming of Knowledge-Based Business," *Harvard Business Review* 72, no. 5 (1994):165–170.

3. A. Farquharson, *Teaching in Practice* (San Francisco, CA: Jossey-Bass, 1995).

4. C. Aguilar, "Patient Education Begins in a Primary Care Setting," *Optimal Health,* January/February 1985, 30–32.

5. *Patient Education.*

6. V. Cason, "Do You Computer Take This Television . . . ?" *Healthcare Informatics,* May 1992, 12–15.

7. "Customized Newsletters Provide Health Care Marketing Tool," *St. Anthony's Managing Community Health and Wellness,* 6.

8. S. Turner, "Plugged In to the Community," *Hospitals & Health Networks,* 20 January 1996, 48.

9. "CHESS™ Helps Patients to Better Care," *Health Commons Update* 3 (Summer 1995):2.

10. S. Sasenick, "Enhancing Health through Technology," *Healthcare Forum Journal* 38, no. 1 (1995):50.

11. "That's Not Peanuts," *Modern Healthcare,* 13 December 1993, 48.

12. E.M. Robertson, "PPO Bets It Can Tame Costs without Coercion," *Managed Healthcare News* 2, no. 3 (1992):6, 7.

13. K. Taylor, "Patient Software: Consultation at the Stroke of a Key," *Hospitals & Health Networks,* 5 September 1994, 72.

14. "U.S. Healthcare Educates Consumers via the Internet," *Inside Preventive Care* 1, no. 10 (1996): 6.

15. S. Nelson and E. Maki, "Marketing and Health Education: A Collaborative Relationship," in *1985 Group Health Proceedings* (Washington, DC: Group Health Association of America, 1985), 172–178.

16. M. Cross, "Weaving Consumers into the 'Net,' " *Health Data Management,* September 1995, 18.

17. L. Harris and C. Crawford, "Electronic Umbilical Cords Bring Healthcare Back Home," *Healthcare Forum Journal* 39, no. 1 (1996):26–31.

18. "Health Promotion for Telecommuters," *Health Promotion Practitioner* 4, no. 12 (1995):5.

19. Taylor, "Patient Software," 72.

20. Farquharson, *Teaching in Practice.*

21. B.A. Webber, "Patient Education: A Review of the Issues," *Medical Care* 28, no. 11 (1993): 1089–1103.

22. Davis and Botkin, "The Coming of Knowledge-Based Business," 165–170.

23. "Learning Styles Determine Counseling Techniques," *Health Promotion Practitioner* 4, no. 11 (1995):6, 7.

24. "Reversing Low Self-Image," *Health Promotion Practitioner* 3, no. 12 (1994):7.

25. M. Baker, "The Chief Scientist Reports . . . Marketing Health," *Health Bulletin* (UK) 46, no. 5 (1988):296–303.

26. "Let's All Talk: Medical Education Is a Team Effort," in *Talk about Prescriptions Planning Guide* (Washington, DC: National Council on Patient Information and Education, 1993), 1–16.

27. Aguilar, "Patient Education," 30–32.

28. "How To Prepare Your Mind and Body for Surgery," *Consumer Reports on Health* 9 (1997):85–89.

29. J. Erfurt, et al., "Improving Participation in Worksite Wellness Programs: Comparing Health Education Classes, A Menu Approach, and Follow-Up Counseling," *American Journal of Health Promotion* 4 (1990):270–278.

30. "Nook and Cranny Wellness," *Health Promotion Practitioner* 3, no. 12 (1994):5.

31. E. Wogensen, "New System Turns In-Room Television into Versatile Patient, Staff Tool," *Strategic Health Care Marketing,* December 1995, 7, 8.

32. "6 Ways To Make Classroom Health Education Better," *Health Promotion Practitioner* 4, no. 12 (1995):4.

33. Webber, "Patient Education," 1089–1103.

34. "Don't Should on Me: Interactive Training Techniques for Health Promotion," *Wellness Management* 11, no. 2 (Summer 1995): 7.

35. B. Hall, *Return-on-Investment and Multimedia Training* (San Francisco, CA: Multimedia, Inc., 1995).

36. "Healthcare on the Superhighway," *Modern Healthcare,* 11 December 1995, 68.

37. G. Cowley, "The Rise of Cyberdoc," *Newsweek,* 26 September 1994, 54, 55.

38. J. Berke and C. Berke, "Disk Doctors: Home Health Software Can Help You Understand What Hurts," *Colorado Homes & Lifestyles Magazine,* October 1995, 165, 166.

39. G. Kahn, "Computer-Based Patient Education: A Progress Report," *MD Computing* 10, no. 2 (1993):93–99.

40. P. Engstrom, "Control in the Balance: How the Net Is Tipping the Doctor-Patient Scale," *Medicine on the Net,* December 1995, 1–4.

41. M. Chamberlain, "New Technologies in Health Communications," *American Behavioral Scientist* 38, no. 2 (1994):271–284.

42. C. Lu, "The E-Mail Edge," *INC. Technology* 4 (1995):39.

43. F. Bazzoli, "The Allure of the Internet," *Health Data Management,* June 1995, 25–32.

44. "Entering a Bright New World," *Intel Healthcare Solutions,* Winter 1996, 7.

45. Harris and Crawford, "Electronic Umbilical Cords," 26–31.

46. M. O'Brien, "Rolling Out SPRINT's Public Health Information Service," *Multimedia Patient Education* (Phoenix, AZ: Institute for International Research, December 1, 2, 1994).

47. T. Ferguson, "Consumer Health Informatics," *Healthcare Forum Journal* 38, no. 1 (1995):28–33.

48. Cason, "Do You Computer," 12–15.

49. P. Amos, "Replacing Medication and Procedures with Information Technology" (Paper presented at a conference sponsored by the Alliance for Healthcare Strategy and Marketing, Las Vegas, Nevada, November 11–12, 1996).

50. "On-Line Information Provides Powerful Patient Education and Self-Care Tools," *Healthcare Demand Management* 1, no. 8 (1995):120.

51. "'Your Modem Has Unexpectedly Disconnected,' " *Health Promotion Practitioner* 5, no. 1 (1996):5.

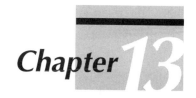

Chapter 13

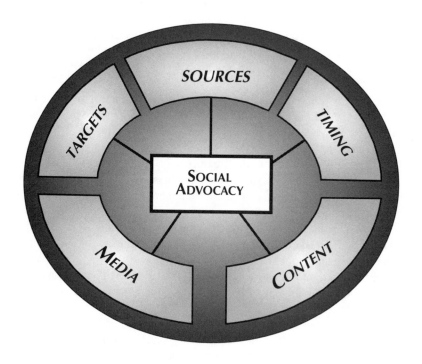

This tactic is commonly termed "social marketing," though it almost always is restricted to the use of publicity and media relations or lobbying to influence policy makers or to mass media advertising and public service announcements to influence the public. By definition, "marketing" should include using the full marketing mix (i.e., product, place, and price factors in addition to promotion). We will discuss true marketing as a tactic for improving consumer health and demand behaviors in Chapter 15.

There are a number of definitions of social advocacy or "social marketing" available, though the term seems to be only a few decades old. After a suggestion for a general broadening of the concept and application of marketing in 1969,[1] the term was coined in 1979 as an approach to planned social change. Its champions argued that social causes can be advanced more successfully through applying principles of marketing analysis, planning, and control to problems of social change.[2]

Andreasen has defined social marketing as a way to "influence the voluntary behavior of target audiences in order to improve their personal welfare and that of society."[3(p.7)] Another definition goes beyond a behavioral focus to refer to social marketing as involving "the design, implementation and control of programs seeking to increase the acceptability of a social idea, cause or practice in a target group or groups."[4(p.49)] In health matters it has been referred to as the use of "mass media aimed at public health and behavior change."[5(p.xiv)]

What generally characterizes the use of social advocacy in aiming for behavior changes among consumers is first a focus on social good rather than commercial gain; this accounts for the "social" part of the term. Second is the use of the concepts and practices of marketing communications, as opposed to public health education or personal counseling in achieving behavior change. It is distinguished from tactics described under the rubric "persuasion" by its use of mass media and a focus on the general population.

Social advocacy may aim to achieve what is called social liberation in the stages of change model if it includes lobbying or public opinion campaigns to promote smoke-free environments, for example. It may also be effective in the consciousness raising technique of the model, awakening consumers to the risks of their current behavior, to social preference for their changing that behavior, and to the advantages to their health or other values they would gain by changing.

Social advocacy may equally well be used to promote the environmental control technique. Lobbying legislatures or supporting public referenda making it illegal, more difficult, or more expensive to buy tobacco products would be examples. Promoting smoke-free worksites and public places helps reduce the environmental stimulus of seeing others smoke. Encouraging restaurants to offer healthier menu items can increase the opportunities for diners to choose them.

Social advocacy is also distinguished from the familiar, commercial advertising by having higher standards and aspirations for success. Where a kick-off advertising effort for a new brand would be ecstatic with the capture of a 5% market share or a campaign for an existing brand delighted with a gain of a percentage point or two, public health media campaigns often hope to convert half or more of their target audiences.

If it were truly marketing, "social marketing" would involve more than talking people into behavior changes using mass media. It would include efforts to change the nature of the desired behavior (and perhaps the undesired behavior as well)—increasing (or decreasing) the benefits thereof, making it easier (or more difficult) to engage in, and decreasing (or increasing) its inherent costs. It would "change the offer" rather then rely on communications alone. (See Chapter 15 for further discussion of this distinction.)

On the other hand, social advocacy might be used to promote "self-marketing" among consumers. It could challenge consumers to find alternatives to their present behavior that would be rewarding, convenient, and low cost, such as choosing their own form of physical activity rather than being persuaded to adopt a specific option. Such an approach would correspond to the countering technique in the stages of change model.

It could as easily be used to promote general self-reevaluation among consumers. Mass media campaigns could challenge consumers to reassess their values in light of their negative behaviors, or the feelings that keep them from adopting more positive alternatives. Such campaigns would strengthen efforts by providers and family members to improve consumer behavior.

What distinguishes social advocacy from education, according to marketers, is first a more thorough grounding in consumer behavior, research into what causes consumers to behave as they do. By focusing on what motivates consumers to behave as they now do, and learning what might cause them to change, sponsors can develop more persuasive communications than can educators, so say marketers.[6]

Marketers can use an explicit focus on the product/place/price marketing mix to develop arguments and facts supporting their promotion of behavior change. Through careful selection and segmentation of targets, setting of objectives, using research to design messages and select media, and stringent evaluation of efforts—plus enlisting peer and community support and feedback from targets—marketers argue their ability to deliver superior results.[7]

Of course, educators, providers, and public health professionals have the ability to employ the same concepts and techniques. And many have expressed concern over the incompatibility of advertising, tainted by its commercial implications, with the worthwhile cause of improving public health.[8] Some see health care as too important for a "customer" focus. Others note that social advertising's track record in eliminating undesirable behavior is far from perfect.[9]

The use of mass media to promote public health through changes in consumer behavior is actually centuries old, going back to the earliest efforts to keep people from using unsafe water supplies.[10] Only the name is new, together with employment of some tricks of the trade perfected in commercial consumer advertising.

Only its more ardent champions would argue that social advertising can do the job by itself. Most see it as a complement to educational and persuasion efforts, needing additional approaches and follow-up to achieve full effect.[11] In many cases it is more effective at reinforcing current behavior patterns than in achieving behavior change. Specific campaigns have often proved to have poor links to demonstrated changes in public behavior.[12]

On the other hand, some see *social* advertising in the mass media as a necessary counterbalance to the *commercial* advertising and promotion of unhealthy products such as alcohol and cigarettes and high-fat foods.[13] If mass media can talk people into behaviors that are intrinsically bad for them, why not use the same vehicles to talk them out of it or into healthier behaviors?[14]

An interesting related approach is that of "behavioral journalism." This tactic employs the same mass media as social advertising and aims at the same kinds of behavior changes for the public good. It simply uses journalists, news stories, and features rather than advertising to do so. Journalism may be more acceptable, perhaps less manipulative than marketing. Examples of campaigns by news media have demonstrated success in Finland, Texas, and New York.[15]

This approach can correspond to the emotional arousal technique in the stages of change model. Stories about admired individuals or friends suffering the negative effects of poor behavior, such as not having a child immunized or not catching a life-threatening condition early enough, can arouse emotions among consumers not yet convinced to adopt such behaviors. Fellow workers who failed to use safety equipment or procedures may prove excellent advocates for their peers.

There are enough examples of successful social advocacy efforts to warrant its inclusion among tactics to be considered for changing or reinforcing consumer health and demand behaviors. As with other tactics, it is more a question of how and how well it is used than whether or not it is applicable.

WHO CAN USE IT?

Most social advocacy efforts have been initiated by government or not-for-profit health organizations. The Stanford program conducted a five-year study on promoting healthier behaviors in the 1970s, for example.[16] The US Public Health Service has long been promoting AIDS awareness, child immunizations, and similar causes. The National Heart, Lung and Blood Institute initiated a campaign promoting awareness and control of high blood pressure in the early 1980s.[17] The State Health Department in South Carolina conducted a five-year health risk reduction campaign, with some success despite limited resources.[18]

Businesses are often involved in social advocacy, though sometimes to help promote their own products (e.g., Kellogg All-Bran, Rockport walking shoes) or simply to stimulate goodwill toward their brand or industry.[19] The Kellogg campaign was conducted in conjunction with and with the blessings of the National Cancer Institute and proved highly successful in alerting the public to the benefits of dietary fiber.[20] Anheuser-Busch has helped reduce drunk driving arrests and accidents with its public service campaigns.

Local businesses can be social advocates as well. Health clubs have good reason to promote exercise in the community. Restaurants offering healthy menu items can benefit from promoting healthy dining. Sporting goods stores gain from promoting participation in both formal and informal sports activities. Businesses can partner with each other to increase their budgets and negotiating strength.[21]

Pharmaceutical companies are increasingly engaging in social advocacy to promote awareness of conditions their products treat and of the availability of treatment for them. While their intention is clearly to promote sales, their efforts have positive social effects as well. Manufacturers of radiology equipment have promoted mammography use, for example.

Hospitals have employed social advocacy to combine image building with promoting public health. St. Joseph's Children's Hospital in Tampa, Florida, promoted public awareness of and screening for sickle cell anemia.[22] St. Anthony's Hospital in Denver, Colorado, has for years conducted a campaign promoting public awareness of chest pain and the need to get immediate care when symptoms arise.

Hospitals have at least two pragmatic motivations for engaging in social advocacy, in addition to their mission commitments. Some types of communications help bring patients their way through a combination of general increases in use of services such as mammography screening and the improved image effects of public service communications. Others help protect not-for-profit hospitals from attacks on their tax-exempt status.

Health plans seem to have done relatively little social advocacy on their own. Considering the growth in managed care bashing, it might be a good idea for HMOs to engage in more public service information efforts in addition to their competitive positioning. The KPS Health Plan (Bremerton, Washington) has engaged in a campaign to promote awareness of health reform issues, wellness, and prevention as part of its enrollment promotion efforts. Rather than respond to media charges such as care denial and excessive profits, HMOs might be better advised to demonstrate their commitment to consumers and health through social advocacy.[23]

All risk-sharing sponsors might try being open and honest about their intentions in improving consumer behavior. Social advocacy communications could start by admitting that sponsors benefit financially when consumers change their behaviors so as to enjoy better health, use the health system more prudently and efficiently, and increase productivity, for example. Since consumers themselves benefit from the same behavior improvements, they should not feel they are being manipulated and may feel greater trust in sponsors that are open about their multiple motives. Of course, such admissions may raise expectations among consumers that they should share in the financial gains their improved behavior produces.

Community-wide partnerships are growing in size, numbers, and efforts at promoting community health. The Kaiser and Lovelace Foundations, Indian Health Service, and local corporations combined to support social advertising efforts aimed at diet and smoking in New Mexico, for example.[24] Local governments, churches, businesses, and providers in Springfield, Massachusetts, partnered in promoting child immunizations.[25]

The national Healthy Communities 2000 program of the US Public Health Service is promoting community-based partnerships throughout the United States.[26] The Healthcare Forum in San Francisco offers Healthier Communities Action Kits for those interested in leading or participating in community health efforts.[27] Health Partners HMO in Minneapolis enlists local businesses and public and private organizations in its Partners for Better Health program, focusing on problems such as domestic violence in addition to traditional health concerns.[28]

To some degree such partnerships represent risks as well as potential benefits for providers and payers interested in changing health behaviors. Community partners may use a wider definition of health in identifying and addressing problems. The Healthcare Forum, for example, found that the public tends to look at crime rates, child abuse, the schools, environment, family values, jobs, and race relations as signs of community health or lack thereof, in addition to conventional health and wellness.[29] Nevertheless community partnerships hold great promise in promoting health and may lead providers and payers to advantageously expand their own notions of what is health.

In Canada, for example, "community-based social marketing" has been used to promote permanent changes in a variety of consumer behaviors. It employs volunteers to make face-to-face contacts with targeted consumers in addition to or instead of mass media. Volunteers seek personal commitments from consumers to make specific changes, exploiting the well-established fact that people will greatly increase their probability of a given behavior when simply asked to do so. Regular reminders are then used to heighten recall of commitments made and suggest self-reminders consumers might use.[30]

TARGETS FOR SOCIAL ADVOCACY

In contrast to persuasion and education efforts, which tend to focus on specific populations at risk, social advocacy almost always aims at the entire community or at least those reached by the mass media. Exceptions can be made for selected advocacy messages when media are chosen to reach specific populations at risk, such as elderly or insomniacs watching late-night television. Of course, messages can be contrived so as to capture the attention of only those intended to be the audience, though advertising costs are based on everyone who is exposed to media communications.

Ideally social advocacy communications should be aimed at people who are most receptive to them at the right stages of readiness to change behavior. Mass media can be effective in consciousness raising for those in the precontemplation and contemplation stages, awakening them to education and persuasion efforts. They can be aimed at opinion leaders in the community who can exert additional motivational impact.[31] Media messages can also reinforce commitments of those in the preparation and action stages, serving as reminders to those who might forget or gentle nudges for those still uncommitted.

Influentials in the community (or at least people who perceive themselves to be so) might be targeted through a headline such as "Do People Look to You for Advice?" Consumers at given stages of readiness might be approached through a headline such as "Thinking about Getting in Shape?" Targets of a specific age, gender, race, chronic condition, or other trait might be differentially attracted to pay attention to the message by using a picture of someone just like them (or just like they perceive themselves to be).[32] If efficiency of communication cannot be increased through media targeting, a qualifying message approach might work.

TIMING

The same rules of timing apply to social advocacy as work for persuasion and education. Some messages may be timed based on seasons of the year: warnings about water safety in the summer and about skiing and avalanche danger in the winter. Others may be timed to coincide with news and feature stories on related subjects. Having close working relations with news media so as to know when they will engage in "behavioral journalism," even influence their choices of timing, can be particularly helpful in achieving optimal timing.

While some times of the year may be particularly good for specific social advocacy efforts, beware of focusing all attention on a short period. Experience has shown that the old adage "out of sight, out of mind" applies to communications as well as people. If messages are not repeated at fairly frequent intervals, public awareness and potential for behavior change can go back to where they started; consumers in the action and maintenance stages of behavior improvement may relapse.[33]

MESSAGE CONTENT

Some social advocates insist on using only factual, objective information and logical and ethical arguments aimed at irreproachable behavior objectives. Since the purpose of mass media health communication is to enable consumers to make the best decisions about their own behavior, messages should focus on their values and needs rather than those of sponsors or society.[34]

Others argue that social advocacy adds to the potential of health education by including emotional appeals as well as purely factual information. Media such as radio and television offer opportunities to suggest images, create moods, and

Exhibit 13–1 Social Advocacy

DEFINITION	✗ MASS MEDIA ADVERTISING TO GENERAL PUBLIC TO CHANGE BEHAVIOR & ATTITUDES ✗ LOBBYING TO INFLUENCE POLICY MAKERS
OBJECTIVE	✗ TO ESTABLISH SOCIAL NORMS FOR HEALTH CARE & BEHAVIOR ✗ THROUGH USE OF PERSUASIVE CONTENT, INCREASE MOTIVATION TO CHANGE BEHAVIOR
EXAMPLES OF TECHNIQUES	✗ ADVERTISING CAMPAIGNS ABOUT CONSEQUENCES OF UNDESIRABLE BEHAVIOR ✗ ADVOCATE FOR LEGISLATION & ORDINANCES THAT DISCOURAGE BEHAVIOR (PUBLIC SMOKING ORDINANCES, PENALTIES FOR DRIVING UNDER THE INFLUENCE OF ALCOHOL) ✗ PROVIDE "HEALTH FAIRS" & OTHER OPPORTUNITIES TO DISTRIBUTE INFORMATION & RECEIVE FREE SCREENINGS
SUGGESTIONS	✗ FOCUS THE CONTENT ON THE VALUES & NEEDS OF THE CONSUMER ✗ ENLIST THE SUPPORT OF BUSINESSES & PUBLIC HEALTH ORGANIZATIONS TO HELP PROMOTE BEHAVIOR CHANGES ✗ TIME THE PRESENTATION TO FIT SEASONS (E.G., SUMMER FITNESS) OR PARTICULAR NEWS & FEATURE STORIES ✗ PROVIDE THE INFORMATION IN PRINT & VISUAL MEDIA THAT CAN BE WIDELY DISSEMINATED

stimulate feelings that will enhance the impact of factual content.[35] Such emotional arousal may prove effective in moving consumers from preparation to action or in strengthening their maintenance.

Social advocacy has demonstrated its potential for achieving dramatic changes in consumer health and demand behavior. It can stimulate consciousness of the value and potential of behavior change. It can increase consumer motivation by dramatizing the advantages of positive behavior and dangers of negative behavior. It can increase consumer capability by enhancing awareness of sources of assistance.[36]

Whether sponsors engage in social advocacy initiatives on their own, in alliance with their risk-sharing partners, or in community-wide coalitions, this tactic has wide applications to demand improvement. It can be used at virtually any of the stages of change and relative to virtually all of the four demand improvement domains. It can motivate, add to capability, and both awaken and reinforce consciousness among consumers (Exhibit 13–1).

REFERENCES

1. P. Kotler and S. Levy, "Broadening the Concept of Marketing," *Journal of Marketing* 32, no. 4 (1969):10–15.

2. P. Kotler and G. Zaltman, "Social Marketing: An Approach to Planned Social Change," *Journal of Marketing* 35, no. 2 (1971):3–12.

3. A. Andreasen, *Marketing Social Change: Changing Behavior To Promote Health, Social Development, and the Environment* (San Francisco, CA: Jossey-Bass, 1995), 7.

4. D. Leathar and G. Hastings, "Social Marketing and Health Education," *Journal of Services Marketing* 1, no. 2 (1987):49.

5. T. Backer, E. Rogers, and P. Sopory, *Designing Health Communications Campaigns: What Works* (Newbury Park, CA: Sage, 1992), xiv.

6. R.C. LeFebvre and J. Flora, "Social Marketing and Public Health Intervention," *Health Education Quarterly* 15, no. 3 (1988):299–315.

7. D.C. Walsh, et al., "Social Marketing for Public Health," *Health Affairs* 12, no. 2 (1993):104–119.

8. J. Mintz, "Social Marketing: New Weapon in an Old Struggle," *Health Promotion,* Winter 1988, 6–12.

9. V.K. Rangan, S. Karmin, and S. Sandberg, "Do Better at Doing Good," *Harvard Business Review* 74, no. 3 (1996):42–54.

10. E. Young, "Social Marketing: Where It Has Come From; Where It's Going," *Health Promotion,* Winter 1988, 2–5, 26.

11. Mintz, "Social Marketing: New Weapon in an Old Struggle," 6–12.

12. Young, "Social Marketing: Where It Has Come From; Where It Is Going," 2–5, 26.

13. C. Lovelock and C. Weinberg, *Marketing for Public and Non-Profit Managers* (New York: John Wiley & Sons, 1984), 567.

14. R. Kimmel, "Fight Ads with Ads on Health Issues," *Modern Healthcare,* 17 February 1992, 34.

15. A. McAlister, "Behavioral Journalism: Beyond the Marketing Model for Health Communication," *American Journal of Health Promotion* 9, no. 6 (1995):417–420.

16. LeFebvre and Flora, "Social Marketing and Public Health Intervention," 299–315.

17. I. Marsh, "Social Marketing," *Marketing News,* 13 May 1983, 26, 27.

18. R. Goodman, F. Wheeler, and P. Lee, "Evaluation of the Heart to Heart Project," *American Journal of Health Promotion* 9, no. 6 (1995):443–455.

19. P. Bloom, P.Y. Hussein, and L. Szykman, "Benefiting Society and the Bottom Line," *Marketing Management* 4, no. 3 (1995):8–18.

20. V. Freimuth, S. Hammond, and J. Stein, "Health Advertising: Prevention for Profit," *American Journal of Public Health* 78, no. 5 (1988):557–561.

21. "Firm Gets More Bang from Small Ad Budget by Value-Added Partnering—Sales Soar 38%," *The Marketing Report,* 7 February 1993, 3.

22. R. Cohen, "Sickle Cell PSA Campaign Meets Community Need," *Healthcare Marketing Report* 11, no. 8 (1993):1, 5, 6.

23. S. MacStravic, "Marketers Can Counter Managed Care Bashing," *Marketing Health Services* 17, no. 1 (1997):49–51.

24. S. Moore, "New Mexicans Take Life Style Changes to Heart," *Business & Health* 6, no. 9 (1988): 36–38.

25. "Public-Private Partnership Tackles Child Health Issues," *Inside Preventive Care* 1, no. 11 (1996):1–3.

26. R. Coile, "Healthy Communities: Reducing Need (and Costs) by Promoting Health," *Hospital Strategy Report* 6, no. 4 (1994):1–7.

27. "A 'Healthier Communities Action Kit,' " *Hospital Strategy Report* 6, no. 4 (1994):5.

28. "Minnesota Prescribes Medicine for Violence," *Modern Healthcare,* 2 December 1996, 24.

29. *What Creates Health? Individuals and Communities Respond* (San Francisco, CA: The Healthcare Forum, 1994).

30. R. Piirto, "The Influentials," *American Demographics,* October 1992, 16–19.

31. C. Schewe and G. Meredith, "Digging Deep to Delight the Mature Adult Customer," *Marketing Management* 3, no. 3 (1994):20–35.

32. T. Albrecht and C. Bryant, "Advances in Segmentation Modeling for Health Communications and Social Marketing Campaigns," *Journal of Health Communications* 1, no. 1 (1996):65–80.

33. S. Ratzan, "Communication—The Key to a Healthier Tomorrow," *American Behavioral Scientist* 38, no. 2 (1994):202–207.

34. C. Nelson, *Integrated Advertising* (Chicago: Bonus Books, 1991).

35. D. Greenberger, "Operating under Reform: The Psychology of Health Care Marketing Communications," *Strategic Health Care Marketing* 10, no. 12 (1993):6–8.

36. E. Crocker, "Go Door-to-Door To Change Behavior," *Marketing News,* 9 June 1997, 4.

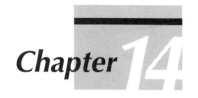
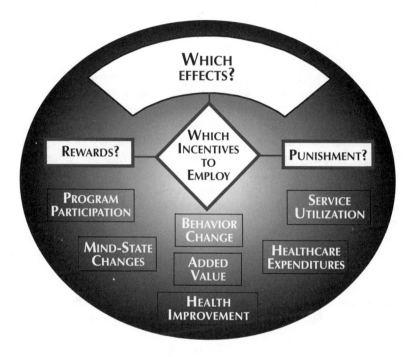

INCENTIVES

Where communications alone will not suffice to achieve consumer behavior change, incentives, including rewards and punishments both promised and conferred, may be used. These are commonly used with respect to health and demand behavior, perhaps because they are familiar tactics to managers, though marketers and demarketers have used them as well. For population control, men in India were offered free portable radios in return for getting vasectomies.[1] Marketers often pay respondents for participating in market research and use promotional items and discount coupons to increase sales.

Rewards and punishments are clearly aimed at motivation of consumer targets, adding new consequences to whatever facts and arguments can be brought to bear. They are based on the "Greatest Management Principle in the World": The things that get rewarded get done[2] and its presumed corollary, what gets punished does not get done. Incentives and disincentives are the simplest ways to alter the behavior experience equation to affect motivation, requiring little understanding of the dynamics of behavior, though they entail significant risks as well and do not always work as intended.

There are two ways in which rewards and punishments can influence behavior. When applied *after* a given behavior, they can promote or diminish its probability of repetition. Hence the "one-minute manager" is always on the lookout to catch employees in the act of doing something good, to be immediately rewarded by anything from a verbal or literal pat on the back to formal bonuses.[3] Enabling a wide range of people, from fellow workers to family and friends, to catch consumers doing something right and immediately rewarding them for it can expand the potential still further. Such an application corresponds to the rewards technique in the stages of change model and is used once people have reached the action and maintenance stages.

We feel that the *promise* of a significant reward, well ahead of the *delivery* of rewards once a behavior change has occurred, can be useful as early as the precontemplation stage, to awaken consumers to a new reason to reconsider their current behavior. It is likely, however, that such promised rewards will have to be more substantial, and thereby more expensive to sponsors, than rewards used to reinforce behavior change among consumers who made their way to the action stage on their own.

The most commonly used rewards and punishments in improving consumer health and demand behaviors have been dollar amounts. Deductibles and copayments have been used for decades to ensure that consumers feel some of the costs of using health services. Health plans "punish" consumers for using the wrong services or for failing to follow preapproval procedures by requiring them to pay the entire bill. They steer consumers to one "preferred" set of providers by paying a higher proportion of the bill than when consumers use "out-of-network" providers.

Dollar incentives in the form of reduced out-of-pocket premium shares are used by employers to stimulate healthier behaviors, while higher shares are used to promote the elimination of unhealthy behaviors. Public agencies have gone so far as to pay teenagers for each week they stay unpregnant.[4] In France women are given subsidies for getting prescribed prenatal care. We seem to have a lot of faith that using bonuses and imposing "fines" are effective in controlling human behavior, generally.

There has been a lot of discussion over the years about the *probability* of rewards and punishments. It is widely accepted, for example, that the *certainty* of punishment has more impact on reducing crime than its severity. If rewards seem too unlikely, as in state lotteries, the amount of the reward has to be enormous to entice participation. At the same time, if rewards are too certain and apply to everyone with little distinction as to individual sacrifice or effort, they lose their impact.

The mere chance at a large reward can often be more effective, and often less expensive, than distributing small rewards to everyone who qualifies. Sunrise Hospital in Las Vegas, for example, offered patients who scheduled their elective admissions for Friday or Saturday a chance at a Monday drawing, the winner to get a free two-week "recuperative cruise." This both evened out the weekly pattern of admissions and increased its market share.[5] In another application, Medicaid mothers were offered a ticket in a $100 raffle for each prenatal visit they made.[6]

In the latter case, the raffle tickets, and for that matter another tactic of paying mothers $5 for each prenatal visit, failed to have the desired effect. This was because the problem was not one of lack of motivation but of capability. Those failing to make prenatal visits were more likely to be sick or to have problems with transportation or difficulties finding day care for their current children. The dollar incentive could not overcome these barriers.

Whenever incentives are to be used, make sure that targets have the capability to behave in the desired fashion. Punishing people for addictive behavior, for example, or promising rewards if they quit runs up against the power of the addiction. Promising rewards for engaging in an exercise program will have little effect on the physically disabled.[7] It may be necessary to eliminate internal and external capability problems before incentives can work.

WHAT SHOULD BE REWARDED OR PUNISHED?

The particular behaviors or achievements to be promoted or discouraged through positive or negative incentives can be found among each of the "set of effects":

1. Participation in some program, class, or activity—getting involved;
2. Demonstrated changes in knowledge, skills, or attitudes;
3. Changes in specific behaviors, lifestyles;
4. Changes in health or functional status measures;
5. Changes in health services utilization patterns; and
6. Changes in health care and disability expenditures.

The effects are discussed in detail below.

1. Participation in educational or training efforts is one of the safest and most equitable bases for incentives. Since the purpose of such efforts includes demonstrable benefit to participants, offering a bonus to employees, patients, or health plan members who register for, attend, or complete a given program will rarely prove controversial. Those who fail to participate may

feel technically "punished," but they were certainly eligible and may qualify in the future. Punishing those who fail to participate through fines or reductions in benefits would be problematic at best, however.

Alliant Techsystems (Hopkins, Minnesota) used a point system to promote desired behaviors among its employees. To those who attended regular "Lunch 'n Learn" sessions, one point was awarded, together with free fruit. Similar points were awarded for attending prenatal classes. Gift certificates were awarded based on accumulation of points.[8] The City of Glendale (Arizona) offered its employees a $150 incentive, with another $150 for spouses to participate in its health screening program.[9]

On the downside, paying targets for showing up at educational or training sessions may encourage "gaming the system." Consumers may be physically present but take no interest in the proceedings. They may already have the desired knowledge, skills, and attitudes and show up just to gain the rewards. Sponsors may find they have spent money but changed nothing.

2. Proven acquisition of knowledge and skills, even demonstrated changes in attitude, can be reasonable bases for rewards. Offering tests or demonstrations may help sponsors learn whether their educational and training programs are successful or which work better than others. They also can help participants' self-efficacy by proving to consumers what they have learned. Rewards for passing, rather than merely for participating, may stimulate efforts to learn.

Of course, failure to pass, combined with not getting a reward, may have significant negative impact on those who do not qualify. They may not only lose confidence in their learning; they may also lose interest in any future opportunities.

Gaming the system is also possible if people already possessed of the desired knowledge, skills, and attitudes attend programs and pass the same tests they could have passed at the outset. On the other hand, if those learnings are valuable, it may make sense to pay everyone who has achieved them on their own, since they can save sponsors the expense of the education and training efforts.

3. Changes in behavior are a little more challenging but are widely used as bases for rewards and punishments. Many employers use positive incentives for nonsmokers or negative incentives for smokers. Baker Hughes (Houston, Texas) charged smokers $10 higher monthly premium costs; the Moore Company (Portland, Oregon) paid 25% more of the premium for nonsmokers.[10] Hershey paid nonsmokers a $48 reward and charged smokers $444 extra in premiums.[11] Some employers simply do not hire smokers, claiming advantages in productivity as well as health and disability cost reductions. Others may not hire people who engage in high-risk activities such as sky diving, mountain climbing, or motorcycling.[12]

Life insurance companies commonly offer lower premiums for nonsmokers. Some accident insurance companies pay victims higher amounts if they were wearing seat belts.[13] Some employers' health plans lower payments to drivers and passengers *not* wearing seat belts when they had an accident.[14] Others pay employees regularly if they do use seat belts or at least say they do.[15]

One of the problems with incentive programs focused on health behaviors is that most rely on self-reporting. When rewarded for doing so, consumers may well change their behaviors, but they may also use "creative reporting" to claim behaviors not fully descriptive of them and obtain rewards to which they are not fully entitled.[16] One employer dealt with the problem by threatening employees with the loss of *all their health benefits* if they lied about their eligibility for healthy behavior incentives.[17]

Rewards may be given for specific *changes* in health behaviors, as well as to consumers who are already "sanitarily correct." Some pay for engaging in exercise programs. Alliant Techsystems pays points for each 30 minutes of recreational activity, with added points for a 10-k run, bike tour, or charity walk.[18] Others subsidize exercise by paying part or all of membership fees in health clubs and fitness centers.

Some pay promised incentives for employees who quit smoking, adopt safer lifting techniques, or begin to wear seat belts.[19] One union/management partnership devised incentives for employees who stopped smoking, increased their exercise efforts, adopted healthier diet habits, and reduced their absenteeism.[20] One must wonder how employees who are already behaving in a healthy manner feel about an unhealthy peer being rewarded for converting to behavior patterns they already follow.

Some combine all health behaviors into a health risk score and reward employees who have low scores or reduce their scores. In most cases, however, such scores combine behavior factors such as smoking and exercise, seat belt use, and so forth, with health status measures such as obesity, cholesterol, and blood pressure.[21]

4. Health status improvements are frequently rewarded when demonstrated. Punishing "bad" health status is already common practice in insurance: denying coverage or increasing premiums for consumers with preexisting conditions. This can include chronic diseases as well as conditions that represent high risk for future problems, such as hypertension and obesity. It is usually not possible, however, to increase premiums to consumers who become obese or hypertensive after the insurance begins.

Many employers reward employees for healthy weight, cholesterol levels, high-density lipoprotein/low-density lipoprotein (HDL/LDL) ratio, and body fat percentages.[22] Alamco (Clarksburg, West Virginia) paid employees $100 for having a cholesterol level under 150 and $50 for blood pressure below 135/85.[23] St. Luke's Episcopal Hospital (Houston, Texas) paid its employees for keeping their blood pressure and cholesterol within normal limits, with levels monitored quarterly.[24]

Others reward improvements in health status measures by those who once had high-risk levels. Blue Cross/Blue Shield of South Carolina found that cholesterol, body fat, and blood pressure levels all improved after introducing an incentive program for one employer.[25] At the Fort Sanders (Tennessee) Health System, employees could get $50 payments for reducing their blood pressure below 130/90 without medication or for reducing their body fat percentage by an agreed-upon amount.[26]

Almost any health status measure *within the control of consumers* could be the focus for an incentive program, paying for good status measures or for improvements in those measures. Some measures, particularly obesity, body fat, and related indicators of weight management seem so subject to recidivism that long-term benefits are questionable. If rewards are to be offered for health status improvements, it makes sense to include programs that will help consumers achieve and maintain them, rather than rely on the incentives alone.[27]

5. Changes in health service use as the focus for incentives have the longest history in consumer demand improvement. Deductibles and copays as well as benefit coverage and exclusions are designed to steer consumers to the right providers and services or away from those that are questionable (at least to payers). PPO, POS, EPO, and HMO plans typically pay less, even nothing if consumers choose some providers, and more or everything if they choose others.

One health plan steers consumers toward using nurse practitioners (NPs) rather than physicians by waiving the copayment requirement when an NP is used.[28] Many employers steer employees toward HMOs versus indemnity plans or toward the cheapest HMO where two or more are offered by paying the full cost of only the cheapest plan, leaving employees to pay any additional premium costs for more expensive coverage.

Deductibles, copayments, and higher premium costs for employees have the added advantage of reducing payer costs in and of themselves. Of course, adding to the employees' burden may result in labor unrest, strikes, or additional costs due to lower morale. And while deductibles and copayment may discourage inappropriate use of services, they tend to discourage appropriate use as well and may delay the seeking of care past the point where the most cost-effective results can be achieved. Unfortunately because they automatically reduce costs to payers, they are increasingly popular.[29]

One study suggested that where payers overly restricted which drugs consumers could get under their health plan, the total costs of care went up because the cheaper drugs were not as effective.[30] In a famous example of pennywise, pound foolish, a New Hampshire Medicaid regulation limiting coverage to three prescriptions for any patient ended up sending droves of elderly into nursing homes and greatly increasing costs instead of reducing them, as intended.

Employers and health plans can promote or discourage routine physicals, screening tests, immunizations, and a variety of health improvement service consumption by deciding to pay for them or not.[31] The Sony Corporation pays 100% of the costs of Pap smears, mammograms, and blood tests for employees meeting eligibility and frequency criteria.[32] One employer goes beyond incentives and makes maternity benefits contingent upon women getting prescribed prenatal care. There may be legal risk in such an approach, since it necessarily discriminates against women.[33]

Employers frequently pay incentives to workers who incur no injury costs over measured periods. They may pay work teams for achieving a quarter or year with no workers' compensation claims. One employer offers a $25 bonus every quarter to each employee who avoided any injury requiring outside treatment.[34]

Some employers discourage use of health services by paying employees bonuses if they use none or so few that their annual deductible is not reached and hence the employer incurs no liability (or even claims handling).[35] Others offer rebates on health insurance premiums for those who use few or no services. One HMO offers incentives to all members who submit no claims during a given year, with the exception of preventive and routine screening. This seems to have little effect, however, as the need for services is often a matter of luck rather than subject to consumer control.[36]

6. Health expenditures not only offer a logical basis for incentives; they provide the dollars to do so. Where any payer (health plan or employer) saves money compared to previous or projected expenditures for health insurance, self-funded care, or workers' compensation, thanks to consumer behavior improvements it has the ability to share those savings with its "partner" consumers. Moreover, it is in a position to know exactly how much of a difference consumers have made through their improved behaviors.

The City of Glendale (Arizona) shares its savings from both workers' compensation and health insurance with its workers in the form of higher salaries and benefits.[37] Medical Plastics Laboratory uses a risk pool approach for its workers' compensation expenditures, refunding to employees any unspent amounts. Its refunds increased from $267 per employee to $600 in just three years.[38] Quaker Oats pays a "dividend" to employees when its health care costs are below budgeted levels.[39]

Almost every type of behavior or achievement seems to have been successfully used as a basis for incentive payments; the choice is up to sponsors. It may be that incentives based on actual savings are the most logical and appropriate, since they come out of the positive consequences of consumer behavior. The closer the behavior to its dollar consequences, the easier it is to calculate and justify the size of the incentive.

On the other hand, there are those who argue that effort ought to be rewarded as well as achievements.[40] Where it is clearly demonstrated or at least confidently believed that participation will produce mind changes, that mind changes will produce behavior changes, that changes in behavior will improve health status and health care demand, and that there is a predictable causal connection across the set of effects to expense reductions, then rewarding each intermediate step makes sense.[41] Particularly where the lag across the set of effects is lengthy, rewarding earlier changes may be the only way to effectively stimulate desired savings.

WHAT KINDS OF INCENTIVES TO USE

Virtually all the examples discussed so far have been financial incentives, specific dollar amounts that consumers could expect and get as rewards or punishments. There are other types of rewards as well, and some would argue that they should be considered as complements to or substitutes for money. Positive incentives can include private and public recognition or symbols such as T-shirts and coffee mugs.

One approach used self-care manuals to reward and recognize participants in wellness activities. The manuals represented value to participants; they would have cost around $10 if purchased and were behavior improvement tools, as well. A similar approach could involve giving those who complete one health education or training class free registration in another class of their choice, combining reward with continuation of the behavior improvement effort.

Point systems used to recognize specific health and wellness efforts could be the basis for contests with trophies or for public posting of progress, recognition letters, and symbols as well as dollar awards.[42] Charts, logs, and diaries that enable participants to record their efforts, measures of weight, blood pressure, strength and flexibility, and other health status indicators can be self-rewarding by showing individual achievement.[43] Team contests can give groups the reward of winning or group achievement.

Recognition may work better if simply delivered rather than used as a promised "carrot" to entice desired behavior. Promising someone a T-shirt or hearty handshake may sound silly, even patronizing, if offered up front. By contrast, using such forms of recognition unexpectedly may be more powerful for some than money rewards. Combining recognition of past effort and achievement with expressions of confidence in future repetition may add a "Pygmalion effect" to the impact. (See Chapter 11.)

Whether reward or recognition or some combination of the two is to be used in promoting (or discouraging) consumer behavior, it is clear that the consequences of behavior have to be understood in terms of consumer values. Whatever is perceived by a consumer as a reward or punishment or any other positive or negative consequence of a behavior will be what determines its effects, regardless of what sponsors might think. Getting some consumer input on proposed consequences, or at least feedback on the ones used, should be part of every program to be sure they fit into targeted consumers' value systems and have the intended effects.

Consequences must be perceived as fair and equitable by consumers if they are to have desired impact and avoid undesired effects on relationships. This means fair in terms of the effort and sacrifice entailed for targets, as they perceive them. If consequences apply to many, particularly where targets are well aware of them, they should be perceived as fair to each in terms of what others get. It also means that consequences should be perceived as fair relative to the value that their behavior delivers to sponsors. Where behavior changes by consumers produce a million-dollar savings to employer or health plan and consumers get a dollar's worth of reward or recognition, the inequity of the exchange will undermine future behavior engineering efforts and relationship retention as well.

Rewards and recognitions will, in most cases, work better if they are tailored to the values of individual consumers (e.g., if they have some choice in the matter). People are sufficiently variable that one form of consequence will work well only on some. Similarly, consequences should be varied over time. We are all so changeable in our perceptions that a consequence that had great impact once "wears out" its effect over time and gets absorbed into the background.

The toughest question regarding consequences is probably that of positive versus negative. Clearly negative consequences work for some people, some behaviors, sometimes. They may be needed to get the attention of some targets relative to well-established, unhealthy habits. Experience with "fear appeals" in persuasion (see Chapter 11) suggests that threats of punishment *when combined with credible and convenient offers of ways to avoid it* can be effective. Thus E.A. Miller (Hyrum, Utah) combined the threat of losing maternity benefits (for those who failed to comply with prenatal visits) with convenient prenatal classes and free babysitting to achieve desired results. Costs and incidence of premature births declined significantly as a result.[44]

In general, the risks of "negative incentives" seem greater than their benefits. Most people do not like being threatened or punished. Relationships are almost sure to be undermined where punishments or threats are employed. Some negative incentives may be illegal and discriminatory. With employee trust already undermined by downsizing, punishments and threats will not help.[45] Their short-term advantages seem always to be overcome by their long-term costs. Wherever possible, accentuate the positive!

WHO SHOULD USE INCENTIVES?

Almost all the examples of rewards and punishments discussed so far have been used by employers relative to their employees and, occasionally, dependents or retirees. Health plans have used incentives to only a slight extent. They may be less sure of the value of incentives or of the value of specific consumer behavior changes. They are more focused on provider behavior, anyway, where they are very much believers in financial rewards and punishments.[46] They may also fear that high turnover among members will deprive them of enjoying the value of many behavior improvements.

There are some exceptions. Group Health of Puget Sound (Washington) uses rebates to low-risk members to encourage healthier behaviors. Their "health pays" program offered 10% to 15% premium discounts to individual enrollees falling within health risk guidelines. Roughly 20% of enrollees qualified. Some HMOs have offered rebates for unspent premiums to individuals.[47]

There seem to be few, if any, examples of providers using incentives to promote changes in consumer behavior. Some may be employing some form of recognition for patient achievements in weight loss or fitness gains, for example, but just are not talking about it. With increasing numbers of physicians and hospitals united in risk sharing for the health of patient populations, their use of incentives, as well as other tactics in reengineering consumer demand, is likely to grow.

Governments have frequently employed incentives to encourage positive health and demand behaviors. Payment for prenatal care, vasectomies, and not getting pregnant have been mentioned. Because of the political influences that apply in government efforts, special care is required to stay away from controversy. On the other hand, governments can require health plans, employers, and providers to offer incentives or certainly encourage them to do so as payers.

TIMING OF INCENTIVES

It is widely agreed that the consequences of behavior should follow as closely as possible to the specific behavior in question. In general, rewards and recognitions are often of the annual meeting variety where a big event is used to recognize common accomplishments, usually of employees. For individuals, celebrating achievements when they happen is often a better approach.[48]

For behaviors that involve doing something once, or only rarely, such as annual screenings, a reward at or immediately after the time of that behavior makes sense. For behaviors that have to be repeated with some frequency, such as attending a series of classes or prenatal care, rewards might be given every time or when the course of action is completed. For behaviors that must persevere for long periods, including a lifetime, such as exercise or not smoking, periodic rewards, perhaps quarterly or annually, may work.

Incentives are clearly aimed at influencing the motivation of consumers and have no impact on capability. The giving and announcement of rewards and recognitions can have consciousness raising and reinforcement effects, as well. For consumers in the precontemplation stage of readiness to change, promised incen-

Exhibit 14–1 Incentives

DEFINITION	✗ OFFERING & DELIVERING EXTERNAL REWARDS OR PUNISHMENTS
OBJECTIVE	✗ TO MAKE DESIRED BEHAVIORS MORE ATTRACTIVE & SATISFYING ✗ TO MAKE UNDESIRED BEHAVIORS LESS ATTRACTIVE & SATISFYING ✗ TO CHANGE CONSUMER MOTIVATION TOWARD SPECIFIC BEHAVIOR
EXAMPLES OF TECHNIQUES	✗ DEDUCTIBLES AND COPAYMENTS ✗ DIFFERENT BENEFIT COVERAGE OR COPAYMENTS FOR SPECIFIC SERVICES ✗ BONUSES, RAFFLES, SHARED GAINS ✗ HIGHER OR LOWER PREMIUMS ✗ RECOGNITION & NONMONETARY AWARDS (T-SHIRTS, MUGS, BOOKS, ETC.)
SUGGESTIONS	✗ DELIVER REWARDS / PUNISHMENTS AS CLOSE TO BEHAVIOR AS POSSIBLE ✗ ENSURE CONSUMERS FEEL INCENTIVES ARE FAIR & EQUITABLE FOR THEIR "SACRIFICE" ✗ CAUTIOUSLY RELY ON EXTRINSIC INCENTIVES FOR LONG-TERM CHANGES ✗ TAILOR INCENTIVES TO INDIVIDUALS WHERE FEASIBLE ✗ BEWARE EFFECTS OF PUNISHMENT ON RELATIONSHIPS

tives may be just the thing to stimulate a new look at the behavior in question. For most, however, it is likely that incentives have their impact at the action and maintenance stages, when they reinforce the intrinsic benefits of improved behavior.

The greatest concern over incentives relates to their long-term consequences. It has been argued that extrinsic rewards drive out intrinsic motivation and make people dependent on repeated, often escalating, rewards to continue what might have otherwise been perceived as continually beneficial behavior if no rewards had ever been used.[49] Because so much of our experience with rewards in improving consumer health and demand behavior has been of the short-term variety, sponsors should carefully weigh the risks when they consider using incentives for populations on a long-term basis (Exhibit 14–1).

REFERENCES

1. M. Konner, *Medicine at the Crossroads: The Crisis in Health Care* (New York, NY: Pantheon, 1993), x.
2. M. LeBeouf, *The Greatest Management Principle in the World* (New York, NY: G. Putnam, 1985).
3. K. Blanchard and S. Johnson, *The One-Minute Manager* (New York, NY: Wm. Morrow, 1982).
4. A. Schrader, "Study: Money Can't Deter Teen Pregnancy," *The Denver Post,* 26 March 1997, 1A, 13A.
5. M.P. Laken and J. Ager, "Using Incentives To Increase Participation in Prenatal Care," *Obstetrics & Gynecology* 85 (1995):326–329.
6. C. Schewe and G. Meredith, "Digging Deep To Delight the Mature Adult Customer," *Marketing Management* 3, no. 3 (1994):20–35.
7. Blanchard and Johnson, *The One-Minute Manager.*
8. "Alliant's Incentive Program Activities," *Employee Health & Fitness* 17, no. 2 (1995):17.
9. S. Caudron, "A Low-Cost Wellness Program," *Personnel Journal* 71, no. 2 (1992):34–38.
10. N. Bell, "From the Trenches: Strategies That Work," *Business & Health* 9, no. 5 (1991):19–25.
11. P. Kenkel, "Companies Sweeten Wellness Plans," *Modern Healthcare,* 23 November 1992, 49.
12. Z. Schiller, "If You Light Up on Sunday, Don't Come In on Monday," *Business Week,* 26 August 1991, 17–21.
13. F. Herzberg, "One More Time: How Do You Motivate Employees?" in *Harvard Business Review Business Classics* (Boston: Harvard Business School, 1991).
14. "More Employers Play Hardball with Staffers' Health," *Business & Health* 14, no. 1 (1996):10.
15. "Healthful Habits Pay Off," *INC.,* April 1996, 111.
16. L. Chapman, *Using Wellness Incentives: Positive Tools for a Healthy Lifestyle,* 2d ed. (Seattle, WA: Summez Corp., 1991).
17. J. Mandelker, "A Wellness Program or a Bitter Pill?" *Business & Health* 12, no. 3 (1994):36–39.
18. "Alliant's Incentive Program Activities," 17.
19. L. Chapman, "Incentive-Based Model Streamlines Activities," *Employee Health & Fitness* 17, no. 1 (1995):10–12.

20. M. Cameron, "Organized Labor's Newest Bargaining Tool: Partnership," *Business & Health* 11, no. 9 (1993):44–47.

21. M. Conklin, "Rural Hospital Forms HMO for Uninsured," *Health Care Strategic Management* 12, no. 10 (1994):14.

22. Chapman, "Incentive-Based Model Streamlines Activities," 10–12.

23. "Healthful Habits Pay Off," 111.

24. "Hospital Pays Employees To Stay Healthy," *Health Care Strategic Management* 11, no. 9 (1993):4.

25. N. Merrill, "Financial Incentives: The Impact on Health Risks and Behavior," *American Journal of Health Promotion* 8, no. 5 (1994):385.

26. "Reward Employees for Effort, Not Just Results," *Employee Health & Fitness* 17, no. 10 (1995):114–116.

27. Chapman, *Using Wellness Incentives: Positive Tools for a Healthy Lifestyle.*

28. Conklin, "Rural Hospital Forms HMO for Uninsured," 14.

29. "Health Care Costs Shared from Employer to Employee," *Health Care Strategic Management* 11, no. 7 (1993):7.

30. "Currents—Quality Watch," *Hospitals & Health Networks,* 5 July 1997, 15.

31. M. Freudenheim, "Patients Pay Price as Health Plans Cut Costs," *The Denver Post,* 13 October 1996, 3H.

32. P. Kenkel, "Financial Incentives in Wellness Plans Aimed at Reducing Insurance Costs by Helping Workers Shed Unhealthy Habits," *Modern Healthcare,* 20 January 1992, 38.

33. Mandelker, "A Wellness Program or a Bitter Pill?" 36–39.

34. "Savings through Self-Funded Workers' Comp?" *Employee Health & Fitness* 17, no. 6 (1995):66, 67.

35. "Cash and Time Off Incentives Increase Wellness Program Participation by 34 Percent," *Inside Preventive Care* 2, no. 11 (1996):6.

36. I. Ritter, "Is a True Wellness Mindset Alive in the HMO Market?" *Strategic Health Care Marketing* 12, no. 1 (1995):7–9.

37. Caudron, "A Low-Cost Wellness Program," 34–38.

38. "Savings through Self-Funded Worker's Comp?" 66, 67.

39. P. Wuest, *The Employer's Health Costs Management Guide* (Wall, NJ: American Business, 1991), 141–158.

40. "Reward Employees for Effort, Not Just Results," 114–116.

41. Chapman, *Using Wellness Incentives: Positive Tools for a Healthy Lifestyle.*

42. "Alliant's Incentive Program Activities," 17.

43. "Incentive Program Design Checklist," *Health Promotion Practitioner* 5, no. 3 (1996):5.

44. Mandelker, "A Wellness Program or a Bitter Pill?" 36–39.

45. "Return-to-Work Program Plagues Denim King," *Business & Health* 15, no. 10 (1997):14.

46. K. Seal, "Health Care Rains Terror on Initiatives," *Managed Healthcare* 6, no. 3 (1996):15, 19.

47. Ritter, "Is a True Wellness Mindset Alive in the HMO Market?" 7–9.

48. "Recognition Reinforces Behavior Change," *Health Promotion Practitioner* 4, no. 5 (1995):6.

49. A. Kohn, "Why Incentive Plans Cannot Work," *Harvard Business Review* 71, no. 5 (1993):54–63.

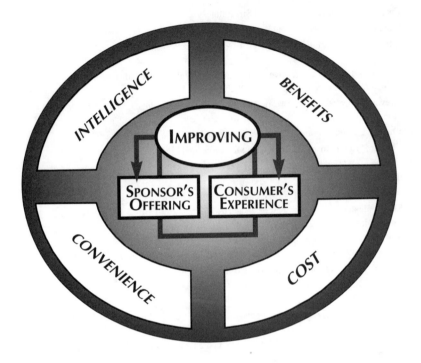

Chapter 15

MARKETING, NEGOTIATION
& EMPOWERMENT

The tactics discussed in Chapters 11 through 14 rely on familiar and relatively simple approaches to improving behavior. Communications are the sole device used in four of the five, and incentives, typically dollar rewards or "fines," are used in the fifth. In this chapter, we will discuss three less frequently employed tactics: (1) marketing, (2) negotiation, and (3) empowerment. Each of the three has wide applications in modifying behavior, generally, though relatively little history in improving consumer health and demand behaviors.

MARKETING

In social advertising, the ideas of exchange and the marketing mix are used as a basis for persuading and thereby motivating consumers to initiate, repeat, and continue desired patterns of behavior. While many marketing concepts and techniques are used in this tactic, it is a communications method based on the mass media. It does not seek to change the nature of the behavior to which it wishes consumers to convert.

A "true," or at least complete, marketing approach looks for ways to "improve the offer" rather than relying on persuading people to buy the present offer. In fact, enticing consumers to purchase what is already on hand is, by definition, a *sales* challenge as opposed to a marketing one. In marketing the idea is to design and deliver an improved offer that will be so attractive and satisfying to customers that it will all but sell itself.

Applied to challenges of converting consumers from bad to good health and demand behaviors, marketing looks for ways to make a desired new or different behavior into an offer that consumers will not refuse. As with other tactics, marketing can be applied to any of the set of effects. It can be used in conjunction with education programs, for example, by making them more attractive and satisfying, more convenient, and less costly to consumers, as suggested in Chapter 12.

Of potentially greater value is the potential for making a specific new or changed behavior, in itself, more likely to be adopted and continued by consumers, making the new health or demand behavior a significantly better value so that more consumers will want to adopt it. The idea is that if we can make a given behavior change sufficiently enticing and rewarding by itself, we need not devote as much attention to persuasion, incentives, or other motivational tactics, though prompting and educational efforts may still be necessary.

Marketing Intelligence

Making a given behavior into a better offer begins with gathering intelligence about selected consumers. The more we can learn about their values, needs, wants, perceptions, and attitudes, the better we will be able to design an offer they will not refuse. By determining where consumers are in terms of stages of readiness, their knowledge, attitudes, and intentions toward their present versus the desired behavior, we can better select who are the most promising targets.

Knowing what mix of motivation, capability, and consciousness is involved in predisposing consumers toward one behavior versus another gives us a place to start. A key requirement in changing consumer behavior is understanding why they are not already behaving in the desired fashion, particularly since the health and demand improvements we are after are supposed to benefit consumers. A second, related requirement is learning what are the "switching costs" that consumers perceive as attending the sponsor-desired behavior change. What will consumers lose by changing behavior?

Using the marketing mix, we need to know how consumers perceive present versus desired behavior patterns in terms of their "product" benefits, the types of basic human values each behavior protects or enhances. We need to understand the "place" convenience, ease, or difficulty and contextual factors that promote the current or hinder the desired behavior. Finally, we want to appreciate the "price" factors, all the negative consequences that consumers perceive relative to both the present and desired behavior.

With such intelligence, we can at least understand the competition (i.e., what we are challenged to surpass with the new behavior offer we are trying to design and deliver). Knowing how tough the competition is will also help in selecting targets; marketers normally prefer going after the easier ones, the "low-hanging fruit" first.[1] This can be essential in what may be the strategic marketing challenge of attracting internal support for consumer behavior improvement per se or in obtaining approval and support from others.

Knowing how consumers perceive the competitive "offer" provides the basis for design, enabling sponsors to select which dimensions (i.e., product, place, or price) to work on and which behavior factors to focus on. It may not be possible to beat the competition on each of its dimensions, nor is it necessary to do so. Offering one or more "competitive distinctions" in the desired behavior that are sufficient to overcome switching costs and convince targets to at least try the desired alternative is the first part of the marketing challenge. Delivering and reminding consumers about enough unique or superior experiences and consequences so that targets will stay converted to the new behavior is the second part.

One of the greatest possible contributions of a marketing approach is the behavior intelligence it may uncover. By discovering that a given set of consumers misperceives the benefits and risks of their present behavior or the advantages of the desired behavior, sponsors may be able to devise a simple persuasion effort that achieves desired changes inexpensively. By learning that targeted consumers have transportation or other capability barriers to adopting the desired behavior, sponsors can avoid spending a lot of time and effort on motivation.

The first contribution of marketing intelligence may be to discover that a full-blown marketing approach is not needed, that some other, simpler and less expensive approach can work. Where this is not the case, marketing intelligence provides the foundation for the full marketing approach, the design and delivery of a better behavior that will attract and satisfy the intended number of consumers. While a comprehensive discussion of marketing intelligence techniques is beyond the scope of this book, we shall briefly describe a few of the more relevant options.

Laddering

One marketing intelligence tool that is likely to be particularly useful in addressing these challenges is called "laddering." The purpose of this technique is to get consumers to "go up the ladder" from factors that represent obvious and meaningful perceptions about a given behavior, their stated reasons for engaging in it, to the basic values that are involved in their attitudes toward it. By identifying which values are involved, marketers can look for better ways to protect or enhance the values that are driving the "wrong" behavior.[2]

For example, consumers may initially be asked: "Why is it that you prefer going to the hospital emergency room for health care?" They might say: "Because it's open 24 hours"; "They have to serve you there even if you're not insured"; They know how to take care of emergencies"; "It's right near where I live"; "I don't have a doctor I can trust," or any number of reasons. To get a list of reasons, the interviewer can ask: "Any other reason?" until consumers shrug their shoulders or otherwise indicate the key reasons have been described.

For each reason, in turn, interviewers then ask: "Why is that important to you?" or "How does that benefit you?" Consumer responses to these questions will tend to move up the ladder toward basic values. Being open 24 hours might be important because consumers have high levels of anxiety about their children and feel they cannot wait for regular office hours. Discovering that emotional security and overcoming anxiety are major drivers of the old behavior can enable sponsors to design ways to deal with the same values and needs through a new behavior, perhaps accessing an urgent care center or being reassured by a nurse counselor through a 24-hour phone triage service, for example.

Knowing the underlying human value or need that is "engaged" in a given behavior can also help sponsors strengthen their communications about it. Being able to cite the human value benefits of a new behavior, perhaps self-esteem or peer respect, can add to promises and reports of more mundane direct benefits such as saving money or avoiding smelly clothes resulting from quitting smoking, for example.

Consumers themselves use basic needs and values in helping to design more attractive offers. Once the basic needs and values involved in motivating the old behavior have been identified, interviewers can ask consumers to suggest other ways those needs and values might be addressed. An anxiety-driven consumer might respond: "If I could at least talk to someone who could tell me if my baby's fever is serious." Such a response could lead sponsors to consider a phone triage option.

The purpose of the laddering exercise is to enable sponsors to focus on the basic needs and values that motivate consumers toward the wrong behaviors, so as to design a better offer that will steer them toward the right ones. Consumers may not always be willing to discuss underlying motivations, and there may be some that are subconscious or unconscious factors they are not even aware of. For that reason marketers cannot totally rely on consumers for insights into what will convert them. Creative imaginations are needed as well as research techniques.

For example, Kotler and Andreasen suggested that as simple a "trick" as employing attractive female nurses in blood drawing might be enough to entice more men to give blood.[3] One might also suggest that using attractive male nurses could do the same for female blood donors. In any case, "laddering" might never turn up such a suggestion. Even where men are conscious of their enjoyment of flirting with or being coddled by attractive nurses, they might be loathe to mention the fact to an interviewer.

For unhealthy behaviors, either consumers or marketers might suggest better options. Nonalcoholic beer could emerge as a way to enjoy the fun and fellowship of the local bar or bowling alley without risking intoxication. Nicotine patches are unlikely to be suggested by smokers, but they might indicate a wish for other ways to get the relaxation or whatever other benefit they derive from smoking. Either consumers or marketers might suggest team sports as an alternative to gang activities, sky diving as an alternative to narcotics.[4]

Naturalistic Observation

Another approach to learning more about consumers is to observe them in their normal surroundings. This is easier when they are in groups, such as participants in an exercise, education, or training program, or at work. Listening in to their conversations and observing their behavior can offer insights into who might be the best prospects for conversion. It can also help identify the social and corporate cultures that influence health and demand behaviors in specific groups of consumers.

One example of this naturalistic observation technique identified three distinct worker segments: (1) a young, fitness-oriented group; (2) an older, even more health-conscious, healthy-behaving segment; and (3) a set of high-risk intransigents who resisted reforming. Analysis of observed behavior led to recommendations for group efforts such as worker committees and task forces to address specific problem behaviors and to the use of peer (coworker and spouse) sources of communications to promote behavior changes.[5]

Feedback

In addition to consumers insights and suggestions at the front end of designing a better offer, getting their feedback on "draft" ideas can help refine designs or at least reduce the risk of implementing ineffective offers. "Test marketing" of a new offer can give consumers another shot at helping marketers come up with the right offer. This may be done at the conceptual stage, asking consumers to react to an idea or a description of the new offer. It can also be done at the "pilot" stage, when the new experience can be delivered at a small scale before widespread implementation.[6]

Pilot testing can help determine how *satisfying* the new offer will be, where concept testing can only address how *attractive* it seems to consumers. Both are essential to success.[7] There is no point in designing and implementing an offer that will attract converts, only to have them go away disappointed and dissatisfied. Even in those rare instances where one trial of the behavior is enough (e.g., a lifetime immunization or end-of-life choice), dissatisfaction with the offer is likely to result in negative word-of-mouth "advertising" to others and the breakdown of trust for any future efforts.

Maximizing target satisfaction with the new offer is the best way to promote its repetition and continuation for behaviors requiring more than a one-time choice. It can also help galvanize delighted consumers into becoming champions of the new behavior among their peers. Since both persuasion and prompting are essential supplements to marketing a better offer, having peers as advocates for the new behavior can be the most powerful source of both.[8]

The marketing mix of product, place, price, and promotion allows marketers to address whatever combination of motivation, capability, and consciousness needs to be improved to make the new behavior both more attractive and more satisfying. Product and price factors are aimed primarily at motivation, enhancing the benefits or reducing the costs of the desired behavior compared to the present competitor. Place factors aim at any capability barriers or enhancements that can make a difference. Promotional communications can then be used to persuade and/or prompt targets into first a trial, then repetition and continuation (i.e., full conversion).

Benefit (Product) Enhancement

Benefit-enhancement possibilities include such examples as nicotine patches or gum and nonalcoholic beer and wine (i.e., ways to deliver many of the same benefits as the "wrong" behavior). A phone triage counseling service delivers the same anxiety-reducing benefit as professional treatment; a 24-hour urgent care center can deliver the same benefits as an emergency department for most non-emergencies. Self-care and self-management of chronic conditions deliver the same benefits as professional services when done correctly.

Knowing what consumers expect and wish from a given experience can enable design and delivery of a superior competitive offer. Building in the communication of a sense of caring, acceptance, and respect (i.e., "stroking") can make the new form of service delivery superior to the old.[9] Adding information to an experience, such as sending a self-care guide to those who call a triage service or including written instructions with a disease management device can also be ways to add to benefits.[10]

One way to improve the benefits of healthier behavior is to build in measuring and reporting systems that permit consumers, their family members, and peers to monitor their accomplishments. Seeing numbers go up or down in response to behavior changes can be reward enough for many; and it can provide the basis for getting praise and recognition from others.[11]

Adding fun and enjoyment to exercise programs, support group discussions, and other group experiences can make them more attractive and satisfying. Consumers themselves may be the best source of ideas for ways to introduce some excitement into a desired behavior.[12] Offering multiple choices of ways to engage in a desired behavior, such as exercise, can help customize the experience to individuals as well as give them a greater sense of control.[13]

Customization to individuals and segments is first a way to gear each desired behavior to the idiosyncratic needs and wishes of different consumers. It gives sponsors a better chance of offering something that consumers will want than a one-size-fits-all approach. It also communicates a commitment to individual and segment interests that will help strengthen relationships. Where it attracts similar consumers to engage in a group activity, such as exercise, it can also add a social participation benefit to the desired behavior.

In many cases, consumers can design their own "product" so as to make it as attractive and satisfying as possible. Encourage them to set their own goals for risk reduction and wellness achievements and devise their own monitoring schedule and system to track their progress. Have them build in their own, self-delivered rewards for benchmark progress and final achievement, such as a vacation trip or a special treat or gift they would not otherwise buy.[14]

Convenience (Place) Enhancements

Making it easier, more convenient for consumers to engage in the desired behavior is one of the most popular approaches to promoting education and training participation. It is also available for any health or demand behaviors that have time and place dimensions. Offering immunizations at the worksite, in shopping malls, or at social gatherings is a common example.[15] Worksite fitness facilities are frequently offered by employers.[16]

Making hours of service more convenient is an equally popular option. The 24-hour accessibility of phone triage and health information makes it competitive with more limited-access providers.[17] Offering blood-sugar testing early in the morning can make diabetes management more convenient for workers; offering devices that enable consumers to perform their own tests at home makes it even more so, combining place and time convenience and enhancing consumer control.

Inviting targets to participate in designing more convenient options is a logical combination of research and customization. Computer-driven "expert systems" can enable consumers to tailor health and wellness programs to their unique values and circumstances. This has the added advantage of promoting their commitment, since they design the new behavior offer themselves. The computer allows them to combine objective information, about what they can and should do, with subjective needs and wishes, about what they want to do, into customized "solutions" that best fit the combination.[18]

In reality convenience factors translate into either benefits or costs. Making it easier for consumers to engage in a given behavior means consumers will save time, "hassle," or some other cost, and having more time for other things or avoiding the stress of hassles is clearly a benefit. What consumers describe as inconveniences are sure to be factors that impose costs—an "inconvenient location" could mean it takes too long to get there, costs too much in gas or bus fares, or is in a high-crime neighborhood causing anxiety, for example. It is worthwhile to probe consumer perceptions relative to the vague concept of "convenience" to learn the specific benefits and costs involved.

Cost (Price) Reductions

There are a variety of ways in which sponsors or consumers themselves can design offers that lower the "price" of new behaviors. Discounts for fitness club fees and free on-site facilities have been commonly offered by employers. Package pricing for completing a program can make it cheaper for consumers to finish the program than to quit in the middle. Employers can make it easier for employees to pay for priced activities such as exercise programs by offering payroll deductions over time.[19]

Making something free is the easiest way to at least eliminate a barrier to a given behavior. This can be done by making sure it is covered under health plan benefit packages or offering it free when not covered. Free public immunizations are a popular example. Free self-care guides can stimulate decision improvements; free monitoring devices such as blood-sugar monitors and peak flow meters can promote their use in disease management.

Free trials are a way to promote consumers trying out a behavior whose full benefits cannot be appreciated except by experiencing them. Such an approach may eliminate the only objective reason consumers can give themselves for not trying it once.[20] The challenge, of course, is to make that trial so overwhelmingly satisfying that it will be repeated even when a price is involved.[21]

Other costs, or negative aspects, of the desired behavior can be addressed as well. Making immunizations painless, or at least less painful, can be a meaningful cost reduction for consumers, as patients and parents. Reducing the time and perhaps lost wages for consumers to obtain desired services or paying them while engaged in health-promoting activities at the worksite are ways to reduce time costs. Ensuring confidentiality of information can avoid embarrassment costs. Just as "product" benefits can only be appreciated and enhanced from the consumer's perspective, so is "price" whatever consumers perceive it to be.

There is a difference between benefits and costs that is important to sponsors aiming for health and demand behaviors that have to be repeated or continued, as opposed to those requiring only one or occasional repetition. A benefit (i.e., positive value) can be noted for each repetition or continuation of the behavior. Exercise can make consumers feel good every time they engage in it; smokers who quit can enjoy their lessened anxiety, money saved, or sense of well-being during every week they remain nonsmokers.

Where some inconvenience or cost represents a barrier to behavior improvement, however, it may have a greatly lessened or no effect on continuing to motivate a behavior once the barrier is overcome. Once a fitness center is made free, for example, consumers are likely not to sense a continuing benefit every time they use it; the being free part can become "background" and a routine aspect of the experience and may not be appreciated anew each time. Where consumers can be reminded of the benefits they gain by exercise (e.g., through measuring their improved lung capacity, weight loss), there is no corresponding potential for measuring and reporting continuing improvement for inconveniences and costs. It is likely to prove more effective in *continuing* improved behaviors if sponsors can offer, measure, and report continuing benefits consumers enjoy as opposed to eliminated costs or inconveniences. (See discussion of how to promote repetition or continuation of improved behaviors in Chapter 16.)

Combining Factors

The fourth component of the marketing mix, "promotion," has already been addressed in chapters on prompting, persuasion, and social advocacy. Promotion can serve an additional function relative to the other three factors, however: it can serve as the basis for designing them. Instead of designing the best product/place/price offer first, then building a promotional campaign based on the offer, marketers might design the most persuasive promotion campaign they can first, then seek to design and deliver the offer accordingly.

For example, sponsors could brainstorm on their own or invite a sample of consumers to help them design a communications campaign aimed at converting people to a desired behavior. They could ask participants what facts and arguments they would find most persuasive in converting them from their present behavior. Based on the promotional theme or "pitch" they identify as most appealing, sponsors can strive to come up with an offer that matches it. Where consumers and sponsors can more readily identify the facts and arguments that will work, this reverse approach can be simpler than starting with the offer as the focus. And it has the advantage of a predesigned promotional campaign if sponsors can deliver the offer in fact.

To get the best results, the full set of product, place, and price factors should be included in offer design efforts. The entire experience that consumers will have while trying, repeating, and continuing the desired behavior should be consciously addressed, from beginning to end.[22] Every opportunity to add value, make new behaviors easier to adopt, and minimize their costs should be considered.

However clever the sponsors assigned to this challenge may be, chances are they are not as clever as the combination of their own and their targets' genius can be. Sponsors should get on the same side of the table as their targets, working to devise a joint solution to the problem, a common approach to their common objectives. This will not only promote finding the most cost-effective and satisfying offers to make; it will enhance relationships with consumers as present and future partners.

For behavior improvement efforts involving large numbers of consumer targets, surveys can be used to obtain their insights and identify their interests up front.[23] Focus groups and depth interviews can be used to learn about motivation, capability, and consciousness avenues to stimulate change. Concept and pilot testing of programs and promotional materials can keep marketers' creative initiatives focused on consumer values.

For smaller groups of consumers, such as patient groups for disease management efforts or employee teams for safety aspects of disability management, the full set of targets can be partners in designing the new offer. Wherever the potential gain is great enough, since gains accrue to consumers as well as sponsors, there is the potential for partnering with consumer targets in devising the offer that will be made. This enables marketing to come close to negotiation as a tactic, achieving something close to a commitment on the part of participating consumers to accept the offer they helped design.

Marketing is primarily a motivational tactic, aiming to design and deliver an improved behavior offer (i.e., greater benefit at lower cost = better value) that will cause consumers to want to adopt and continue the very behavior pattern that sponsors wish. It can also contribute to enhancing capability by identifying internal or external capability barriers to the desired behavior. Moreover, it can enhance external capability factors by making the behavior more convenient through the design process.

While the promotional component of the marketing mix has been mentioned, it is often true that marketing communications have more impact on already committed "customers," reminding them of facts they already know and attitudes they already have. In this sense, it serves as a consciousness reinforcement agent as well (Exhibit 15–1).

Exhibit 15–1 Marketing

DEFINITION	✗ ENTICING CONSUMERS TO ADOPT DESIRED BEHAVIOR BY ENHANCING ITS BENEFITS, REDUCING ITS COSTS, AND/OR MAKING IT EASIER TO ADOPT
OBJECTIVE	✗ TO INCREASE CONSUMER MOTIVATION CAPABILITY BY MAKING DESIRED BEHAVIOR MORE ATTRACTIVE & SATISFYING AND/OR MORE CONVENIENT, LESS COSTLY
EXAMPLES OF TECHNIQUES	✗ ADD VALUE SUCH AS SOCIALIZATION THROUGH GROUP SESSIONS, INTERNET CONTACTS, ETC. ✗ REDUCE PRICE VIA SPONSOR DISCOUNTS / FREE PROGRAMS ✗ MAKE DESIRED BEHAVIOR MORE CONVENIENT VIA ON-SITE FITNESS CENTERS, SCREENING PROGRAMS, ETC.
SUGGESTIONS	✗ USE MARKET RESEARCH TO LEARN ABOUT CONSUMER VALUES, BARRIERS TO DESIRED BEHAVIOR; OBTAIN FEEDBACK ON PROBLEMS ✗ COMBINE "PRODUCT" ENHANCEMENTS, "PRICE" REDUCTIONS, "PLACE"IMPROVEMENTS WHERE FEASIBLE ✗ CUSTOMIZE OFFER TO SPECIFIC SEGMENTS OR INDIVIDUALS ✗ COMBINE WITH PROMPTING & PERSUASION TACTICS

NEGOTIATION

Negotiation is a logical extension of marketing as a means to engineering behavior change. Instead of marketers designing an exchange offer they hope targets will "buy," negotiators sit down with targets and work out an exchange agreement that both will sign or otherwise commit to. Like marketing, it tends to focus on motivation, discussion of what it will take to get targets to commit to changing their behavior, but it can include capabilities and consciousness as well, perhaps specifying the education or training and prompting that sponsors will contribute as their part of the deal.

Negotiation may take place one-to-one, as when a physician, nurse, or other provider works out a contract for a patient's health and wellness plan. It may involve representative groups, as when union negotiators hammer out an arrangement whereby employees agree to a nonsmoking workplace or to sharing cost-savings resulting from better health and demand behavior. In some cases it may include all consumers targeted for behavior change, as when a group of patients discusses making a commitment to a disease management effort.

There are two advantages to negotiation as a tactic in bringing about behavior change. First, it involves the direct participation of the very consumers targeted for behavior improvement in determining what it will take to get them to change their behavior. This can make what sponsors have to offer both more effective and more efficient than what marketers might come up with on their own. Overzealous marketers might design an offer that is much more elegant and expensive than would be needed to convert targets. Or they might misconstrue research results and end up with an offer that consumers reject, once apprised of it.

Negotiation should produce the most acceptable offer from the perspective of both parties. Ideally it will produce a win-win outcome that delights both parties. At a minimum it should produce a compromise both can live with. And as its main contribution, it should produce an agreement, a commitment on the part of both sponsors and consumers to do what they agreed to. People tend to do what they have agreed to, particularly if the agreement is public, in writing, and is legally enforceable.

Negotiation, by placing both parties in the same room together, is also helpful in identifying common values, goals, and aspirations. Where sponsors might otherwise have to guess or conduct research to learn consumer perspectives, negotiation encourages consumers to disclose them. Similarly, where consumers might otherwise wonder what motivates sponsors to aim for a given behavior change, negotiation encourages sponsors to divulge what their interests are. Such mutual disclosure promotes trust, which, in turn, facilitates negotiation and good relationships.[24] These, in turn, promote future success in behavior improvement efforts.

Agreements need not require extensive negotiation, nor even concessions or commitments on the part of the sponsor. Physicians have often obtained patient and family-member agreement to "contracts" that are legally unenforceable and commit the physician to nothing, but that formally and publicly express patient/family commitment to playing their part in managing an acute or chronic condition.[25] Similar contracts make sense when dealing with health and wellness behavior.

There are a host of helpful works on the subject of how to negotiate successfully. Fisher and Ury's *Getting to Yes*[26] and Ury's *Getting Past No*[27] are popular examples. Beale and Fields' *The Win/Win Way,*[28] the Albrechts' *Added Value Negotiating,*[29] and Mayer's *Power Plays*[30] are three more, though the last has a sales/persuasion focus on winning that threatens its value in promoting trust and lasting relationships. We will not attempt to offer a comprehensive discussion of negotiation here, in light of the excellent works already available.

There are some tricks of the trade in negotiation that may prove helpful, however. Knowing as much about targets as is helpful in marketing is a sound basis for negotiation.[31] Knowing what Ury calls their Best Alternative to Negotiated Agreement (BATNA; i.e., what their other best option would be) is especially helpful. Using a joint problem-solving approach that focuses on values, how each would like to gain, as opposed to positions, where each is now, is also recommended.[32]

Another recommendation is to bring to the table a "Chinese menu" of options for targets to choose from, rather than have a single objective in mind.[33] Letting individual targets design their own commitment from among options already acceptable to the sponsor can facilitate reaching agreement by preserving targets' sense of control and autonomy. By contrast, hammering out an agreement based on the sponsor's single behavior objective may make consumers feel manipulated.

Another suggestion is to "get into the other's shoes" by challenging each other to state the other party's position and reasons for it to the point of mutual satisfaction. This may help determine whether any disagreement is based on differences in value versus different perceptions of reality. It can also give each party an understanding of the other's position not achievable otherwise.

One employer found that simply getting employees to agree to the idea that cutting health care costs is a worthwhile goal helped in negotiating specific commitments. By recognizing how both parties would benefit by achieving the goal, labor and management could get on the same side of the table in working out ways to achieve it.[34]

At the individual level, the challenge in improving consumer health and demand behaviors is first to get consumers to assume "locus of control," to recognize and commit to their being in charge of their own behavior and the consequences thereof. Using a workable integrated negotiation process to achieve specific commitments can help achieve or reinforce consumers' sense of responsibility and power over their own behavior, as opposed to passivity and helplessness.[35]

Negotiation is not without risk as a behavior improvement tactic. Assuming that sponsors engage in good-faith negotiation, they must enter discussions with less than full control over what agreement will be reached. They may well end up investing more than they intended to achieve the desired behavior change. Sponsors should have a clear and accurate estimate of the value of the behavior change they are after so that they still end up with a worthwhile outcome, even if not precisely the outcome they intended.

While sponsors may start with a specific goal as to what behavior change they seek, they should be at least open to considering alternatives if consumers participating in the negotiation process come up with an acceptable approach. Sponsors may aim for obtaining a weight reduction commitment from consumers, for example, yet be willing to accept a fitness improvement commitment, instead, if it will produce essentially the same desired outcomes (Exhibit 15–2).

EMPOWERMENT

In a sense, our entire discussion of tactics is based on "empowerment" (i.e., encouraging and enabling consumers to take control over their own behavior for their own good). As a specific behavior modification tactic, however, empowerment has a narrower meaning. Essentially it means turning over the challenge and the power to achieve a given objective to consumers, standing back and letting them see what they can do.

Empowerment relies on consumers being already motivated by at least the outcomes desired by sponsors (e.g., better health and use of health services). It also assumes that capability is not a problem and that, at a minimum, consumers empowered to find their own path to desired outcomes can do so. It may later prove that empowered consumers ask for the sponsor's help in carrying out the solution they devise, however.

All the other tactics start with a specific behavior objective in mind: consumers should initiate, repeat, or continue some desired behavior or should reduce or quit some undesired pattern. Sponsors then look to prompt, persuade, educate, communicate, market, or negotiate a way to get them to comply. Empowerment leaves the selection of a behavior objective up to consumers. If sponsor and consumers can agree on a common goal, then consumers can take charge of identifying what they will do to achieve it.[36]

There is no exchange necessarily involved, unlike marketing and negotiation. Consumers decide how they will change their own behavior to achieve some goal they commit to. Sponsors can introduce a reward or exchange, of course, by volunteering to provide a bonus or share savings if the goal is achieved. Consumers still have the power to decide how best to achieve it.

Empowerment rests on the fact that there are significant shared values and goals between consumers and sponsors, whether payers or providers. Acceptance of the commonality of goals may be mutual and clear at the outset, or it may take some

Exhibit 15–2 Negotiation

DEFINITION	✗ Sponsor & consumer jointly designing a behavior experience
OBJECTIVE	✗ To increase consumers' motivation and/or capability by involving them in design process & addressing their values & barriers ✗ To obtain their commitment to changing behavior
EXAMPLES OF TECHNIQUES	✗ Employers negotiate with workers individually, in teams, with union ✗ Providers negotiate with patients ✗ Consumers negotiate with family members, friends, coworkers
SUGGESTIONS	✗ Seek a formal, public commitment even if not legally binding ✗ Be willing to accept behavior change different from initial objective if same outcomes will be achieved ✗ Be careful not to reach agreement that costs more than its value

persuasion or education to achieve. In some cases commonality may be negotiated, as when employers and unions work out a sharing of the savings realized if employees can devise and implement successful methods.

If this commonality exists and commitment to common goals and objectives is strong enough among consumers, as individuals or groups, then empowerment may be an acceptable, if not preferred tactic. Consumers may not only come up with better ways to achieve the common goals (i.e., a more effective or efficient behavior change than sponsors might identify). They are also more likely to commit to investing the effort required in achieving the specific behavior change they identified because it was their idea.

Empowerment may be thought of as a kind of leadership, helping consumers manage themselves by challenging them to come up with specific objectives, programs, rewards, and punishments, whatever it will take for them to achieve those objectives.[37] Since all management is ultimately self-management, empowerment may both promote success in achieving individual objectives and enhance consumer motivation and capability to manage other behaviors in future.[38] It tends to promote self-efficacy, where it produces successful behavior change, though it can also undermine self-efficacy, where empowered consumers come up with an approach that does not work.

A comprehensive approach to empowerment applied to consumer health and demand behavior would include acquainting consumers with a variety of tactics available for influencing each other's behavior (e.g., give them a copy of this book) and letting them choose which they can use in improving their own behavior. Where they ask for support, resources, changes in benefit plans, or similar sponsor assistance in achieving their goals, sponsors can decide where the investment promises a good return in specific behavior changes and relationship benefits.[39]

Empowerment is likely to be more risky than other tactics or certainly to seem more risky since sponsors give up control over what consumers will decide. Where consumers are well-motivated to seek the same outcomes as desired by sponsors, however, and well-informed as to the kinds of behavior changes that can lead to such outcomes, they may well prove better at devising successful initiatives than sponsors are. Where this happens, sponsors stand to gain a better working relationships with the consumers involved and thereby improved prospects for future success than are likely to be available through most of the other tactics.

Combining Marketing, Negotiation, and Empowerment

A special form of empowerment can be called "self-marketing." Sponsors can empower targeted consumers, encourage them to set their own behavior improvement goals, and design their own behavior change experiences. These would include whatever changes in the "product" or benefits each consumer considers at-

Exhibit 15–3 Empowerment

DEFINITION	✗ TURNING OVER TO CONSUMERS THE RESPONSIBILITY FOR DECIDING ON AN APPROACH TO CHANGING BEHAVIOR OR A WAY TO ACHIEVE A VALUED OUTCOME (E.G., HEALTH STATUS, UTILIZATION, EXPENDITURES)
OBJECTIVE	✗ ENHANCE CONSUMERS' MOTIVATION AND/OR CAPABILITY BY GIVING THEM THE POWER TO DECIDE FOR THEMSELVES
EXAMPLES OF TECHNIQUES	✗ EMPLOYERS & EMPLOYEES AGREE ON VALUE OBJECTIVE; *THEN* EMPLOYEES CREATE COMMITTEES / TEAMS TO PURSUE NEEDED BEHAVIOR CHANGES ✗ PROVIDER AND PATIENT AGREE ON HEALTH STATUS OUTCOME; *THEN* PATIENT TAKES RESPONSIBILITY FOR IDENTIFYING & MAKING BEHAVIOR CHANGES
SUGGESTIONS	✗ ENSURE CONSUMERS VALUE OUTCOMES, HAVE INFORMATION & RESOURCES TO IDENTIFY & MAKE WORTHWHILE CHANGES ✗ PROMOTE FORMAL, SIGNED / PUBLIC AGREEMENT EVEN IF NOT LEGALLY ENFORCEABLE

tractive, perhaps socializing with others or engaging in a competition, for example. "Place" factors such as location and timing, as well as "price" factors such as out-of-pocket costs and paid or unpaid time would also be designed as a draft self-offer by each consumer. "Promotion" would be chiefly focused on prompting systems, from self-promoting via calendar or computer to using buddy systems or other external reminders.

Having designed a customized marketing offer, each consumer can then approach the sponsor to negotiate whatever support is required. Sponsors might have to put up the money to subsidize out-of-pocket costs, to pay for time away from work, to cover costs of reminder systems. Consumers might ask for specific rewards or recognitions from sponsors. Such an approach entails all the risks of empowerment (i.e., that consumers may ask for more than sponsors wish to pay or can justify given the value of the behavior changes to which consumers commit).

On the other hand, it also contains the built-in control of negotiation, whereby sponsors can cite the "natural" limits of budgets or estimated value, offer alternatives, and otherwise work toward win-win resolution of unreasonable demands. By empowering consumers in the first place and employing a self-marketing approach to designing the behavior change experience, sponsors are likely to secure consumers' commitment to their self-designed change. Consumers' own designs may well be less expensive than what sponsors would have come up with on their own. If they are more expensive, sponsors always have the option of negotiating a lower cost alternative.

Marketing, negotiation, and empowerment are by no means the last resorts for sponsors to consider, though they may involve the greatest investment or risk and least sponsor control. Because each more fully involves consumers in designing initiatives, each necessarily undercuts sponsor control. At the same time, such greater involvement stands to improve the chances for success in particular initiatives and to enhance long-term working relationships with consumers for future efforts (Exhibit 15–3).

REFERENCES

1. B. Gelb and J. Bryant, "Designing Health Promotion Programs by Watching the Market," *Journal of Health Care Marketing* 12, no. 1 (1992):65–90.

2. J. Myers, *Segmentation and Positioning for Marketing Decisions* (Chicago, IL: American Marketing Association, 1996), 263–282.

3. P. Kotler and A. Andreasen, *Strategic Marketing for Nonprofit Organizations,* 3d ed. (Englewood Cliffs, NJ: Prentice-Hall, 1987).

4. Gelb and Bryant, "Designing Health Promotion Programs," 65–90.

5. D. Leathar and G. Hastings, "Social Marketing and Health Education," *Journal of Services Marketing* 1, no. 2 (1987):49–52.

6. A. Andreasen, *Marketing Social Change* (San Francisco, CA: Jossey-Bass, 1995), 223–250.

7. M. Baker, "The Chief Scientist Reports . . . Marketing Health," *Health Bulletin* (UK) 46, no. 5 (1988):296–303.

8. "Drip Marketing—or How To Cultivate High Potential Patients or Clients," *The Practice Builder* 12, no. 2 (1994):1–3.

9. R. Conklin, *How To Get People To Do Things* (New York, NY: Ballantine Books, 1979).

10. "Boomers Hit Middle Age," *Health Promotion Practitioner* 4, no. 12 (1995):2.

11. L. Chapman, *Using Wellness Incentives: Positive Tools for Healthy Lifestyles,* 2d ed. (Seattle, WA: Summex Corp, 1991).

12. J. Rippe, "Seduce Yourself into Shape," *Heart Health,* Special Advertising Section Published by *Newsweek Magazine,* 1991, 12–16.

13. "10 Ways To Get New Participants . . . And Keep Them," *Health Promotion Practitioner* 4, no. 5 (1995):1.

14. Rippe, "Seduce Yourself," 12–16.

15. W. Novelli, "Applying Social Marketing to Health Promotion and Disease Prevention," in *Health Behavior and Health Education,* eds. K. Glanz et al. (San Francisco, CA: Jossey-Bass, 1990), 342–369.

16. C. Petersen, "Employers, Providers Are Partners in Health," *Managed Healthcare* 5, no. 1 (1995): 36–38.

17. "Healthcare on the Superhighway," *Modern Healthcare,* 11 December 1995, 68.

18. D. Straus and D. Yen, "How an Expert Corporate Fitness Program Might Be Designed," *Health Care Supervisor* 10, no. 3 (1992):40–55.

19. "Boosting Volume Participation," *Health Promotion Practitioner* 4, no. 7 (1995):6.

20. "Free Prospecting Seminars Boost Health Promotion Participation All Year," *Health Promotion Practitioner* 5, no. 1 (1996):1.

21. S. Fine, ed., *Social Marketing* (Boston, MA: Allyn & Bacon, 1990).

22. Petersen, "Employers, Providers," 36–38.

23. "Use of Survey Data in Corporatewide Health Promotion Program," *Metlife Statistical Bulletin* 73, no. 2 (1992):28–38.

24. L. Crosby, et al., "Relationship Quality in Services Selling," *Journal of Marketing* 54, no. 3 (1990):68–81.

25. "Form Alliance with Community Mental Health Program," *Healthcare Demand Management* 1, no. 9 (1995):129–132.

26. R. Fisher and R. Ury, *Getting to Yes: Negotiating Agreement without Giving In* (New York, NY: Penguin Books, 1983).

27. R. Ury, *Getting Past No* (New York, NY: Bantam Books, 1991).

28. L. Beale and R. Fields, *The Win/Win Way* (New York, NY: Harcourt Brace Jovanovich, 1987).

29. P. Albrecht and S. Albrecht, *Added Value Negotiating* (Burr Ridge, IL: Irwin Professional, 1994).

30. R. Mayer, *Power Plays* (New York, NY: Random House, 1996).

31. B. Elms, "Six Winning Negotiation Strategies," *Personal Selling Power* 13, no. 8 (1993):70.

32. Ury, *Getting Past No.*

33. Albrecht and Albrecht, *Added Value Negotiating.*

34. B. Posner, "Preventive Medicine," *INC.* 11, no. 3 (1989):131, 132.

35. H. Ratzan, "Health Communications as Negotiation," *American Behavioral Scientist* 38, no. 2 (1994):224–247.

36. "Participant Partnerships Get Results," *Health Promotion Practitioner* 4, no. 2 (1995):5.

37. C. Manz and H. Sims, *Super-Leadership* (New York, NY: Berkeley Books, 1990).

38. W. Weijts, "Responsible Health Communication: Taking Control of Our Lives," *American Behavioral Scientist* 38, no. 2 (1994):257–270.

39. J. Allen and R. Bellingham, "Building Supportive Cultural Environments," in *Health Promotion in the Workplace,* 2d ed., eds. M. O'Donnell and J. Harris (Albany, NY: Delmar, 1994), 204–216.

PART IV

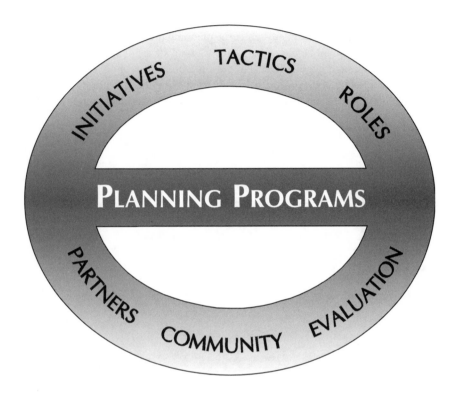

Part IV covers tactical or programmatic planning for Demand Improvement initiatives. It is intended primarily for those with programmatic responsibilities. Strategists may wish to at least review its contents as a means of ensuring that their strategies provide the basis for making the best tactical decisions and designing the most successful programs.

Chapter 16 offers a recommended format for planning specific programs, based on our value-adding Demand Improvement paradigm and our Motivation, Capability, and Consciousness factors for changing behavior. Chapter 17 addresses the challenge of choosing tactics from the wide range of options presented in Part III.

Chapter 18 discusses a key issue relative to the planning and implementation of Demand Improvement initiatives: who can and should be involved? While recognizing the at this issue applies differently to the many potential sponsors of such initiatives, it addresses the key considerations each sponsor might consider in choosing partners for particular efforts. Chapter 19 discusses and recommends community-wide options for improving demand, as a favored strategy or complement to sponsors' proprietary efforts.

Chapter 20 covers the last key step in the planning process, deciding how strategies and programs will be evaluated. This is a vital step, not simply as a way for sponsors to determine if their efforts have borne fruit, but to supply both strategists and program planners with information for improving their future planning and implementation. We strongly urge all readers to include this chapter in their list of readings.

Chapter 6

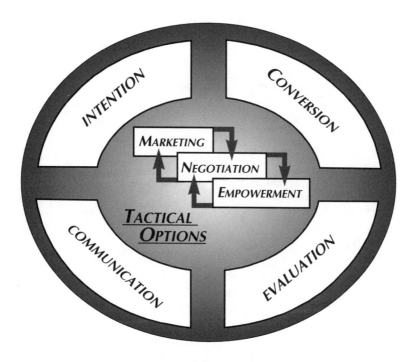

**PLANNING DEMAND
IMPROVEMENT INITIATIVES**

In this chapter, we will describe a 12-step process for planning particular demand improvement initiatives, once the strategic decision has been made as to what specific outcomes are to be sought. This process can be used with any of the tactics described in Chapters 11 through 15, though it is designed to best accommodate the marketing tactic.

For communications tactics alone, sponsors will use all 12 steps, though will emphasize steps 7 through 9. For negotiations, they can skip the three communications planning steps (steps 7 through 9) using the negotiation process itself to reach consumer commitment to behavior changes, rather than communications. For empowerment, sponsors may use just the first five steps, relying on targeted consumers themselves to carry out the next four, then combining with consumers for the last three. The 12 steps fall into four categories: A. Intention; B. Conversion; C. Communication; and D. Evaluation, as follows:

A. Intention
     1. Select consumer behavior change targets.
     2. Formulate behavior change objective(s).
     3. Estimate value of achieving objective(s).
B. Conversion
     4. Develop tactical behavior change intelligence.
     5. Design behavior change tactic(s).
     6. Plan and budget implementation of tactic(s).
C. Communication
     7. Formulate communications objectives.
     8. Develop media plan.
     9. Develop message plan.
D. Evaluation
     10. Assess results and return.
     11. Plan determination of impact on relationships.
     12. Plan learning for subsequent initiatives.

The emphasis in this process is on accountability; identifying specific, measurable outcomes to be achieved; determining reasonable effort based on the value of such outcomes; and efficient and effective initiatives to achieve them. The planning process may begin anywhere, not necessarily at the first step; sponsors of initiatives may have an inspiration about a particular tactic they wish to employ or a message they think will be persuasive and may develop a plan retrofitted from there.

In any case, the plan should be developed with each step considered as a draft until the entire plan is completed. Sponsors may realize or decide something at step 7 that causes them to revise what they planned in step 2 and should feel free to make whatever changes they wish in prior steps as they go along. It could be that by the time they estimate the costs of tactics designed in step 5 or communications efforts in steps 7, 8, and 9, they will discover that the costs of the effort far exceed the value of the behavior change objective and decide that the entire plan should go back to the drawing board. Or they may realize as they develop the evaluation plan in steps 10–12 that there is something they meant to add to the objectives in step 2 or even other targets they should have included in step 1.

OUTCOMES CHALLENGE

The outcomes challenge is the general statement of what motivates the development of the plan in the first place. Ideally the outcomes will reflect clear value through improved health status, use of care or expenditures, quality of life, loyalty, organizational performance, or other added value effects. In a health improvement situation, the challenge may be to decrease the number of people afflicted with communicable disease or the number of auto accident injuries. In decision improvement the desired outcomes might be to reduce total health care expenditures, inappropriate ED utilization, or futile care. A disease management challenge might be to reduce expenditures for ED care for patients with asthma and diabetes. In disability management the challenge might be to reduce unsafe lifting, to steer employees with low back pain toward chiropractors, or to increase participation in work-hardening programs.

While changing consumer behavior is always a component of demand improvement initiatives, the challenge should be stated in terms of specific results desired. Sponsors may begin planning with the determination to reduce the incidence of low-birth-weight babies in the population of concern. They may intend to cut back on rising workers' compensation costs or ED expenditures. As long as the desired results can be translated into specific behavior changes among specific target populations or segments thereof, those results can serve to initiate the planning process.

The challenge may be stated in fairly general language, outlining roughly what is to be accomplished in terms of the direction of change desired in some parameter considered important by the organization or community (e.g., "Decrease adverse fetal outcomes"). It may also be stated in traditional planning terms with a measurable outcome and time frame for its achievement (e.g., "Increase the proportion of normal newborns from 95% to 97% within two years"). Since it is written as a draft to stimulate and guide other steps, either approach will do.

CHALLENGE

THE STATEMENT THAT STIMULATES & GUIDES PLANNING FOR THE PARTICULAR BEHAVIOR CHANGE INITIATIVES

(The outcomes challenge normally emerges from the strategy development process described in Chapter 10. Sponsors may wish to make the outcomes more precise, however, as they begin planning for specific interventions. Where multiple outcome challenges are to be pursued simultaneously, separate plans should be prepared for each. The plans can then be combined for synergies and economies of integration later.)

SPECIFY INTENTION

Select Targets

The first step is to specify the people whose behavior is to be changed. Where some general notion may serve as a challenge statement, the specification of targets should be precise and numerical: exactly which individuals are to be approached by the behavior change initiative; how many of them are there? Are the targets the employees, dependents, or retirees of a given employer, or all three? Are they the entire enrolled population of a health plan or just those identified as high risks? Are minority members of the community to receive special attention? Are only the new patients in a practice to be targeted for effort?

Targets may be the entire set of people answering a particular description, or the set may be divided into subsets or segments for differentiated attention. If women are to be approached differently from men, children differently from adults, and Medicare and Medicaid and commercial enrollees differently from each other, a segmented approach may apply. If so, each segment represents a different target group for planning, and each should have its own plan. Once the separate plans are complete, behavior change sponsors can look for economies of scale or synergies through combining the implementation efforts.

The number of targets selected for attention needs to be specified. Effort needed to convert 10,000 people from one behavior to another is likely to be far greater

TARGETS

THE PRECISE NUMBER & ACTUAL IDENTITIES OF THE PERSONS TO BE APPROACHED FOR BEHAVIOR CHANGE

than that needed to convert a dozen; even if not, the value of the two accomplishments will be different. The precise numbers are needed, not proportions or percentages. Sponsors may decide that it is only possible to contact 50% of a given population of interest, but the plan should be based on what that 50% represents in hard numbers: 100 or 1,000 or 10,000 people. The value of objectives and costs of tactics can only be estimated based on hard numbers.

For many purposes the actual identities of targets should be specified, in addition to their numbers. In health improvement, for example, the names of people with particular health risks need to be identified to send correct risk assessments and appropriate health behavior change recommendations to the right people. Identities are often needed so results of efforts can be tracked and evaluated and subsequent initiatives planned. In decision improvement, names of individuals are needed to make follow-up calls after phone triage and to monitor what choices of therapy are made with what results.

In disease management the names of people and their chronic conditions must be matched to focus initiatives and in many compliance cases to determine if drug prescriptions have been filled. In disability management the names of employees targeted for safety promotion, as well as those in case management, must be known. In general, health plans and employers will have all names of targets available to them, and hospitals or physicians will have the names of all patients. Confidentiality and privacy of information will complicate targeting in many cases. (See Chapter 8.)

Objective(s)

Once consumer targets are specified, the next step is to describe exactly what change is to be achieved among exactly how many of those targets and how many are to be "converted" from one behavior to another. Precision is needed in specifying the change, both to plan and to evaluate the effort. Where the challenge might have been stated in terms of simply reducing smoking among employees, for example, the conversion objective should clearly state if the intent is to convert a given number to nonsmokers, to reduce the average number of cigarettes some number smoke per day, or simply to shift them to lower tar/nicotine brands. If quitting is the desired behavior, is it to be abstaining from smoking for a week, a month, a year?

If so many targets are to obtain all needed immunizations, the precise number of immunizations must be described. If advance directives are to be signed, the types of advance directives deemed acceptable need to be spelled out. If participation in a work-hardening program is desired, is initiation enough, completion, or ability to take a new assignment the definition of success?

While the number of consumers targeted for attention is specified under "targets," the number intended to actually convert to a different behavior is specified in the objective. Often the number intended to convert will be a small proportion of those targets approached by a given initiative. The behavior change may be difficult to accomplish, or take a long time, so that a one-year objective may aim for a small percentage of those approached. In some cases only a hard-core of consumers may remain unconverted. In other cases, for a new behavior such as self-care or use of a triage service, a high proportion of those approached may be expected to convert.

An objective might be stated in terms of any one of the set of effects that can result from demand improvement efforts:

- Increased participation in some activity (e.g., getting immunized or screened, engaging in an exercise program, attending a class);
- Improved awareness, knowledge, attitudes, intentions—any mind state that is expected to result in improved behavior;
- Improved behavior—adopting a better lifestyle, increasing use of self-care, controlling one's chronic condition, complying with treatment or rehabilitation;
- Improved health status—any specific measure or indicator of health whose improvement is intended;
- Improved use of services—the right amount, right type, in the right place at the right time, from the right provider;
- Improved expenditures for health care—typically lower expenditures but perhaps increased expenditures of one type versus another; and
- Added values of other kinds, including value to sponsors. For employers: worker morale, productivity, retention, lower absenteeism; for health plans: higher member satisfaction, loyalty, word-of-mouth "advertising"; for providers: higher patient satisfaction, retention, volunteering, for example. Added value to consumers may be enhanced quality of life, longevity, or both.

Any one of these factors in the set of effects may be chosen as the parameter to be changed in a targeted population. Sponsors may select a parameter among the early factors, in the confident expectation that an increase in participation or

OBJECTIVE

DETERMINING THE NUMBER OF CONSUMERS & THE SPECIFIC CHANGE IN BEHAVIOR SOUGHT

change in mind-states will surely result in improvements in health status, services utilization, expenditures, or some added value. They may aim specifically for a change in consumer behavior or pick an objective related to health status, expenditures, or added value—and leave it to consumers how they will change their own behavior so as to accomplish the resulting outcome.

For the most effective and efficient planning, however, objectives should be stated in terms of behavior change. Such changes can be used as a basis for estimating value far more easily than can participation or mind-state changes. They can be used to develop intervention tactics far more easily than health status, utilization, or expenditure changes. Demand improvement requires changes in consumer behavior, and these should be specified in planning.

It would be wise for sponsors to identify as many sources of value in their behavior change objectives as possible. Where a health plan aims for improved fitness, for example, and expects to save on expenditures as a result, if it cites added employer value such as higher employee productivity, added provider value such as their own reduced risk under capitation, and added consumer value such as better health, energy, and well-being, it is likely to enhance the level of cooperation it achieves. Moreover it may avoid the kind of "HMO bashing" and distrust that could be promoted if it aims only at increasing its own profits.

The *precise numbers* of targets who are to be converted should be stated. The number of converts desired out of those targeted for the effort should be a reasonable proportion; 100% conversion is rarely achievable, and a 10%, 30%, or 60% conversion may produce as much value as is likely in the time frame selected. Where percentages may be used to select the conversion objective, however, the objective must be stated in numbers (e.g., a 30% conversion of 1,000 smokers means that the objective is to get 300 people to quit).

The *time frame* for accomplishing the objective should be included: within a year, by December 1, in six months. In many cases the time frame for the objective will not match the time frame for expenditure of effort. Effort may take place in the next few months, with results expected months or even years later. Results may be modest in the first year and grow thereafter, while effort is greatest in the first year and reduced thereafter. Given the realities of budgeting, it makes sense to state objectives for fiscal periods covered by budgets and expenditures.

For example, it may be that the heaviest expenditures for a smoking cessation campaign are planned for the upcoming year but that only 150 targets are expected to quit (the average person who quits tries three times before succeeding) in the first year, with 450 the second. It would be wise to set an objective of 150 the first year and 450 the second rather than simply set an objective of 600 over two years, risking disappointment and perhaps reduced funding when only 150 quit the first year.

Objectives may also be set in terms of specific results to be achieved by targets, rather than specific changes in behavior. For weight management or exercise initiatives, for example, objectives may be stated in terms of weight loss to be achieved, resting heart rates, or other health status measures. For targets with a given chronic condition, the objective may be stated in terms of reductions in ED use or better control of blood sugar levels, for example. For workers, objectives may be reductions in accidents, injuries, or lost work days.

Where consumers respond better to results desired and are offered total freedom or multiple options as to how they will be achieved, objectives based on results are preferable. Relationships with targeted consumers may be enhanced by giving them the freedom to choose how the results are to be achieved. This empowerment tactic may reinforce their sense of self-responsibility and self-efficacy in managing their own health and consumption of services in general.

On the other hand, where they may have great doubts as to their ability to achieve results, objectives may be better stated in terms of specific behavior change. In weight management, for example, consumers may have had repeated unsuccessful attempts at losing weight and keeping it off. Sponsors may find it works better to state objectives in terms of achieving and maintaining new nutrition and exercise habits among targeted consumers, rather than weight loss. Consumers may find it easier to believe in their ability to achieve behavior changes than specific results.

Sponsors should choose objectives that will motivate and be perceived as achievable by targeted consumers, as well as valuable to the sponsor. Where consumers see objectives calling for changes in their behavior as beneficial to them, in addition to sponsors, they are less likely to feel manipulated and will be more receptive to specific sponsor initiatives.

Estimate Value of Change

If the behavior change objective is achieved, what will be the value of the consequences of that change? As will be discussed further in Chapter 20, the effects of demand improvement initiatives can be *tracked* in terms of any one or more of the links in the chain of effects. However, it is when dollar amounts can be attached to such changes that true *evaluation* is possible. Since conversion initiatives will cost dollars, it is always helpful to be able to estimate value in dollar terms.

To estimate dollar value, it is usually necessary to estimate effects on health service use and expenditure or added value such as absenteeism, productivity, or retention, which can readily be translated into dollar terms. Even though the purpose of specific demand improvement initiatives per se is to improve the quality of demand, its dollar value will be measured in terms of reduced expenditures in most cases. Where greater appropriateness of demand is the intended result or where no estimate can be made of the intended behavior change on health expenditures, assigning a dollar value to the conversion objective may prove problematic.

If a dollar estimate of value cannot be made based on the objective (e.g., if the objective is expected to improve health status and quality of life, with uncertain effect on demand for health services), the value can be estimated after the plan is completed. Since at that point the costs of the initiative will have been estimated, planners need only satisfy themselves, and anyone else who must approve the effort and expenditures, that the value of the objective is greater than the estimated costs of achieving it.

Having to wait until the end of the planning process before addressing the question of whether the behavior change is worth the cost of achieving it is by far the lesser of the two options in estimating value. Having an estimate at step 3 will help greatly in considering tactics and communications efforts by setting a clear upper limit on what expenditures would make any sense. As soon as it is clear what the effort will cost compared to the value of the objective, a sound financial decision can be made. If no estimate of value is possible at step 3, it may not be feasible to make such a decision until the entire planning process has been completed.

Where the behavior change objective is stated in terms of using health services (e.g., reducing the use of ED services by patients with congestive heart failure), the estimation of value may be fairly simple: the saved costs of whatever number of visits it is that will not take place. If the objective is stated in terms of some numbers of consumers using self-care instead of professional services, it will be necessary to estimate how many occasions will arise where such a substitution is possible, then translate into reduced use of services and saved expenditures. Where the objective is stated in terms of some number of people quitting smoking or using safety equipment, the "causal chain" connecting the behavior change and health status improvements, reduced utilization, and savings in health care expenditures will be both longer and more difficult to use in estimating value.

If it is known that smoking is a risk factor that produces, on average, annual health care expenditures $500 higher than for nonsmokers, then a simple estimate of value in getting some number of smokers to quit might be reducing expenditures for that number by $500 per year. Yet recent smokers may take some time before the health consequences are felt. Studies may be available that show a gradual reduction in expenditures for those who have quit, providing a more real-

ESTIMATED VALUE

THE RETURN ON INVESTMENT (ESTIMATED) PRIOR TO PLAN DESIGN (IF POSSIBLE) OR AT THE END OF THE PLANNING PROCESS, BUT BEFORE IMPLEMENTATION

istic basis for estimating value. Similarly, wearing a seat belt may make drivers more safety conscious and reduce the number of accidents as well as their seriousness and costs or, conversely, may make drivers feel they are better protected from injury and cause them to drive more recklessly.

The estimated value of achieving the behavior change objective is merely an estimate. If later on in the planning process, the costs of the planned effort begin to approach the original estimate of value, it may be necessary to do more work on the estimate. Perhaps further analysis of published studies may reveal a more reliable estimate. More careful calculations of current employer or health plan costs may contribute to a better estimate. As long as costs of planned efforts are well below the estimated value, a rough guess should serve, provided it is reasonable and on the conservative side. When initiating demand improvement efforts, there are likely to be many opportunities for interventions that will have returns on investment in the five- or ten-to-one range, so rough estimates will be safe enough. Over time, when the best opportunities have been exploited, the need for more precise estimates is more likely.

CONVERSION OF CONSUMER BEHAVIOR

Develop Tactical Intelligence

There are many steps in the planning process where gathering, analyzing, and employing information is useful, if not essential. Targets may be better identified by first learning which individuals are at greatest risk or which ones are in certain stages of change, for example. Objectives may be set based on the estimated receptivity of targets, how many are very likely to change, or are at least receptive to the idea of change. Value may be estimated based on cross-sectional comparisons between those already evidencing the desired behavior and selected targets or on longitudinal tracking of previous consumers who changed their behavior.

Similarly, information on present states of mind among targets will be useful in setting communications objectives. Data on media reach and preferred sources of information can be helpful in selecting media. Pretesting of message content can frequently improve the effectiveness and efficiency of communications efforts. And collecting new information is essential in evaluation, then planning subsequent efforts.

If there is one stage in planning where additional information is most important, yet least likely to be sought, it is in selecting tactics, the basis for enticing targets into changing their behavior. Ideally such information should help make the new behavior irresistible to targets. Since consumer targets have not adopted the desired behavior already, it has to be accepted as at least very likely that there is some problem of motivation, capability, or consciousness that stands in the way.

If research into the current motivation of targets indicates that they are undermotivated, then tactics should be designed so as to increase their motivation. New information may persuade them, or incentives might be added to make a more attractive behavior. Targets might be asked what it would take to make them want to adopt the desired behavior, and tactics may be designed through a "virtual" negotiation. Alternative tactics might be tried on a pilot basis to test which have the best results.

Where research indicates that the problem is one of capability, lack of self-efficacy, or some barrier in the environment, a quite different tactic would be designed. Education, rather than persuasion or incentives, would make sense. A financial barrier to participation in exercise programs could be overcome by making it free, partially subsidizing the costs. Transportation problems could be overcome by providing a van or taxi vouchers.

In those situations where targets are sufficiently motivated and capable of adopting the desired behavior, but need some consciousness raising to remind them when and where to do it, then prompting may suffice. Even when research suggests some combination of motivation and capability will have to be addressed, prompting is still likely to help. By obtaining information from targets or enlisting their help directly in designing tactics, both the effectiveness and efficiency of the behavior improvement effort should be enhanced.

At a minimum, sponsors of behavior change initiatives should have a reasonable idea why targeted consumers are not already manifesting the desired behavior. In some cases, where only a small proportion of targeted consumers need respond to tactics for the initiative to be successful, sponsors may design the tactics based on some loose assumptions about what will motivate or enable some to respond. In effect, sponsors will be counting on having enough consumers out there who will be motivated/enabled by the tactics they choose.

Where high proportional response is needed for success, as is true for most health and demand improvement initiatives, sponsors would be well advised to

TACTICAL INTELLIGENCE

BARRIERS TO CHANGE
MC² FACTORS
INFORMATION, INCENTIVES

learn more about the targeted consumers' status and reasons for motivation and capability and level of consciousness. Every once in a while, by chance, sponsors may design tactics that optimally match what will most effectively and efficiently elicit the desired response among targeted consumers. Even though the vast majority of initiatives have had comfortable return on investment (ROI) ratios in the past, however, it would be far wiser to invest in a little learning rather than rely on chance.

Designing Tactics

Four of the tactical options described in Part III rely on communications alone to bring about behavior improvements in consumers. Where communications alone will do the trick, sponsors may achieve results at relatively low cost. Where information gathered in step 4 suggests that enough consumer targets will respond favorably to prompting, persuasion, education, or social advocacy, sponsors may decide on one or more of these tactics and move directly to step 7.

Whenever sponsors discover they will have to do more than talk targets into changing their behavior, it is helpful to consider ways in which the experience of the new behavior can be made more attractive and satisfying, through incentives, marketing, negotiation, or empowerment. The four pure communications techniques rely on the desired behavior being already attractive and satisfying as is.

Even in education or persuasion efforts, however, it may be necessary to improve a behavior in order to get targets to participate in the effort. An educational/persuasion program that is intended to convince targets to change their behavior may be easier if the program, itself, is made as attractive, convenient and low cost as possible. Trying to talk consumer targets into participating in a program that will attempt to talk them into changing their behavior, with no consideration as to how attractive, easy, and low cost either the program or the new behavior is, may be relying overmuch on communications.

Sponsors can use the marketing mix to consciously address how the desired behavior or participation in a program designed to change behavior can be made more attractive and satisfying, more convenient and less costly. Adding to attrac-

DESIGNING TACTICS

THE NEW, MORE ATTRACTIVE & SATISFYING BEHAVIOR EXPERIENCE

tion and satisfaction power amounts to working on the "product" aspects of the desired behavior. Adding incentives is a simple and obvious example, but there are other possibilities. Making participation more socially enjoyable, for example, by making it fun, including health status measures that are expected to improve so as to give participants a sense of accomplishment, adds consumer benefit or product enhancements.

The "place" component of a behavior includes everything about it that makes it easier or more difficult to adopt. Developing a fitness center on site is one way an employer could make worker exercise behavior more convenient. Ensuring that phone counseling lines are staffed 24 hours a day and are rarely if ever busy when called is a way to make it easier for targets to call. Providing a weight management/nutrition class just before or after work or during lunch hour may make it easier for consumers to participate. Location, hours, rules of eligibility, registration process, parking availability—all can be designed so as to make the desired behavior more convenient to adopt.

The "price" component of the marketing mix covers everything that targets are likely to perceive as negative or annoying, unattractive, and unsatisfying about the desired behavior. It includes any out-of-pocket costs for a program or behavior change, such as costs for belonging to a health club to promote exercise. Subsidizing such costs is a simple and common approach to improving the price aspect of the offer. Other costs may be the time it takes to participate in a program or engage in an activity, the physical pain or discomfort involved, even psychological costs such as fear of being alienated from one's peers if one stops smoking, drinking, or engaging in some other dangerous but popular behavior.

The idea of including a tactic devoted to redesigning the desired behavior is to make the behavior change more probable. This should include deliberately addressing "switching costs," the perceived negative consequences of changing behavior, the loss of whatever benefit targets see themselves as gaining from their current behavior. This is particularly true for health improvement, where targets will almost always have an existing motivation for their current unhealthy behaviors and often a powerful one. Either switching costs have to be reduced or switching gains must be so motivating as to overcome the costs.

The traditional approach to using the marketing mix involves sponsors thinking of ways to improve the offer. The thinking, expertise, and experience of sponsors or consultants can be supplemented by market research aimed at discovering what people feel and think, why they engage in current behaviors, and what would make alternative behaviors more attractive. The theory has always been that if the behavior is made to better meet consumer needs, expectations, and wishes, then "selling" the behavior will be a piece of cake.

In improving health and demand, we can actually go one step further: we can involve consumers in designing the behavior directly, including them as active partners in developing an offer they will not refuse. This "partnership marketing" approach is possible because of the clear and significant benefits to consumers of engaging in the very behaviors that will achieve the desired improvement. Where most marketers are faced with the challenge of promoting purchases of goods and services that are barely better, and sometimes worse than competing options, sponsors are promoting behaviors that represent significantly better value to consumers than the behaviors they are currently practicing.

This being the case, sponsors can be absolutely open and honest with targets, can sit on the same side of the table and address behavior change objectives as common goals and current behavior consequences as common problems. Having close, personal participation of targets in designing the offer has all the advantages of conventional market research, plus the added benefit of eliciting target commitment. People who design the offer that is to be made to them are far less likely to refuse it once made; after all, it is "their" offer. It can turn a marketing approach into a negotiation process: "What will it take to get you to want to change your behavior?" Participants are likely to feel honor bound to accept the offer once it has been specifically made to their liking. Where the outcomes of behavior change can be achieved through a number of different behaviors, sponsors may choose an empowerment tactic, relying on consumers to choose a behavior improvement that will have worthwhile results. As in the negotiation tactic, it is expected that consumers who come up with their own ideas on how to achieve results they value will tend to be more committed to changing their behavior than if the pressure for change came from external sources.

(The selection of tactics for specific behavior change objectives is sufficiently complex and important to warrant a chapter of its own, that being Chapter 17.)

Implementing and Budgeting Tactics

Designing a behavior change or program participation tactic is one thing; delivering it may be quite another. In any case, implementing tactics is where costs are incurred over and above any time and effort spent in the design process. Designing an incentive program needs to be followed by estimating how much it will cost to provide rewards if the intended number of targets (or perhaps more) accept the offer and change their behavior. Delivering value-adding components of experience to an educational/persuasion program so as to increase participation will add to the costs of the program. Making exercise easier to adopt by offering an on-site fitness facility will involve quite an investment. Subsidizing costs, such as through free parking, means shifting costs from targets to sponsors.

In some cases implementing a tactic may prove legally risky for the sponsor. There may be physical or financial barriers to implementing the design: lack of land for an on-site fitness facility, lack of capital for construction. The people needed to conduct an educational program may not be available; qualified nurse

IMPLEMENTATION / BUDGET

DETERMINING HOW THE OFFER WILL BE IMPLEMENTED, FEASIBILITY & COST

counselors for guiding consumer decisions may be hard to find or may take months to train. A full implementation plan for chosen tactics, or as close to it as is feasible, needs to be developed—both as a guide to those who will implement the plan and as a basis for determining its feasibility and costs.

Both costs and feasibility should fully recognize the staff time and effort that will be included in implementation. Even if no additional staff will be hired, the salary/benefits costs of current staff *attributable* to the initiative should be included in delivery costs and their availability in feasibility considerations. At a minimum, using them in any behavior change effort means opportunity costs to the sponsor. If their time and effort are not included in calculations, all programs relying on inside staff will appear to be free, and there will be no realistic basis for comparing make versus buy options. In addition, ROI amounts and ratios will tend to be overstated.

COMMUNICATION

Communications Objectives

Despite the maxim: "Build a better mousetrap and the world will beat a path to your door," no sponsors should rely on simply designing and delivering a better behavior; it is necessary to tell people about it! Even in cases where sponsors aim to realize changes in targets' behavior through communications alone, it is useful to plan such communications based on two specific responses.

For almost all health and demand improvement behaviors, communications objectives, as well as the media and message plans for achieving them, are best organized around two distinct responses that consumers are intended to make: (1) adopting, quitting, or changing the behavior in question; and (2) repeating or continuing in the new behavior. The first can best be achieved by *promising* or otherwise creating confident expectations on the part of consumers as to what value they *will gain* as a result of converting to the new behavior. The second is achieved by *reporting* (i.e., *reminding*) consumers of the value they *have gained*.

Just as there tends to be more attention to gaining new customers in marketing and not enough to keeping them, so is it usually the case that more attention is given to converting consumers to improved behavior than to keeping them converted. Most demand improvement objectives are written in terms of getting consumers to change, and most evaluation is aimed at determining if they have changed after a few months or a year, for example. This is understandable given the short-term financial objectives of many sponsors, but it means that not enough attention is paid to, nor enough known about, long-term persistence in improved behavior, in the states of maintenance or termination (Prochaska's term; i.e., "Permanence" [our term]).

As we mentioned in Chapter 15, achieving persistence in a desired behavior, whether through frequent or occasional repetition or daily continuation, is a separate problem from achieving conversion to the behavior in the first place. If consumers do not perceive the value they expected, such persistence is unlikely to be achieved or maintained. Communications can be used to promote persistence as well as initial conversion, but the two challenges are different.

The first communications plan, with separate communications objectives, media, and message plans, is aimed at the first response: conversion. The knowledge, attitude, and intention mind-state objectives for this plan are geared to converting to the new behavior—promoting confident expectations of benefit and low costs (motivation), supplying information needed to adopt the behavior (capability) and reminding consumers of where and when the behavior is to begin (consciousness).

The second communication plan, with its separate objectives, media, and message plan is aimed at the second response: achieving repetition or continuation of the new behavior. Its knowledge, attitude, and intention objectives are based on persistence: raising consciousness of the value already gained and attribution of that value to the particular behavior change made. By measuring and reporting on value gained by *individual* consumers through the new behavior, sponsors can both inspire persistence (motivation) and enhance it through promoting consumers' sense of self-efficacy (capability).

There are two basic approaches sponsors can take to reminding consumers of value gained: (1) using their own objective measures, and (2) relying on reports by consumers themselves. Sponsors may develop databases that will enable them to report improvements in health status measures, performance on tests, for example, which consumers may not even be aware of until reported or may be aware of but can have their awareness enhanced through sponsor reporting. Sponsors can remind consumers of incentives they have received or out-of-pocket costs avoided, for example, in addition to health benefits.

For many types of value received, and often the most important, such as quality of life, reduced stress, sense of well-being, and greater energy, the only source of measures is the perceptions of consumers (and perhaps their parents or caregivers) themselves. In such cases, by checking on such benefits in terms of whether and to

COMMUNICATIONS OBJECTIVES

- CONVERSION & PERSISTENCE
- NEW & DIFFERENT KNOWLEDGE, ATTITUDE & INTENTION TO BE ACHIEVED THROUGH COMMUNICATION

what extent consumers *perceive* them, sponsors awaken consumers' awareness just by asking about them. (And asking about perceptions of value received is part of evaluation step 11). Just asking can also remind consumers about where the benefits came from (i.e., promote their attribution to the behavior change), and promote their giving credit for the value to the sponsor!

Sponsors can combine their own objective measures of consumer value added with a summary of consumer-reported subjective measures of added value to further remind individual consumers of how they have benefited. They can also use the summary information in communications aimed at unconverted consumers as evidence of the benefits available to them. And, with permission, sponsors may use comments of individual consumers as testimonials to further add to the credibility of promises being made to the unconverted.

The entire process of promoting persistence in behavior can add to the value that sponsors gain from demand improvement initiatives. Promoting awareness of benefits gained can only enhance the positive impact on the already reported (see Chapter 5) consumer satisfaction with the sponsor (i.e., employee morale and retention, patient loyalty, or member reenrollment). In turn, such increases in satisfaction and retention add marketing, operations and revenue/profit value to sponsors over and above what they gain through demand improvement per se.

Communications objectives for improving consumer behavior may include any combination of desired changes in (1) awareness, knowledge, and beliefs; (2) perceptions, attitudes, and feelings; (3) intentions, commitments, and plans; and (4) actual behavior. Where an intermediate objective is to entice a certain number of targets to participate in a stress management or caregiver education program, for example, communications objectives for an advertising campaign might include making targets aware of the program, its duration, times and locations; getting them to feel that the program promises significant benefit to them; getting them to commit to attending, and getting them to sign up for the program and come to the first meeting. After that the experience of the program and any actual benefits they perceive from its participation will determine if they continue to participate.

The communications objectives should be explicit, specific, and measurable. A good set of objectives is invaluable in designing media and messages to accomplish them. The objectives may also be translated into early indicators as to whether the initiative is working, particularly where there is a built-in time lag between communications and measurable behavior change. Counting the numbers of consumers who sign up for an educational program can be done well before the program begins or is completed and certainly before checks are made as to whether any behavior changes have occurred, for example.

A key decision is setting communications objectives is what motivation, capability, and consciousness are to be addressed. Is motivation assumed, so that targets need only be told how, when, and where to change behavior or reminded on occasion with some modest cues, or is it necessary to point out the advantages of the new offer to persuade targets to change their mind about a desired behavior? In most instances some combination of motivation and capability focus will be useful, and cues to stimulate or reinforce consciousness of a desired behavior will almost always improve results.

Media Plan

Once communications objectives have been formulated, the media or communications channels to be used for achieving them can be selected. Where the names of targets are available, some form of personal contact may be used, such as one-to-one counseling, group education, or direct mail. Where social advocacy is to be used to modify the attitudes and behavior of an entire community, options can include newspapers, magazines, radio, television, and billboards. In some cases incentives can serve as communications devices, as when participants in a wellness program receive free T-shirts extolling the program or their involvement; by wearing them participants help entice their peers to join in.

Whatever channel is to be used, a key question involves who will be the source of the communications. Using celebrity spokespersons can be effective in mass media campaigns, for example. Having messages come from the CEO of the company can have powerful impact, though messages from peers are often more persuasive for employees. An expert authority may be the preferred source where factual materials such as research results are to be communicated. Generally, people respond best to sources they admire, respect, want to be like, or see as like themselves. Research into target attitudes toward alternative communications sources, pretests of different sources, and past experience should help sponsors make source decisions.

Both media and source choices affect the costs of sending messages. Physicians in one-to-one counseling are one of the most effective source-media combinations for health communications, but also one of the most expensive. Using a celebrity

MEDIA PLAN

(1) THE SOURCE OF COMMUNICATION
(2) FORM OF MEDIA
(3) COST OF PRODUCTION & DELIVERY OF MESSAGES TO EFFECTIVELY ACHIEVE COMMUNICATION OBJECTIVE

spokesperson may improve impact but may cost a lot, though many celebrities have volunteered their time for health-related communications. Using the CEO to give multiple talks to employees can be expensive. Mass media can involve large production costs to produce a message for television or to design a print ad, for example. A key component of the media plan is an estimate of the costs of conveying messages.

Media vary widely in their "targetability," their potential for delivering messages to all members of their target audiences without wasting messages on nontargets. Personal contact and direct mail, for example, can be highly targetable, reaching almost everyone they intend to and nobody else. Mass media tend to be poor on this dimension, unable to reach all targets and reaching a lot of unintended people as well. Sponsors have to look for the best combination of a medium's ability to reach as many of the intended targets as possible while not wasting too much money reaching unintended audiences.

Media also vary in their ability to convey messages and have impact. A billboard normally can accommodate only five to ten words, for example, and still be read by motorists driving by. Postcards cannot contain as much information as letters; letters and flyers typically rely on words alone, whereas brochures and pamphlets can include visual materials, though they lack the personal touch. Television is respected as the most intrusive and flexible medium, given its ability to combine words, pictures, and action, though it is not always the most trusted medium.

Costs will also be affected by the number of different media to be used and the number of times targets are to be exposed to messages. Many campaigns fail because they rely on one exposure or one medium, where multiple exposures may be needed to have any effect, and communications through multiple media tend to have greater impact. The media plan should outline exactly when and how often messages are to be sent to targets. Production costs may occur only once, while delivery costs increase with every repetition.

Message Plan

The message plan specifies exactly what will be contained in communications, that is, just how the knowledge, attitude, intention, and response objectives will be achieved. When aiming at converting consumers, sponsors should consider what *evidence* or other basis for credibility they can include to achieve particular confident expectations of benefit on the part of consumers. They may use data from past initiatives, testimonials from past converts, case histories, perhaps even guarantees. The communications objectives describe what consumers are intended to know, perceive, and intend; the message plan specifies the content that will persuade them.

For those consumers already converted, the message plan need only list the types of benefits and their objective or subjective measures sponsors will include in their measurement and reporting. Credibility will not normally be an issue, since the messages will contain individual data on each consumer, including information consumers supplied, themselves.

For conversion, as opposed to persistence response messages, we recommend a headline, or "grabber"; body content; "hook," or response request; and signature. Each element is discussed in detail below:

- Grabber. The first and most essential purpose of a message is to grab the attention of intended targets. Any combination of verbal, visual, and aural content may be used to gain and hold attention (e.g., get direct mail recipients to open the envelope, television viewers to wake up or stay in the room, newspaper readers to read, or radio audiences to listen). Given the media clutter that affects almost all of us, it is an increasingly difficult challenge merely to get targets to "attend" the messages we send them.

    Grabbers can also be used to promote selective attention by exactly the targets sponsors want to reach. A message aimed at people we wish to invite

MESSAGE PLAN

PERSUASIVE CONTENT
EVIDENCE OF PROMISED BENEFIT
REPORTS OF DELIVERED BENEFITS

to a weight management program might begin with the headline: "OVER-WEIGHT?" A message promoting fitness for seniors might use a visual of a senior proclaiming: "I CLIMBED A MOUNTAIN AT AGE 70; SO CAN YOU!" One aimed at asthma sufferers could assert: "I HAVEN'T HAD AN ASTHMA ATTACK IN MONTHS, THANKS TO MY SELF-MANAGE-MENT TRAINING!"

- Body. The body of the message is everything after the "grabber" that is not hook or signature. It could be a description of the content of an educational session, a script for a counseling interchange, a CD-ROM or software disk, an Internet Web Page, a letter, or phone call. It could be a strictly planned script, a protocol or algorithm for an interaction, or a loosely outlined set of ideas for personal counseling or group discussion. It should be designed to interest the target audience in whatever mind-state changes or reinforcements are set as communications objectives. Any of the types of evidence previously mentioned as ways to achieve credibility could be used.

  There is no useful rule or guideline as to the proper length of messages, except that they should be long enough but not too long. If the message is interesting enough, targets may stick with it for pages and minutes; if not, they may be lost after the first few words or seconds. For complicated objectives, or where significant mind changes are intended, a series of long messages may be needed. For simple reminders or cues, a word or two can do the trick. Message design is an art that needs constant practice and frequent testing to promote effectiveness.

- Hook. The hook in a message is an explicit request for a response, exactly what targets are intended to do after exposure to the message. It may be something like "Step on the scale and ask yourself if you like what you see" for a message aiming at leading consumers toward interest in a weight management program; or "Count up how much you spent this week for cigarettes" to promote interest in a smoking cessation program. In most cases, however, the requested response is one that message senders can track and one that should lead targets toward a specific desired behavior.

  A sponsor's message may contain a request that targets "call 555-5555 for more information" or "Send in this coupon for a free self-care book." Such responses first give sponsors a way of tracking the effects of their communications, of measuring the differential impact of different media and messages. To test which of two messages has the greater impact, for example, sponsors could offer different phone numbers to call or use different coupons and see which generates the greater number or percentage of responses. The same sort of "split-test" can be used to determine which newspapers, radio stations, television channels, or other media produce the best response.

Another purpose of a hook is to start targets on what may be a longer process of communications for effect. Callers to a suggested number may be given a sales talk about participating in a program, which is where the "real" message will be delivered. The hook may ask consumers to make an appointment with their personal physician to discuss the problem addressed in the body copy. It may invite targets to ask for another type of message, such as a self-care book, which is part of the overall communications campaign to get targets to replace professional care with self-care for selected, self-limiting medical conditions.

In many cases the hook will be asking consumers to adopt the desired change in behavior for the first time, to try it: for example, make an appointment for prenatal care, initiate a mall-walkers exercise program, use a peak flow meter. In others the hook will be asking them to repeat or continue the desired behavior: for example, make an appointment for an annual mammogram, remain abstinent from smoking. In such cases the hook corresponds directly to the respective conversion or persistence response objective.

Where intermediate response objectives such as attend a class or call for more information are involved, it is wise to develop a separate set of communications objectives, media, and message plan for each. Employees may be enticed to come to a meeting about the employer's plans for a fitness program through posters on bulletin boards (medium) announcing the meeting and mentioning only that employees who attend could be winners of a free vacation trip and barely mentioning the fitness program (message), for example. The meeting itself would be the medium for convincing them to try the program.

- Signature. The signature is a legally required component of advertising messages, clearly indicating the name and usually the address of whoever sent the message. In other media the signature may be a reminder or the only indicator of who the source for the message is. In phone communications the signature may come at the beginning of the message, as callers introduce themselves to targets. It indicates who is responsible for the message and shows who the targets should contact if they have any questions, comments, or complaints about the message.

Where the signature is that of an organization—for example, the health plan, physician group, vendor, hospital, or employer—it may also include a slogan or "tag line" that is intended to make or reinforce an identity for the sender. A campaign promoting self-care, for example, might include a motto such as "The one person you can always manage is yourself" in each signature used in a series of messages. A health plan, physician practice, or hospital might put a tag line such as "Your Health Partner" on all its messages.

EVALUATION PLAN

Any behavior improvement effort worth planning and executing is worth evaluating. In many cases, starting with an evaluation plan is a good way to promote accountability of efforts; in all cases, evaluating efforts should be routine. There are three steps in an evaluation plan, each addressing a separate and important question: (1) What results and return did we get? (2) What effects did we have on key relationships? and (3) What did we learn from the experience? Each step is discussed in detail below.

Assessment of Results and ROI

The results of the effort should be measured and reported in terms of what specific conversions have been achieved. How many of the intended targets adopted, repeated, continued the desired new behavior? What impacts were identified on health status measures, health services utilization, and expenditures? What added value was achieved? Initial effects such as changes in awareness levels or attitudes or numbers of participants in a program may be used as well for monitoring purposes, but results are better stated in terms of measures that clearly suggest value, in terms of dollar savings where possible. The plan must specify how results will be measured.

Just as there are strong relationship reasons for stating objectives in terms of value to everyone affected, so too should evaluation of results address everyone who benefited. If objectives are stated in broad terms of employer and provider gains and consumer benefit, but evaluation focuses exclusively on how much the health plan saved, most people are likely to assume that the health plan's profits were the only *real* value intended to be improved.

The ROI is calculated by comparing the costs of the effort with the value of the results. This comparison can be stated in terms of the *difference* between cost and value (e.g., an $85,000 reduction in health care expenditures minus $40,000 in program costs = a *return* of $45,000); or, in terms of the benefit/cost *ratio* of the two, $85,000 divided by $40,000 = 2.125; so every dollar invested returned $2.125 in savings, an ROI *ratio* of $2.125:1. In most cases the amount of value received will be the telling measure, though ROI ratios are helpful in comparing different approaches to the same problem or in comparing demand improvement investments to other things sponsors might have done with the same amount of money.

Where results cannot be stated in dollar terms, sponsors can repeat the approach they used in estimating whether the expected results looked to be worth the estimated costs during the planning process. The only difference is that they will be using actual costs and results rather than estimates. In many cases, added value,

MEASUREMENT OF RESULTS

WHAT RESULTS WERE ACHIEVED; WERE THEY WORTH THE EFFORT; WAS THE VALUE RECEIVED ENOUGH GREATER THAN THE COST TO MAKE THE EFFORT WORTHWHILE

such as consumer quality of life, which cannot be translated into dollar amounts, may prove to be the reason for continuing an effort whose dollar ROI is modest, even less than $1.00:1.

The standard for evaluation, for determining if the effort succeeded or not, is not whether the original objective was achieved. Only an extremely lucky sponsor will find that exactly the results planned were achieved. The object is to determine if the results achieved were worth the effort or if the value was greater than the costs—or enough greater to make the effort seem to be at least a good investment, and perhaps an excellent one.

Effects on Relationships

The effects of the effort on relationships can be equally important as the financial or other value received. Utilization (i.e., supply) management programs have frequently succeeded in reducing health care utilization and expenditures by far more than the cost of the effort involved, but have in many cases so angered physicians, consumers, and legislators that the efforts could hardly be considered a success. By checking on how such relationships are affected, sponsors can get a truer picture of the full effects of their efforts, and perhaps avoid disastrous side effects in the future.

A key component of evaluation is checking on targeted consumers' perceptions of benefits gained. Learning whether and to what extent consumers feel they have benefited from programs offered and changes they have made will help sponsors understand their overall attitudes toward programs, sponsors, and the new behavior. And, as mentioned in the response objectives discussion, checking on such perceptions provides sponsors with information they can use in a variety of ways to further their success.

The impact on relationships can be measured through routine tracking systems such as annual health plan member, employee, and patient surveys. Questions in the surveys can ask not only how consumers feel about the specific behavior improvement experience they had, but how they feel about the plan, physician, hospital, or employer responsible for it. Participants in education or counseling programs can be surveyed during as well as after a series of encounters, in addition to any regular attitude survey. Positive responses indicating both satisfaction with the experience and an improved perception of its sponsors will indicate added value. Where negative results are found, they represent added costs that may cause reconsideration of whether the program was a success.

It may well be that relationships other than those with consumers will have been affected. Family members may be happy or not with the impact of disease management programs or health behavior changes made by targets. Physicians may object to the way a triage or treatment counseling program in a decision improvement effort is being handled or may be delighted with a reduction in inappropriate visits. All of the stakeholders who are involved in or affected by demand improvement efforts should be checked, both to show sponsors' interest in the relationship and to find out if their efforts had added value or costs that should be recognized.

Learning

Every evaluation effort should be thought of as an opportunity to learn more about demand improvement, in addition to a test of results, return, and relationships. One of the reasons for suggesting that a plan might begin with the evaluation planning step is that if learning is seen as an added outcome for specific efforts, those efforts can be planned from the outset so as to promote optimal

---

IMPACT ON RELATIONSHIPS

EVALUATION OF THE IMPACT OF THE INITIATIVE ON STAKEHOLDERS TO DETERMINE WHETHER THE EFFORTS HAD ADDED VALUE OR COSTS THAT SHOULD BE RECOGNIZED

learning, rather than hoping to squeeze some learning out of the experience after the fact.

For example, if sponsors are torn between two different behavior change tactics, they might decide to use both in a controlled experiment design to see which works better, rather than try to pick only one. They can design alternative messages or media approaches to communications in hopes of learning more about what works. Otherwise, if only one approach is used, sponsors can only learn whether or not it works, not how it compares to alternatives they might have tried. If we are sufficiently convinced that one approach is far superior to all other possibilities, such split-testing may have no appeal, but we will also never find out if we were wrong.

(Evaluation of demand improvement efforts is sufficiently complex and important to warrant a more comprehensive treatment. For this discussion, see Chapter 20.)

As shown in Exhibits 16–1 and 16–2, there are at least 11 planning choices that typically must be made in planning particular initiatives: who will participate in sponsoring them, what will be invested, who will be targeted, what objectives, how intelligence will be gathered, where initiatives will be carried out, what tactics will be used, what value delivered, what value gained, which media, and what message content to use. If there were only four options for each choice, there would be $4^{11} = 4,194,304$ possible combinations, once all choices were made.

With so many possibilities, and there are really far more, since more than four options are available for most choices, it is no wonder that there is no agreement on what is the best way to approach particular demand improvement challenges. In fact, there can never be one best way, given the variability of challenges and consumers. Some extrapolation from others' experiences and results may be possible, suggesting more promising options for particular choices, but the likelihood of finding that one, or even a handful of combinations, that consistently works best is probably infinitesimal.

LEARNING

ONGOING OPPORTUNITY FOR LEARNING ABOUT HOW TO MORE EFFECTIVELY DEVELOP FUTURE BEHAVIOR CHANGE INITIATIVES

Exhibit 16–1 Planning Choices

SPONSORS:
HEALTH PLANS, PROVIDERS, GOVERNMENTS, COMMUNITIES

INVESTMENT:
MONEY (AMOUNT?), STAFF TIME, SPACE, EQUIPMENT, INFORMATION, COMMUNICATIONS MEDIA

TARGET POPULATIONS:
EMPLOYEES (DEPENDENTS, RETIREES), MEMBERS, PATIENTS, RESIDENTS

BEHAVIOR CHANGE OBJECTIVES:
LIFESTYLE, SAFETY, PREVENTION, SYMPTOM RESPONSE, TREATMENT CHOICE, CONDITION SELF-MGMT.

MODES OF GATHERING INTELLIGENCE:
INTERVIEWS, FOCUS GROUPS, SURVEYS, RECORDS, PUBLISHED ARTICLES & REPORTS

SETTINGS FOR INITIATIVES:
WORKSITE, HOME, PUBLIC, COMMUNITY

Exhibit 16–2 Planning Choices

TACTICS:
PROMPTING, PERSUASION, EDUCATION, SOCIAL ADVOCACY, INCENTIVES, MARKETING, NEGOTIATION, EMPOWERMENT

VALUE DELIVERED:
QUALITY OF LIFE, HEALTH OUTCOMES, DOLLAR SAVINGS, PRODUCTIVITY, EFFICIENCY, MORALE, RECRUITMENT, RETENTION, MARKET SUCCESS, PROFITS

VALUE GAINED:
PRIDE OF ACCOMPLISHMENT, DOLLAR SAVINGS, PUBLIC RELATIONS, PRODUCTIVITY, EFFICIENCY, MORALE, RECRUITMENT, RETENTION, MARKET SUCCESS, PROFITS

COMMUNICATIONS MEDIA:
ONE-ON-ONE, PERSONAL PRESENTATIONS, DIRECT MAIL, PHONE, FAX, INTERNET, TELEVISION, RADIO, NEWSPAPERS, DISPLAYS

MESSAGE CONTENT:
(WHATEVER WORKS)

Sponsors need not make choices by chance, however. By combining information about their own situation and consumer targets with published benchmarks, and particularly through careful evaluation of and learning from their own experiences, they can aim for at least continuously improving their success. In the following chapters in this part, we discuss options on information, tactics, and partners to consider in strategic and programmatic planning and evaluation. In Chapters 21 through 24 we provide examples of successful efforts to aid sponsors in making choices.

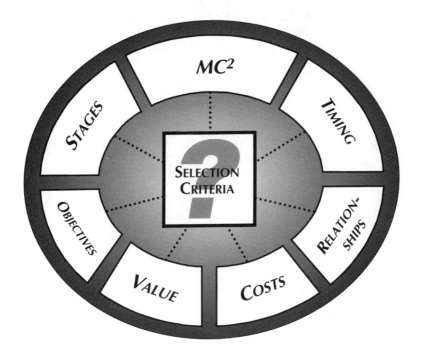

Chapter 17

CHOOSING TACTICS

Deciding which tactics to employ for which consumer targets and which behavior objectives is a complex process. The best tactics are those that produce the greatest success at the most reasonable costs (i.e., are both effective and efficient). Moreover, they should promote or maintain, and certainly not endanger or harm, the relationship between the sponsors of specific initiatives and the consumers whose behavior they are trying to improve.

The criteria that are useful in making tactical choices include:

- How consumers are to be approached
- Where targeted consumers are in stages of change
- What specific $I = MC^2$ changes are sought
- How quickly changes in behavior are desired
- How high a success rate is intended
- How much the behavior conversion is worth to sponsors
- How much tactics will cost to implement
- How well tactics fit the sponsor's (or sponsors') values and position
- How tactics will affect relationships with consumers

BASIC APPROACH

The first decision in tactical planning is that of the basic approach to be taken in approaching the challenge of improving consumer behavior. Consumers may be thought of and treated as (1) objects whose behavior is to be managed, (2) people to be make their own best choices, or (3) partners in a common effort. The determination of philosophical approach will make the biggest difference in selecting the proper tactic.

Where consumers are approached as objects for behavior improvement, tactical choices will tend toward those that can be used with the greatest confidence that they will have the intended effect. Prompting or social advocacy for consciousness awakening or reinforcement; persuasion, marketing, or incentives for motivation; education and training for building or reinforcing self-efficacy would be logical choices. Behavior research, pilot testing, and experience over time will help in identifying the tactics that will be most effective and efficient.

In an arm's-length approach, consumers would be informed and enabled to make and carry out their own decisions. Emphasis is on education, with prompting a natural adjunct. If persuasion is used, it employs only objective, factual information, avoiding emotional appeals. Peer pressure would not be appropriate, since it relies on emotional rather than rational impact. The preferred tactic would be empowerment.

If sponsors of demand improvement initiatives are willing to shoot for specific *outcomes* or effects of behavior change (i.e., health status, utilization or expenditure improvements, perhaps value-adding outcomes such as productivity, retention, return to work), they may leave it up to consumers to choose and adopt behavior changes that will achieve those outcomes. In such cases sponsors do not choose the tactics; consumers do. They are empowered to select whatever tactical support they require from sponsors but make their own choices, as individuals or groups.

In a partnership approach, negotiation is preferred, with both parties working from the same side of the table in a common effort to solve a problem or achieve a goal. The partnership may choose any of the tactics as devices to achieve a specific purpose, once the purpose has been jointly agreed upon. The difference is

that rather than the sponsors alone choosing how best to change consumers' behavior, consumers and sponsors together make the choice, with consumers agreeing to have the tactics applied to them.

STAGES OF CHANGE

As discussed in Chapter 6 among the models related to improving behavior, the
stages of change model offers both a way of looking at how people change their
behavior and a way of selecting tactics for encouraging and enabling them to do
so. The authors of *Changing for Good*[1] cite their own experience and research
indicating which tactics work best for which stages in the change process. Suggestions for specific tactics are presented here for each of the six stages.

Precontemplation

The challenge when people targeted for behavior improvement are in the
precontemplation stage is first to whack them aside the head with a two-by-four to
get them to wake up! In this stage they see no reason to change, are unaware of or
not interested in the benefits of changing, or think the risks of maintaining their
present habits are not applicable to them.

Prochaska et al.,[1] in describing the techniques that people use to change themselves, recommend the tactics of consciousness raising and social liberation for
use at this stage. Consciousness raising can mean uncovering people's own hidden
thoughts, feelings, and past experiences, such as would occur in counseling, or
supplying them with new information, facts of which they were previously unaware. Social liberation means creating new opportunities or dynamics in the environment—nonsmoking legislation and smoke-free facilities, for example.

Motivation is the main challenge at this stage—making it easier (capability)—
or simply prompting (consciousness reinforcement) will have little effect on
someone totally disinterested in changing. Some significant incentive, such as a
bonus for changing or penalties for continuing bad habits, may serve. Social advocacy may arouse awareness and interest in specific problem consumers, while also
stimulating their peers and significant others to press them toward making
changes. New rules on the job or new laws (e.g., making the wearing of motorcycle helmets mandatory) can awaken interest, so social advocacy can help in that
way as well. Any dramatic development that would startle people out of their
complacency can help at this stage.

Contemplation

Once consumers targeted for behavior improvement have reached at least the
contemplation stage, where they are thinking about changing, they are receptive to

additional tactics. Consciousness raising and social liberation are useful at this stage as well, but so are emotional arousal and self-reevaluation. Emotional arousal normally takes place within a person's own private life (e.g., the death of a friend). It can be stimulated through devices such as psychodrama, role playing, and confrontation (e.g., in peer or family contexts). Self-reevaluation of one's situation and self can be stimulated through counseling to promote recognition of conflicts between one's avowed values and one's behavior or the effect one's behavior has on others and oneself.

Peer efforts are likely to be effective here. Where professional counseling might be overkill or too expensive, peer volunteers may stimulate reevaluation or arouse emotions by demonstrating their concern about family, friends, or coworkers with problem behaviors. Sponsors can stimulate peer pressure through group efforts, organization, and education of volunteers, such as employee group contests and group incentives. Social advocacy, including "social journalism," may help by stimulating or reinforcing awareness of the consequences of behavior.

Preparation

When people have moved from thinking about it to planning a specific change (e.g., setting a date to begin a new habit or end an old one), emotional arousal and self-reevaluation are still useful. Social liberation can provide a constant reminder and can stimulate the number of peers who model the desired behavior, such as coworkers using an onsite fitness center or talking about their use of a triage phone line.

The challenge at this stage is to get people to make a firm commitment to change, and that is the new technique recommended for this stage. Promote self-responsibility and self-efficacy through training, for example. Encourage people prepared to change to make a public commitment or sign a "contract" with themselves, their coworkers, family, or friends formalizing their intention to begin or end a habit on a specific day. In some cases, actual negotiation of an agreement, with family, physician, employer, for example, may work.

For simple, specific behavior change (e.g., quit smoking, install a smoke detector) the commitment may be to the behavior itself. For other behaviors that must be continued to be effective (e.g., exercise, diet, use of a blood glucose monitor or safety equipment), the commitment may be to achieving a goal (e.g., weight loss, blood pressure reduction, injury-free workplace). The commitment to an outcome rather than a specific behavior may be more powerful, since it preserves individual choice and is likely to feel less invasive or manipulative.

All three of the MC² tactics can apply here. Internal and external sources of motivation can promote commitment. Internal and external capability barriers should be reduced or eliminated, making the execution of a commitment easier in practice. Internal and external cues, such as notes on their calendars, can prompt people prepared to change to do so at the time they committed to doing so.

Action

As consumers initiate the new behavior, a mostly new set of tactics takes over. Social liberation tactics such as environmental facilitators and reminders will still help, as will the existence of a formal (preferably public) commitment. In addition, countering, or counterconditioning, may be needed. This tactic involves reducing risks of old behavior (e.g., staying out of bars to avoid alcohol abuse) and finding substitutes for former habits (taking a short walk when feeling hungry, perhaps).

Another tactic is environmental control, eliminating opportunities and reminders of former behaviors in the environment, plus inserting reminders of the new behavior. Eliminating cigarette machines in the building and supplying phone stickers or refrigerator magnets to remind people to call a triage phone line would be examples. Posters at the worksite or calls from a volunteer "buddy" when periodic screenings are scheduled are others.

Rewards and punishments (i.e., incentives) are also recommended tactics at this stage. Incentives may be promised as part of encouraging contemplation, preparation, or commitment, but administering them once action is initiated can confirm a new behavior. The incentives may apply to a specific behavior change or to achievement of a goal that will result from changed behavior. When an external agent employs incentives, as opposed to individual consumers deciding to reward or punish themselves, incentives based on outcomes are likely to be seen as less manipulative.

Both positive and negative incentives may work to promote action (i.e., changes in behavior). Punishments, however, tend to suppress problem behavior rather than promote permanent conversion. Those subject to punishment are more likely to hide the "bad" behavior than abandon it. And if the punishment is lifted or its threat becomes less credible, it is likely to lose its effect altogether. Rewards also have the tendency to promote dependence, to reduce intrinsic motivation, and to create reliance on continuation of the reward to continue the desired behavior.

In addition to incentives, helping relationships are a recommended tactic at this stage. Such relationships may involve personal physician, counselors, family, friends and coworkers, formal support groups, clergy, or anyone who can motivate, assist, or remind consumers involved in improving their behavior. Sponsors of behavior improvement efforts can refer targeted consumers to sources of support, help organize support groups, and encourage family and friends. They can educate others to be effective sources of support, encouraging and recognizing supporters just as they do the targeted consumers.

Maintenance

For behaviors (or abstinence) that must be continued for a long period, even a lifetime, continued interventions are likely to be needed. Lapses in adherence to new habits or compliance with medical regimens are common. They should be treated as such when they occur, with targeted consumers "recycled" back to preparation and action stages if necessary to repeat the conversion. Neither the consumer nor supporters (or, for that matter, sponsors) should think of or treat lapses as failures but merely as predictable "looping" through the stages of change.

Formal and public commitments and reminders thereof can be both motivators and prompters in maintaining new behavior patterns. Countering and environmental controls will reduce the incidence of relapsing. Frequent rewards for small achievements and regular progress can help the converted persevere when the ultimate goal seems far away. These tend to work more in the early stages of maintenance. Supportive behaviors and continued/renewed commitment are the tactics that apply throughout.

Termination

The sixth stage is defined as one in which no further interventions of any kind by anyone, even the consumer, are needed. (We prefer calling this stage "permanence.") The new behavior is so firmly entrenched in the mind and habits of the individual that no one need reinforce it. The consumer has changed for the better—and for good (i.e., permanently).

Given the propensity of humans to lapse, however, the only way we can be sure any particular consumers will not revert to a previous stage is to wait till they die, or "defect," from the employee, enrollee, patient, or community resident relationship that created our concern with their behavior in the first place. Sponsors can never completely write off consumers as permanently "reformed" as long as they still have a relationship with them.

For behaviors that must first be remembered to be repeated, however, and which are called for so infrequently that memory may not be reliable, prompting for consciousness reinforcement (i.e., reminding consumers) may still be a useful tactic. Given the number of such behaviors applicable in improving demand (e.g., mammograms every one or two years, pneumonia vaccination every five, tetanus every ten), simple reminders are likely to be useful if not necessary, so even permanently improved consumers may require some attention.

Recommendations for specific tactics are based on what has worked best at specific stages. Other tactics still have some effect and may be tried in conjunction with those recommended. Those recommended have simply proven more cost-effective in practice. Given the variability and changeability of populations, sponsors must always be ready to change tactics to match what particular consumers respond to and to keep specific programs from getting old.

It has been demonstrated that people are differentially responsive to specific behavior change techniques depending on where they are in the stages of change. Any particular consumer may respond to or use any of the techniques at any stage, but some techniques work better than others across populations. Greater efficiency and effectiveness can be achieved by tailoring the technique to the most common stage in a population, by focusing on those at stages closer to the desired behavior, or by using different techniques for those at different stages (see Table 17–1).

I = MC² CHANGES DESIRED

Just as form is supposed to follow function, so tactics should fit the reasons that consumers are not already behaving as desired. The specific change in consumer behavior that is desired, the objective of the tactical effort, should guide the choice of tactics intended to achieve the change, depending on what mix of motivation, capability, and consciousness represents the barrier to or avenue for the improved behavior.

If the change desired is in motivation, tactics such as persuasion, social advocacy, incentives, marketing, negotiation, and empowerment may all be appropriate. If a change in capability (i.e., self-efficacy) is needed, one of the education modes would fit, or perhaps a marketing effort focused on "place" factors. If consciousness is to be created or raised, prompting, social advocacy, or marketing promotion would be useful (Fig 17–1).

To select the best tactic and to design its specifics, the current states of motivation, capability, and consciousness among targeted consumers must be known or reasonably estimated. Where the differences between present and necessary states are small, relatively modest amounts of new information, incentives, or improvements on the behavior may suffice. Where differences are great, significant additions to knowledge, incentives, and the natural attractions of the desired behavior will be needed.

If they are open and receptive to the idea of changing their behavior, consumers may be excellent prospects for negotiation and empowerment tactics. They may be able to articulate specific changes in the desired behavior (marketing) or its consequences (incentives) that would make the desired behavior irresistible or at least more attractive and easier to adopt. They may have ideas on ways to reduce the "switching costs" of changing from their present behavior. If a specific health status, health care use, or expenditure outcome is set as a goal, consumers may be empowered to select their own way of accomplishing it, rather than complying with sponsor-selected behavior.

If already favorably disposed toward the desired behavior, consumers may be receptive to simple prompting by their peers, specific capability-raising programs, or marketing initiatives that make the desired behavior easier to adopt and continue. At this stage no dramatic initiative should be needed, merely enough intervention to encourage and enable the motivated consumer to put plans into action.

Once having tried the new behavior, consumers are likely to be most receptive to prompting and incentives or marketing support for behaviors that must continue. Employers, health plans, and providers can be sources for such tactics.

Table 17–1 Tactics & Stages of Change Model

STAGE OF CHANGE ▼	TACTIC	PURPOSE
PRECONTEMPLATION	PROMPTING SOCIAL ADVOCACY EDUCATION (TEACHING) PERSUASION	RAISE CONSCIOUSNESS PROMOTE SOCIAL PRESSURE FOR CONSEQUENCES ASSIST IN MAKING CHANGING BEHAVIOR ATTAINABLE PROMOTE RECONSIDERATION OF POSITIVE/NEGATIVE CHOICES
CONTEMPLATION	INCENTIVES (PROMISED) EDUCATION (TRAINING) EDUCATION (INFORMATION)	CHANGE BALANCE OF CONSEQUENCES PROVIDE SKILL / INCREASE SELF-EFFICACY REINFORCE TEACHING, ENABLE INFORMED CHOICE
PREPARATION	EMPOWERMENT NEGOTIATION	ENABLE CONSUMERS TO OWN CHOICE OF BEHAVIOR ACHIEVE COMMITMENT
ACTION	INCENTIVES (DELIVERED)	REWARD, REINFORCE BEHAVIOR CHANGE
MAINTENANCE	PROMPTING /INCENTIVES	REMIND/REWARD TO CONTINUE BEHAVIOR
TERMINATION (PERMANENCE)	PROMPTING	REMIND TO REPEAT BEHAVIOR

Figure 17–1 The I = MC² Model & Related Tactical Options

CONSCIOUSNESS
EDUCATION
REMINDING
PROMPTING

MOTIVATION
PERSUASION - INCENTIVES
MARKETING - NEGOTIATIONS
SOCIAL ADVOCACY

GOAL:
HEALTH
&
MEDICAL
SELF-EFFICACY

CAPABILITY
INFORMATION
TRAINING
EDUCATION
EMPOWERMENT

Peers can provide both prompting and support, together with the added motivational impact of their modeling and stated expectations.

For continuing behavior, sponsor recognition and rewards, peer recognition, self-monitoring, and self-rewarding can help maintain motivation levels. Regular prompting in newsletters, posters, public service announcements, as well as personal contact will also be helpful in reminding consumers of intermittent or occasional behavior, such as periodic screening or using triage counseling.

The specific new behavior can also make a difference to which tactic is used. For one-time behaviors such as installing smoke or carbon monoxide detectors in the home, resetting the water heater to a safe temperature, lowering the height of the bed of an elderly person, prompting or social advocacy may be all that is needed. To increase compliance, sponsors might facilitate the behavior by offering free or discounted devices or advice on installation and use. Contests that reward employee groups for one-time safety steps can combine incentives and peer prompting. Social advocacy may serve the same purpose for community populations.

For regular, repeated behavior such as exercise, once begun, regular prompting and sponsor, peer, or self-recognition/rewards are advisable. Both should be altered before they get stale, particularly the recognition/rewards. For irregular, occasional (i.e., required for the occasion) behaviors, such as practicing safe sex or avoiding drinking and driving, social advocacy and peer support are likely to be most effective.

Behaviors that are to be repeated regularly but infrequently, such as annual screenings, may need only prompting among the already motivated and capable. Prompting by a peer, such as "buddy-system" reminders for annual mammograms or checkups, can be promoted by sponsor communications. Worksite screenings, where employers improve the offer by giving employees time off, making screening free and more convenient, and promoting them through internal communications, are good examples of applying the marketing tactic.

Where the desired behavior involves quitting a dangerous practice, such as smoking or alcohol abuse, a full array of tactics may be needed. Often the tactic must be customized to the individual, combining a unique set of motivating, capability-enhancing, and prompting tactics. Some smokers may be able to quit "cold turkey"; others may be weaned slowly; some may require nicotine patches or gum to enable them to overcome their addiction. Work environment (e.g., smokeless workplaces) and public efforts (e.g., antismoking legislation, social communications campaigns, higher taxes) may be the tactic of choice or may be used to supplement other tactics (see Table 17–2).

HOW QUICKLY CHANGE IS DESIRED

Some tactics are likely to have earlier impact than others or can be implemented so as to achieve early response. Simple, one-time danger-reducing behaviors may

Table 17–2 Tactics & MC² Model

TACTIC ▼	OBJECTIVE	MC² FOCUS
PROMPTING	TO RAISE CONSCIOUSNESS, REMIND OF CONSEQUENCES OF BEHAVIOR	CONSCIOUSNESS / MOTIVATION
PERSUASION	TO GIVE COMPELLING REASONS TO CHANGE BEHAVIOR	MOTIVATION
EDUCATION	TO IMPROVE KNOWLEDGE & SKILLS, PROMOTE SELF-EFFICACY	CAPABILITY
SOCIAL ADVOCACY	TO RAISE GENERAL AWARENESS OF PROBLEM, PROMOTING PEER PRESSURE FOR CHANGE	CONSCIOUSNESS / MOTIVATION
INCENTIVES	TO CHANGE BALANCE OF POSITIVE VS. NEGATIVE CONSEQUENCES OF BEHAVIOR	MOTIVATION / CAPABILITY
MARKETING	TO MOTIVATE TO CHANGE BEHAVIOR & MAKE CHANGE EASIER	MOTIVATION / CAPABILITY
NEGOTIATION	TO CHOOSE AMONG TACTICS FOR BEHAVIOR CHANGE	MOTIVATION / CAPABILITY
EMPOWERMENT	TO ENABLE CONSUMERS TO MAKE OWN CHOICES	MOTIVATION / CAPABILITY

be promoted early by combining incentives, prompting, and social advocacy. Getting consumers to consider self-care and call a triage phone line before seeking emergency medical care may be promoted by mass distribution of self-care guides together with incentives (e.g., lower copays if okayed by phone counselors) and education/persuasion campaigns.

Education, persuasion, or social advocacy alone may take longer to achieve desired changes in behavior than incentives and marketing, for example. Negotiation (e.g., with individual patients or a unionized employee group) may achieve very quick response if agreement can be reached right away, or it may take years. Empowerment tactics depend on how long it takes consumers to decide on the behavior change they will make, as well as figure out how to make it.

WHAT PROPORTION OF RESPONSE IS DESIRED

Simple prompting, asking and reminding consumers to adopt or change a specific behavior, is likely to have the lowest proportional response. Only those already motivated, capable, and conscious of the desired behavior are likely to respond. Adding in educational initiatives can increase response by enabling those with capability barriers to respond. Including persuasion, social advocacy, incentives, or marketing tactics can add those at low levels of motivation. Negotiation and empowerment may be needed to get the more resistant members of a population to respond.

In some cases gradual response may be desirable. In testing an initiative whose results are uncertain, for example, sponsors may simply invite consumers to participate in a pilot program rather than aiming to get all or a majority. Some programs may have limited capability, or the budget may dictate that only some be enticed into changing behavior where incentives are offered or programs are expensive. Tactics may be chosen to promote or limit the numbers who respond.

VALUE OF THE BEHAVIOR CHANGE

The estimated value of the intended behavior change, together with the probability and timing of that value, should greatly influence the choice of tactics. Where the value is substantial, certain, and immediate, sponsors should feel comfortable in choosing tactics that are expensive to use. As previously argued, when the ROI amount is significant and the ratio high, sponsors can afford to borrow the money needed to finance these tactics, knowing that they will be better off doing as much as they can.

The estimated amount, probability, and timing of the value expected from a particular initiative normally sets the upper limit for the investment in that initiative. Total value, in expenditure savings, side effects, and health/quality of life should be included, of course. Tactics can be selected based on their particular ROI amounts, just as in selecting strategies.

COSTS OF TACTICS

The costs of particular tactics will determine their ROI, once the value of their impact is calculated. Costs may also limit which tactics can be chosen, where budgets are limited, or where sponsors are uncertain of the value they will gain in return. Smaller investments may seem more advisable as sponsors experiment with the idea of improving consumer behavior. Toe-in-the-water investments may doom initiatives to failure, of course, or guarantee suboptimal and incremental success while competitors achieve more dramatic returns.

EFFECTS ON RELATIONSHIPS

The choice of tactics has great potential impact on relationships with consumers and with other stakeholders who are party to or affected by that choice. Incentives, for example, are often criticized as promising only short-term impact and driving out intrinsic motivation, making consumers expect rewards for everything. Persuasion, social advocacy, or marketing efforts that are seen as manipulative can destroy trust. Educational programs that are seen as patronizing can do the same.

Negotiation can undermine relationships if sponsors fail to find win-win solutions (preferably WIN-WIN versus WIN-win) or acceptable compromises and break off negotiations. Empowerment may fail to achieve the results intended by sponsors and may undermine the use of that tactic in future. Social advocacy and government sanctions (e.g., higher taxes on cigarettes, guaranteed confidentiality for HIV/AIDS patients) may be seen as oppressive or in violation of prevailing values or personal freedom.

There is no way to say that a particular tactic will undermine or strengthen relationships or have the same impact on all relationships. Empowering consumers via nurse phone counseling, for example, may be seen by some physicians as undermining the patient-physician relationship. Some stakeholders may object to the use of incentives or marketing tactics to elicit behaviors they feel consumers should adopt on their own responsibility for their own good.

The challenge is to keep in mind the potential impact of a tactic and of the particulars of how it is implemented on important relationships. Both the duration and potential mutual contributions of stakeholder relationships determine their importance. In turn, the length of those relationships may be affected by the tactics chosen and by the results achieved in using them. Consumers are likely to become more loyal to employers, plans, and providers who demonstrate commitment and contributions to their personal health and well-being. Employers are likely to prove more loyal to plans or providers who achieve significant cost savings through improving consumer behavior, especially if they share those savings with the employer.

REFERENCE

1. J. Prochaska, et al., *Changing for Good* (New York, NY: Avon Books; 1994).

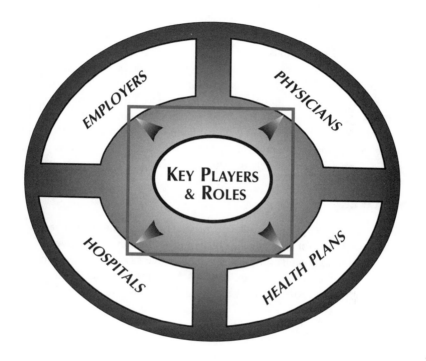

DECIDING WHO DOES WHAT

As discussed in Chapter 10 and Chapter 16, a key question in planning and implementing programs to improve consumer health and demand behaviors relates to who can do what—which stakeholders are best equipped to play which roles. This question applies to each of the risk-sharing partners of interest in managing consumer demand: governments, employers, physicians, hospitals, and insurers. It also extends to a wide variety of other possible partners, and particularly to consumers themselves.

In identifying who is best suited to what role, *their* capability and motivation are critical, just as with consumers. Who has the knowledge, skills, resources, and access to consumers to influence which consumer behaviors? Who has the trust and credibility to be accepted by consumers? Who can carry out which tactics for which targets and what behaviors? Who has the information needed to identify the most promising targets, set objectives, and track results?

Motivation to engage in demand improvement is a criterion that can help identify a wider range of potential partners. Employers, physicians, hospitals, and insurers have clear, financial reasons for doing so, even under fee-for-service, financing but particularly under capitation. So may nurses, schools, churches, businesses, suppliers, labor unions, pharmacists, governments, and a wide variety of organizations with interests in health. Added to the list may be vendors of particular demand improvement services and, perhaps most importantly, consumers as active partners in, not merely objects of, demand improvement programs.

EMPLOYERS

As payers for the costs of health care utilization under commercial or self-insurance and taxpayers for much of the costs of utilization by those covered by government insurance as well as the uninsured, employers have long had a stake in the quality and quantity of health care demand. Until recently most were passive, if loudly complaining participants in enduring the health care cost crisis. Now employers are growing in power as lobbyists for reforms, customers of health insurance, and, increasingly, as instigators of and partners in efforts to manage consumer demand.

Health Improvement

Many employers have for years, sometimes decades, engaged in efforts to promote their employees' health. Coors Brewing Company in Golden, Colorado, is an excellent example. Faced with liability for paying the health care costs of a largely older, male, blue-collar work force with some of the worst health habits imaginable, Coors has long promoted better fitness, with its own on-site fitness center and smoking cessation and similar health improvement programs.

At one time Coors was among the few employers actively involved in attempting to influence consumer health behaviors, though it has been actively promoting the idea among its peers. Now it is unusual for a large employer not to be involved, and even midsized employers are joining in. In a 1995 survey, 40% of responding companies in the midsize to large category reported sponsorship of at least one employee wellness program.[1]

The Dow Chemical Company promotes employee wellness by encouraging physicians to write "prescriptions" for their patients calling for wellness program participation. These are then "filled" by wellness staff at Dow. Employers throughout the country, such as Dean Foods[2] and HealthTrust[3] subsidize costs or reduce health insurance premiums for their employees who participate in outside wellness and fitness programs.

The involvement of employers in promoting their employees' health and otherwise improving their demand for health services was threatened by one component of the Clinton health reform proposals. Had community rating become standard for health insurance, employers who were not self-insured could lose their motivation to worry about their own employees' health behavior. All employers would pay the same premium rates, regardless of how healthy their employees were or how low their use of health services.[4]

To counter the potential impact of community rating, it was suggested that employers who met some requirement for promoting employee health be given discounts from prevailing rates.[5] Even without special consideration, however, employers might continue involvement in wellness and fitness efforts in order to promote better worker morale, productivity, and safety, for example.[6] With no stake in improving demand, however, due to not benefiting from any health insurance savings that resulted, employer involvement might be severely limited.

Decision Improvement

Employers are also engaging in efforts to guide or at least influence employee choices of health plans. They are demanding HMO inclusion in what they offer to employees[7] and working to steer employees, even retirees, toward HMO plans.[8] Through their own selection of which health plans to offer their employees, which often turns out to be one option, employers dictate the selections of millions of employees.

Even where they offer multiple choices, employers can greatly influence how consumers decide. Employers are forming powerful alliances, such as the National Federation of Independent Business, demanding that provider and health plans address their needs.[9] They are using their collective market power in regional coalitions to standardize health plan benefit packages and increase the number of employee health plan choices.[10]

In addition to influencing what health plans offer, employers are engaging in direct contracting with providers, steering their employees, dependents, and retirees to selected providers for special "carve-out" services or the full range of health care. Direct contracting has become popular for high-cost, tertiary services such as heart surgery, neurosurgery, and transplants, for example.[11] It has also been used to steer employees toward a selected group of providers for all physician and hospital services, as TWA did in St. Louis.[12]

In other cases employers have used direct contracting to expand rather than restrict employee choices. The Business Health Care Action Group in the Twin

Cities, Minnesota, contracts with integrated provider networks as well as health plans, giving employees vouchers they can use to select from among all contracting parties. The group also supplies employees with data on prices, quality, patient satisfaction, and related provider performance to help in the selection process.[13]

Experience suggests that direct contracting can save employers significant expense. The Bariod Corporation in Houston has enjoyed annual increases in expense roughly half those of other area businesses since implementing direct contracting in 1987.[14] Though employers who engage in direct contracting are decidedly in the minority, there is growing interest in at least considering the idea.[15]

Disease Management

We found few examples of employers taking an active role in disease management. Perhaps they feel such efforts are best left to professionals. On the other hand, large employers who have significant numbers of workers with the same condition could gain substantially from some involvement. Chronic conditions such as arthritis[16] and depression[17] are among the most frequent causes of worker disability. Large employers may contribute by sponsoring support groups and education programs on-site for a variety of common chronic conditions. The First National Bank of Chicago has partnered with the local March of Dimes to improve access to and use of prenatal care by its pregnant employees, including free, on-site care by physicians.[18]

In addition, employers' influence on health plan coverage and processes can greatly influence the success of disease management efforts by providers. Minnesota's Business Coalition has proposed that specialists, such as endocrinologists for patients with diabetes, cardiologists for chronic heart disease, and nephrologists for end-stage renal disease, serve as "gatekeepers" rather than conventional primary physicians.[19]

Employers can play a significant role in the development of disease management strategies. The Business Health Care Action Group is working with providers to develop clinical guidelines for management of selected diseases; Deere & Company is working with Mayo Clinic in developing specific disease-focused strategies.[20] The national Foundation for Accountability, which includes 30 large employers as well as government agencies, is working to develop "benchmark" guidelines for the best treatment of high-severity, pervasive conditions.[21]

Disability Management

Employees have a clear interest in doing whatever they can to reduce rapidly escalating workers' compensation expenditures. Disability costs are rising toward $200 billion a year, including the costs of income replacement, replacing or retraining workers, and reduced productivity as well as health care—from 8% to 10% of total payroll costs.[22] Employers in high-risk industries such as construction, manufacturing, agriculture, and transportation have higher than average costs, while others in financial and other services industries enjoy lower than average costs.[23]

In attempts to reduce costs at the upstream stage, employers are striving to get employees to adopt safer patterns of work behavior. Identifying those at high risk of injury and focusing behavior change efforts accordingly can eliminate the causes of many injuries.[24] Comprehensive programs of "medical event management" can minimize costs for disability episodes once injury has occurred.[25]

Some employers are steering injured employees to their own occupational medicine clinics on site, providing both emergency intervention and follow-up care.[26] Others are contracting with health plans, such as Kaiser, that offer special occupational medicine clinics off site.[27] Such steering is not always accepted by employees, however. In states where employees are forced to use providers selected by their employers, there have been charges that providers serve employers' interests at the expense of employees.[28]

Business groups are also urging legislative consideration of what is called "24-Hour Coverage," which would combine workers' compensation with employee health insurance. Health plans currently offering both types of insurance promise better coordination and greater continuity of care for employees.[29] Estimates are that combining the two forms of insurance would save billions of dollars in employer costs for workers' compensation. It could also cost billions of dollars by mandating health insurance coverage for employees not now covered[30] (Exhibit 18–1).

Advantages-Disadvantages of Employers

Employers are, in many ways, natural choices for participation in health and decision improvement and disease and disability management programs. They have the advantage of high motivation, as long as they incur significant effects from health insurance and disability costs. They have the greatest access to consumers, at least to employees, on a day-to-day basis. They can offer on-site programs in wellness and fitness that greatly increase participation because of their convenience. If employees trust their employer and feel a sense of community in the employer's success and survival, they may be strongly motivated to cooperate in activities aimed at improving their health and demand for services.

Employers may have valuable information about their employees' health status, from preemployment and routine physicals or from claims data where they are self-insured. They must be extremely careful about using such data, of course, given the risk of violating the Americans with Disabilities Act or of leaking confidential information about employee problems cared for through employee assistance programs.

Exhibit 18–1 Employer Roles in Improving Demand

Domain	Roles
Health Improvement	X Provide on-site fitness and wellness centers X Encourage physicians to "write prescriptions" for wellness activities X Subsidize the costs / reduce premiums for those who participate
Decision Improvement	X Negotiate with HMOs as to benefits covered X Steer employees to HMO X Form purchasing coalitions to standardize benefit packages X Contract directly with providers
Disease Management	X Sponsor support groups and on-site education programs X Pioneer efforts for specialists to be "gatekeepers" X Work with providers to develop clinical guidelines and benchmarks
Disability Management	X Support employees in adopting safer work habits X Develop comprehensive programs of "medical event management" X Provide on-site occupational medical clinics

There are issues related to whether or not employers have the legal right or practical ability to verify health behavior information useful in health improvement, such as which employees smoke, use seat belts, exercise regularly, or comply with dietary advice. Will prospective employees be honest and forthcoming in preemployment physicals or discussions about their health if they fear it will affect their hiring prospects? Are employer incentives or disincentives regarding health and demand behaviors coercive?

In addition, employees may not trust employer efforts, particularly where there has been a history of labor-management strife. They may be concerned that if they do not behave in a "sanitarily correct" manner, management will get back at them somehow. Employers who have, in the past, attempted to reduce health care costs by shifting the burden to employees, by steering them to providers that employees do not trust, or by severely restricting their health plan choices may find their credibility legitimately doubted when they shift to promoting programs they claim are in the employees' best interests.

Employers may not have a long-term interest in their employees, where they are totally focused on this quarter's financial performance or are used to and content with high worker turnover. They may rely on health plans and providers to worry about consumer health, much like consumers may feel no responsibility for their own health. Their employees may not want them to get involved or may fear their knowing private details about themselves and their dependents.

Employees may not want to participate in worksite health and fitness activities, feeling they spend enough time at work already. Even where an employer has a large number of employees, they may be spread out across a wide range of locations; besides, convenience for employees does not always mean the same for retirees and dependents.

Clearly employers can play a significant role in a wide variety of programs that can reengineer consumer health behaviors. At the same time, they are not necessarily the best choice for some roles and some efforts. A challenge in all efforts aimed at employees, dependents, or retirees will be to identify the best role for employers to play in particular programs and to get them to accept and enthusiastically perform that role (Exhibit 18–2).

PHYSICIANS

Physicians can also play a key role in managing consumers' health behavior as well as in controlling their demand. The American Academy of Family Physicians has espoused what they refer to as "patient education" as a vital part of patient care and promotes the idea that family physicians should play a leadership role in this effort.[31]

Exhibit 18–2 Strengths & Limitations of Employers in Improving Demand

STRENGTHS	LIMITATIONS
✗ CAN PROVIDE CONVENIENT ON-SITE SERVICES ✗ CAN SELECT HEALTH PLANS THAT PROMOTE HEALTH IMPROVEMENT ✗ CAN PROMOTE SAFER PATTERNS OF WORK BEHAVIOR ✗ ARE HIGHLY MOTIVATED TO CONTAIN HEALTH CARE COSTS	✗ WORKERS MAY NOT TRUST EMPLOYER EFFORTS ✗ EMPLOYERS MAY NOT HAVE LONG-TERM INTEREST IN EMPLOYEES ✗ EMPLOYEES MAY NOT WANT TO SPEND MORE TIME AT WORK IN FITNESS PROGRAMS

Their level of involvement, however, tends to be fairly low. In a 1995 survey, even among large medical groups, only 35% reported currently offering or planning to offer health promotion and wellness programs.[32] Among solo practices and small groups, the proportions are no doubt even lower, despite the built-in advantages physicians enjoy when it comes to influencing the health behavior of their patients.

Physicians normally enjoy far higher levels of trust compared to health plans and most employers, though this trust may be diminishing with concerns that the new health care system provides too many incentives for physicians to minimize their patients' use of health services, even when necessary.[33] The family or personal physician is likely to know facts about consumers as patients that are too sensitive for consumers to divulge to anyone else. Because of their expertise, authority, and commitment to patient welfare, physicians can be powerful sources of influence on consumer behavior.

They have the opportunity of one-on-one contact with consumers, often at times when patients are highly susceptible to suggestions for behavior change in order to prevent recurrence of an immediate problem, achieve an early cure, or minimize the effects of a chronic condition just diagnosed. They may also have the chance, during periodic checkups, to address dangerous behaviors before they produce symptoms and to promote early detection and intervention.

Like employers, physicians have limitations as well as strengths in managing consumer health behaviors. They are not, for the most part, trained in wellness promotion and the full range of prevention. While the average consumer would welcome greater activity by physicians, they tend to rate both the importance of and their training in such activities far below the ratings given by their patients[34] (Exhibit 18–3).

When physicians have taken on the risks of caring for a specific population under capitation financing, they have tended to adopt precisely the same kind of emphasis on managing provider behavior as did insurers and HMOs.[35] They appear to lack belief in the importance of managing consumer behavior or perhaps lack confidence in their ability to do it well, compared to managing the behavior of their peers.

Under capitation, primary physicians are expected to act as "gatekeepers," managing consumer utilization directly through controlling referrals, tests, and treatments. This may well seem an easier, more effective and efficient approach than empowering patients to become better self-managers of their own health and utilization. Physicians may define their role more as that of a manager than as a coach and enabler.

The very thing that makes physicians potentially most powerful in influencing consumer behavior, their authority, expertise, and personal relationship, tends also to make them the least efficient. Paying the cost of a physician's one-on-one counseling of a patient would be enormously more expensive than using nurses, health educators, social workers, and other behavior engineers in group sessions or classes. Under capitation, primary physician income is determined by how many patients they are responsible for. Coping with their demands for reactive treatment will severely limit the time available for proactive behavior management.

Primary care physicians may lack a full picture of the care their patients are already getting and the reasons for it. Under traditional indemnity insurance, their patients may be self-referring to a variety of specialists, even using another primary physician without their regular physician's knowledge. They may be seeking alternatives to medical care, paying out of their own pockets, with neither physician nor health plan aware of it. They may be taking prescriptions that other prescribers are unaware of, to say nothing of over-the-counter medications.

With employers and health plans sometimes "carving out" components of patient care, primary physicians may be out of the loop in terms of control, even awareness of what patients are doing and getting in the way of treatment. In many cases decision improvement programs sponsored by health plans, employers, or hospitals can triage patients to other providers without the primary physician's permission or even knowledge. Outsourcing disease management programs may give the responsibility for managing chronic patients to a pharmaceutical firm or benefit management company, with minimal involvement of the primary physi-

Exhibit 18–3 Physician Roles in Improving Demand

DOMAIN	ROLES
HEALTH IMPROVEMENT	✗ EMPLOY COMMUNITY NURSES & HEALTH EDUCATORS
DECISION IMPROVEMENT	✗ PROVIDE / SPONSOR TRIAGE, INFORMATION PROGRAMS ✗ OFFER SELF-CARE MANUALS / ADVICE
DISEASE MANAGEMENT	✗ USE GROUP SESSIONS TO EDUCATE LARGE NUMBER OF PATIENTS WITH SAME CONDITION
DISABILITY MANAGEMENT	✗ PROVIDE WRITTEN MATERIALS, INSTRUCTIONS ✗ ENLIST PATIENT AS PARTNER IN RETURN TO WORK

cian. Outside health risk management firms may take full responsibility for assessing, reporting, and modifying consumer health behaviors, with no physician involvement.

Physicians may even prefer to be left out, where keeping up with ongoing demands for care is sufficiently onerous. Relying on an outside triage firm can make more of physicians' time their own, though a large segment of physicians object to "nine-to-five medicine." For dozens of conditions, outside firms may be more effective and efficient at disease management, while physicians still benefit from reduced demand and expenditures. Other agencies, including public health and mass media, may be far more efficient and effective in achieving widespread immunization, early detection, healthier behaviors, and similar components of health improvement.

Yet physicians can also find ways to improve their effectiveness and efficiency. As medical schools and residency training programs shift more toward preparing physicians for careers as health managers as well as sickness treaters, the effectiveness of physicians may be greatly increased. Physicians have used group sessions for disease management where they have a large number of patients with the same condition and can employ community nurses and health educators to supplement their own efforts.

As with employers, physicians should always be included in planning and implementing demand reengineering efforts. Their particular roles will depend on what they, themselves, can and will take responsibility for and what their other partners decide. The key is to exploit their strengths while recognizing and accounting for their limitations. With the growing threats to the patient-physician relationship, physicians may find that engaging in efforts to improve consumer health and use of services is one way to strengthen that relationship, in addition to controlling their risk under capitation payment systems.[36]

In general, the role of physician versus patient can be viewed along a continuum—from activities that can be carried out by consumers independently, with no physician involvement, to activities carried out by physicians with essentially no consumer involvement. There are no activities across the health, decision, disease, and disability categories that necessarily fall into a specific point on this continuum; it is a matter for physicians and their patients to work out.

In addressing specific health improvements, for example, consumers may decide to improve their lifestyle behavior entirely on their own, without any mention of the challenge or support from a physician. Or the physician may be the principle instigator, bringing up a recommended behavior at every opportunity, referring patients to classes, counseling, screening, or whatever intervention is appropriate and acceptable to the patient. For one-time interventions such as immunizations (though most have to be repeated eventually), the physician may achieve acceptance by the patient and give the shot with little fuss. For lasting behavior changes subject to lapses (e.g., exercise, smoking), regular reminders, rewards/recognition, and recommitment may be necessary.

To improve health care decisions, consumers may find their own information via the Internet, library reference searches, condition-specific interest groups, support groups, or friends and family. They may be guided and assisted in their search by their physician, who may also supply materials directly. For some patients, the physician may be the only source of information even considered.

In improving the management of disease, consumers may also go off pretty much on their own, from testing and diagnosing themselves to finding out what sorts of treatment are available and what lifestyle changes necessary. More likely, they will at least seek physician confirmation of their diagnosis, and expect guidance, if not explicit direction in how to cope with their condition. In many cases, such as emergency situations where the patient is unconscious, the physician exercises absolute power in managing the condition.

For disability challenges, prevention, and risk reduction efforts are often in the hands of the employer, though personal physicians and occupational medicine specialists may be involved as well. Workers may adopt their own behavior improvements or select their own treatments and providers without professional advice or with it. Some form of partnership with the physician responsible for their case is likely, with the physician almost never completely dictating the process and outcomes of care.

Physicians, consumer groups, and a variety of policy leaders have joined in advocating a true partnership between physicians and patients. They expect this partnership to improve the process and outcomes of care and to improve the quality of life for both patients and physicians. To a great extent consumers are demanding—though many physicians are resisting—this new relationship; it appears certain, however, that partnerships will eventually become the norm[37] (Exhibit 18–4).

HOSPITALS

American hospitals have a long history of engaging in activities designed to promote both patient and public health, in addition to their more obvious role in caring for disease and injury. From a purely business perspective, at least under fee-for-service payment systems, this is often against the hospital's best interests, since such activities tend to reduce the need and demand for hospital services. With only a minority of hospitals receiving any capitation payments—less than 25% of HMOs paid hospitals by capitation in a 1995 report[38]—there are clearly other motivations involved.

Much of hospitals' effort is attributable to the missions of their sponsoring organizations, including religious orders, church congregations, and voluntary, not-for-profit organizations. Much may also be attributed to the fact that nurses have

Exhibit 18–4 Strengths and Limitations of Physicians in Improving Demand

STRENGTHS

✗ ARE USUALLY TRUSTED
   BY PATIENTS

✗ HAVE OPPORTUNITY TO
   DETECT PROBLEMS EARLY

✗ HAVE IMPRIMATUR OF
   AUTHORITY AND EXPERTISE

LIMITATIONS

✗ NOT TRAINED IN WELLNESS PROMOTION
   & FULL RANGE OF PREVENTION

✗ APPEAR TO NOT BELIEVE THAT MANAGING
   CONSUMER BEHAVIOR IS IMPORTANT

✗ MAY CHAFE AT THE "GATEKEEPER" ROLE

✗ ARE INEFFICIENT IN DELIVERING HEALTH
   IMPROVEMENT PROGRAMS

always been key components of hospital operations, bringing with them a commitment to community and patient health beyond the walls of the facility. Growing concern over maintaining tax-free status undoubtedly has some effect as well.

Health Improvement

A major focus for hospital effort has traditionally been health promotion, prevention, and early detection. St. Francis Hospital in Roslyn, New York, carries out mobile screening for cardiac illness using outreach vans, as well as worksite programs, cardiopulmonary resuscitation training, a fitness center with education, and exercise promoting cardiac health.[39] St. Vincent Medical Center in Toledo, Ohio, offers a wide variety of screening programs, including glaucoma, blood pressure, pulmonary disease, anemia, cholesterol, and diabetes, with a special focus on ethnic minorities, the poor, and migrant workers.[40]

Hospital fitness centers have developed throughout the country, often as profit centers in addition to mission services. A 1996 report found that over 250,000 people were members of such centers, up 773% since 1983. Through programs in "integrated lifestyle management," hospitals are teaching consumers how to improve their own health, as well as attracting customers to their sports medicine, cardiac rehab, and physical therapy programs.[41] Studies have found that patients coming to hospital emergency departments, particularly those patients without a personal physician, had high levels of interest in health and prevention care and information, yet reported failure to obtain such information from their providers.[42]

Promoting the use of early detection services, such as mammography screening, has been common to most hospitals. This is good business where it results in direct revenue for the service itself and indirect revenue when patients whose conditions were detected are referred to medical staff physicians. It is also a service to the community and to the patients whose conditions are detected at a stage where better outcomes can be achieved and also for consumers found to be healthy.

The Flagstaff (Arizona) Hospital Medical Center encourages and enables its nurses to volunteer in community and school programs, offering first aid training, wellness education, immunization, and other health enhancing programs.[43] Overall, according to a 1996 survey, 80% of hospitals are involved in some health promotion/prevention effort, from exercise/fitness to smoking cessation to stress management.[44] Hospitals are redesigning and reconstructing spaces to fit a shift to more of a wellness/health role in addition to their sickness/injury role.[45]

Decision Improvement

Hospitals have invested heavily in physician referral programs, though mainly with a view to steering callers to their medical staff and use of their own services.

They have long offered general disease and treatment-specific information to help consumers make health care decisions through phone-accessed audiotapes and nurse information lines such as "Ask-a-Nurse." More recently hospitals such as the Sutter system have moved into the phone triage field, offering conventional "emergency" advice plus counseling on treatment options, referrals, access to its medical library, and advice on prescriptions, for example.[46]

The Planetree Model of empowered patient and family involvement in their own care originated in 1981 at Pacific Presbyterian (now California Pacific) Medical Center in San Francisco. It gives patients and family members ongoing access to their medical records and to its medical library and resource center and generally aims at empowering patients to be full participants in making treatment decisions, as well as in carrying them out. This model has since spread to other hospitals throughout the country.[47]

Efforts by hospitals to steer patients in their direction have been a major emphasis of their marketing and managed care contracting efforts. These have not always succeeded, of course. One instructive example was that of St. Francis Medical Center in Monroe, Louisiana, which signed discount contracts with local employers so they would steer patients their way. Unfortunately they failed to include their medical staff physicians in the strategy and found that the disgruntled physicians were steering patients in the opposite direction, thereby angering employers who were not getting what they had bargained for. A "back-to-the-drawing-board" restart, with full involvement of medical staff as well as employers and insurers worked a lot better[48] (Exhibit 18–5).

Disease Management

Promoting better management by consumers of their chronic conditions is a logical focus for hospital demand improvement efforts. Hospital emergency departments and inpatient units see the results of patients' poor self-management and devote a large portion of their resources to caring for avoidable crises. They have had significant impact through simply providing discharged patients with written instructions on follow-up and contingency care.[49]

The Washington University School of Medicine and its affiliated hospital focused disease management efforts on congestive heart failure patients. Education and counseling on diet and nutrition while treating them as inpatients, plus follow-up phone monitoring postdischarge by nurses, significantly reduced the rate of rehospitalization among these patients.[50]

Hospitals have taken advantage of new technologies, employing video presentations of clinical pathways on consumer roles in inpatient care; coordinated, one-stop-shopping information lines; and Internet access so that patients can obtain helpful advice at home.[51] Celebration Health, a futuristic hospital in Disney's

Exhibit 18–5 Hospital Roles in Improving Demand

DOMAIN	ROLES
HEALTH IMPROVEMENT	X PROVIDE MOBILE VANS & OTHER OPPORTUNITIES FOR SCREENING X DEVELOP FITNESS CENTERS AS PROFIT CENTERS AT HOSPITALS X PROMOTE USE OF EARLY DETECTION SERVICES X ENCOURAGE NURSES & STAFF TO VOLUNTEER IN COMMUNITY & SCHOOL PROGRAMS
DECISION MANAGEMENT	X OFFER TELEPHONE TRIAGE & GENERAL DISEASE INFORMATION TO PATIENTS X GIVE PATIENTS & FAMILIES ONGOING ACCESS TO RECORDS & RESOURCES
DISEASE MANAGEMENT	X PROVIDE WRITTEN INSTRUCTIONS FOR FOLLOW-UP CARE X PROVIDE EDUCATION & COUNSELING WHILE PATIENTS ARE INPATIENTS X PROVIDE FOLLOW-UP MONITORING BY NURSES AFTER PATIENT DISCHARGE X EXPLOIT NEW INFORMATION TECHNOLOGY TO PROVIDE EDUCATION
DISABILITY MANAGEMENT	X REHABILITATION & WORK-HARDENING PROGRAMS X OCCUPATIONAL MEDICAL CENTERS WITH OT & PT PROGRAMS

model community near Orlando, Florida, uses the Internet to monitor blood sugar levels in diabetic patients in a joint venture with two Eli Lilly subsidiaries.

Hospitals have a number of natural advantages in particular consumer behavior reform efforts. They have potentially greater credibility as being committed to patients' and public health than do most health plans, though hospitals too are suffering from declining public trust.[52] Hospitals often catch consumers when they are most receptive to health behavior improvement: right after a heart attack or an asthma or diabetes crisis. They often have enough patients suffering from the same condition to offer support programs, training, education, and counseling activities more efficiently than physicians could.

On the other hand, hospitals lack a comprehensive database about their patients; they only know about encounters in the hospital. They often lack a convenient location and can offer far fewer locations than there are physician practices. If they experience a high turnover among their patients, through medical staff, or more likely health plan deselection, they may lack both the motivation and ability to influence their patients on a long-term basis. With declining utilization and payment levels, they may not be able to afford to keep up even what they are doing already, much less expand into new possibilities (Exhibit 18–6).

HEALTH PLANS

Health plans, particularly HMOs, have advertised their commitment to prevention and promotion for decades in keeping with the spirit of the designation "health *maintenance* organization." On the other hand, there has often been more rhetoric than substance in their claims. As long as they could reduce their liability through combinations of provider discounts and utilization management efforts aimed at providers, they seem to have paid mostly lip service to improving consumer health behaviors.

Considering that it is the nature of insurance to recompense people damaged by unexpected events, it has been essentially a reactive industry.[53] Early on in health insurance there was great debate over whether maternity care should be included, since it was not an unexpected disaster, was the direct result of chosen behavior, and people had nine months to save up for its expense.

Insurers have found other ways of dealing with the unfortunate tendency of many people to get sick and incur covered expense. They have used coverage limits, precertification requirements, and other rules and regulations to control their liability for patient disease and injury. They have employed the device of "underwriting" to exclude from coverage those consumers who might need the most care.

The more reputable and progressive health plans have gradually moved to the consumer demand half of the equation, though often only after exhausting the provider supply side. A 1996 report on managed care plans found 50% offering or

Exhibit 18–6 Strengths & Limitations of Hospitals in Improving Demand

STRENGTHS

✗ Have always had health promotion, prevention & early detection as part of mission

✗ A few have pioneered efforts to empower patients to be full participants in health care decisions

✗ Can access resources to make delivery of health improvement services efficient & effective

✗ Have relatively high credibility in the community

LIMITATIONS

✗ May lack comprehensive database about their patients

✗ May not have convenient location

✗ May lack motivation & ability to influence patients on long-term basis

✗ Have difficulty affording what they already provide much less expanding into new market areas

✗ Dominated by physicians with acute inpatient focus

✗ Conflicting financial incentives (need to fill beds and retire debt)

at least planning health and wellness activities, though this was far less than the 80% found for hospitals and health systems. They offer programs to add value to their competitive offering or to match their competition, as well as to reduce their risks, control demand, and improve the health of their members.[54]

Health plans are in a strong position to influence consumer health behavior through coverage for prevention and promotion programs, incentives such as lower premiums and copayment for consumers practicing healthy behavior, and disincentives such as higher premiums and copayments for those with high-risk behaviors. They already provide incentives for consumers to select preferred providers through preferred provider organization and point of service coverage. Growing numbers of plans are investing in disease management efforts, with most reporting positive results.[55]

Health plans may have the best databases, through their claims information, for identifying which consumers and which behaviors are best prospects for interventions. Larger plans are likely to have enough consumers with similar behaviors, conditions, and interests to provide the critical mass for efficient interventions. They can use their claims data to track the impact of specific interventions over time, trying various experiments to learn what programs are most effective and efficient (Exhibit 18–7).

In many cases plans may contribute most to demand improvement efforts through their sharing of data. By opening their claims data to perusal by employers, physicians, and hospitals, they may fill in the gaps that prevent these partners from maximizing their effectiveness. By sharing what they learn about what works best, they may be able to contribute more as guides and advisors for their partners than as direct providers of behavior change interventions.

Unfortunately health plans have suffered a lot of "managed care bashing" in recent years. Their often heavy-handed, sometimes outrageous efforts to minimize their expenditures have created media heydays and fodder for politicians. Low proportions of expenditures for care (i.e., medical loss ratios), coupled with sometimes outrageously high profits and executive salaries, may prompt consumers to wonder whose side they are on. They are likely to be fairly low on the credibility ladder if they claim a disinterested commitment to promoting consumer health.

Health plans, unless they are also service delivery providers such as Kaiser, also lack any natural, ongoing personal contact with consumers. Interactions with insurance companies are likely to be about benefits and claims and are often adversarial. Many plans offer periodic newsletters and health hints, but such communications are impersonal.

Of course, health plans can use demand reform efforts to create opportunities for more personalized communication. Health risk management programs include customized assessments or analyses followed by personalized improvement plans and follow-up efforts. Disease management programs can also be personalized to

Exhibit 18–7 Health Plan Roles in Improving Demand

DOMAIN	ROLES
HEALTH IMPROVEMENT	**X** SUPPORT EFFORTS AT PREVENTION **X** PROVIDE HEALTH & WELLNESS ACTIVITIES **X** PROVIDE COVERAGE FOR PREVENTION & PROMOTION PROGRAMS **X** PROVIDE INCENTIVES FOR THOSE PRACTICING HEALTHY BEHAVIOR
DECISION IMPROVEMENT	**X** NURSE COUNSELING & EDUCATION PROGRAMS **X** TELEPHONE TRIAGE & SHARED-DECISION–MAKING PROGRAMS
DISEASE MANAGEMENT	**X** CASE MANAGEMENT BY DISEASE TYPE **X** INFORMATION MANAGEMENT FOR POPULATION-BASED PROGRAM PLANNING **X** IDENTIFY MEMBERS AT RISK
DISABILITY MANAGEMENT	**X** SOME HAVE VERY STRONG CASE MANAGEMENT SYSTEMS OR CONTRACT OUT TO VARIOUS SPECIALTY VENDORS AND PROVIDERS **X** "24-HOUR" COVERAGE

individual families and can include personal contact by nurses and educators employed by the plan.

Health plans may lack a long-term relationship with consumers if their employer clients and members have a tendency to change plans at every opportunity. In fact, plans that invest in long-term-payoff health improvement efforts may find themselves at a price disadvantage when trying to retain their employer clients long enough to see the investment pay off.

Like their other three risk-sharing partners in managed care, health plans have both strengths and limitations when it comes to managing consumer health behavior and use of health services. Plans should carefully consider and discuss how to work closely with those partners to identify their most effective role and coordinate their efforts as they carry out that role (Exhibit 18–8).

OTHER STAKEHOLDERS

One of the most serious limitations of most current demand improvement initiatives, even those where employers, physicians, hospitals, and health plans are working together, is that they omit other stakeholders who may be able to contribute in ways that sponsors never dreamed of. These other stakeholders may not share the financial risks of full partners in an integrated health system; they may not have a financial stake in improving consumer demand for health care. But they may have significant value to offer, providing competitive advantage to sponsors that exploit their potential compared to those that fail to even recognize that potential.

The examples described in the following pages represent cases where other stakeholders have contributed significantly to one or more aspects of demand improvement. They by no means circumscribe the potential such stakeholders represent; in almost all cases they made such contributions on their own, without being asked by or coordinating with payers of providers. Eleven groups of stakeholders will be discussed. To avoid any suggestion of their relative importance or potential value, they will be presented in alphabetical order.

Businesses

In one sense businesses have already been mentioned as employers, hence payers, in the risk-sharing partnership. Here they will be discussed as playing a different role, unconnected with their health insurance liability. One national example has been the involvement of private firms in promoting healthy behavior together with their own products. Kellogg has had significant impact on public awareness of the value of dietary fiber and on public consumption of such fiber, enjoying along the way significant increases in the sale of its oat bran cereals. Rockport has promoted and sponsored a wide range of exercise walking programs, while enjoying increased sales of its walking shoes.[56]

Exhibit 18–8 Strengths & Limitations of Health Plans in Improving Demand

STRENGTHS

✗ CAN INFLUENCE CONSUMER HEALTH BEHAVIOR PATTERNS THROUGH FINANCIAL INCENTIVES

✗ CAN INFLUENCE PURCHASING PATTERNS THROUGH "PREFERRED PROVIDER" COVERAGE

✗ HAVE GOOD DATABASES THAT CAN ASSIST IN PLANNING AND PROGRAMS

✗ GUIDE & ADVISE PROVIDERS IN PLANNING EFFECTIVE PROGRAMS

LIMITATIONS

✗ EFFORTS TO MANAGE USAGE MAY BE PERCEIVED AS HEAVY-HANDED & SELF-SERVING

✗ HIGH PROFITS & SALARIES BREED DISTRUST AMONG CONSUMERS & EMPLOYERS

✗ LACK ONGOING CONSUMER CONNECTIONS

✗ CONSUMERS FEAR BREACH OF CONFIDENTIALITY, LOSS OF COVERAGE, REPORTS SENT TO EMPLOYERS

✗ INTERFERENCE WITH PHYSICIAN-PATIENT RELATIONSHIP

✗ PROGRAMS MAY COMPETE WITH THOSE OF OTHER HEALTH PLANS & PROVIDERS

In a more indirect public relations effort, Anheuser-Busch has for years promoted responsible drinking and the use of a designated driver. Whatever the impact of these efforts on beer sales, they have had significant impact on drunk-driving accidents, reported as a 62% reduction the last time this was reported on television. Auto manufacturers have installed both front and side air bags to reduce bodily injury in accidents and have used this to improve their sales as well.

In Toledo, local supermarkets and the Big Boy restaurant chain joined with a local hospital to promote healthier eating, including offering more healthy options to their own customers.[57] In Minneapolis, grocery stores, restaurants, and health clubs partner with the HMO Health Partners to promote healthier behaviors by consumers. Health Partners sponsored contests, with entries judged by its members, to identify the tastiest healthy food items.[58]

Another business category that offers significant potential is the mass media. In Southern California, CareAmerica Health Plans joined with KABC Talkradio in a six-month campaign to promote consumer awareness of health issues and specific programs such as nutrition education and stroke risk screenings.[59] The Calhoun County (Alabama) Medical Society enlisted local television, radio, and newspaper help in promoting general health awareness and preference for local providers versus those in the competing big city.[60]

Churches

Churches have strong interests in spiritual health but also contribute to the physical, mental, and social health of their congregations and their neighborhoods. Many sponsor parish nurse or neighborhood nurse programs, wherein nurses contribute to community health. A survey of Chicago churches found over 80% of Catholic churches sponsoring at least one health activity, with significant though smaller proportions in other denominations. These activities covered the gamut, from AIDS to prenatal care and education to mental illness, substance abuse, flu shots and child immunizations, early detection screenings, and fitness programs.[61]

In Hollywood, California, the Queen of Angels-Hollywood Presbyterian Medical Center created a "health partnership" with local churches to promote screening activities, prenatal care, and health education through their parish nurse programs.[62] While church-sponsored efforts cannot be targeted to benefit only members of specific risk groups, they have advantages of geographic convenience and credibility and often reach poor and minorities that are the most difficult to include in payer/provider-sponsored programs.

Community Organizations

This category is really a catch-all for organizations that simply do not fit into the other categories. It may include private foundations or fund-raising entities like the American Red Cross or March of Dimes. The national arms of these organizations may offer literature for distribution to consumers, advice on public awareness programs, and health promotion activities, in addition to the contributions they make to public awareness through their national fund-raising, advertising, and media relations efforts.

Local arms may contribute as direct partners in specific programs and events. The Williamsport (Pennsylvania) Hospital & Medical Center worked with local chapters of the American Cancer Society, Heart Association, Lung Association, Red Cross, and the American Association of Retired Persons (AARP) to create a shopping-mall-based LifeCenter™ program to promote community health awareness and participation in wellness activities. It reported such participation up 15-fold in two years.[63]

A 1995 survey found 29% of the health plans responding had partnered with community organizations such as the YMCA to promote consumer wellness and health.[64] Group Health of Puget Sound (Washington), the state's largest HMO, partnered with local community health centers to provide a comprehensive continuum of mental health care for its members and to minimize recidivism.[65]

Aside from their frequently free contributions to general health, community-based organizations may offer advantages as options or additional sites for payer/provider-sponsored programs. They may be more convenient for dependents and retirees than worksite locations, for example. Employees and consumers may feel more autonomous participating in community-based activities, rather than complying with the expectations of employers or health plans.[66]

Governments

As payers through Medicare, Medicaid, CHAMPUS (Civilian Health and Medical Program of the Uniformed Services), and other insurance programs, governments have a great deal to do with what types of prevention and promotion services are covered. As providers, through Veterans Affairs and Defense Department hospitals and clinics, they can engage in any of the demand improvement activities already described for hospitals and physicians. In addition, governments can play a vital role in affecting the health of the general public.

In Hawaii, for example, the state government passed the Prepaid Health Care Act, mandating employer health insurance coverage for workers, plus the State Health Insurance Program for unemployed, resulting in Hawaii's having the highest proportion of its residents insured among the 50 states. In addition, it has promoted health education in schools, needle exchange programs to reduce risk of AIDS among drug users, and gun control laws to reduce damage from violence.[67]

The federal CDC sponsors and conducts studies into best practices for preventing sexually transmitted disease and for reducing smoking and teenage pregnancy.

It promotes child immunization and publishes the definitive work on which preventive services are cost-effective, *Guide to Clinical Preventive Services*.[68]

Experience suggests that government-sponsored public health agencies can do better at some disease management challenges than can private providers. In New York City, for example, when the management of TB patients was turned over to private clinics, the success rate for completing treatment regimens fell to only 10%.[69]

As private providers and health plans move to cover Medicaid beneficiaries, they would be well advised to look for partnership opportunities with the public clinics and hospitals that have long served these populations. As payers and providers look for ways to minimize disease and injury, they may find public health programs among their most effective allies.

Nurses

As employees in hospitals and physician practices, nurses are already playing a key role in caring for patients. Because they are trained in and motivated toward promoting health as well as treating disease and injury, nurses are also potentially powerful allies in reengineering consumer demand for health services.

The federal government (i.e., HCFA) sponsors demonstration projects called community nurse organizations (CNOs) in which nurses improve the health and demand behavior of Medicare-insured seniors. Each nurse is responsible for between 100 and 200 seniors, depending on their health status. Nurses provide regular health assessments, manage chronic conditions, and refer for medical and home health care. Experience suggests that nurses perform these functions most cost-effectively.[70]

In Arizona the Carondelet Health System operates a CNO for 3,000 Medicaid risk enrollees, with 2,000 participating in the nurse management program and 1,000 as controls getting conventional medical care.[71] It also uses the same approach to nurse management for the seniors served by its 19 senior community health centers.[72]

In payer and provider organizations, nurses are often best suited to promote health and manage demand for consumers. They are automatically more economical than physicians and have formal training in counseling and educating patients, plus their credibility has yet to be attacked, as has that of physicians and payers, in the "bashing" aimed at managed care. By enlisting their ideas as well as services, payers and providers may discover a wide variety of innovative ways that nurses can contribute[73] (Exhibit 18–9).

Pharmacists

Pharmacists often play a modest role in health care, filling prescriptions for patients and little more. Yet they could play a far greater role. Pharmacists may be

Exhibit 18–9 Other Stakeholder Roles in Improving Demand

STAKEHOLDER	ROLES
BUSINESSES	✗ PROMOTE HEALTHY PRODUCTS & RESPONSIBLE BEHAVIOR ✗ JOIN WITH INSURERS / PROVIDERS IN MEDIA EVENTS TO RAISE AWARENESS
CHURCHES	✗ SPONSOR COMMUNITY NURSE PROGRAMS & HEALTH ACTIVITIES ✗ CREATE HEALTH PARTNERSHIPS WITH PROVIDERS TO PROMOTE SCREENING & HEALTH CARE EDUCATION, ESPECIALLY AFFECTING SPECIFIC POPULATIONS OR MINORITIES
COMMUNITY ORGANIZATIONS	✗ PROVIDE EDUCATION & INFORMATION ABOUT SPECIFIC DISEASES ✗ PARTNER WITH PROVIDERS IN SPECIFIC PROGRAMS AND EVENTS ✗ PROVIDE SITES FOR PROVIDER-SPONSORED PROGRAMS
GOVERNMENTS	✗ ENGAGE IN ACTIVITIES TO REDUCE COSTS TO THEIR POPULATIONS ✗ PROMOTE EDUCATION & MEDIA SUPPORT FOR RESPONSIBLE BEHAVIOR ✗ PROMOTE COMMUNITY-WIDE HEALTH & PREVENTION EFFORTS
NURSES	✗ ALIGN WITH PATIENTS TO DEMAND PREVENTIVE & PROACTIVE HEALTH SERVICES ✗ PROVIDE COST-EFFECTIVE HEALTH & DECISION IMPROVEMENT SERVICES ✗ PROMOTE HEALTH & MANAGE DEMAND FOR CONSUMERS ✗ UTILIZE PATIENT EDUCATION SKILLS

best qualified to identify situations where consumers are using outdated or contraindicated medications, for example. They can add significantly to instructions about medications, both oral and written, compared to the brief discussion commonly offered by physicians.

Clinical pharmacists are participating as active care team members in hospitals, for example. They are promoting questions by and discussions with consumers about specific medications and promoting compliance with medication orders by physicians. As they refill prescriptions, they can check the timing to see if it indicates proper compliance and check for any problems consumers are having. They can supply helpful aids such as unit doses and day-of-the-month pill holders to help consumers comply properly.[74]

Schools

Neighborhood schools are natural locations for health education, immunization, and screening efforts aimed at students and parents. They can offer a variety of health education, first aid, and CPR training as parts of their curricula. School nurses can provide care and counseling to students. Providers may partner with them in any number of health promotion, prevention, and early detection efforts.[75]

Suppliers

Suppliers of products and services in the health care industry are increasingly getting more involved in the operations of provider organizations. Pharmaceutical companies are developing programs and operating subdivisions devoted to managing the use of medications by enrolled populations (e.g., pharmacy benefit management). They are offering comprehensive disease management services for a variety of patients with specific chronic conditions.[76]

For example, pharmaceutical firms are offering guaranteed lifetime prices for some medications where lifetime use is likely (e.g., hypertension prescriptions). They are sending instructions and follow-up reminders directly to patients or supplying them to pharmacists for use in patient encounters.[77]

Unions

Employers are normally identified as the initial sources of payment for health insurance, though often unions serve this function. Through contracts, they may serve as the intermediary, responsible for administering trust funds that are the repositories for employer fringe benefit payments. Moreover, unions may make the health plan or direct contracting decisions for employees. As such they can exert the same influences as employers on health and demand improvement.

In Chicago, for example, the Truck Drivers, Helpers and Warehouse Workers Union selects benefit plans and programs that promote prevention and wellness among its members and employee selection of economical, effective medical care providers. It does its own case management for acute and chronic disease patients and offers health screening and education programs, using the money it saves through reducing the use of health services to augment fringe benefits for its members.[78]

Vendors

We have used the term "vendors" to distinguish firms that offer specific demand improvement services from "suppliers" of other products and services already discussed. Representative lists of vendors offering a variety of health and decision improvement and disease and disability management services are offered in Part V. For this discussion, let it be recognized that outside vendors may have distinct advantages for some situations.

Many of these vendors have had years of experience in delivering a service that may be totally unfamiliar to payers or providers. By serving multiple clients they can frequently offer economies of scale unavailable to providers and payers because of the number of consumers involved. As outside agents they may be able to offer privacy and confidentiality that would otherwise be a problem for consumers concerned about employers and insurers having access to sensitive information. One survey found that only 46% of consumers trust their employers and only 39% trust insurers with medical record information.[79]

In many cases vendors work closely with providers and payers as "partners" rather than arm's-length vendors. For example, Greenstone Healthcare Solutions (vendor) contracts with Lovelace Healthcare System (integrated delivery system) in the development and testing of disease management programs to be sold to other provider and payer clients.[80]

At the same time outside vendors may have drawbacks. They may aim for the easiest targets to change, for example, rather than those whose behavior change may be harder to achieve but would produce greater value. If vendors are paid based on, for example, their costs or amount of time they spend or based on getting consumers to participate, they may devote their energies to maximizing the measures that will promote their revenue and profit rather than emphasizing impact on consumer health or demand. Growing numbers of vendors are sharing risks and rewards or guaranteeing results, however.[81]

Consumers

While this is a violation of the alphabetical order used in discussing the roles of other stakeholders, it is done deliberately. Consumers are clearly the *objects* for demand improvement efforts, but they should also be considered as potential partners therein.

In many instances, consumers can be the most powerful sources of influence on their peers. Parents and children can be influential in promoting healthier behaviors and better use of services within families. Friends, relatives, and coworkers can be sources of peer pressure in promoting healthier behavior and reducing health risks. Fellow sufferers from chronic conditions can be the most credible sources of advice on how to manage disease or make treatment decisions.

Fellow consumers can be used in "testimonial" videos, for example, describing their experiences with managing a chronic condition or selecting a particular procedure for treating an acute condition. Reformed smokers, drinkers, and drug users may be the most effective spokespersons for educational efforts. Support groups of consumers suffering the same problems can help each other—in group sessions, on phone crisis lines, on the Internet.

Consumers should also be thought of as potential partners in designing specific demand improvement programs. They can supply suggestions on what types of information, what kinds of experiences, and what rewards and incentives are likely to be most effective in enticing them to participate in programs or change specific behaviors. They can help providers lobby payers and vice versa to promote better coverage of prevention and promotion services to stimulate the development of specific programs.

The great advantage available in health and decision improvement and disease and disability management is that consumers independently gain from their success, over and above the advantages to payers and risk-sharing providers. Because of this, consumers should be strongly motivated to participate in a variety of ways as full partners rather than merely as arm's-length targets for particular efforts. We may have no idea as to their potential for contribution until we ask them (Exhibit 18–10).

PARTNERSHIPS

A common theme running through these discussions and examples of specific stakeholders' roles, as well as through the references at the end of this chapter, is the value of partnerships. Champions of health system integration argue that having insurers, hospitals, and physicians integrated, with their incentives properly aligned, is key to achieving health care reform.[82] Having each of the partners select its best role, coordinating efforts, and sharing gains is essential to creating the "Grand Alliance" we need to solve the health cost crisis.[83]

Beyond this limited partnership lies the potential for inclusion of other stakeholders. Programs for "healthy communities" require the cooperation of insurers, physicians, hospitals, local businesses, schools, governments, and community organizations—essentially everyone motivated and capable of helping.[84] Programs

Exhibit 18–10 Other Stakeholder Roles in Improving Demand

STAKEHOLDER	ROLES
PHARMACISTS	X IDENTIFY WHEN PATIENTS USING OUTDATED / CONTRAINDICATED MEDICATION X PROVIDE CLEAR, COMPREHENSIVE INSTRUCTIONS FOR CONSUMERS X ASSIST IN ENSURING COMPLIANCE WITH MEDICATION REGIMENS
SCHOOLS	X PROVIDE LOCATIONS FOR HEALTH EDUCATION & PREVENTIVE PROGRAMS
SUPPLIERS	X DEVELOP PROGRAMS DEVOTED TO MANAGING USE OF MEDICATIONS X OFFER COMPREHENSIVE DISEASE MANAGEMENT SERVICES
UNIONS	X EXERT INFLUENCE ON HEALTH & DEMAND IMPROVEMENT PLANS X PROMOTE SELECTION OF ECONOMICAL, EFFECTIVE MEDICAL CARE PROVIDERS
VENDORS	X PROVIDE ECONOMIES OF SCALE IN DELIVERING DEMAND IMPROVEMENT SERVICES X PARTNER WITH PROVIDERS IN DEVELOPING & TESTING DISEASE MANAGEMENT PROGRAMS
CONSUMERS	X INFLUENCE BEHAVIOR OF CHILDREN, SPOUSES, FAMILY MEMBERS & FRIENDS X PROVIDE CREDIBLE SOURCE OF ADVICE ON HOW TO MANAGE DISEASE & MAKE DECISIONS X PROVIDE "TESTIMONIALS" THAT ENCOURAGE BEHAVIOR CHANGE X PARTNER IN DESIGNING PROGRAMS THAT WILL ENHANCE OWN HEALTH & IMPROVE OWN DEMAND

such as the National Chronic Care Consortium engage providers and community organizations across the country in active partnership.[85]

In any instance, stakeholder partners will have to be carefully selected for specific efforts; their potential contributions and ongoing relationships will have to be carefully managed. Involving them will complicate as well as potentially strengthen particular demand improvement programs. But we will not truly have an integrated health system and enjoy all its benefits until all the stakeholders who can contribute meaningfully to the effort are included (more on this subject in Chapter 19).

REFERENCES

1. "Health Promotion and Wellness Climbs Higher on the Strategic Agendas of Healthcare CEOs," *The Alliance Report,* March/April 1996, 16.

2. C. Petersen, "Employers, Providers Are Partners in Health," *Managed Healthcare* 5, no. 1 (1995):36–38.

3. C. Petersen, "Companies Find Wellness Efforts Bring Health to Their Bottom Line, Too," *Managed Healthcare* 4, no. 2 (1994):24–25.

4. "Deductions Urged for Companies with Wellness Programs," *Business & Health* 11, no. 12 (1993):12.

5. "Industry Alliance Makes Wellness a Player in Health Reform Debates," *Employee Health & Fitness* 16, no. 8 (1994):101–104.

6. A. Peck, "Reform Could Cool Off Those Sweating for Fitness," *Managed Healthcare* 3, no. 11 (1993):34–36.

7. W. Nelson, "Customers Demand Managed Care," *Healthcare Financial Management* 49, no. 8 (1995):10.

8. "HMOs Ally with Employers To Boost Medicare Business," *Managed Care Outlook* 8, no. 1 (1995):5.

9. Peck, "Reform Could Cool," 34–36.

10. "Currents—Employers," *Hospitals & Health Networks,* 5 January 1997, 10, 11.

11. J. Drobny, "Cardiac Hospitals Offer Savings through Carve-Out Program," *Managed Care Outlook* 5, no. 21 (1992):5, 6.

12. "TWA Implements Direct Contract Network in Seven Months," *Direct Contracting & Hospital Managed Care* 2, no. 1 (1992):6, 7.

13. D. Borfitz, "Twin Cities Coalition Creates Competing Care System Model," *Strategic Health Care Marketing* 12, no. 9 (1995):1–6.

14. "A Case Study in Direct Contracting," *Direct Contracting & Hospital Managed Care* 1, no. 9 (1992):4, 5.

15. "Direct Contracting in the Heartland," *Hospitals* 20 March 1992, 22.

16. P. Greenberg, et al. "Calculating the Workplace Cost of Chronic Disease," *Business & Health* 13, no. 9 (1995):27–30.

17. "Caught in the Middle," *Hospitals and Health Networks,* 20 July 1997, 68.

18. E. Zicklin, "Prenatal Teamwork Fosters an Employer/Employee Partnership," *Business & Health* 10, no. 3 (1992):36–40.

19. "Specialist Gatekeeper Model Aimed at Cutting Demand among Chronically Ill," *Healthcare Demand Management* 1, no. 2 (1995):22–23.

20. K. Terry, "Disease Management: At These Companies, the Future Is Now," *Business & Health* 13, no. 4 (1995):73–76.

21. "FAcct Targets 'Best Treatment' Subjects," *Business & Health* 13, no. 10 (1995):10.

22. K. Robbins, "The Growing Costs of Disability," *Business & Health Special Report: The Advantages of Managed Disability* 11 (1993):8, 9.

23. H. Pipkin, "Estimating Market Size for Work Related Injuries," *The Alliance Report,* January/February 1996, 1, 2.

24. M. Fruen, "Disability Management Focuses on Prevention," *Business & Health* 10, no. 12 (1992):24–29.

25. E. Lipson, "Medical Event Management Moving to Forefront of Cost Containment," *Managed Care Outlook* 8, no. 25 (1995):5–10.

26. E. Meszaros, "Cheaper by the Dozen, Cheaper On Site," *Managed Healthcare* 4, no. 11 (1994): 24, 25.

27. M. Edlin, "Kaiser OM Clinics Help Curb Calif. WC Costs," *Managed Healthcare* 4, no. 10 (1994):10.

28. S. Steers, "Still Hurting," *Westword* 19, no. 31 (1996):14–21.

29. C. Petersen, "Is 24-Hour Care an Empty Promise?" *Managed Healthcare* 5, no. 4 (1995):62–64.

30. I. Kertesz, "Costs Outweigh Savings of 24-Hour System—Study," *Modern Healthcare,* 24 July 1995, 22.

31. *Patient Education: A Leadership Role for Family Physicians and the AAFP* (Kansas City, MO: American Academy of Family Practice, 1993).

32. "Health Promotion and Wellness," 16.

33. H. Anderson, "New Guide Offers Planning Tips for Preventive Care," *Hospitals,* 5 June 1992, 68–70.

34. C. McBride, et al., "The Physician's Role: Views of the Public and the Profession on Seven Aspects of Patient Care," *Archives of Family Medicine* 3, no. 5 (1994):948–953.

35. E. Kerr, et al., "Managed Care and Capitation in California: How Do Physicians at Risk Control Their Own Utilization?" *Annals of Internal Medicine* 123 (1995):500–504.

36. D. Beckham, "The Engine of Choice," *Healthcare Forum Journal* 39, no. 4 (1996):58–64.

37. J. Heymann, *Equal Partners: A Physician's Call for a New Spirit of Medicine* (Boston, MA: Little, Brown, 1995).

38. J. O'Malley, "Reducing Healthcare Costs with Demand Management," *The Alliance Bulletin,* August 1995, 3, 5.

39. R. Weiss, "A Hospital That Is All Heart," *Health Progress* 74, no. 9 (1993):60, 61.

40. R. Weiss, "Promoting Community Health," *Health Progress* 74, no. 5 (1993):62–64.

41. J. Bensky, "Quickening the Pulse of Health and Quality," *Managed Healthcare* 6, no. 2 (1996):24, 25.

42. R. Rodriguez, et al., "Need and Desire for Preventive Care Measures in Emergency Department Patients," *Annals of Emergency Medicine* 26, no. 5 (1995):615–620.

43. "Nurses Go Back to School," *Modern Healthcare,* 4 December 1995, 72.

44. "Health Promotion and Wellness," 16.

45. L. Carlson, "Designing Healthy Spaces," *Healthcare Forum Journal* 37, no. 2 (1994):37–39.

46. "Sutter Redirects Referral Center To Serve Managed Care," *Physician Referral Update* 9, no. 1 (1996):4.

47. D. Weber, "Planetree Transplanted," *Healthcare Forum Journal* 35, no. 5 (1992):30–37.

48. F. Cerne, "Local Alliance Calms Tempers and Tackles Health Costs," *Hospitals & Health Networks,* 20 November 1993, 54.

49. Anderson, "New Guide," 68–70.

50. "Quality Watch," *Hospitals & Health Networks,* 5 February 1996, 14, 15.

51. M. Magee, "Information Empowerment of the Patient: The Next Payer/Provider Battlefield," *Journal of Outcomes Management* 2, no. 3 (1995):17–21.

52. "Selling Wellness to a Suspicious World," *Health Care Advertising Review,* March/April 1996, 1–8.

53. J. Goldsmith, et al., "Managed Care Comes of Age," *Healthcare Forum Journal* 38, no. 5 (1995):14–24.

54. "Health Promotion and Wellness," 16.

55. "HMOs Aggressively Developing Disease Management Programs: Cost Reductions Reported," *Healthcare Demand and Disease Management* 3, no. 6 (1997):94–96.

56. P. Bloom, et al., "Benefiting Society and the Bottom Line," *Marketing Management* 4, no. 3 (1995):8–18.

57. Weiss, "A Hospital," 60, 61.

58. "Community Partnerships a Key Piece of the Demand Management Puzzle," *Healthcare Demand Management* 1, no. 7 (1995):101–104.

59. "Talkradio Talks Healthcare," *Profiles in Healthcare Marketing* 11, no. 6 (1995):27–30.

60. W. Koehler, and N. van Marter, "Turning Media Gatekeepers into Advocates," *Journal of Health Care Marketing* 15, no. 3 (1995):59–63.

61. L. Ramsdell, "Church-Based Health Promotion," *American Journal of Health Promotion* 9, no. 5 (1995):333–336.

62. "Putting Faith in Religion and Medicine," *Hospitals & Health Networks,* 5 September 1995, 22, 23.

63. W. McClain, and B. Stratton, "Planning and Partnering for Healthier Communities," *Journal of Health Care Marketing* 14, no. 4 (1994):10, 11.

64. "Health Promotion and Wellness," 16.

65. "Form Alliances with Community Mental Health Programs," *Healthcare Demand Management* 1, no. 9 (1995):129–132.

66. "Organizational Health through Community Programming," *Health Promotion Practitioner* 4, no. 10 (1995):1.

67. J. Levin, "Prevention in Paradise," *Healthcare Forum Journal* 36, no. 6 (1993):22.

68. J. Wechsler, "A Pound of Prevention, But Just a Pinch of Guidelines," *Managed Healthcare* 6, no. 2 (1996):16, 45, 46.

69. J. Smith, "Can Managed Care Do It All?" *Health Systems Review,* November/December 1994, 34–37.

70. "CNOs Help Define Top Demand Management Strategies," *Healthcare Demand Management* 1, no. 1 (1995):1–7.

71. M. Hey, "Nursing's Renaissance," *Health Progress* 74, no. 8 (1993):26–32.

72. "Pilot DM Projects May Not Fly with Cost-Driven MCOs," *Healthcare Demand Management* 1, no. 5 (1995):65–68.

73. "Take the Outbound Approach To Enhance Your Call Center," *Healthcare Demand & Disease Management* 3, no. 5 (1997):65–68.

74. "Let's All Talk: Medical Education Is a Team Effort," in *Talk about Prescriptions Planning Guide* (Washington, DC: National Council on Patient Information and Education, 1993), 1–16.

75. Weiss, "A Hospital," 60, 61.

76. L. Muir, "Disease Management," *Hospitals & Health Networks,* 5 June 1997, 24–30.

77. "Let's All Talk," 1–16.

78. "Chicago Union Saves $2 Million on Health Care Costs without Copayments," *Business & Health* 10, no. 5 (1992):22–24.

79. "Currents—Who Do They Trust?" *Hospitals and Health Networks,* 5 October 1997, 30.

80. "Greenstone and Lovelace To Develop 30 Disease Management Programs," *Health Care Strategic Management* 14, no. 3 (1996):4, 5.

81. J. Burns, "DM Vendors Talk the Talk and Walk the Walk—And They Guarantee Their Results," *Managed Healthcare* 7, no. 8 (1997):18–21, 25.

82. D. Coddington, et al., *Making Integrated Health Care Work* (Englewood, CO: Center for Research in Ambulatory Health Care Administration, 1996).

83. R. Coile, "HMO/Insurer-Provider Partnerships: Creating the 'Ultimate Model' for Hospitals, Physicians and HMOs/Insurers," *Hospital Strategy Report* 6, no. 6 (1994):1, 3, 6.

84. "Passport to Health™ Reaches Kids at Risk," *Wellness Management* 11, no. 2 (1995):1, 5, 6.

85. "Consortium Develops Tools for Use in Risk Identification Efforts," *Healthcare Demand Management* 1, no. 5 (1995):69, 70.

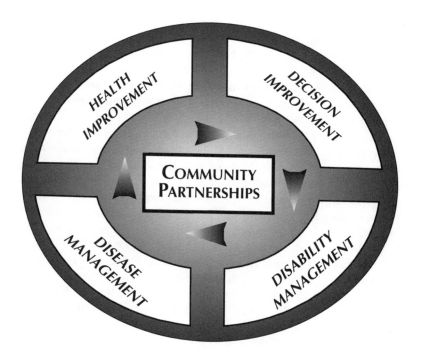

Chapter 19

COMMUNITY-BASED INITIATIVES

While any of the organizations at risk, payers or providers, may sponsor demand improvement initiatives, there is a growing movement toward collaborative efforts involving two or more organizations. Hospitals are collaborating with their peers, health plans with their peers, and employers with theirs, for example. In addition, at-risk organizations are developing and participating in community-wide coalitions including government agencies, community groups, schools and churches, and a wide variety of interested parties to promote improvements in health and in the use/cost of health services.

PROBLEMS AND POTENTIAL

Many have argued that health and demand cannot be successfully improved by focusing solely on individuals or population segments such as employees, health plan members, or the patients of specific providers. Health is a community phenomenon as well as a personal one. As long as there is poverty, crime and violence, homelessness, drug and alcohol abuse, unemployment, illiteracy, and similar "sociomas," efforts at improving health status will fall short.[1]

Significant and growing problems among seniors have been noted: abuse and abandonment by their children and spouses, depression, malnourishment (which adds to the cost of health care when needed), and growing threats to their independence, placing them at risk of requiring nursing home services for many years at public expense.[2] At the other end of the spectrum, adolescent suicide and homicide rates have more than doubled and poor health habits are on the rise.[3] The "health gap" between the poor and the affluent is growing, despite decades of social programs.[4] Environmental problems like smog affect everyone in the community, and smog has been found linked to 26% higher mortality, controlling for other health variables, comparing the smoggiest to the cleanest cities.[5]

People want to be able to control their own health along with other major life quality factors.[6] According to surveys, the public favors greater spending on prevention and health improvement, though little effect has been noted.[7] Our Canadian neighbors spend $.70 per citizen per year to improve health habits, hardly an impressive sum, while Americans spend $.06, less than a tenth as much.[8] We spend less than 4% of health dollars on prevention versus 96% on treatment.[9]

Some readers may recall the optimistic efforts of comprehensive health planning begun in the mid-1960s, when the federal government attempted to galvanize community efforts to improve health and health care delivery. While a few vestiges of that movement remain, it was largely unsuccessful.[10] At the same time, new efforts with broader business, provider, and community support, such as the Community Health Information Network movement[11] and Healthy Communities 2000,[12] have emerged.

Efforts of single sponsors often fail, such as the minimal effects on health achieved by the Florence, South Carolina, Health Department, acting alone.[13] By contrast, collaborative efforts have frequently achieved impressive results. A combined effort of the Harvard School of Public Health and television media organizations achieved a 10% increase in the use of designated drivers.[14] Collaboration between employer and health plan reduced disability costs by 77.5%.[15] Community immunization programs for measles, mumps, and rubella save an estimated $1.4 billion each year.[16]

As the interests of physicians at risk, hospitals committed to health as well as sickness, and employers and health plans converge, improving health and demand becomes a common necessity.[17] It has been estimated that 20% to 30% of all health expenditures could be eliminated if everyone's health behaviors were ideal.[18] Reforms in the health behaviors of populations can best be achieved through collaborative efforts among all interested parties.[19]

Awareness of the advantages of promoting community health is growing. A survey of hospitals found that two thirds were engaged in specific health improvement efforts.[20] In Los Angeles, reduced funding of public clinics has forced them to look for private partners to continue serving Medicaid and indigent patients.[21] Canada has demonstrated how much can be achieved in promoting public health awareness through community efforts.[22] Most reported community efforts seem to have had significant positive impact.[23]

ADVANTAGES TO SPONSORS

The advantages of investing in community efforts are many (Exhibit 19–1). Hospitals can achieve significant public relations/reputation enhancement as well as protection of not-for-profit tax exemption by investing in community health improvement.[24] Health plans can counter the currently popular "managed care bashing" by visibly committing themselves to community health.[25] (In Minnesota, it is a requirement of state law that they do so.[26]) Employers in San Jose, California, realizing that workers change jobs frequently, collaborate on improving employee health, whereby all benefit.[27]

Community health assessments, a common starting point for community-wide collaborations, can provide information to providers on new business opportunities.[28] Simply conducting such assessments and publishing the results for interested community groups to read may be enough to promote coordinated efforts. The results of assessments may provide or at least reinforce the rationale behind provider alliance efforts.[29] The same assessments can be repeated at regular intervals to track accomplishments and maintain enthusiasm.[30]

Community efforts can greatly increase the investment in improving health and utilization. Financial support from foundations such as the Robert Wood Johnson Foundation may be obtained where community-wide efforts are proposed.[31] An army of volunteers may be recruitable when initiatives have a community focus. Mass media may be recruited to contribute public service announcements and feature items in support of such efforts.

Economies of scale are frequently achievable by focusing efforts on larger populations and combining sponsors. Health plans can achieve efficiencies by collaborating on phone call centers and triage/counseling programs, for example. Immunization programs that are community-wide can benefit from both economies of scale and government funding. Getting automakers to install airbags and water heater manufacturers to set temperatures lower may prove far more effec-

Exhibit 19–1 Community-Focused Initiatives

PROBLEMS / POTENTIAL	ADVANTAGE: SPONSOR	CONCERNS	ADVICE
X SOCIAL PROBLEMS SUCH AS POVERTY & ENVIRONMENTAL CONCERNS ARE GROWING X AFFLUENCE GAP BETWEEN RICH & POOR SPREADING X COLLABORATIVE EFFORTS HOLD MORE PROMISE FOR PROMOTING EFFECTIVE HEALTH INITIATIVES	X IMPROVE REPUTATION IN THE COMMUNITY X INCREASE RETURN ON INVESTMENT FOR PROGRAMS WHERE HIGH TURNOUT IS DESIRABLE (IMMUNIZATION) X ACHIEVE ECONOMIES OF SCALE FOR HIGH-TICKET INVESTMENTS	X MAY HAVE DIFFUSED RESULTS SO SPONSORS MAY BE RELUCTANT TO INVEST X MAY HAVE FOCUS BROADER THAN TRADITIONAL HEALTH-RELATED ISSUES (CRIME, FAMILY STRUCTURE) X DETERMINING WHO SHOULD TAKE THE LEAD MAY BE PROBLEMATIC X EVALUATING EFFECTIVENESS IS DIFFICULT	X WORK WITH SMALL GROUP TO TARGET COMMON INTERESTS & BUILD TRACK RECORD OF SUCCESS X COMBINE PERSPECTIVES & INTERESTS OF THE COLLABORATORS X CAREFULLY SET PARAMETERS & STANDARDS FOR EVALUATION X MAKE A PUBLIC COMMITMENT TO THE EFFORT & SOLICIT INPUT FROM MANY SOURCES

tive than changing the behaviors of millions of consumers. Increasing state taxes on cigarettes may prove to be a powerful deterrent to smoking.

Many health utilization problems may be beyond the power of individual sponsors to correct. Hospitals may find themselves unable to discharge patients as early as appropriate due to the lack of nursing home beds, home care systems, competent caregivers at home, or adequate transportation. Public apathy or ignorance about prevention and early detection potential may hamper every sponsor's efforts. Where individual sponsors plan to use mass media to reach their populations of interest, they will also be reaching other populations and may as well seek partners to share in the costs as well as benefits: "The rising tide raises all boats."

CONCERNS, LIMITATIONS, AND ISSUES

While many problems may be best addressed at the community level, taking such an approach is by no means trouble free. Inviting in other organizations automatically introduces new and potentially conflicting interests and perspectives. It complicates efforts by requiring that sponsors spend time, energy, and resources on building and maintaining new relationships, in addition to whatever specific initiative they undertake. It may delay action by requiring a lengthy decision-making process before partners can agree.

Other stakeholders may insist on investments and activities that run counter to the values of some sponsors, or prevent initiatives that sponsors would prefer. The community-wide effort may end up having far less impact on a sponsor's population or problem of interest than the sponsor could have achieved with the same investment as an individual organization. Interested parties may have narrow interests, interests in specific populations, or interests in diseases or programs that complicate or even prevent collaborative efforts.

To secure the cooperation of a commercial organization (e.g., in a safety feature or health-promoting investment) it may be necessary to recruit all its competitors, lest the cooperation of one put it at a competitive disadvantage. If the community tried to get one television channel or movie-production company to reduce the showing of violence or unhealthy behavior in a positive light, it is likely to find each unwilling to take the risk of financial damage unless everyone plays by the same rules.

One of the characteristics of community-wide efforts is a far broader definition of "health" than payers and providers are used to. The problems identified may relate to crime, violence and domestic abuse, homelessness and unemployment, or education and racial intolerance, with little foreseeable impact on traditional health status, utilization, or expenditures of interest to at-risk sponsors. The payoff from initiatives aimed at social problems may be significant but far off. Efforts may end up being focused on what most concerns the community rather than what can be successfully improved.

With so many interested parties, who should *lead* community-wide efforts? Will there be a battle of egos over that question? Will the community health assessment process end up being a substitute for rather than prelude and stimulus to action? How do different stakeholders define the "community"? It is clear that people vary widely in their definition, from as narrow as "my friends"—people with similar values, race, religion, age, profession, socioeconomic status, residence—to as broad as one's country and the world.

Which problems should be addressed and who should decide? Should we rely on experts or popular opinion? Shall we choose the worst problems or the ones where we see a strong probability of quick and visible success? Should we invest based on "need" or potential return on investment? Shall we be limited by where consensus is achievable? Will "political" issues cloud judgment and force grand gestures that are doomed to minimal success?

How will community-wide efforts be evaluated? Can we use a rigorous experimental/control design with random assignment without charges of discrimination or consumer objection to not being included?[32] Can sponsors agree on what outcomes should be sought and measured and what value can be placed on them? Will sponsors be willing to gamble on a single intervention to learn what works or insist on a shotgun approach to be sure that something does?

RECOMMENDATIONS

Based on the substantial experience communities have had in collaborative effort, there are some suggestions that seem at least promising. One is that sponsors hire/assign staff specifically to building, maintaining, and exploiting (in the sense of "getting the most out of") community collaboration. Riverside Methodist Hospital in Columbus, Ohio, has a director of community partnerships, for example, and many hospitals have created positions of community health coordinator, community action coordinator, and the like. (The job title community health planner appears to be out of date and overly analytical versus action oriented.)

Sponsors might try starting small, working with one or a small group of collaborators to learn how and demonstrate the value of this approach, rather than aiming for an alliance with practically everybody. This may permit them to focus on precisely their population of interest. Collaborations among health plans, employers, and providers may easily be focused on specific employees or members, for example, rather than encompass the entire community. LifeGuard Health Plan in San Jose, California, partnered with the local diabetes society in its efforts to better manage diabetic patient enrollees.[33]

Sponsors may select partners to increase the likelihood that collaborative programs will focus on problems and goals they are most interested in, even if the programs affect the entire community. An employer, health plan, or provider system may discover high levels of cardiac risk in its population of interest and choose to work with the local heart association to ensure the problem will be addressed. Employers, providers, and plans may agree up front on partnering with a specific vendor so as to achieve economies of scale in a particular effort, such as call center/triage.

Some partners may be sought specifically because they have a strong interest in a problem or goal of concern to sponsors. Kellogg cereal company and Rockport shoe company proved powerful partners in community national promotions of increased dietary fiber and walking programs, for example.[34] The more partners selected for collaborative efforts share strong common goals and values, the greater the chance for both successful initiatives and lasting relationships.

By starting small, sponsors can learn how to conduct collaborative efforts before committing to full-scale, community-wide initiatives. They can also build up a track record of success that will be helpful in achieving internal commitment to the idea and in recruiting additional partners. Specific problems and programs may be selected for their contributions to building and maintaining relationships as well as their impact on community health.

In selecting problems it is probably best to combine the perspectives of consumers with those of interested stakeholders, with some "expert" advice on what is likely to work. It may be advisable to work on many problems rather than a single problem or objective so as to maintain the coalition and improve the chances of some success. If a single outcome is chosen, it should be one that has a high probability of prompt, visible, and valuable success. Child immunization has frequently been chosen and succeeded, for example.

Whatever problems or goals are selected for immediate attention, a careful measurement of the current state of the parameter to be changed should be made, with careful evaluation of impact on that parameter planned for as soon as a significant change is likely.[35] Regularly repeated community health assessments may serve this purpose for a number of parameters.[36]

One of the most valuable components of community health efforts may be the sharing of experiences, both successes and failures, with the public. Just as clinical treatments are now being carefully scrutinized to improve the quality of medical care, so should community interventions be evaluated and reported to identify best practices in improving community health and utilization. A national clearing-house for such information should be developed so that communities may learn from each other and promote the selection and adoption of the most successful (effective and efficient) initiatives.[37]

(Ideally a similar approach should be used for sponsor-specific initiatives. This is true in sharing outcomes of medical treatment, but competitive realities may prevent cooperation that might be construed as sharing competitive secrets.)

In general, sponsors considering community-wide, collaborative initiatives are advised to make a clear and public commitment to their collaborative role and to the specific outcomes intended for specific initiatives. They should listen to all their "customers," from consumers targeted for interventions to all collaborating parties. Welcome and commit to the broader definition of health embedded in the notion of community health and build on all community assets as well as problems in planning interventions. Be willing to work with competitors as well as natural allies. Use hard data in selecting problems and setting priorities, and be sure to measure and report results.[38]

Some questions suggested for selecting problems for attention include:

- How compelling, or commitment arousing, is the problem?
- How identifiable and reachable is the population of interest?
- How great are the present gaps between what is and is not possible?
- How much change in the problem can be achieved in the short term?
- How much planning and groundwork has already been accomplished?
- How measurable is the change in the short term?[39]

COMMUNITY HEALTH EXAMPLES

Health improvement is easily the most popular area for attention in community-wide efforts. Promoting better health, preventing disease and injury, and detecting conditions when they can be most effectively treated is enough to galvanize a wide range of stakeholders. Hospitals, physician groups, health plans, and employers have partnered with schools, governments, churches, media, and community neighborhood organizations in a wide range of initiatives.

Community Health Assessments

Crozer Keystone Health System in Chester, Pennsylvania, conducted a community health assessment (CHA) on a community-wide basis in its service area.[39] Six towns in Connecticut collaborated on a CHA for a population of 96,000.[40] The province of Ontario has conducted a province-wide assessment.[41] The state of Illinois sponsors the Illinois Program for Local Assessment of Needs (IPLAN).[42] Spokane, Washington, used the SF-12 survey form to capture citizens' perceptions of their health problems and needs.[43] The Baton Rouge (Louisiana) Health Forum combined the efforts of 10 local provider organizations in conducting interviews and focus groups to identify needs.[44] The VHA sponsored a CHA pilot project for its 1,300 member hospitals, including Butler (Pennsylvania) Memorial, Lutheran Medical Center (Denver), and Riverside Methodist (Columbus, Ohio).[45]

Health Improvement Initiatives

We examined 44 references to community-wide initiatives aimed at reducing health risks and promoting wellness, prevention, and early detection. Participants included churches and media,[46] city government,[47] hospitals,[48] HealthPartners (Minnesota HMO), Partners for Better Health,[49] California's Healthy Cities Project,[50] the BJC Health System in St. Louis,[51] neighborhood organizations in metro Boston,[52] Kmart, SelectCare (HMO), schools in the Detroit area,[53] public health agencies, and six hospitals in Montana.[54]

Community-wide coalitions have been created in Chicago (Swedish Covenant Hospital), Pittsburgh (Allegheny General), and Columbus, Ohio (Riverside Methodist).[55] PacifiCare Wellness Company conducted a community-wide wellness program in Wellsburg, West Virginia.[56] St. John Health System, Anderson, Indiana, worked with the local YMCA and YWCA.[57] Health partnerships have been created in Austin, Texas; Phoenix; Anchorage, Alaska; Camden, New Jersey; Edmonton, Alberta, Canada; Kingsport, Tennessee; London, Ontario; Monroe, Louisiana; and Twin Falls, Idaho.[58]

There seems to be no end to the list of potential partners, given the vast number of organizations concerned about and committed to health. The challenge is to identify the right partners for specific problems and initiatives and resources that can help in building, maintaining, and energizing community-wide coalitions. Some resources that may prove useful in such efforts include:

- The American Association of Health Plans;
- The American Hospital Association's Hospital Community Benefits Standards Program—Chicago;
- CDC's *Guide to Clinical Preventive Services,* 2d ed. (Baltimore, MD: Williams & Wilkins, 1995)—authoritative reference on what works;
- The Healthcare Forum (San Francisco) Healthier Communities Action Kit, Healthier Communities Project, and Community Builder software simulation program that simulates the effects of possible interventions;
- Innovation Associates (Waltham, Massachusetts)—planning simulation;
- The National Civic League (Denver);
- The Robert Wood Johnson Foundation; and
- United States Public Health Service's Healthy Communities 2000 Project (Washington, DC).

Managing Disease

In contrast to the vast number of community efforts aimed at improving health, there seem to be relatively few devoted to managing disease where it already exists. The few examples we have found involve limited partnerships, typically one at-risk sponsor and one other organization.

The US Health Corporation (Pennsylvania) collaborates with schools, for example, in pregnancy testing and care for teenagers, where many more community programs limit themselves to efforts aimed at preventing teenage pregnancies.[59]

Riverside Methodist Hospitals in Columbus, Ohio, also spearheads a community-wide program that includes prenatal care.[60] The National Cancer Institute is working with HMOs to enlist consumers in clinical trials.[61] Aiken (South Carolina) Regional Medical Center works with the local county health department to promote healthy outcomes of pregnancy.[62] As mentioned, Lifeguard Health Plan works with the local diabetes society in helping diabetic patients manage their condition.[63]

Decision Improvement

We found roughly the same small number of community-wide initiatives aimed at improving consumer health care decisions. Community-wide phone triage programs are being tried in Boise, Idaho,[64] and in Rochester, New York, with a multi-HMO collaboration program in Washington, DC.[65] In the Rochester example, experimental and control groups numbering 80,000 people are being compared.[66] In Los Angeles, public clinics hope to be able to steer Medicaid and indigent patients to private providers.[67] Baton Rouge (Louisiana) Health Forum has published a health resources directory to help consumers locate providers.

Disability Management

As might be expected, we found no community-wide efforts in the area of disability management, understandable since employers have the risk and responsibility. We did find two examples of collaborative effort, however. PacifiCare Wellness Company worked with an employer on a job performance testing program to reduce workers' compensation claims.[69] In San Jose, California, employers collaborate on a general worker health promotion program that should affect both workers' compensation and health insurance costs.[70]

REFERENCES

1. D. Tong, "Beyond Prevention: Healing the Sociomas," *Healthcare Forum Journal* 39, no. 3 (1996):39, 40.
2. R. Addleman, "Eldercare: Out of the Institution and Into the Community," *Healthcare Forum Journal* 38, no. 3 (1995):58–64.
3. "Young Adolescents at Health Risk Crossroads," *Health Promotion Practitioner* 4, no. 12 (1995):6.
4. T. Hancock, "Seeing the Vision, Defining Your Role," *Healthcare Forum Journal* 36, no. 3 (1993):30–35.
5. "Smoggy Days Shorten Lives," *Health* 7, no. 5 (1993):8.
6. L. Breslow and T. Tai-Seale, "An Experience with Health Promotion in the Inner City," *American Journal of Health Promotion* 10, no. 3 (1996):185–188.

7. H. Taylor, "Prospects for Prevention," *Health Management Quarterly* 14, no. 2 (1992):21–24.

8. M. Bricklin, "The Power of Proactive Prevention," *Prevention* 46, no. 2 (1994):45, 46, 116.

9. "Continuum of Care," *Hospitals & Health Networks,* 5 August 1993, 21, 22.

10. T. Hudson, "Make No Little Plans," *Hospitals & Health Networks,* 5 May 1996, 47–50.

11. Hudson, "Make No Little Plans," 47–50.

12. E. Wogensen, "Participation in Healthy Communities Movement Entails Patience, Listening, Shared Responsibility," *Strategic Health Care Marketing* 12, no. 2 (1995):1–4.

13. R. Goodman, et al., "Evaluation of the Heart to Heart Project," *American Journal of Health Promotion* 9, no. 6 (1995):443–455.

14. "TV Promotes Designated Drivers," *Medical Self-Care* 54 (1990):12.

15. "Positive Return on Investment Demonstrated from HMO/Wellness Merger," *St. Anthony's Managing Community Health and Wellness* 2, no. 2 (1995):6.

16. K. Pallarito, "Spending on Preventive Care Urged," *Modern Healthcare,* 19 September 1994, 18.

17. L. Kaiser, "Beyond Boundaries, There Are Healthier Communities," *Healthier Communities Direct,* Summer 1995, 3, 4.

18. *Health Gains: Improving the Health of Communities through Integrated Health Care* (Minneapolis, MN: Allina, 1994).

19. W. Pidgeon, "Motivating an Individual To Use Preventive Health Services," *Medical Interface* March 1992, 59–62.

20. "Toward Healthier Communities," *Hospitals & Health Networks,* 5 July 1994, 18.

21. L. Kertesz, "L.A.'s Plan for Clinics Stalled; Public Health Cuts Raise Fears," *Modern Healthcare,* 27 May 1996, 19.

22. "Tracking Canada's Health Promotion Campaigns," *Health Promotion,* Winter 1988/1989, 22–26.

23. P. Terry, et al., "Does Health Education Work?" *The Bulletin* 37, no. 2 (1993):95–109.

24. "Emphasis Is No Longer on Just the Bottom Line!" *Inside Preventive Care,* Special Report 1995.

25. R. Coile, "Healthy Communities: Reducing Need (and Costs!) by Promoting Health," *Hospital Strategy Report* 6, no. 2 (1994):1–5.

26. S. Mitchell and S. Mosow, "Promoting Population Health: Minnesota's Public-Private Initiative," *1996 Healthier Communities Summit Report* (San Francisco, CA: The Healthcare Forum, 1996).

27. "Wellness Veterans Share Their Knowledge in Mentor Program," *Employee Health & Fitness* 18, no. 2 (1996):13–15.

28. J. Thalhuber, "Social Entrepreneurship: The Promise and the Perils," *The Alliance Report,* May/June 1996, 5–7, 11, 12.

29. "Three VHA Institutions Find Community Assessment Strategy Facilitates Integration," *Health Care Strategic Management* 14, no. 4 (1996):12.

30. G. Dobbins, *Mid-Michigan Medical Center* (Midland, MI: personal report 1995).

31. "Early Report: 'Smarter' Patients Lower Health Care Costs" (News Release, Boise, ID: The Healthwise Community Project, March 18, 1997).

32. W. Lear, "Needle Test Trial Criticized," *The Denver Post,* 18 October 1996, 2A.

33. "How To Improve Your Diabetes Management Program," *Inside Preventive Care* 2, no. 5 (1996):1–4.

34. P. Bloom, et al., "Benefiting Society and the Bottom Line," *Marketing Management* 4, no. 3 (1995):8–18.

35. "Community Values Can Be Used To Measure Health and Well-Being," *St. Anthony's Managing Community Health and Wellness* 2, no. 2 (1995):1, 2, 8.

36. Dobbins, *Mid-Michigan Medical Center.*

37. J. Flower, "Sound Mind, Sound Body?" *Healthcare Forum Journal* 37, no. 5 (1994):78–86.

38. E. Zablocki, "Improving Community Health Status: Strategies for Success," *The Quality Letter* 2, no. 2 (1996):2–20.

39. "Assessment Process Helps Turn Broad Community Goals into Targeted Initiatives," *Healthcare Demand Management* 1, no. 4 (1995):52–57.

40. "Connecticut Coalition Aims To Achieve Healthy Community," *St. Anthony's Managing Community Health and Wellness* 2, no. 9 (1996):2–4, 8.

41. M. Cousins and I. McDowell, "Use of Medical Care after a Community-Based Health Promotion Program," *American Journal of Health Promotion* 10, no. 1 (1995):47–54.

42. Hudson, "Make No Little Plans," 47–50.

43. "Spokane Health Partnership Brings Together Diverse Interests," *Inside Preventive Care* 2, no. 1 (1996):7, 8.

44. "Ten Health Providers Band Together in Louisiana To Conduct Community Assessment," *Inside Preventive Care* 1, no. 9 (1995):1–3.

45. "Three VHA Institutions," 29.

46. E. Chapman and T. Wimberly, "Looking Upstream," *Healthcare Forum Journal* 37, no. 3 (1994):18–21.

47. "Citywide Program Has Something for Everyone," *Employee Health & Fitness* 18, no. 2 (1996):19–21.

48. Coile, "Healthy Communities," 1–25.

49. "Community Partnerships a Key Piece of the Demand Management Puzzle," *Healthcare Demand Management* 1, no. 7 (1995):101–104.

50. M. Coye, "Can Public Health Lead the Way?" *Healthcare Forum Journal* 36, no. 3 (1993):39–44.

51. J. Hotze and R. Ward, "Making Community Health Work in a Stage Two Market," *The Alliance Report,* March/April 1996, 11, 12.

52. T. Landsmark and J. Mogul, "Building Community Partnerships for Urban Change," *The Boston Sunday Globe,* 14 May 1995, 79.

53. "Detroit HMO's School-Based Wellness Programs Target Kids," *Healthcare Demand Management* 2, no. 4 (1996):57–59.

54. B. Pfingsten and L. Matison, "Using Collaboration To Implement a Healthier Community Marketing Plan," *The Alliance Bulletin,* February 1995, 1, 2, 5.

55. T. Smith, "Urban Hospitals Use Community Business Ties To Improve Public Health, Reduce Violence," *Health Care Strategic Management* 14, no. 8 (1996):16, 17.

56. "Positive Return," 6.

57. R. Weiss, "Organizations Collaborate To Provide Wellness Programs to Area Businesses," *Health Progress* 78, no. 3 (1995):60, 61.

58. Zablocki, "Improving Community," 2–20.

59. Chapman and Wimberly, "Looking Upstream," 18–21.

60. Coile, "Healthy Communities," 1–5.

61. L. Kertesz, "NCI Seeks Partnerships with HMOs," *Modern Healthcare,* 24 June 1996, 12.

62. K. Lumsdon, "Breaking Down Barriers, Building Up Hopes," *Hospitals & Health Networks,* 20 January 1996, 33–38.

63. "How To Improve," 1–4.

64. "Early Report."

65. "Health Plans Form Alliances To Promote a Mutually Beneficial Demand Management Agenda," *Healthcare Demand Management* 2, no. 6 (1996):93–96.

66. "Leading Business, Health Care, Insurance Organizations Jointly Sponsor Pilot Health Care Program" (Press Release, Rochester, NY: Jay, Inc., April 18, 1996).

67. Kertesz, "L.A.'s Plan," 19.

68. "Ten Health Providers," 1–3.

69. "Positive Return," 6.

70. "Wellness Veterans," 13–15.

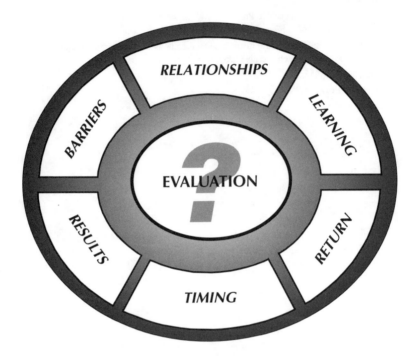

Chapter 20

**EVALUATING DEMAND
IMPROVEMENT INITIATIVES**

The evaluation of interventions is a complex challenge about which there are many differences of opinion. The essential purpose of evaluation is to place a value upon (i.e., determine) the net worth of the effects of an intervention. Whenever value is involved, differences in values among people and organizations are likely to be reflected, hence differences in evaluative judgments. Evaluation is, therefore, a subjective process, though it can be aided by objective measures and analysis.

In this chapter we can but scratch the surface of the full extent of knowledge and opinion about evaluation. Our intent is to offer a basic overview of the issues and some suggestions for dealing with them. Our emphasis will be on using the evaluation process as a means to learn how to improve future overall efforts and specific initiatives, as well as to judge past activities.

Ideally a well-developed plan for specific interventions for improving consumer health and demand behaviors will lead directly and easily into evaluation. As described in Chapter 16, an evaluation plan is the last of the 10 components of an intervention plan, addressing three questions:

1. Results and return—How much change in desired behavior has been achieved (or avoided) and how great a return on investment has been accomplished?
2. Relationships—What positive and negative effects on relationships with targets and other stakeholders has the intervention had?
3. Learning—What have we learned about changing consumer behavior that will help us be more effective and efficient next time?

RESULTS

As discussed in Chapter 5, results of particular interventions may be measured in terms of any one or mix of the seven items in an intervention's set of effects: participation, mind-state, behavior, health status, service use, expenditure, or value-adding effects. Where the intent is to prevent change (i.e., preserve, protect, or maintain one of these effects), results should reflect minimal or no change in such parameters; where the intent is to change them, results should reflect the amount and direction of change.

Results should always mean the DIFFERENCE that an intervention has made, what the situation turns out to be compared to what it would have been without the intervention. This is not the same as the difference between what is and what was; reality is a moving, changing phenomenon. The difference that an initiative makes should be estimated in terms of what the original parameter(s) would have become without the intervention, compared to what it does become with it.[1]

WHAT RESULTS?

Just as it is wise in planning for "political" as well as consumer relationship reasons to focus on consumer benefit as well as sponsor financial effects, so it is equally recommended for evaluation. If the only effects sponsors look at in evaluating initiatives are financial, they can easily be accused of attempting to manipulate consumer behavior for their own good versus improving consumer behavior for the benefit of all.

Evaluations should routinely include consumer satisfaction with the intervention as a process and a personal experience, as well as quality-of-life outcomes perceived. Since perceived health benefits and satisfaction enhance employee morale and patient, enrollee, and employee retention, these measures of results add to the understanding of the *value* achieved, which is the purpose of evaluation.

EVALUATION TIME FRAMES

It is often tempting to evaluate an intervention as early as possible. In reviewing published examples, we found many cases in which sponsors or vendors report on the implementation of a particular initiative before any results have been determined. In such cases the authors exude confidence in their interventions and may have some anecdotal indication of good results but clearly are suffering from a rush to judgment.

In other cases sponsors and vendors have taken results found at three, six, or nine months and have extrapolated them to estimate a year's impact. Only time will tell whether such extrapolations are accurate; in particular cases, results may encounter diminishing returns over time or, conversely, may see growing impact and diminishing costs. A year is probably the minimum time period for getting a decent picture of the effects of an intervention. Early impact such as participation and mind-state changes may occur sooner, but those effects that demonstrate value are likely to be detectable later, and a full fiscal year may be needed to discover total financial impact.

Ideally multiyear evaluations should be made and published so that sponsors of initiatives and those considering similar investments can learn the pattern of effects over the long run. Will results or return on investment (ROI) increase as consumer trust and self-efficacy increase, or will early success tail off as the few tractable consumers are reformed early on and the rest prove unreceptive to the chosen initiative? Most of the examples followed and reported over a multiyear period show increasing results and returns over time, but there are so few such examples that it is risky to generalize.

When evaluations are planned and executed only after an intervention, they may reach erroneous conclusions. After a fitness program has been implemented, for example, a "post-hoc" comparison of program participants to nonparticipants will often discover that participants have lower utilization and costs, probably lower absenteeism and turnover as well. This does not mean that the program made any difference, however. Participants may well have *always* had lower utilization, costs, and absenteeism because they were healthier to begin with. The only way to detect a difference is to collect data on parameters of interest before the program is implemented.

COMPARISONS

An estimate should be made of what present reality will become without intervention as part of planning to estimate the difference that the planned intervention will have. To do better than an estimate in evaluating results, a comparison group should be used to track what happened to the parameter of interest in a population or segment without the intervention but reflecting the effects of the passage of time or other factors in the environment.[2]

A simple before-and-after comparison of health care expenditures, for example, may suggest that an intervention has been successful. But a drop in total health care costs may have been caused by a decline in the numbers of people in the population: downsizing of employees, disenrollment in a health plan. Measuring results in costs per employee or member will take care of such possibilities.

To check on the possible impact of other factors, comparisons may be made to other populations unaffected by the chosen intervention. Comparisons to other employee groups or health plan enrollees may prove that the reduction in health expenditures set as an objective occurred elsewhere without any intervention; perhaps inflation rates declined everywhere or a weak flu season this year reduced health care costs for almost everyone. In such cases it may prove difficult to claim that any RESULTS have actually occurred.[3]

For a more scientific approach, sponsors may use an experiment/control group comparison within their population of interest. A common problem in many evaluations of health improvement efforts, for example, arises from comparing the health status, service utilization, or expenditures of participants in a fitness or

COMPARISON GROUPS

TRACK THE EFFECTS OF PASSAGE OF TIME OR OTHER UNRELATED FACTORS

CONTROL GROUPS

HELP DETERMINE WHETHER CHANGE IS DUE TO INTERVENTION

wellness program to those of nonparticipants. When participation is voluntary and participants are self-selected, it must be wondered if they are not so much healthier and more careful about their health behaviors that their status, use, and expenditures have always been lower than their less health-conscious peers.

A split comparison of before and after parameters for participants versus nonparticipants will address this problem, where looking only at "after" differences will not. A fully scientific approach would randomly assign members of a population to an "experimental treatment" (i.e., to experience a chosen intervention), with other members assigned as "controls" getting no such experience. Such an approach eliminates the effects of self-selection, the differences that may have preexisted in participants versus nonparticipants. In such a way the differences found in parameters of interest after an intervention can more confidently be termed the results of the intervention.[4]

USING STATISTICS

Statistics and evaluation may seem inseparable; the use and abuse of statistics in evaluating interventions are certainly widespread. One type of statistics (i.e., descriptive statistics) is virtually inescapable (see box entitled "Descriptive Statistics"). Having information on particular parameters (i.e., measures of a population) is essential in planning and evaluation, regardless of which links in the chain of effects are of interest. The other type, inferential statistics, may or may not be useful.

Inferential statistics look at measures in a *sample* of the population of interest and make inferences to the entire population. Hence we are familiar with terms such as "statistical significance," referring to the probability that differences or changes found in a sample are attributable to chance or are "real." Using strict standards of statistical significance (e.g., insisting that the probability of chance can be no greater than 5%) is essential in good science whenever samples are involved.

In many cases, however, health and demand behavior reforms are implemented in entire populations, not samples. If the "treated" group, perhaps the entire employee or health plan member population, is given a self-care guide and shows a 5% reduction in health care use and expenditure as compared to a comparison or control group, is such a difference statistically significant? The question is irrelevant; no inference from a sample is involved. For that population, at that time, the difference actually happened—it is real.

Whether the difference is *practically* significant (i.e., represents a worthwhile opposed to merely a measurable difference) is a judgment call. It can be addressed best in terms of return on investment rather than inferential statistics. If an em-

DESCRIPTIVE STATISTICS

**ESSENTIAL FOR TRACKING ACTUAL
RESULTS OF INTERVENTIONS**

INFERENTIAL STATISTICS

**UNLESS STUDY VERY CAREFULLY
MANAGED, OF LIMITED HELP IN
DETERMINING VALUE OF INTERVENTION**

ployer or health plan saved $250,000 one year by implementing a self-care program, it saved the money; statistical significance is not an issue.

It is an unfortunate artifact of inferential statistics that "statistical significance" can be *calculated* even where it has no meaning. If 35% of the members in a given population smoked before an intervention and 25% smoked after the intervention, for example, the statistical significance of that difference can be calculated simply by inserting the size of the population. In a population of 25 workers, the difference would be found to be "not statistically significant." It would be assigned a higher than 5% probability as "having occurred by chance." In a population of 100 workers, the difference would be labeled statistically significant; in a population of 500, perhaps "highly significant."

The point is, however, that some number of workers did quit smoking. Whether they did so because of whatever smoking cessation program was implemented is an entirely separate question that cannot be answered based on how many in the population quit or how large the population was. A chance probability refers to the probability that chance variations in samples produce differences in sample statistics as opposed to population parameters (e.g., that the average age of a sample might be some years above or below the mean for the population). Statistically calculated chance probabilities do not indicate whether a *change* in a *population* is attributable to luck. Only careful examination of events, perhaps surveys of those who changed, will divulge such information.

If some "experts" argue that a given employee or enrollee population is too small to use in evaluating a program (i.e., that the results of the evaluation would not be statistically significant), they may be misconstruing and miscommunicating the meaning of statistical significance. The effect of "sample size" on the reliability of results relates to using such results to extrapolate conclusions to a larger population. If the "sample" is the entire population you are concerned with, its size is not the problem. If you are inferring from the results in that population to what can be expected with the same population next year, the uncertainty of that inference is not a function of the size of the population. It is the inherent uncertainty of extrapolating from the past to the future. The members of the population may change; their attitudes may be altered; many factors may make predicting the future unreliable.

Where sponsors might wish to extrapolate results from one population to another, sample sizes can make a difference but so can other factors. Rules of statistical inference apply to extrapolating results that occur within a sample of a given population to all the members of that population. If the sample is well chosen so as to be statistically representative of the entire population, the inference should be reliable, within the limits imposed by sample size.

If sponsors wish to extrapolate from what happened with one population in order to predict what will happen with an entirely different population, however, it is not sample *size* that is the problem but its *representativeness*. Unless the population or sample from which the extrapolation is made is representative of the new population, the extrapolation is dangerous because of the differences between the populations, not simply the sample size.

Sponsors should recognize that extrapolation from results that are found in one population at one time and place to another population in another time and place will always be risky, in spite of sample size. Differences in populations in time and place can always confound extrapolation or inference, though unless such differences are large and have great impact, such extrapolation may be the best basis for making estimates.

In general, where evaluations include data on the entire population of interest (i.e., where no sampling is involved), it may be wise to avoid inferential statistics. Calculating statistical significance of results may make results appear more reliable or evaluation methodologies more rigorous. But when the inference is not from a sample to a population from which it was drawn but from one population, time, and place to another, measures of statistical significance may overstate the reliability of the inference and thereby mislead sponsors. Judgment will always be needed to address possible population, time, and place effects on inferences.

Some might argue that the experience of a given population in one year is a "sample" that has to be extrapolated to other years in order to be evaluated. This is at least a strong argument, where decisions based on one year's experience will affect future years. However, one year's experience cannot be treated as a statistically reliable sample of other years in the same way that a random sample of a population is treated as representing the entire population. There are simply no inferential statistical rules that govern how one year is treated as a sample of all years.

Far from being a random sample of all years, one year's experience will surely change all future years, for example. Results in future years may be greater than in the first, as cumulative effects increase the impact or reduce the cost of interventions. They may also be far less if early efforts achieve changes in the most receptive audiences and later efforts must be aimed at increasingly recalcitrant groups. A given year's results may or not be an accurate indication of what repetition of the same effort in the same population will produce in another year. Inferential statistics are not designed to tell what the future will be like.

SUCCESS: REACHING OBJECTIVES?

It is a standard but unfortunate characteristic of many evaluation discussions to focus on the question of whether or not results match objectives. Did the intervention produce the results specifically called for, the precise change described in the objective? It makes more sense to think of the objective as a rough expression of intent, used in planning to estimate the value of an initiative to design and justify an intervention. An initiative is not a failure because it does not meet an objective nor a success because it does meet it; an intervention should be judged by whether it achieves worthwhile results at acceptable costs.

Where a particular effort achieves 50%, 80%, or 90% of the predetermined objective and thereby a significant benefit to sponsors, it should not be construed as a failure. If it achieves such success at significantly less than the anticipated cost or has significant positive side effects (e.g., impact on key relationships, learning for next time), it may be more valuable to sponsors than full achievement of the original objective. If it returns a net savings of $150,000 instead of an estimated $200,000, or an ROI ratio of 2.5:1 instead of 3.0:1, how can it be deemed a flop?

SUCCESS

IF PERCENTAGE OF DESIRED RESULTS IS REACHED WITH:
- ✗ **LESS THAN ANTICIPATED COST**
- ✗ **SIGNIFICANT POSITIVE SIDE EFFECTS**
- ✗ **BETTER THAN ANTICIPATED ROI**

FAILURE

IF DESIRED RESULTS ARE REACHED BUT WITH:
- ✗ **GREATER COSTS THAN ANTICIPATED**
- ✗ **MORE NEGATIVE SIDE EFFECTS THAN ANTICIPATED**
- ✗ **NO SIGNIFICANT LEARNING ADDED**
- ✗ **WORSE THAN ANTICIPATED ROI**

Similarly, if a program achieves the original objective, but with greater costs and/or negative side effects than anticipated and no significant learning to add value to future efforts, it may well be a failure in spite of making its goal. The net value may prove to be less than anticipated, and if costs are greater, the ROI ratio may end up less than 1:1, or at least far less than a number of other initiatives that might have been implemented with the same resources.

Where the objective was expressed in terms of one of the early stages in the set of effects (e.g., participation, mind-states, or behaviors), it may turn out that the impact of changes in these effects on health status, utilization of services, expenditures, or side effects was significantly greater or less than anticipated. In other words the VALUE of the objective might be far different from the estimate. In such cases achieving an objective may prove to be worth less than the cost of the initiative or achieving less than the objective may prove to be worth far more than the cost.

This is not to denigrate the value of objectives. Without a clear notion of what effects are desired, it would be difficult to justify an intervention or to select one over another. Moreover, having objectives can help to eliminate one of the most common flaws in evaluation: drawing the target around whatever the arrow hits. Looking for results after an intervention, with no clear picture of what results were intended, is usually a challenge to find ways to make it look good and may lead to fictional results or questionable attribution.[5]

ATTRIBUTION

A significant question applicable to almost every evaluation challenge is that of attribution: can the results noted be attributed to the intervention or were other factors at work? As with most evaluation issues, the question of attribution has to be addressed in the planning and implementation of an initiative; it cannot be handled after the fact anywhere near as well as before.

To make a case for attribution, it is first essential to be able to link changes in any of the set of effect measures to sponsor interventions *by individual*. Sponsors should be able to show that the specific consumers who participated in a program were the ones whose mind-states and behavior were improved and that it is, for example, *their* health status, utilization, and expenditures that were improved or *their* morale, satisfaction, retention, and productivity that were improved.

Population-based measures may suggest that positive results have been achieved, but only linkages of measures to interventions by individuals will show that apparent improvements are truly *results* of interventions rather than chance events. If the percentage of smokers declines in a work force, for example, it might be that turnover and replacement have reduced the number of workers who smoke, but that no one has actually quit. Improvements in health behavior or utilization patterns might have been greater or as great among nonparticipants in a program as among participants. The only way to tell is to be able to track each individual in both the intervention population and any comparison group examined.

A sound basis for attribution can be created by tracking each stage in the set of effects that should have been influenced by an intervention. If distribution of a self-care guide is expected to reduce the use of ED care, for example, and such a reduction is noted, it would be worthwhile to check if people who received the guide actually used it, if they felt it was useful, and if it made a difference to their decisions when confronted with particular symptoms. Did a disease management effort aimed at consumers with asthma actually improve their self-management of asthma and reduce the number of crises, in addition to their overall use of health care? Did a safety education program improve workers' knowledge of safety issues and increase use of safety equipment as well as apparently result in a reduction in injuries?

Attribution can also be argued where comparison groups have been used in evaluation. Ideally the only difference between the experiences of intervention versus comparison group, experimental versus control, should be that one had the

TRACKING ATTRIBUTION

✗ ASK IF PEOPLE WERE INFLUENCED BY INTERVENTION
✗ COLLECT DATA ON INTERVENTION AS WELL AS
  COMPARISON GROUPS
✗ UTILIZE MULTIPLE CONTROL GROUPS WITH
  MULTIPLE INTERVENTIONS

chosen intervention and the other did not and one's behavior, status, utilization, or expenditures, as well as side-effect measures, changed in a better way. If arrangements are not made to selectively assign consumers to experiment versus control groups or to collect data on both intervention and comparison groups before the intervention is implemented, it may prove impossible to do so later.

Attribution may also be a problem when results might have come from any one or a combination of interventions. In clinical paths and case management, for example, while most emphasis is on provider behavior, patients may play a significant role.[6] In managing chronic conditions, patients and family members are aided by providers. If efforts are underway to modify behaviors of both providers and consumers, who gets the credit for any improvement in outcomes?

Where multiple programs simultaneously address multiple actors and behaviors, comparison groups may be used to isolate the effects of individual efforts. If it is important enough to learn, clinical paths and case management may be tried in some facilities without including patients, for example, with results compared to those in facilities where patients were included. Diabetes management interventions may focus exclusively on consumers in one experimental group and include providers in a second, with yet a third used as a control group having no intervention.

Where there are no experimental versus control or other comparison groups so that the effects of one versus another intervention can be isolated, then sharing the credit may be the only reasonable as well as possible option. As long as the return on investment is admirable, after accounting for the costs of multiple interventions, no further attempt at attribution may be needed. If it is a key question, then a control/comparison trial can be used to settle the issue.

RETURN

The most challenging issue in evaluation is assigning dollar values to results. Where the intended change (or no-change) objective is stated in terms of participation, mind-states, behavior, even health status and utilization, can specific savings in health care expenditures be attributed to them? Where the objective is stated in dollar savings, the challenge is simpler, as long as savings can be attributed to the intervention.

If "side effects" such as productivity improvement, absenteeism and turnover reduction, or improved retention of health plan members are included in evaluation, they should be translatable into at least well-informed estimates of dollar value. There is often a snag with assigning dollar value to absenteeism reductions, however. When workers are absent, what do employers actually lose? Therefore what do they gain if absenteeism is reduced?

It is obvious that employers pay for most worker absences, though not all. But do they *lose* that payment? When a worker is absent, if coworkers make up for that absence by simpy working harder or more efficiently, then no production may be lost and no costs added. If coworkers have to work overtime or temporary replacements have to be used, then the cost of that overtime or replacement worker is real added cost and there are therefore real savings if absences are reduced. But only in unusual coincidences will the added cost of absences be exactly the cost paid to the absent workers, yet that is the usual measure of the cost of absences.

For the true added-value dollar impact of reduced absences to be used in evaluation, the true costs of doing without the workers involved must be used, not the costs of paying the absent workers. In many cases salaried employees may simply make up for their own absences by working longer hours when they get back to work, and the employer incurs no added salary costs. Reducing such absences may help morale or quality of performance, but the dollar savings will not be accurately expressed as days of salary replacement saved.

When effects involve quality of life, worker morale, and satisfaction and other psychosocial factors, the translation is problematic. It is common to express health risks in health improvement in terms of years of remaining life expectancy compared to what could be expected in a riskless life. How much are added years of life expected (or even actually enjoyed) worth?

In a comparison of public health interventions, childhood immunization was estimated to cost virtually nothing per year of life "saved," while flu shots cost $600 per year; construction safety rules $38,000; kidney dialysis $46,000; heart transplants $104,000; and radiation controls $27.4 million.[7] Such data may help in deciding where and how to intervene, but what should we decide in evaluating such programs after the fact? How much is too much to pay for adding a year to someone's life?

In a study of the effects of participation by women in a cardiac rehabilitation program, levels of anxiety, depression, hostility, pain, and psychosomatic symptoms were found to have been significantly reduced. Mental health, energy, general health/well-being, and daily functioning were improved.[8] What dollar value can be assigned to such results?

There may be many ways to measure the quality of life, but no consensus exists as to the best approach. How can sponsors incorporate the value of quality-of-life improvements when evaluating demand improvement results without a valid and reliable measure? One discussion suggests that quality of life is too vague and immeasurable, though subjectively perceived health status might work. It would at least be a means whereby the consumer perspective could be incorporated into evaluations.[9]

How long should we wait to detect results? Interventions such as self-care promotion, prenatal care, and chronic condition/case management have been shown to produce results in the same year as the intervention. This is particularly handy for budget makers whose perspective may be circumscribed by the fiscal year. But since budgets are often prepared many months before the beginning of a fiscal year, budgeters may want to see results only a few months after an intervention has been implemented, well before any are likely to show up.[10]

For most behavior change interventions, it takes some time to detect even the behavior change desired or to demonstrate its permanent adoption. Smokers must abstain for a lengthy period, often a year, to be considered as having truly quit. Exercisers must get by the three or six months when so many "experimenters" drop out to be considered as having truly reformed. Pregnant women must begin prenatal care in the first trimester and continue it for up to nine months before it can be said they complied with a desired behavior pattern. If it takes that long to detect even the desired behavior, how can later effects on health status, use of services, and expenditures be detected except by waiting even longer?

If it takes years for some results to show up, even longer for interventions aimed at reducing cholesterol or blood pressure levels or increasing bone density to prevent osteoporosis, how do we assign dollar values to the intervention or to health status improvements whose impact on service use and expense may be so far in the future? On the other hand, to not assign a dollar value may mean defining such interventions as failures and reducing or eliminating investments therein.

Discounted future value of estimated utilization and expenditure effects may be made where credible translations of the effects of changes in health status are available. Discounted value of future years of life or quality of life versus quantity are another question entirely. Only human judgment can be used to estimate the value of such improvements, and probably the combined judgment of payers, providers, and consumers is needed rather than reliance on payers alone.

Many health promotion and prevention efforts tend to extend life when successful, for example. This will add to the numbers of people experiencing the unavoidable effects of aging and can add to lifetime costs of health care.[11] It may also shift responsibility for paying such costs from employers to government, of course, though consumers, as either customers or taxpayers, are ultimately responsible either way. Should such added costs be considered as offsets to added years of life?

PROBLEMS WITH DETERMINING RETURN

HOW DO WE VALUE:
- ✗ A "RISK-FREE" LIFE?
- ✗ AN ADDED YEAR OF LIFE?
- ✗ SIGNIFICANT IMPROVEMENTS IN WELL-BEING?

PROBLEMS WITH DETERMINING ROI

HOW DO WE COST OUT:
  ✗ FUTURE RESULTS
  ✗ DIFFERENCE BETWEEN QUALITY AND QUANTITY OF LIFE
  ✗ SHIFT OF RISK TO OTHER PAYERS BECAUSE OF
    AGING POPULATION

Since the costs of interventions should be accurately countable or at least estimable in almost all cases, calculating return on investment when results cannot be stated in dollar terms is problematic. It is not essential to calculate an actual net return or ROI ratio, however. We need only decide if the value of what has been accomplished is at least as great as the cost of accomplishing it. When value cannot easily be stated in dollar terms, it is only required that we achieve consensus among those concerned that it is greater than the cost.

COSTS

One of the most common problems in evaluation is the undercounting of costs. This most frequently occurs when interventions are planned, implemented, and evaluated by staff within the sponsoring organization. The undercounting occurs because staff do not count their own time and effort or that of other employees of the organization, arguing that they are expenses already being borne and therefore not attributable to the intervention.

It may well be true that a sponsor incurs no additional expense in the course of a specific initiative; it merely represents a new challenge for existing staff, a different way for them to spend their time. This certainly does not mean the initiative has no cost, however; it has the costs of the time and effort and salary plus benefits of all staff working on it. If such costs are not recognized, there is no way to account for the "opportunity costs" involved (i.e., what else might have been accomplished with the same expenditure of time and effort). Without accurate and complete staff salary and benefit costs reflecting the time they spend in an initiative, there is no basis for comparing alternative initiatives that sponsors might choose in planning or in evaluating which ones deserve continuation.

For both planning and evaluation purposes, staff time and salary/benefit costs, at a minimum, should be "charged" to initiatives as if they were additional expenses (i.e., as if staff were external vendors). Whether overhead costs, for ex-

DON'T FORGET TO ACCOUNT FOR

✗ **INTERNAL STAFF SALARIES & BENEFIT COSTS**
✗ **OVERHEAD COSTS**
✗ **PLANNING COSTS FOR DETERMINING WHETHER OR NOT TO OUTSOURCE THE INITIATIVE**

ample, for facilities, maintenance and support services, and depreciation should also be counted is best answerable by the organization. If the costs would be incurred whether or not the employees involved in the initiative were on staff, then perhaps they should not be counted. Where they represent costs of having the employees on staff, they probably should.

Outsourcing specific interventions is almost always a possibility in reforming consumer behaviors, so an accurate and complete accounting for internal staff costs is equally essential in judging whether to make or buy specific initiatives. If such costs are hidden as already existing or "sunk" costs, it will tend to make internal implementation the preferred option when it should not be.

It must be noted that evaluation itself will cost money in staff resources as well as possible outside services. If a given intervention is to be implemented only once, during one fiscal period, the full costs of evaluation should be charged to the intervention. If it is to continue for a longer, perhaps indefinite future, the costs may be applied to the next fiscal period as an investment in planning or split between the current and subsequent periods as applicable to both. Particularly where evaluations contribute significant learning, they can reasonably be considered as delivering future value.

ROI

ROI is an important consideration in evaluation in both absolute and relative terms. The absolute ROI is the total amount of money saved or nondollar value realized after accounting for all attributable costs (i.e., the net return). This is an amount of value, presumably a positive amount, except where a given intervention failed to produce positive results or costs were greater than the value achieved.

The ROI ratio is simply the relationship between the total value achieved and the total costs of achieving that value, the quotient of value divided by costs. As is discussed in Chapter 10 on strategy, this ratio provides important but limited insight into how successful a given intervention has been. Anything other than a positive ratio suggests failure; anything less than the return ratio that could be achieved through prudent investment in stocks and bonds (e.g., 1.10:1 or a 10% return) could be thought as a poor return.

When the ROI ratios for a number of initiatives are both positive and above acceptable money market levels, they have limited worth. The ratios of different approaches to achieving the same results can be compared so as to choose which deserves preference. But when the results are different in value, it is the net value, the absolute net return, that should guide future investment rather than the ratio.

If the ratio described an unlimited reality—for example, if a 5:1 ratio meant that we could invest any amount of money and it would always produce a net value of $4.00 on top of each $1.00 invested, a 400% interest rate—we might wish to devote all available dollars to an effort with such a ratio. In reality such ratios apply to situations in which usually only a limited amount of money can be invested for a return. There is no point in buying two or 10 self-care guidebooks for employees in the hope that such an investment will double our return or increase it by an order of magnitude.

Each possible intervention must be evaluated at the planning stage in terms of how much investment is possible or reasonable as well as the ROI ratio it promises. Evaluation can include the ROI ratios for limited future use but should focus more on net return as the truest reflection of how much value has been achieved at what cost.

ROI ratios have frequently been found to increase over time. Sometimes this results from decreasing costs of interventions, such as self-care manuals that are distributed in the first year to all consumers but only have to be distributed to those added to the population in subsequent years. In other cases the effects take time or are cumulative and so build up over time. Whichever applies, it suggests watching ROI over many years rather than relying on results in a single year or less to reach strategic conclusions.

VALUE OF ROI ESTIMATIONS

✗ ABSOLUTE ESTIMATIONS . . . AMOUNT OF MONEY SAVED
. . . VALUABLE FOR DETERMINING COST-EFFECTIVENESS
✗ RELATIVE ESTIMATIONS . . . AMOUNT OF MONEY THAT
COULD BE EARNED IF INVESTED ELSEWHERE . . . OF LIMITED
VALUE IN PLANNING & EVALUATING

EVALUATION BARRIERS

Achieving an accurate and complete evaluation of results and return is a significant challenge. There are many barriers to good evaluation of health and demand improvement initiatives. It is impossible to use the classic double-blind technique in assessing interventions, since consumers will necessarily know whether they are being "treated" by any initiative. Hence the "Hawthorne effect" of responding to the fact that someone is paying attention may account for some changes in behavior, rather than the specific initiative. Similarly, there is no way to eliminate the potential for a "placebo effect" caused by participants believing that the initiative will help them, since no control group can get just a placebo.

Self-selection, rather than random assignment to experiment versus control comparison groups, is a frequent problem. Consumers who select themselves to participate in a given program have to be suspected to differ from those who elect not to participate, and that difference, rather than the program, may account for some, even all of the differences in behavior, health status, use of services, expenditures, and side effects noted later.

Employers may find it difficult to restrict their interventions to half their employees, especially if they believe wholeheartedly in the intervention they initiate. Union agreements may preclude "discriminating" against one group of employees by treating them differently, even though that is essential to controlled evaluations. Employees themselves may refuse to accept random assignment as an infringement of personal freedom.

In one case, an experimental versus control group study that was to provide five years of comparison data was cut short because of the success of the experimental intervention. Sponsors found so much success after the first year that they extended the initiative to the entire population, thereby eliminating the control comparison group.[12] In another case consumer groups insisted that members of a proposed control group should not be denied the benefits of the experimental treatment, making comparisons impossible.[13]

Attrition is likely to be a considerable hindrance to evaluation in long-term evaluations. Consumers may drop out of participation and end up representing a special intermediate group of people who have experienced part but not all of the intervention. They may drop out of the population through leaving employment, disenrolling from the health plan, or leaving the community. Attrition may reduce the numbers of consumers below a level where significant differences can be found or may make the experimental versus control groups less comparable.

Another form of attrition occurs when members of control groups change their behavior on their own, perhaps as a result of a·Hawthorne effect, and reduce the apparent effects of the intervention. Consumers are subject to advice in the media and pressure from friends and family on health and utilization of services, so may quit smoking, initiate an exercise regimen, or seek decision or disease-related information on their own, reducing the differences between them and the experimental group.

Still another type of attrition occurs when participants in an experimental initiative partially comply. They may engage in some exercise but not the level recommended, for example, or reduce smoking but not quit altogether. Consumers may call a triage phone line some of the time but not in all recommended situations. Results from partial compliance may accurately reflect the results of the intervention but understate the effects of the desired behavior change. It may lead sponsors to give up on achieving a specific behavior change, where better marketing and greater acceptance (i.e., a better program) would have proven highly successful, abandoning the end when only the means had failed.

In addition to the attrition problem is the fact that new people may join the population of interest over the evaluation period. New employees may be hired, new members join the health plan, or new patients enter the practice. Unless data are tracked by *individual* participant and nonparticipant, population-based data may reflect changes in the membership of both groups rather than changes in behavior made by those members.

Sponsors of initiatives can only hope to minimize these barriers. They can start with large enough numbers to anticipate the effects of attrition and strive to minimize attrition itself. They can hope to achieve random assignment versus biased self-selection of control versus experimental groups by explaining the importance of good evaluation and obtaining union and/or employee approval of the evaluation plan.

Since the Hawthorne effect applies to both participants and nonparticipants alike, it can be factored into evaluations by pretesting and posttesting of both control and experimental groups, with any overall effect on both groups enjoyed as a windfall. To guard against being misled by partial conversion, sponsors may check the results among those fully converting separately, comparing them to partial converts to identify the difference that a better program might achieve.

RELATIONSHIPS

Interventions aimed at reforming consumer health and demand behaviors are sure to have some impact on some relationships. Such effects may have been identified as specific objectives, value-adding side effects, since they can almost always represent benefit to consumers, improving satisfaction and retention, for example. At a minimum, the possibility of negative impact on relationships should be considered during planning and addressed in evaluation.

Heavy-handed efforts to reform consumer behavior may have the kinds of negative impact on relationships with employees, enrollees, and citizens described in Chapter 3. The use of disincentives to achieve healthy behavior, such as penalties for not using seat belts or denial of coverage for maternity if women fail to comply with prenatal care rules, may produce as much of a backlash as "drive-through deliveries" and ED permission requirements. On the other hand, if selected with employee participation and approval, such devices may be less of a threat to relationships.

Relationships with providers are also potentially affected by interventions of payers. Steering consumers to "carve out" providers (e.g., for high-cost centers of excellence procedures or specialist groups for an entire category of services such as orthopaedics and ophthalmology) may anger primary physicians over loss of their referral role. Using triage phone services that refer callers directly to specialists may be perceived as destroying continuity or undermining the primary physicians' gatekeeper role. No intervention should be labeled successful if it produces the intended return in cost savings but also incites a riot among physicians.

Consequences of specific interventions in relationships with other stakeholders should also be addressed. Significant improvements in employee or enrollee health and certainly improvements in citizen health can produce positive impact on relations with the public, with media, and with governments. Interventions that increase sales of drugs or devices for disease management may open up opportunities for closer working relationships with suppliers.

The key is simply to consider which relationships might be affected by particular interventions, and then to look for what the effects might be. Looking might involve something as simple as a phone call to an interested party or as complex as a full-scale survey of public, employee, or enrollee opinion. Both positive and negative effects should be sought, since both are possible, with special emphasis on positive effects, since outraged stakeholders are likely to report their ire, where their mildly pleased counterparts may keep silent (Table 20–1).

LEARNING

Every intervention experience, whether success or failure, should be treated as a learning experience. As in addressing results, attribution, return, and relationships, opportunities for learning are greatly improved if planned in advance rather than left for retrofitting. If sponsors are uncertain which of two possible messages will achieve higher participation response, they may try both in a split-test approach and check which generated the greater response.

Two (or more) competing self-care guides may be tried, though this may add to costs if smaller orders of each mean lower volume discounts and the lower performing guides have to be replaced with the higher. Payers may try both primary physicians and specialists to learn which group does better in particular disease management initiatives or may send half of employees with back injuries to physicians and the other half to chiropractors.

Exhibit 20–1 Possible Impacts on Relationships

RELATIONSHIPS ▶	POSITIVE IMPACTS	NEGATIVE IMPACTS
CONSUMERS	✗ IMPROVED HEALTH & SERVICE RESULTING IN SATISFACTION & RETENTION	✗ PENALTIES FOR NONCOMPLIANCE MAY RESULT IN CONSUMER BACKLASH
PROVIDERS	✗ SATISFACTION & RETENTION ✗ COOPERATION IN FUTURE EFFORTS	✗ STEERING CONSUMERS TO "CARVE-OUT" SPECIALTIES MAY RESULT IN ANGRY PHYSICIANS; ✗ TRIAGE THAT DIRECTS PATIENTS TO SPECIALISTS MAY THREATEN REFERRAL ROLE
PUBLIC & MEDIA	✗ IMPROVEMENT IN COMMUNITY HEALTH RESULTING IN GOOD REPUTATIONS	✗ FAILURES = SCANDALS OVER WASTED MONEY

It will always be a temptation to select what seems to be the most promising option and focus all investment on that one. Where there is sufficient uncertainty about the merits of competing options or even curiosity about other possibilities, dual or multiple alternatives may be tried, with careful evaluation used to determine which ought to be preferred in the future. This is one case where inferential statistics will be essential, by the way, since subsets of the population will be used as samples, and differences between samples rather than changes over time will be the focus of the evaluation. Statistics will be needed to determine if differences detected are attributable to differences in interventions or to chance differences between the samples studied.

Where multiple interventions are to be pilot tested, care must be taken that enough energy and resources are devoted to the test to enable it to succeed. There is always the risk that a toe-in-the-water approach will be so tentative and unenthusiastic that it will produce mediocre results through a self-fulfilling prophecy. Pilot testers should want all options being tried to succeed and should act accordingly, ensuring that each alternative is tested exactly as it would be used in full-scale application.[14]

The same techniques as are used in gathering information for strategic and tactical decisions are applicable to specific intended learning (see Chapter 8). By consciously aiming to learn from each reform intervention experience and planning the implementation and evaluation of each accordingly, the evaluation process can add greatly to, in addition to determining the value of, the experience itself.

PREDICTED EFFECTS

All previous discussion has focused on evaluations of program efforts and interventions after they have been made. In some cases evaluators may wish to make an evaluation based on future projections of effects based on effects thus far. Evaluators have been known to extrapolate from one year's cost savings to many years in the future. While such extrapolations are risky, including future savings may be the only fair and complete basis for evaluation of programs that have long-term results.

The problem is that projections of future effects are guesses, even if carefully calculated extrapolations from results already achieved. Projecting the effects of changes in health behaviors may ignore the fact that the population in question will be getting older over the projection period and may experience new morbidity simply as a consequence of aging. Or it may fail to include the future expenditures that will be needed to reinforce and maintain behavior changes, projecting only the savings.

In general, if future savings are needed to justify continuation of an intervention (i.e., if results thus far show greater costs than savings for sponsors), the evaluation should look only as far into the future as is needed to find a positive and attractive ROI. Moreover, the costs of continuing the intervention, presumably at lower costs since it has only to maintain changes rather than initiate them, should be included along with estimated savings. The purpose of evaluation should always be to *discover* the effects of an intervention, not to prove it was a good thing.

REFERENCES

1. J. Burns, "The Need for More Rigor When Measuring and Reporting Results," *Business & Health* 13, no. 1 (1995):8.
2. J. Fries, et al., "Randomized Controlled Trial of Cost Reduction from a Health Education Program," *American Journal of Health Promotion* 8, no. 3 (1994):216–223.
3. "2 Rights Don't Make a Right," *Health Promotion Practitioner* 4, no. 6 (1995):2, 8.
4. G. Guyatt, et al., "Users' Guide to the Medical Literature II: How To Use An article about Therapy or Prevention A. Are the Results Valid?" *JAMA* 270, no. 21 (1993):2598–2601.
5. "With Program Evaluation, Don't Close Barn Door after the Horse Is Out," *Employee Health & Fitness* 17, no. 11 (1995):121–126.
6. K. Knudsen, "Scott & White Measures 'Quality of Health' in Outcome Studies," *Health Care Strategic Management* 11, no. 3 (1993):7–9.
7. "Sick Care and Preventive Health Care Are Bargains," *Health Care Strategic Management* 12, no. 8 (1994):3.
8. "Cardiac Rehab for Women: A Solid Investment," *Business & Health* 13, no. 5 (1995):19.
9. A. Leplege and S. Hunt, "The Problem of Quality of Life in Medicine," *JAMA* 278, no. 1 (1997): 47–50.
10. S. McBride, "Don't Let the Short-Term Wolf Blow Your Long-Term Objectives," *Managed Healthcare* 6, no. 3 (1995):16–18.
11. "Can Prevention Lower Health Costs by Reducing Demand?" *Hospitals & Health Networks,* 4 February 1994, 10.
12. *An Absolute Success: The Taking Care® Program at the WEA Insurance Trust* (Oakton, VA: Center for Corporate Health, undated).
13. W. Lear, "Needle Test Trial Criticized," *The Denver Post,* 18 October 1996, 2A.
14. L. Scott, "Looking Beyond Cost," *Modern Healthcare,* 28 February 1994, 36–40.

Technical Addendum

For those interested in the design of "scientific" evaluations, there are a number of models for measuring results so as to be confident that true changes have occurred and can be attributed to the efforts undertaken.

Without Comparison Group

The simplest model for evaluation is Intervene, then Observe (I,O). To get a better idea as to whether the intervention made a difference, however, it is essential to Observe, then Intervene, then Observe again (O,I,O). To protect against the possibility that things were changing already in the measure of interest, multiple observations should be made before the interventions—or past measures collected rather than delay the intervention (O,O,O,I,O). To find out if the effects of the intervention last, multiple observations are made after the intervention (O,I,O,O,O). If both checks are desired, multiple observations both precede and follow the intervention (O,O,O,I,O,O,O). The intervention may be repeated to see if it works more than once (O,O,O,I,O,O,O,I,O,O,O).

With Comparison Group

Having a comparison group means repeating observations in both the group experiencing the intervention and the comparison group experiencing no intervention. These observations should be made in the same way at the same time so as to ensure as much as possible that only the intervention differentiates the groups, hence the results that show up in observations. If more than one intervention is to be tested, separate intervention groups are needed for each, while a single, no-intervention control or comparison group will suffice for all.

Essentially the same models of observation and intervention are used in comparisons, except that two or more sets are used to compare those with versus without the intervention(s). Thus the simplest (and least reliable model) is Intervention, Observation (I,O) compared to No Intervention, Observation (–,O). Then comes (O,I,O) compared to (O,–,O); (O,O,O,I,O) compared to (O,O,O,–,O); (O,I,O,O,O) compared to (O,–,O,O,O); (O,O,O,I,O,O,O) compared to (O,O,O, –,O,O,O); and (O,O,O,I,O,O,O,I,O,O,O) compared to (O,O,O,–,O,O,O,–,O,O,O).

For a more detailed discussion of these observation/intervention models, see R. Goetzel, "Program Evaluation" in M. O'Donnell and J. Harris, eds. *Health Promotion in the Workplace,* 2d ed. (Albany, NY: Delmar, 1994), 118–159.

PART V

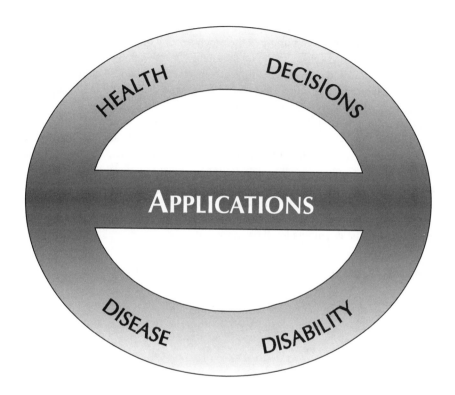

The four prior parts have addressed general concepts and suggestions for improving consumer health and care-seeking behaviors. In this part, we discuss each of the four different domains of demand improvement individually and separately. Sponsors who have already decided where to focus their attention may choose to devote their reading to the specific chapter addressing their chosen domain. Program planners may prefer an even narrower focus on one of the particular challenges within a given domain. We recommend that both strategists and tactical planners skim the other chapters, and parts thereof, at least for future reference.

Chapter 21 addresses the domain of health improvement, offering a wide-ranging discussion and numerous case examples in the areas of health risk management and illness/injury prevention, which are the basic approaches to avoiding the need for care, and early detection, which is one of the means of reforming demand. Chapter 22 covers decision improvement, including the replacement of care-seeking through self-care and the achievement of demand reform through informed consumer decision making.

Chapter 23 discusses disease self-management, addressing acute and chronic conditions, behavioral health, and pregnancy in terms of how consumers and their family/friend caregivers can improve the processes and outcomes of care through their own efforts. It emphasizes the replacement of care-seeking by the empowerment of consumers to care for conditions themselves. Chapter 24 applies the discussion of avoiding, replacing, and reforming demand to the particular challenges of the workplace through disability management.

Chapter 25 wraps up the book's coverage of demand improvement with both a summary of key points and issues and some specific suggestions for improving the discipline itself. Demand improvement is an emerging discipline with widely varying terminology and practitioners from a wide variety of training and experience backgrounds, and there is a long way to go and much we can all learn from each other. This chapter is recommended to all readers as a stimulus for their personal growth, for the further development of the discipline, and for the enhancement of the value it delivers to all concerned.

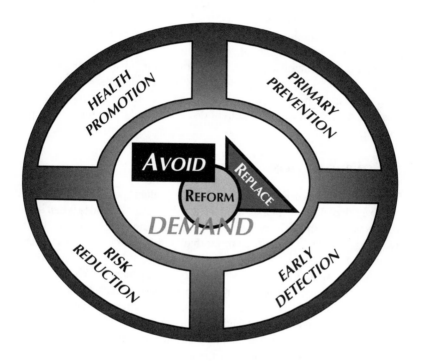

HEALTH IMPROVEMENT

It is at least arguable that the first place to begin efforts aimed at improving demand is with health improvement. By enhancing a population's overall health, reducing or eliminating risky behaviors, preventing preventable disease and injury, and catching conditions early, many of the demand problems needing attention can be eliminated or at least reduced. By devoting resources "upstream," before symptoms drive consumers toward demanding some sort of provider attention (i.e., by avoiding avoidable morbidity), we can reduce the size of the inappropriate utilization problem.

It is widely held that anywhere from 50% to 70% of all health problems and 20% to 30% of all health care expenditures can be avoided through some combination of health improvement activities.[1] This is an estimate because we have no examples of anyone applying all possible efforts simultaneously or longitudinally to a population. We think that because such proportions of morbidity and utilization arise from conditions we can do something about, we can achieve the full effects by doing something about all of them.

We divide the general topic of health improvement into four categories: (1) health promotion, (2) primary prevention, (3) risk reduction, and (4) clinical detection (secondary prevention). While these categories are somewhat fluid and imprecise, we feel they at least help in discussing and planning specific possible interventions.

HEALTH PROMOTION

It has long been argued that there is something called "positive health" in addition to the absence of disease, injury, and specific risks thereof. The idea is that if consumers can achieve optimum levels of physical, mental, and spiritual health, they are not only better protected against risks of morbidity, they also enjoy high levels of life quality. In addition, sponsors who achieve improvements in positive health can enjoy added value from increased employee, member, and patient satisfaction and loyalty and reduced costs that flow therefrom. In turn, increased satisfaction and loyalty help promote the success of other health improvement efforts, as well as decision improvement, disease management, and disability management efforts.

The initiatives we shall discuss under this category address overall health rather than specific risks and aim for distinct quality-of-life enhancement, in addition to whatever specific risks they may affect. The distinction between health promotion and risk reduction is somewhat arbitrary and fuzzy, but we believe it is also useful, with risk reduction aimed primarily at specific risks and reducing identified morbidity, while health promotion aims at general wellness and promoting life quality.

The definition of health in health promotion includes physical, mental/emotional, and spiritual dimensions. The programs and interventions we will discuss under this rubric include physical fitness, stress management, and spiritual health initiatives. While complete health promotion includes a wide range of environmental factors and programs, we are focusing on the consumer behavior factors of health promotion, so will not be addressing environment.

Physical Fitness

Problems and Potential

It is recognized that physical fitness, promoted via exercise programs and activities, has a wide variety of positive effects on health risk conditions such as blood pressure, weight and body mass, cholesterol, and blood sugar. It also tends to make those who are fit feel better, have more energy and enthusiasm about life, perform better on the job, and have fewer absences from work.[2] Although studies consistently show that participants in exercise and fitness programs incur far lower health care expenditures than nonparticipants,[3] such findings are typically confounded by the fact that consumers self-select participation, and participants tend to be fitter and more health conscious to begin with (Exhibit 21–1).

One of the more positive aspects of fitness is that it can be improved fairly dramatically in a relatively short time, and most dramatically among the least fit. The elderly can regain the strength and flexibility they enjoyed in their youth, though not the aerobic potential. People who are in poor physical shape make faster strides in fitness programs than those who start out fairly fit.[4]

Recently it has been discovered that fitness helps people maintain or recover mental acuity, in addition to its physical effects. While aging commonly slows mental processes, high levels of fitness can greatly reduce aging effects.[5] Fitness reduces risks of osteoporosis, back injury, cancer, and cardiovascular disease and promotes mental health. It adds to employers' disability management efforts by promoting safety and reducing work injuries.[6]

Concerns and Barriers

Given the wide-ranging and dramatic benefits of fitness, it would seem that virtually everyone would be avidly striving to achieve and maintain this wonderful state. This, however, is far from reality. Americans are among the least fit people on earth, suffering from high levels of obesity and low levels of strength, flexibility, and aerobic capacity. The "Baby Boomer" generation seems to have more sedentary lifestyles than the one that preceded it.[7] When worksite fitness programs are offered, only 10% to 20% of workers, and mostly the already fit, take advantage of them.[8]

Aside from inertia or plain laziness, people cite factors such as lack of time, difficulties in access to facilities or programs, dollar costs, pain and discomfort, age, and physical difficulty as reasons for not engaging in fitness programs.[9] Employees are commonly unaware of the fitness programs their employer offers, with only 44% of employees aware in one study.[10] Some forms of exercise, such as in-line skating, create their own added risk of injury.[11]

Sponsors frequently lack long-term experience with fitness, so are not sure which programs are likely to both attract the most participants and achieve the greatest benefit.[12] Because the benefits of fitness in terms of health status, health care use, and expenditures are harder to trace, being so general, sponsors may be hard pressed to justify them, as compared to the more easily attributed effects of prevention, risk reduction, and early detection.

Examples

Despite these difficulties, fitness efforts, particularly by employers as part of worksite wellness initiatives, are among the most common health improvement

Exhibit 21–1 Fitness

PROBLEMS / POTENTIAL	✗ PARTICIPANTS (ALTHOUGH SELF-SELECTING) TEND TO HAVE LOWER HEALTH CARE COSTS ✗ CAN SEE DRAMATIC RESULTS RATHER QUICKLY ✗ BENEFITS INCLUDE INCREASED MENTAL ACUITY, FEWER INJURIES, & FEWER DEBILITATING DISEASES
EXAMPLES	✗ ON-SITE FITNESS CENTERS MAKE PROGRAMS EASILY ACCESSIBLE ✗ SOCIAL ADVERTISING & PARTNERSHIPS MAKE EXERCISE ACCEPTABLE
CONCERNS	✗ CONSUMERS HAVE PLETHORA OF EXCUSES FOR WHY THEY DON'T EXERCISE & AREN'T FIT ✗ SPONSORS LACK LONG-TERM EXPERIENCE SO CAN'T CHOOSE AMONG OPTIONS WISELY
ADVICE	✗ PROMOTE & MARKET EXERCISE TO ACHIEVE HIGH LEVELS OF PARTICIPATION ✗ PROVIDE INCENTIVES TO PARTICIPATE IN SPECIFIC PROGRAMS ✗ MAKE PROGRAMS FLEXIBLE SO THEY CAN BE CUSTOMIZED TO INDIVIDUAL NEED ✗ MAKE PROGRAMS EASILY ACCESSIBLE, PROVIDE VARIETY & PEER SUPPORT

activities. This may well be due to the wide range of value-adding benefits achieved through improving fitness, aside from direct effects on health care utilization and costs. In addition to employer-sponsored programs, there are examples of virtually every imaginable sponsor having invested in fitness efforts.

Hospital fitness centers, with over 300,000 members, are an example of investments originally promoted as sources of additional fee-for-service (FFS) revenue but easily convertible to use in helping to manage capitation risks.[13] Health plans such as CareAmerica 65 Plus and Kaiser K-Plus offer senior fitness programs.[14] Simply by promoting fitness benefits, plans may attract healthier seniors, in addition to improving the health of seniors who become members.

Aside from sponsors with a direct capitation stake in the health of consumers, community efforts have focused on fitness as well as other ways of improving health. Social advocacy and a variety of partnerships have stimulated interest in exercise and activity.[15] Mall walker and zoo walker programs are often used to stimulate healthy, though less demanding activity.[16] The Marriott hotel system offers guests guides to simple exercises they can perform in their rooms, and promotes its program to encourage businesses to use its hotels.[17]

Suggestions

It seems clear that simply making fitness activities available is not enough; they must be promoted and/or marketed to achieve high levels of participation. An employer who invited employees to participate but did nothing to promote response found little effect.[18] All three of the $I = MC^2$ factors—motivation, capability, and consciousness—should be addressed, or as the National Institutes for Health refer to them, rewards, opportunities, and reminders.[19]

Incentives are widely used to at least promote participation in specific sponsored activities, both education and exercise.[20] The natural benefits of fitness—from improved immunity to fewer, shorter colds[21]—can be promoted as well as its benefits to appearance, energy, performance, and general quality of life.[22] Specific measures of these effects should be tracked and reported to participants so they have heightened awareness of the benefits and avoid the danger zone of 3 to 6 months after embarking on a fitness program, when a high proportion of participants quit.

Fitness promotion programs should be flexible, with potential for customizing activities to individual or at least varying tastes and preferences. Computer-based "expert systems" can be used to both design regimens[23] and act as "personal trainers" for participants.[24] A wide variety of rewards and recognitions, from employers, physicians, family, and friends, will tend to work better than one incentive for all. Encouraging consumers to participate in designing programs and incentives is likely to help.[25]

Fitness activities should be made as easy and convenient as possible. Worksite programs may involve a five-minute exercise break every hour. Numerous, short efforts, such as 10-minute mini-exercises three or more times a day, may be easier for some than the typically recommended 30-minute commitment.[26] On-site fitness centers make exercise convenient for workers,[27] or subsidies may be offered so they can use nearby health clubs.[28]

Research into what barriers consumers perceive and their suggestions for overcoming them can help sponsors design programs. Learning what would make fitness fun rather than a demanding strain is likely to help achieve long-term participation.[29] Combining aerobics, weight training, and flexibility activities can ensure variety as well as promote a wider range of benefits.[30] Charging something for programs may help consumers feel they have made an investment in something worthwhile, provided the charge is not so high as to be too great a barrier.[31]

Rather than use "experts" or teachers to stimulate participation, it may serve better to have peers who have recently improved their fitness tell their stories. Testimonials from peers are often more credible in convincing consumers that they can achieve fitness than the exhortations of fitness gurus.[32] Reminders should be continuous rather than relying on a one-time "blitz."[33] Both programs and messages can be pretested before full implementation to help pick the most promising approaches.[34]

Variety should be built in over time, in addition to flexibility for different individual preferences. Any program or set of incentives is likely to wear thin over time. A wide variety of choices and changing options over time can help maintain interest.[35] On the other hand, sponsors should not change successful programs or appeals just for variety; if something is still working, it may be the best approach to keep using it.

Because fitness has so many value-adding side effects, it makes sense to include fitness initiatives as part of comprehensive health promotion efforts that address mental and spiritual health and as parts of overall health improvement efforts. Include as many partners as possible, so that employers, health plans, and providers, as well as family, friends, and community can reinforce each other's efforts. Having physicians write "prescriptions" for fitness participation can stimulate participation as well as serve as a control on whose participation is subsidized.[36]

Stress Management

Stress is widely recognized as one of the most prevalent and dangerous risk factors for both physical and mental health. If there were some way to prevent or reduce stress, it would belong under risk reduction discussions. However, the chief aspiration relative to stress is to empower consumers to manage it, to cope with it, and even to use it to their advantage, as an inevitable reality of modern life. Moreover, its widespread effects separate it from the more common risk factors. Besides, risk reduction will be defined as changing risky behavior, where stress management involves adopting positive behavior; it aims at mental fitness (Exhibit 21–2).

Exhibit 21–2 Stress Management

PROBLEMS / POTENTIAL	✗ MOST COMMON PROBLEM FOUND IN HEALTH SCREENINGS, GENERALLY ATTRIBUTED TO WORK ✗ STRESS MANAGEMENT PROGRAMS ARE HIGHLY EFFECTIVE IN PROMOTING GOOD MENTAL HEALTH AS WELL AS PHYSICAL HEALTH
EXAMPLES	✗ EMPLOYEE ASSISTANCE PROGRAMS MAY OFFER STRESS MANAGEMENT CLASSES ✗ SUPPORT GROUPS REDUCE STRESS
CONCERNS	✗ FEW PEOPLE ARE AWARE OF THE POTENTIAL FOR STRESS REDUCTION ✗ MANY WHO ARE AWARE OF PROGRAMS DON'T AVAIL THEMSELVES OF THEM BECAUSE OF FEAR OF REPERCUSSIONS
ADVICE	✗ OFFER PROGRAMS THAT COMBINE RELAXATION AS WELL AS COPING SKILLS ✗ OFFER A WIDE VARIETY OF PROGRAMS THAT INCREASES CHANCE OF SUCCESS ✗ ENCOURAGE PARTICIPATION IN THE PROGRAMS ✗ EMPOWER EMPLOYEES TO TAKE STEPS TO REDUCE STRESS ON THE JOB, PERHAPS BY GIVING SOME AUTONOMY OVER TIME DEMANDS ✗ PROMOTE SOCIALIZATION AS ADDED BENEFIT

Problem and Potential

Stress is probably the most common problem found in health screenings and health risk assessments. In health fairs conducted at worksites in Denver, between 30% and 60% of workers reported that they experienced high levels of stress in their lives.[37] Stress from job, personal finances, responsibilities, divorce, sex, in-laws, and other causes were cited by workers, 43% of whom perceived themselves to be under above average stress. They reported an average of five stress episodes a month, with half having less than one a month but 10% reporting daily crises.[38]

Work appears to be the number one source of stress, cited by 52% in one study, compared to 37% citing money, 25% family, 18% life changes, and only 2% fear of unemployment.[39] It significantly reduces productivity, creates accidents, and promotes health care utilization, fatigue, headaches, and anxiety attacks that feel like heart attacks. It is a major cause of social ills such as domestic violence.[40]

While initiatives aimed at empowering consumers to better manage stress are far less common than physical fitness programs, they have been shown to have significant impact when used. A review of studies of stress reduction programs found that they reduced physician visits by 35% to 50%.[41] One application based on transcendental meditation reduced health insurance claims between 5% and 7% each year for seven years. It also reduced blood pressure, smoking, alcohol and drug use, and anxiety-related illnesses, producing significant quality-of-life enhancement for consumers.[42] Employers have found that stress management programs reduce both on-the-job accidents and overall physician visits.[43]

Negative stress reactions are typically physical/somatic overreactions to "dangers," manifestations of the fight-or-flight responses we needed in more primitive days.[44] Stress at the worksite has been primarily attributed to the combination of excessive demands for attention and lack of control over coping with such demands.[45] Stress can be lessened by reducing demands, virtually the opposite of what popular downsizing efforts achieve, or increasing workers' ability to control responses to that demand.

Examples

Offering employee assistance programs (EAPs) to help employees cope with all forms of stress and many of their manifestations is common.[45] Providing effective mental fitness or stress management training is relatively rare among other potential sponsors, however. Not only the uninsured but retirees and dependents as well as Medicare and Medicaid beneficiaries are unlikely to have access to stress management programs.

Employers who have offered stress management programs have reported generally favorable results. One combined exercise programs with training in coping skills, time management, and relaxation, enjoying reductions in physician visits ranging from 35% to 50%, in addition to fewer accidents.[46] Another found workers' compensation costs reduced almost 60%.[47]

Concerns and Barriers

Like physical fitness, stress management programs often suffer from lack of employee awareness. Where employers offered interventions, only 30% of employees were found to be aware of their stress management programs, 16% of their EAP, and 12% of other mental health programs.[48] In another study, while 60% of employees complained of stress-related problems, only 30% had used services offered by their employer.[49]

In the worksite, where work is the major source of stress, it is often difficult for employees to identify problems, particularly when they arise from their superiors. Employees may fear complaining of stress will jeopardize their advancement, even their jobs. They may be unwilling to share concerns over their home life, alcohol or drug abuse, for fear of job consequences. Similar concerns may apply if health plans were to enter the field.

Suggestions

There are a wide variety of stress management/coping techniques that can be effective. Offering a variety of options in stress management, such as relaxation techniques, controlled breathing, meditation, time management, and guided imagery, can promote participation and increase the likelihood that consumers will find one or more that work for them. Combining stress management with fitness and spiritual health programs is also recommended, since they have greatly overlapping effects.

Just as with fitness, encouraging participation will achieve greater impact than simply offering programs. The positive impact that stress management programs have on worker productivity and health care expenditures should provide the resources and return employers need to justify programs, with enough left over to promote participation via incentives and shared savings.

Giving workers the right to stop or at least to interrupt demands (e.g., on the assembly line), to take time out when stress gets too much, can combine the benefits of reduced demand and increased perceptions of control.[50]

Spiritual Health

While promoting spiritual health is recommended by many, it appears to be practiced by few. In contrast to hundreds of examples of physical fitness and dozens of examples of stress management, we found only a handful of discussions of spiritual health and no operational examples. Partly the problem may be uncertainty over what is meant by "spiritual," particularly the perception that it involves religion, which is bound to make any effort controversial (Exhibit 21–3).

Exhibit 21–3 Spiritual Health

PROBLEMS / POTENTIAL	✗ SPIRITUAL HEALTH LINKED TO BETTER PHYSICAL & MENTAL HEALTH ✗ INCREASED SELF-RESPONSIBILITY ESSENTIAL TO IMPROVING HEALTH & DEMAND
EXAMPLES	✗ SOME PRIVATE, RELIGIOUS SPONSORED ORGANIZATIONS COMBINE THE SPIRITUAL & MENTAL ASPECTS OF HEALTH
CONCERNS	✗ CONCERN ABOUT "PROMOTING" RELIGION IN WORKPLACE MAKES SPONSORS RELUCTANT ✗ DIFFICULT TO SEPARATE SPIRITUAL HEALTH FROM STRESS MANAGEMENT
ADVICE	✗ SUPPLY TIME & FACILITIES FOR CONSUMERS TO CONDUCT OWN SPIRITUAL ACTIVITIES, SUCH AS A CHAPEL OR CLASSES EXPLORING THE INTERSECTION OF HEALTH AND SPIRIT ✗ SET SPECIFIC OBJECTIVES FOR FUNDAMENTAL MEASURES LIKE SELF-RESPONSIBILITY

While most writers on spiritual health appear to come from religious backgrounds, "spiritual" is by no means the same as "religious" and is certainly not restricted to one religion. One defined spiritual as "that aspect of our well-being which organizes the values, the relationships and the meaning and purpose of our lives."[51] Another defined spiritual health in terms of connectedness, a sense of being unconditionally loved and accepted (by family, friends, society, perhaps, in addition to a deity)—including self-responsibility and self-reliance, a sense of self-worth, self-acceptance, and confidence.[52]

Victor Frankl boiled down the essence of spirituality to the ultimate recognition that we are responsible, that even in a Nazi concentration camp, we are ultimately responsible for how we react to what happens and to what others do.[53] Spiritual health is a sense of self-health; of love, hope, and charity toward and connectedness with others; of purpose and meaning.[54] The qualities that are cited as part of spiritual health are, in many ways, the fundamental qualities needed for consumers to play an optimal role in demand improvement: self-responsibility and self-efficacy, especially.

It is difficult to completely separate stress management from spiritual health, particularly since they share many of the same techniques. Discussion groups, support groups, and prayer groups have similar dynamics and effects. Meditation, holistic contemplation, and prayer are closely related. Promoting self-awareness, perceptions of purpose and meaning in life, and connectedness to a larger reality has been found in systematic research studies to improve compliance with medical advice, to reduce anxiety and to improve outcomes of health care and perceived quality of life.[55]

Sponsors can promote spiritual health and enjoy its direct and value-added effects in improving health without transforming themselves into churches or religions. One simple approach is to sponsor, perhaps merely supply the time and facilities for consumers to conduct their own spiritual activities. Consumers empowered to select their own approach to promoting their spiritual health gain the added value of choice and control, whether or not they select a religious approach. Sponsors can set specific objectives for fundamental measures such as self-responsibility and self-efficacy, perceived health, and related constructs to evaluate and justify their efforts.

Recently a growing number of employers have begun hiring ministers, priests, or rabbis to serve as worksite chaplains. These chaplains can be especially useful to employees and their families in crises. One vendor has supplied 300 contract chaplains to 160 companies and 110,000 employees, though it is estimated that several thousand chaplains are employed at worksites.[56]

PRIMARY PREVENTION

While all health promotion efforts aim at preventing avoidable morbidity as well as improving quality of life, primary prevention focuses on using specific interventions to prevent specific diseases and injuries. Since the focus of this discussion is on what consumers can do to prevent morbidity, there are but two primary prevention behaviors that fall under this category: immunization and personal (as opposed to public and worksite) safety.

Immunization has long been a performance measure for providers. The National Council for Quality Assurance's Health Plan Employer Data and Information Set (HEDIS) measures have included such measures as the proportion of children fully immunized among indicators of health plan quality, with health plans, in turn, expecting high levels of compliance among their physicians.[57] Yet unless consumers go to their providers for flu shots, measles, mumps and rubella, polio, whooping cough, and other vaccines, there is little physicians can do. It would be illegal for physicians to forcibly inoculate consumers and outrageously inefficient to chase consumers around looking for the right opportunity.

Personal safety, from having smoke and carbon monoxide detectors in the home; to setting water heaters at safe levels, to wearing auto seat belts and bicycle and motorcycle helmets; to otherwise eliminating or at least reducing risks of injury and disease could as easily be included among risk reduction efforts. The only reason for including them here is that they involve taking positive steps rather than the elimination or changing of negative (i.e., risky) behaviors. And since we will discuss risk reduction behavior as well, in the next section of this chapter, it should not make a great deal of difference in which category we put it.

Immunization

Problem and Potential

Immunizations are frequently touted as the most cost-effective approaches to avoiding demand and improving health available. While a measles outbreak in Dallas, Texas, cost an estimated $3.5 million and infected 500 children, resulting in 12 deaths, it was argued that an immunization effort costing as little as $200,000 could have prevented it, with an return on investment (ROI) ratio of 25:1.[58] The incidence of measles, polio, and other immunizable diseases is down 99% since vaccines became available, with ROI ratios for different vaccines ranging from 6:1 to 30:1 and averaging 10:1[59] (Exhibit 21–4).

Yet children being incompletely immunized is the rule rather than the exception. One study found only 60% of children with all their shots[60]; another found only 45.2% fully immunized at age two, and 53.3% at age six.[61] The very infrequency of what were traditionally childhood illnesses everyone worried about has apparently

Exhibir 21–4 Immunization

PROBLEMS / POTENTIAL	✗ MOST COST-EFFECTIVE INTERVENTION TO REDUCE COST & AVOID DEMAND
EXAMPLES	✗ CHILDHOOD IMMUNIZATION PROGRAMS WORK WELL FOR COMMUNITY COLLABORATION ✗ ANY EMPLOYER OR PROVIDER CAN PROVIDE INEXPENSIVE IMMUNIZATIONS ON SITE
CONCERNS	✗ STILL HAVE MANY CHILDREN & ADULTS WHO ARE NOT IMMUNIZED ✗ IMMUNIZATION PROGRAMS IN MULTIPLE SITES COMPLICATES RECORD KEEPING
ADVICE	✗ OFFER VACCINATION PROGRAMS FREQUENTLY IN EASILY ACCESSIBLE LOCATIONS TO MAXIMIZE PARTICIPATION

reduced parents' anxiety levels below the point where they are sure to have their children vaccinated.[62] And physicians often see children when they are sick, making the physician less likely to choose that as the best time for immunizations.

Adults are not better off.[63] Flu shots are recommended for the elderly and for younger adults with histories of respiratory problems, yet are obtained by a minority. The fact that a shot has to be obtained every year for the particular strain at risk means that this vaccine is more challenging to market than one-time or occasional booster shots. People vary widely in their attitudes about flu shots, where childhood immunizations are almost universally accepted.[64]

In general, adults are poorly aware of what immunizations or boosters they need, and providers are spotty at checking and reminding them.[65] Many adults have little or no established relationship with a physician, though a survey of ED patients found them very interested in prevention.[66] Managed care, by promoting stronger relationships with primary physicians, can greatly improve on past track records in immunization of adults.

Yet adults who were immunized in one case were found to have 43% fewer sick days, with ROI ratios of $1.60:1 based on saved medical expenses and $4.69:1 based on less absenteeism, for a total ROI ratio of $6.29:1.[67] Another employer saved $117 per employee per year, reducing influenza and pneumonia hospitalizations by 48% and 57%.[68] Another reviewed national studies and found an average ROI ratio of $8.80:1, with its own program achieving a ratio of $48.00:1.[69]

Examples

On the plus side, childhood immunizations have been a popular subject for community collaborations. In one case a hospital, physician, and insurer coalition significantly increased immunizations through a direct mail and media campaign.[70] A door-to-door campaign involving neighborhood volunteers increased the proportion of children immunized by 150%.[71] CIGNA offered parents an incentive and increased the proportion of children with all immunizations from 65% to 80% among HMO members, from 15% to 51% among indemnity insurance members.[72]

Making it easier for parents to get immunizations also helps. A mobile van bringing immunization to where children lived helped in one case.[73] Giving shots in schools and community centers helped in another.[74] In Tampa, Florida, Kiwanis and public health departments combined to bring shots to children in public housing.[75] Hospitals have achieved high immunization rates by offering shots at the worksite; one achieved 95% to 100% success.[76]

Checking records and reminding parents of immunizations due (and reminding their physicians as well) worked for LifeGuard Health Plan in California.[77] Harvard Community Health Plan (Massachusetts) increased immunization penetration from 24% to 83% with a combination of reminder postcards and notes on patient charts.[78] MetLife used a six-year schedule of immunizations sent to parents to promote immunization levels.[79] In a community-wide effort, a collaboration of HMOs, hospitals, health departments, and pediatricians, with the help of McDonald's, promoted child immunization.[80]

Concerns and Barriers

Aside from hindrances already mentioned, there are relatively few difficulties in the idea of immunization. Some health plans' benefit packages fail to cover all immunizations, though in one case getting a vaccine covered increased immunizations by only 17%.[81] One HMO was the subject of "bashing" for refusing to *promote* the use of a new chicken pox vaccine. It argued that it was better for people to get chicken pox as children and gain natural immunity rather than rely on unproved vaccine that might lead to them catching the disease as adults when it is much more serious. Critics insisted the plan was simply trying to save money.[82]

Suggestions

As with other health promotion efforts, immunizations need a combination of motivation, capability, and consciousness raising. While they are simple enough and low cost, often free, the general motivation level seems low, and modest barriers, as well as forgetfulness, conspire to hold down success rates.[83]

Virtually everyone can help: hospitals can ask patients in the ED, outpatient departments, and inpatient units to raise their awareness and can offer shots to the general community. Health plans can at least include immunizations as covered benefits and should find ways of working with other interested parties, including their competitors, to promote higher immunization levels.[84] By multiplying the locations where consumers can get vaccines, sponsors can greatly increase success, though this may complicate recordkeeping.

Safety

Safety covers a wide range of behaviors, from one-time steps such as turning down the thermostat on the water heater to repetitious and continuing habits such as wearing cycle helmets, seat belts, and life jackets. In some cases these steps are truly primary prevention, avoiding morbidity altogether. In many cases, they merely reduce the seriousness of injury, more like secondary prevention.

Safety at work technically falls under disability management and is certainly a major focus for employers and workers compensation insurance companies. Safety on the highways is a major public focus. Safety in the home and in recreational activities is primarily the responsibility of consumers. One of the greatest challenges in safety is the enormous number of behaviors that can be either safe or unsafe. It is virtually impossible to list them, much less remember them when appropriate (Exhibit 21–5).

Problem and Potential

The National Health Interview Survey identified a rate of 23.8 "injury episodes" per 100 people per year, a total of 58.6 million such episodes in the United States, leading to 672 million restricted activity days, an average of 2.7 per person per year. Of these episodes, 39% occurred at home, 19% on the road, 11% at work, and the remainder in a wide range of locations.[85] Home risks are found in every room, on stairs, in electrical equipment, in the yard, and in the garage.[86] Roughly one child in five experiences an injury requiring medical attention each year; children are involved in roughly 400,000 bicycle accidents a year.[87]

Safe behavior can make a significant difference. The wearing of motorcycle helmets, mandated by law in California, cut fatalities by 37.5% among drivers and 69.7% among passengers.[88] In Texas, a similar law cut head-related injuries by 52.9% and fatalities by 57.0%.[89] Training consumers in safe driving has substantially reduced accidents, in one case cutting claims from 2.8 million to 1.3 million with the same number of drivers.[90]

With an estimated 2.3 million hospital admissions due to trauma each year in the United States, and 142,500 deaths, providers have long been aware of the costs of unsafe behavior.[91] Auto accidents alone cost $53 billion a year in health care and lost/replaced productivity. Estimates are that truly safe driving could save $50,000 for every million miles driven.[92]

Concerns and Barriers

With enormous potential for savings in health expenditures and both quantity and quality of life available through safety, we are far from realizing much of it. Providers have certainly lacked the financial incentive to prevent trauma in the past under FFS financing, though they have been active in promoting safety as part of their mission. Payers have always been at risk but have concentrated more on worker safety, by and large, where their risk and potential savings are at least more concentrated.

Many safety promotion ideas run up against champions of personal freedom, as with motorcycle helmets, where one of Colorado's US Senators refused to wear a helmet. People find it difficult to remember all the safe things to do or may feel that the risk to them is too low to worry about. Teenage males are easily the worst offenders in recognizing or at least preparing for danger. There are many activities that we engage in so rarely that we are simply not prepared; others we engage in so often that we may forget the risks.

Safety is also subject to one of the fundamental problems in demand improvement—the tendency of many people to see bad things that happen as purely a

Exhibit 21–5 Safety

PROBLEMS / POTENTIAL	✗ NUMBER OF OCCURRENCES & COST OF ACCIDENTS A SIGNIFICANT COST
EXAMPLES	✗ HOSPITALS CAN CONDUCT SAFETY PROMOTION PROGRAMS ✗ COMMUNITY EFFORTS (SUCH AS MADD) CAN INCREASE AWARENESS AND REDUCE ACCIDENTS ✗ TRAINING PROGRAMS IN USE OF EQUIPMENT CAN REDUCE ACCIDENTS
CONCERNS	✗ FEE-FOR-SERVICE ARRANGEMENTS NOT CONDUCIVE TO PROMOTING SAFETY ✗ SAFETY OFTEN CLASHES WITH DESIRE FOR PERSONAL FREEDOM (E.G., MOTORCYCLE HELMETS) ✗ ACCIDENTS SEEN AS RANDOM AND BEYOND PERSONAL CONTROL, SO PEOPLE DON'T ENGAGE IN SAFE BEHAVIOR
ADVICE	✗ CONSISTENTLY REMIND PEOPLE TO BE CAREFUL IN THEIR WORK ✗ COMMUNITY PARTNERSHIPS ARE OFTEN EFFECTIVE IN PROMOTING SAFE BEHAVIOR

matter of chance, totally beyond their control. The more we attribute injuries to external factors, the less we will do to prevent them. The combination of self-responsibility and self-efficacy is at least as important to safety as it is to good health and utilization in general.

It is also subject to the same infrequency effect that applies to immunizations. Having engaged in a familiar activity so long without mishap, we may underestimate the risk. In one sense the public media attention given to accidents may counteract this tendency, though it may also make accidents seem inevitable to some.

Social advocacy campaigns promoting awareness of safety issues do not always change behavior. A campaign promoting turning down settings on water heaters to prevent scalding produced demonstrably higher awareness, but very few people did anything about it.[93] It may be more effective to pass a law requiring lower settings on water heater thermostats, making manufacturers responsible versus consumers.[94]

The issue of who should take responsibility is common in safety. Auto makers can install seat belts, but consumers must still put them on; air bags demand nothing of consumers, though they have caused serious injury to children not properly prepared. As legal liability is increasingly extended to manufacturers and commercial establishments, consumers may be getting the message that others are responsible for ensuring their safety and that they can sue whenever they are injured because someone else is bound to be responsible.

Examples

Hospitals have long been promoters of safety in the media, perhaps combining mission and public relations intentions. One rehabilitation hospital promoted water safety, including warnings against unsafe diving that too often results in serious head injury.[95] Kaiser and Group Health of Puget Sound have promoted summer safety, warning against bee stings, poison ivy, sunburn, Lyme disease, fireworks, and the variety of hazards encountered in warm weather when school is out.[96]

In one city, Mothers against Drunk Driving, local churches, police, and media implemented a campaign against auto and bicycle accidents as well as guns and domestic violence after a 38% increase in trauma cases at the local hospital in just one year.[97] Employers and insurers have promoted the wearing of seat belts by reducing the benefits for those involved in accidents who were not wearing them. Generally education in specific safety skills, such as driving or social advocacy to promote safe behaviors, are the preferred approaches.

Suggestions

As with immunization, safety appears to need a full-fledged $I = MC^2$ approach. Even with the clear personal advantages to consumers, they seem to require added motivation. Safe behavior should be made easier than unsafe behavior, wherever possible. Consumers may need to be researched to discover why they find unsafe behavior more convenient, or even more enjoyable, with steps taken to reverse the competitive advantages that unsafe behavior enjoys.

Constant reminders are likely to be even more necessary in safety, given the myriad of things to remember and the frequency with which some behaviors must be practiced.[98] As with immunization, a wide variety of partners ought to be available for specific initiatives—not only all risk-sharing stakeholders but police and fire departments, public health and community organizations, media, and social service organizations. The benefits to consumers and society are so great that many should be willing to help.

RISK REDUCTION

In most cases the "risk" that is to be reduced is a health risk, hence health risk assessments or appraisals (HRAs) are commonly available products (the questionnaire or survey form) and services (which include analysis of the survey and reports of results). It is equally important, however, particularly for sponsors, to think in terms of utilization risks and expenditure risks.

Health risks relate to the risks of certain behaviors to the health status and life expectancy of consumers; reducing those risks may also reduce utilization and expenditures, though that may take a long time, up to decades for some risks. Utilization risks involve behaviors that are associated with higher probability of utilization of services by an individual and higher actual use in the population segment characterized by those behaviors. Expenditure risks address the same behaviors but look at the relative costs of such utilization as well.

There are typically two distinct factors covered in risk appraisals/assessments: risky behaviors and dangerous health status measures. It is wise to address both when determining risk, since both separately affect the likelihood of mortality and morbidity, utilization, and expenditure. For this discussion, however, we will address only health, utilization, and expenditure risks that arise from consumer behaviors. Risks related to health status measures, including specific diagnoses, will be addressed in the final section of this chapter on early detection.

(It should be noted that health risk measures have an equally important role in determining capitation payment levels. While payments are typically adjusted for age and sex, they would be better if adjusted for health status and risk. This would eliminate built-in incentives for health plans and providers to seek to avoid attracting sick members and patients. It would also provide incentives and resources useful in disease management for sicker members of populations.)

Problem and Potential

When HRAs are used for consumer populations, they typically find that a significant portion of that population is at risk. In most cases the more risk factors that are addressed, the more risks are found. It has been argued that 50% to 70% of all diseases are caused or at least stimulated by poor health behaviors, such as smoking, poor diet, sedentary lifestyles, and alcohol and drug abuse.[99] On the plus side, it has also been argued that the risks of heart disease can be reduced to virtually zero by eliminating risky behaviors[100] (Exhibit 21–6).

In practice, one employer was able to cut its medical insurance claims in half by reducing risky behaviors.[101] Another was able to increase the portion of its employees in the low-risk category from 73% to 85% in just six months.[102] The 3M Company found that reducing health risks also increased productivity.[103] When consumers reform their health risk behaviors and maintain healthy behaviors instead, the payoff continues indefinitely, while sponsor investment is likely to lessen.[104]

When it used risk assessment and followed it up with efforts to reform members' behaviors, Group Health Management Association (GHMA) found it saved $65 for every member screened.[105] A large financial firm compared two groups of its employees, one having received a risk appraisal, a computer-generated report and recommendations, and personal counseling on better behavior, while the other was "untreated" as a control group. The "treated" group significantly improved on most risk measures, far more than the controls.[106]

While utilization and expenditure risks are addressed far less often, it has proven possible to identify those whose behavior or condition makes them more likely to use expensive services in the near term. One analysis identified in one year the 30% of the population who would cost 60% of health care expenditures in the following year.[107] Another traced low- and high-risk segments and found that when low-risk consumers stayed low, their expenditures increased only $72 per year; when low risks reverted to high, their expenditures went up by $530. If high risks stayed high, their expenditures increased $789 per year, while if they reformed to low risk, their expenditures dropped by $781.[108]

Concerns and Barriers

Reforming consumer health behavior is by no means a simple matter. Teenagers and many adults are likely to view many unhealthy behaviors as manifestations of individual freedom and rebellion against authority. Many men may feel that certain unhealthy behaviors are proof of their macho masculinity and that healthy behaviors are for wimps.[109]

A study by the University of California at Los Angeles (UCLA) Center for Health Care Policy Research found that physicians rarely even ask patients about unhealthy behaviors, much less aggressively strive to reform them.[110] When Kaiser of Colorado sent out HRA surveys to its members, many argued that this violated their privacy, fearing the information would be used by the plan or their employers against them.[111]

Consumers are often unsure what is risky and what is healthy behavior. The labels seem to change by the minute as new studies are published. They may ob-

Exhibit 21–6 Risk Reduction

PROBLEMS / POTENTIAL	X WHEN HEALTH RISK APPRAISALS USED, FIND THAT SIGNIFICANT PORTION OF POPULATION AT RISK X OFTEN SMALL LIFESTYLE CHANGES REAP GREAT REWARDS IN TERMS OF DELAYED HEALTH CARE COSTS
EXAMPLES	X HEALTH RISK APPRAISALS VERY USEFUL TO BRING INFORMATION TO CONSUMERS X SCHOOL PROGRAMS CAN MAKE HEALTHY LIVING HABITUAL EARLY SO DON'T HAVE TO REFORM
CONCERNS	X CONSUMER LACK OF AWARENESS & UNCONCERN GREATEST BARRIERS TO CHANGING BEHAVIOR X PROVIDERS OFTEN DO NOT AGGRESSIVELY TARGET CONSUMER BEHAVIOR CHANGE AS GOAL X SOCIAL ADVOCACY VERY EFFECTIVE IN CHANGING ATTITUDES BUT NOT BEHAVIOR
ADVICE	X HRAS USEFUL IN IDENTIFYING AREAS THAT NEED ATTENTION X INCENTIVES ARE EFFECTIVE IN ENCOURAGING BEHAVIOR CHANGE X SPONSORS SHOULD PAY ATTENTION TO THE "PAY-OFFS" FOR RISKY BEHAVIOR, THEN TAILOR INCENTIVES X DIARIES, PERSONAL COMMITMENT & OTHER VOLUNTARY PARTICIPATION IN PROGRAMS EFFECTIVE IN SUPPORTING BEHAVIOR CHANGE

tain great enjoyment from the most unhealthy behaviors and feel that healthy alternatives are difficult or simply no fun. They may not understand the risks of present behaviors or the advantages of new behaviors or may not believe the risks and rewards apply to them.[112]

Many social advocacy and health communications efforts have been shown to have significant impact on consumer knowledge and attitudes toward specific behavior but little impact on the prevalence of the behavior itself.[113] For many of the unhealthiest behaviors, such as smoking and alcohol abuse, there is more advertising that promotes the "bad" behavior than communications that promote the "good."[114]

Reforming health risk behavior means making permanent changes in habits that may have persisted for decades. Relapse is common (e.g., 90% to 95% of consumers who reform their dietary habits so as to lose weight relapse and gain back the weight within a few years, many in one year or less).[115] Smokers wanting to quit average three unsuccessful tries before succeeding.[116]

For sponsors, the return on investment from health behavior improvement tends to be far into the future compared to the effects of many other demand improvement efforts.[117] The attention given to health risks can increase the use of health services by raising consumer sensitivity to their health.[118] Society has been trying to eliminate some behaviors, such as drug use, violence, and crime, for generations, and has failed. Do we know well enough how to achieve behavior improvements?

Examples

Health, utilization, and expenditure risks must first be identified in the population of concern. CIGNA has conducted HRAs for its employees, for example.[119] Computers have been used to conduct interviews, though participants failed to respond by changing their behavior.[120] The CDC offers a standard HRA survey form.[121] Checkup Centers of America conducts surveys, sending out reports and advice to participants.[122] Physicians or their office staff can use hand-held computers with built-in HRA software to survey their patients.[123] Hospitals survey their patients and the general public.[124]

Health risk behaviors have been the subject of school-based programs to get children started off on the right foot rather than try to reform them later.[125] The SeniorFit program uses the SF-36 survey form to obtain seniors' perceptions of their overall health and functional status.[126] The Palo Alto Medical Foundation used a restricted access web site for its health risk surveys.[127] The Child Health and Illness Profile Adolescent Edition includes questions on 20 domains relevant to younger populations.[128]

The Healthtrac program combines HRA items with stages of readiness questions to identify those who are ready to reform, as well as those who should.[129] Customer Potential Management calculates "health age" versus chronological age to give consumers a measure of how they compare to their peers.[130] Other HRAs include questions to identify consumers' health interests as well as behaviors.[131]

Suggestions

The purpose of programs that identify health, utilization, and expenditure risks in populations is not simply to gain knowledge. The HRA is only the first part of initiatives that aim to stimulate improvements in consumer behavior. The HRA should also be used to determine the types and amounts of change achieved over time. Utilization and expenditure changes should be tracked so as to help sponsors determine their return on investment, while reports of health behavior and status changes, life expectancy, or health age tell consumers how they have benefited.

Incentives are frequently used in risk reduction to encourage consumers to complete and return HRA surveys[132] as well as to reduce specific identified risks.[133] One program found that getting consumers to make a bet with themselves or a friend of as little as $40 achieved 97% success in risk reduction compared to only 20% success without the bet.[134]

Sponsors interested in reforming consumer behavior are advised to learn what it is that consumers gain from unhealthy behaviors, so as to have a basis for devising a better offer. Including questions that indicate consumer interests, capabilities, and readiness to change can help sponsors focus on those most likely to respond.[135] Personal counseling, in addition to printed reports and recommendations for change, helps to achieve new behavior patterns.[136]

Consumers may gain additional motivation for behavior change by appealing to their desire for better control over their health, as well as better health, per se.[137] Programs should be tailored to specific lifestyle segments[138] or, ideally, should be customized to individuals, rather than using a one-size-fits-all approach to specific behavior changes; customized communications achieved a 23% success rate in one case versus 9% for mass communications.[139]

Changes in behavior can be made easier by promoting perceived self-efficacy in general and by reducing "triggers" in the environment.[140] Making healthier foods more available in the company cafeteria can help promote better diets, for example.[141] Offering multiple options for better behavior, as well as multiple approaches to behavior change, can improve overall success rates.[142] Preserving in consumers the sense that they have choices and are in control can reduce concerns that they are being manipulated or coerced.

Consumers who commit to reducing their risks should be encouraged to set realistic goals, with frequent monitoring of stages of success.[143] Substitutes for enjoyable activities should be sought rather than force the giving up of enjoyable but unhealthy habits.[144] Support groups and family involvement can help make changes easier, as well as add peer influence.[145]

Personal diaries can be useful in reminding consumers of the changes they are trying to make, maintaining their consciousness as well as giving them a basis for evaluating and rewarding themselves.[146] Sponsors can partner with each other and with community organizations and media to promote healthier behaviors for everyone.[147] They can use triage/call center programs to conduct surveys and remind consumers of specific behavior changes they should make.[148]

Participation in both assessments and specific behavior change efforts should be voluntary. Frequent, short communications to promote and remind consumers of behavior changes are likely to work better than one-time, lengthy "lectures."[149] Combining specific changes with efforts to promote self-efficacy and physical, mental, and spiritual "fitness" can add to the effects of both.[150]

EARLY DETECTION

Here we define early detection to include all efforts aimed at identifying conditions among consumers that can be better managed by themselves and by sponsors if known as early as possible. Efforts to identify such conditions may include HRA surveys, where they ask consumers to report conditions already diagnosed that sponsors may not be aware of or symptoms that could lead to an earlier diagnosis. Health fairs and screening events addressing multiple conditions as well as disease-specific checkups and screenings are part of early detection as well (Exhibit 21–7).

While most discussions of early detection focus on a single condition (e.g., mammography for breast cancer; weight, body mass, and skinfold tests for obesity), we will discuss the problem and potential, concerns and barriers, and suggestions in general terms, counting on what has been learned in specific examples to have wider applicability.

Problem and Potential

Just as there is a wide variety of risky behaviors that can be reduced, so there is a myriad of conditions that might be detected through self-reporting or clinical testing. The first challenge is to identify those conditions whose identification by sponsors can make a significant difference to subsequent developments affecting the health of consumers and use of or expenditures for health services.

In general, the identification of chronic conditions such as hypertension, diabetes, and asthma, which are good prospects for disease management, may be achieved through self-reporting in HRA surveys, through sharing of medical record information by providers, or through early detection via clinical screening. With many conditions likely to be unknown to consumers who have them (e.g., diabetes, hypertension), it is probable that a combination of approaches will be needed to get a complete picture of the incidence and prevalence of important conditions in any given population.

Identifying consumers with chronic conditions should always be accompanied by referral to providers for their part in disease management, in addition to empowering consumers to carry out their role. Detection can only begin the process, and it does not automatically follow that consumers will seek provider attention,

Exhibit 21–7 Early Detection

PROBLEMS / POTENTIAL	X Number of conditions can be discovered through simple clinical testing
	X Early detection of chronic conditions can enhance health as well as save resources
	X Clinical screenings increase consumer awareness of possible conditions and risks of unhealthy behavior
EXAMPLES	X Mobile vans & on-site screening makes the process easy & accessible
	X Insurance packages as well as gift certificates help people get past cost barrier
	X Multi-media as well as specific prompts for checkups increase response
CONCERNS	X Risk of false results increases concern about efficacy of inexpensive tests
	X Professionals not in agreement about how often screening should be performed
	X Consumers are often undermotivated to get screenings done
ADVICE	X Restrict to those at high enough risk to make worth time & resource investment
	X Use "buddy systems" to encourage people to participate
	X Promote general awareness through community partners & social advocacy

much less change their lifestyle appropriately. In one case consumers picked up 57,000 colorectal cancer detection kits but returned only 29,619 (53%) for analysis. While 3.9% of the analyses identified and reported problems, only 93% of the notified consumers sought attention for them.[151]

Early detection can make a significant difference for most conditions commonly identified through screening. Breast cancer caught early, for example, averaged $10,000 to $15,000 in health care costs, where caught late it averaged $150,000 to $175,000. A mammography promotion effort increased the proportion of cases caught early from 48% to 70%.[152]

When Bull Information Systems of Billerica, Massachusetts, conducted a survey of its employees, it found that 39% had high cholesterol levels, 20% were overweight, 15% had high blood pressure, 19% of women had abnormal Pap smears, 21% had diabetes, and 26% reported low back pain.[153] Each sponsor must conduct its own analysis to learn the prevalence and distribution of problems it must deal with, but chances are there are many. Such analyses can be used to identify positive health (e.g., fitness, stress management, spiritual health) as well.

Some may argue that some of the conditions identified through surveys and screenings are properly called "conditions" (e.g., obesity, high cholesterol, hypertension) rather than "diseases." Such a distinction is only useful if it makes a difference to how sponsors and consumers respond to them. One difference may be whether medications are useful in controlling them, or whether consumers must change their behavior to reduce their impact, or both. With medications possible allies in weight management, smoking cessation, and other health risks, this distinction may not always make a real difference.

Most clinical screenings discover a number of conditions previously unknown to consumers, as is their purpose.[153] The challenge to sponsors is to complete the "conversion chain": consumers participate in screening, return surveys or specimens, obtain reports of results, read and understand them correctly, seek follow-up care where indicated, and comply with medications and lifestyle changes as appropriate. Providers, in turn, must play their essential roles in providing, prescribing, and promoting.

Unlike most of the other health improvement initiatives, early detection has been used by providers to generate additional FFS volume. Problems detected by mammography generate biopsy and surgery volume as well as radiation and chemotherapy utilization, for example. As with fitness centers serving dual purposes, providers have found that health fairs and other screening programs serve equally well under capitation payment.

Examples

Making screening convenient has helped increase the numbers of consumers screened. Employers have made screening available at the worksite, for example.[154] Hospitals have developed mobile vans that can bring screening to where consumers live or worship.[155] Making screening convenient by placing a permanent facility in a shopping mall has also helped.[156]

Reducing the costs of screening also helps. Mammography prices were cut to as low as $39, for example, which together with an ad campaign boosted the number of women getting mammograms from 4,199 to 11,651 in one case.[157] Offering gift certificates is a way that people can encourage friends and family members to get specific tests.[158] Covering all useful screening under health plan benefit packages is certainly a good way to eliminate financial barriers.

Enhancing the value of screening to consumers is another approach. In mammography, for example, providing prompt reports when no problems are found or combining with stereotactic biopsy capability can significantly reduce the anxiety of the women screened. Providing results of screening immediately can greatly magnify perceived value among consumers.[159]

Prompting consumers to get general or specific tests is almost always an essential part of early detection. In one case a statewide health communications effort increased the proportion of eligible women getting a mammogram from 58% to 81%.[160] The use of multiple media and frequent repetition helps, with targeted follow-up for those who fail to respond to initial prompts.[161] In one case, repeated reminders, including postcards and phone calls to nonresponders, increased response from 28% to 42%, with phone calls doubling the impact achieved by mail.[162]

Concerns and Barriers

The two biggest concerns with early detection are the risks of false results and of useless findings.[163] Some screens, such as exercise/stress tests for cardiac problems and mammography, have false positive rates as high as 80% among low-risk populations, meaning that large numbers of consumers will be frightened and will use unnecessary health services in follow-ups to confirm the diagnosis or to treat the nonexistent problem. The prostate-specific antigen test for prostate cancer has a 60% false positive rate and a 20% false negative rate, creating problems both ways.[164]

Useless results are those that can make no difference to the progress or outcomes of the condition found because they were detected early. For sponsors, problems that will cost more when detected early add to their financial risks. Genetic conditions, HIV/AIDS, and other conditions may be detected, for example, but create risks that consumers will be unable to find insurance or fears that employers will discharge them.[165]

There is anything but unanimity of opinion among providers and payers as to who should be screened and how often or even who should do the screening.[166] Should mammograms be given to women when they reach 40 or not until they reach 50; annually or every other year? Should women past 70 years have them at all? For providers who invested in their own equipment to do screening, having too much capacity can lead to higher prices, since volume per machine will be less, and perhaps of poor quality as well, where providers do not get enough practice.[167]

Consumers are often undermotivated to be screened. They may have low levels of anxiety regarding the likelihood of finding anything or such high levels that they would rather remain ignorant. They may fear X-rays or blood sticks, for example, or the pain, discomfort, or embarrassment of some tests.[168] The most frequently cited barriers are the lack of referral or encouragement by their physicians[169] and out-of-pocket costs.[170] These may be more rationale than reason, of course.

Suggestions

Screenings of many kinds have to be restricted to those at high enough risk to make them worthwhile. Mammography and prostate screens are recommended only for those whose age or family history puts them at above-average risk. Some tests make sense as routine requirements for those of a given age and gender (e.g., Pap smears, blood pressure, bone density), while others are aimed at those whose lifestyles or living conditions put them at high risk (e.g., HIV/AIDS, blood lead levels for children in poor housing). The federal government has published a resource book describing which screening tests make sense under what circumstances.[171]

Address each of the $I = MC^2$ factors, as with other health improvement initiatives. Enhance value to consumers, where possible, to improve motivation, primarily through prompt reporting, especially of negative results, which are often left for last.[172] Make obtaining screens as easy and convenient as possible, such as the osteoporosis screenings offered at Walgreens Drug Stores.[173]

Enlist everyone who can help motivate and prompt consumers. "Buddy systems," where friends remind friends, have worked in many cases.[174] Asking those who have been screened before to bring a friend who has not can motivate both.[175] Securing the cooperation of physicians in reminding, even writing a prescription for screens, can play a major role.[176]

Using community partners to promote general awareness, in addition to focused efforts, can achieve synergies and economies. In one case Blockbuster Video agreed to carry free breast cancer videos in its stores to aid in a community campaign.[177] Health plans and providers can promote covered checkups in their newsletters. Employers have easy access to employees to prompt them toward clinical detection efforts.

REFERENCES

1. R.W. Whitmer, "Why We Should Foster Health Promotion," *Business & Health* 11, no. 13 (1993):74, 68.
2. D. Anspaugh, et al., "Risk Factors for Cardiovascular Disease among Exercising versus Nonexercising Women," *American Journal of Health Promotion* 10, no. 3 (1996):171–174.

3. "Exercise for the Ages," *Consumer Reports on Health* 8, no. 7 (1996):73–76.

4. C. Bailey, *Smart Exercise: Burning Fat, Getting Fit* (Boston, MA: Houghton Mifflin, 1994).

5. P. Jaret, "Stay Physically Active To Keep Brain Drain at Bay," *The Denver Post,* 12 August 1996, 1F, 2F.

6. T. Collingwood, "Fitness Programs," in *Health Promotion in the Workplace,* 2d ed., eds. M. O'Donnell and J. Harris (Albany, NY: Delmar, 1994), 240–270.

7. T. Pipp, "Lazy Lifestyle May Affect Boomers' Future Health," *The Denver Post,* 31 January 1997, 27A, 30A.

8. "How To Start an Exercise Habit You Can Stick With," *Consumer Reports on Health* 5, no. 7 (1993):69–71.

9. G. Godin, et al., "Differences in Perceptual Barriers to Exercise between High and Low Intenders," *American Journal of Health Promotion* 8, no. 4 (1994):279–285.

10. "Address Awareness Issues To Improve Wellness Program Use, Value," *Wellness Program Management Advisor* 1, no. 3 (1996):5.

11. The Health Project, *1993 Awards* (New York, NY: Tenneco Life Gain, 1993).

12. J. Robison and M. Rogers, "Impact of Behavior Management Programs on Exercise Adherence," *American Journal of Health Promotion* 9, no. 5 (1995):379–382.

13. "Focus on Fitness," *Modern Healthcare,* 8 April 1996, 38–42.

14. P. Gapen, "But Wait, There's More . . ." *Managed Healthcare* 4, no. 6 (1994):48–51.

15. B. Marcus, et al., "Using the Stages of Change Model To Increase the Adoption of Physical Activity among Community Participants," *American Journal of Health Promotion* 6, no. 6 (1992):424–429.

16. J. Pickens, "'Health Steps' Valuable Lesson in Fitness Programming," *Health Care Marketing Report* 11, no. 12 (1993):12, 13.

17. "'Inn Shape' Program Takes Fitness on the Road," *Employee Health & Fitness* 17, no. 2 (1995):19, 20.

18. M. Battagliola, "One Company on the Wellness Frontier," in *The State of Health Care in America* (Montvale, NJ: Business & Health Magazine, 1995), 18.

19. "Panel Pushes Exercise," *The Denver Post,* 21 December 1995, 12A.

20. R. Naas, "Health Promotion Programs Yield Long-Term Savings," *Business & Health* 10, no. 13 (1992):41.

21. "Does Exercise Boost Immunity?" *Consumer Reports on Health* 7, no. 4 (1995):37–39.

22. "Why Do We Exercise?" *Quirk's Marketing Research Review* 9, no. 8 (1995):30–32.

23. R. Strauss and D. Yen, "How an Expert Corporate Fitness Program Might Be Designed," *Health Care Supervisor* 10, no. 3 (1992):40–55.

24. "Putting Wellness on the Fast Track for the Info Highway," *Employee Health & Fitness* 16, no. 7 (1994):92–94.

25. "Name the Champion . . . and Other Fin Stuff To Keep Participants Motivated," *Health Promotion Practitioner,* February 1996, 3.

26. "Short Exercise Routines Add Up," *Employee Health & Fitness* 18, no. 2 (1996 Supplement).

27. *1993 Awards* (New York, NY: The Health Project, Coors Brewing Co., 1994).

28. D. Andrus and R. Paul, "The Challenge of Marketing Wellness Programs to Small versus Large Firm Employees," *Health Marketing Quarterly* 13, no. 1 (1995):87–103.

29. M. Bricklin, "Better than a Sweatband, Wear a Smile," *Prevention* 48, no. 4 (1996):21, 22.

30. G. Gutfeld, "60 Days to a New Shape," *Prevention* 46, no. 2 (1994):48–54, 117, 118.

31. Naas, "Health Promotion Programs," 41.

32. M. Bricklin, "The Power of Proactive Prevention," *Prevention* 46, no. 2 (1994):45, 46, 116.

33. E. Brown, "How Cost-Effective Are Wellness Programs?" *Managed Healthcare* 5, no. 1 (1995):40–42.

34. *1993 Awards* (New York, NY: The Health Project) Ventura County, CA.

35. *The Little Black Book* (Boulder, CO: Bottom Line Personal, 1996).

36. C. Petersen, "Employers, Providers Are Partners in Health," *Managed Healthcare* 5, no. 1 (1995):36.

37. Program at Provenant Health Partners with Channel 9 TV Station, Denver, CO.

38. M. Golen and T. Hanlon, "Yearning To Be Stress-Free," *Prevention* 47, no. 3 (1995):74–81.

39. "Work Is World's No. 1 Stressor, But Here Are Suggested Strategies," *Employee Health & Fitness* 17, no. 2 (1995):13–16.

40. Golen and Hanlon, "Yearning," 74–81.

41. "Saving Money by Reducing Stress," *Harvard Business Review* 72, no. 6 (1994):12.

42. R. Herron, "The Impact of the Transcendental Meditation Program on Government Payments to Physicians in Quebec," *American Journal of Health Promotion* 10, no. 3 (1996):208–216.

43. C. Scott and D. Jaffe, "Stress and Stress Management in the Workplace," in *Health Promotion in the Workplace,* 2d ed., eds. M. O'Donnell and J. Harris (Albany, NY: Delmar, 1994), 390–427.

44. E. Brown, "Stress Test," *Managed Healthcare* 4, no. 11 (1994):28–30.

45. M. Bryant, "Testing EAPs for Coordination," *Business & Health* 9, no. 8 (1991):20–24.

46. "Saving Money," 12.

47. Scott and Jaffe, "Stress and Stress Management," 390–427.

48. "Address Awareness Issues," 10.

49. "Personal Problems: Employee Snapshots," *Business & Health* 14, no. 2 (1996):64.

50. "These 'Stressbusters' Fight on Two Fronts at Once," *Employee Health & Fitness* 16, no. 8 (1994):106–108.

51. L. Seidl, "The Value of Spiritual Health," *Health Progress* 74, no. 7 (1993):48–50.

52. B. Seaward, "Reflections on Human Spirituality for the Worksite," *American Journal of Health Promotion* 9, no. 3 (1995):165–168.

53. V. Frankl, *Man's Search for Meaning* (Boston: Beacon Press, 1959).

54. M. O'Donnell, "Dimensions of Optimal Health" (Paper presented at The Art and Science of Health Promotion Conference, Colorado Springs, CO, February 27–March 2, 1996).

55. S. Hawks, et al., "Review of Spiritual Health," *American Journal of Health Promotion* 9, no. 5 (1995):371–378.

56. D. Abu-Nasr, "Workplace Chaplains in Demand," *The Denver Post,* 3 February 1997, 1A, 12A.

57. M. Grobman, "Calling the Shots," *Managed Healthcare* 4, no. 5 (1994):34–36.

58. R. Anderson, "Investment in Prevention Is a New Idea in Our 'Pay-Me-Later' Society," *AHA News* 28, no. 20 (1992):6.

59. E. Meszaros, "Safeguarding Our Future," *Managed Healthcare* 5, no. 5 (1995):S10–S15.

60. "Be Wise and Immunize," *Profiles in Health Care Marketing* 56 (1993):40–45.

61. "Benefits Do Not Ensure Immunization," *Health Progress* 75, no. 3 (1994):12.

62. G. Poland, "The Immunization Imperative," *Hospitals & Health Networks,* 20 November 1993, 60.

63. "Programs Give Shot in the Arm to Vaccination Efforts," *Healthcare Demand Management* 2, no. 3 (1996):46–48.

64. R. Oliver and P. Berger, "A Path Analysis of Preventative Health Care Decision Models," *Journal of Consumer Research* 6, no. 3 (1979):113–122.

65. D. Fedson, "Adult Immunization: Summary of the National Vaccine Advisory Committee Report," *JAMA* 272, no. 14 (1994):1133–1139.

66. R. Rodriguez, et al., "Need and Desire for Preventive Care Measures in Emergency Departments Patients," *Annals of Emergency Medicine* 26, no. 5 (1995):615–620.

67. "Flu Shots Make Sense for All Ages," *Business & Health* 13, no. 11 (1995):14.

68. "Mayo Clinic Develops Disease Management Strategy To Handle Capitation," *Healthcare Leadership Review* 14, no. 7 (1995):9, 10.

69. "Issue: Childhood Immunization in Colorado," *Hospitals for Healthy Communities* 2, no. 2 (1995):1, 2.

70. "Be Wise," 40–45.

71. C. Chappell, "Mission Denied, Mission Restored," *Health Progress* 75, no. 1 (1994):68, 69.

72. "CIGNA of Arizona Uses CQI Approach to Immunizations," *Managed Care Quality* 1, no. 9 (1995):108–111.

73. T. Defino, "MCOs Join Health Care Officials To Provide a Shot in the Arm," *Managed Healthcare News* 3, no. 5 (1993):20, 21.

74. D. Kim, "Providers Boost Immunization Efforts," *Modern Healthcare,* 12 September 1994, 76–78.

75. "Mobile Immunity," *Modern Healthcare,* 20 July 1992, 40.

76. R. Brawley, "Improving the Compliance of Military Hospital Staff with Immunization Requirements," in *Clinical Practice Improvement,* eds. S. Horn and D. Hopkins (Washington, DC: Faulkner & Gray, 1994), 247–252.

77. "Immunization Tracking and Reminder System Raises HEDIS Indicator 7 Percent in One Year," *Inside Preventive Care* 2, no. 2 (1996):1, 2.

78. "Incremental Changes Help Flu Shot Program," *Managed Care Quality* 1, no. 10 (1995):124, 125.

79. *MetLife HMO Health Reminder* (Fairfield, CT: Managed Care Services Group, 1993).

80. "A Shot in the Arm," *Profiles in Healthcare Marketing* 11, no. 6 (1995):15–18.

81. P. Short and D. Lefkowitz, "Encouraging Preventive Services for Low Income Children," *Medical Care* 30, no. 9 (1992):766–780.

82. L. Kertesz, "Potshots over Pox Shots?" *Modern Healthcare,* 5 August 1996, 104–106.

83. Brawley, "Improving the Compliance," 247–252.

84. "Programs Give Shot," 46–48.

85. K. Brandenburg, "Nearly 60 Million Injuries Reported in 1990," *The Numbers News,* February 1992, 3.

86. L. Chapman, "Affecting Safety and Risk-Taking Behavior through Wellness," *Employee Health & Fitness* 16, no. 5 (1994):74–76.

87. "Children," *Speaker's Idea File* (Chicago, IL: Ragan Communications, 1993), 2.

88. "Consumers," *Hospitals & Health Networks,* 20 January 1995, 12.

89. N. Fleming and E. Becker, "The Impact of the Texas 1989 Motorcycle Helmet Law on Total and Head-Related Fatalities, Sever Injuries and Overall Injuries," *Medical Care* 30, no. 9 (1992):832–845.

90. "Working Well at CIGNA," *C. Everett Koop National Health Awards 1995* (New York, NY: The Health Project, 1995).

91. M. Levy, et al., "Educating Our Youth To Prevent Central Nervous System Injuries," *American Behavioral Scientist* 38, no. 2 (1994):323–340.

92. "What Car Crashes Could Be Costing You," *Business & Health* 13, no. 9 (1995):10.

93. M. Katcher, "Prevention of Tap Water Scald Burns," *American Journal of Public Health* 77, no. 9 (1987):1195–1197.

94. S. Webne and B. Kaplan, "Preventing Tap Water Scalds: Do Consumers Change Their Present Thermostats?" *American Journal of Public Health* 83, no. 10 (1993):1469, 1470.

95. "3 Seconds from Now . . ." Advertisement by Mississippi Methodist Rehabilitation Center, Jackson, MS, 1992.

96. D. Coleman, "Sun, Fun and Wellness," *Managed Healthcare* 4, no. 7 (1994):36–38.

97. "Injury Prevention Centers Focus on Traffic, Bicycles & Guns," *Inside Preventive Care* 2, no. 3 (1996):1–4.

98. V. Rezis and N. Rezis, "An Analysis of the Value of Marketing to Non-Profit Organizations: The Case of Child Safety," *Health Marketing Quarterly* 11, no. 1/2 (1993):163–189.

99. Whitmer, "Why We Should Foster Health Promotion," 74, 68.

100. K. Napier, "Your Game Plan for Life," *Prevention* 48, no. 4 (1996):101–111.

101. J. Flory, "Employers Explore New Ways To Manage Managed Care," *Strategic Health Care Marketing* 11, no. 7 (1994):8–10.

102. J. Norvell, "Behavioral Health Risk Rating: Health Care Cost Management That Works," *AAPPO Journal* 4, no. 1 (1994):15–19.

103. E. Brown, "How Cost-Effective Are Wellness Programs?" *Managed Healthcare* 5, no. 1 (1995):40–42.

104. J. Leutzinger, et al., "Projecting the Impact of Health Promotion on Medical Costs," *Business & Health* 11, no. 4 (1993):40–44.

105. "GHMA Finds Health Assessment Is Key to Lowering High-Risk Enrollee Costs," *Report on Medical Guidelines & Outcomes Research* 6, no. 13 (1995):5–8.

106. D. Gemson and R. Sloan, "Efficacy of Computerized Health Risk Appraisal as Part of a Periodic Health Examination at the Worksite," *American Journal of Health Promotion* 9, no. 6 (1995):462–466.

107. W. Lynch, et al., "Predicting the Demand for Healthcare," *Healthcare Forum Journal* 39, no. 1 (1996):20–25.

108. W. Lynch, *Demand Management for Healthcare* (Chicago, IL: Strategic Research Institute Conference, 1996).

109. M. Lipman, "Why Men Don't Get It," *Consumer Reports on Health* 8, no. 6 (1996):71.

110. "Women's Health Marked by Their Own High-Risk Behavior and Provider Negligence," *Health Care Strategic Management* 14, no. 1 (1995):8.

111. "Survey by Kaiser Raises Eyebrows," *The Denver Post,* 21 December 1995, 1A, 12A.

112. "25 Trends Shaping the Future of American Business," *The Public Pulse* 8, no. 5 (Special Edition 1993).

113. "For the Record," *Modern Healthcare,* 17 January 1994, 16.

114. C. Goerne, "Don't Blame the Cows," *Marketing News* 26, no. 13 (1992):1, 2.

115. J. Foreyt and G.K. Goodrick, "Impact of Behavior Therapy on Weight Loss," *American Journal of Health Promotion* 8, no. 6 (1994):466–468.

116. N. Sofian, et al., "Tobacco Control and Cessation," in *Health Promotion in the Workplace,* 2d ed., eds. M. O'Donnell & J. Harris (Albany, NY: Delmar, 1994), 342–366.

117. Brown, "How Cost-Effective," 40–42.

118. J. Fries, et al., "Predication of Medical Costs for the Following Year" (unpublished manuscript) (Palo Alto, CA: Stanford University School of Medicine), available through Healthtrac, Palo Alto, CA.

119. S. Aldana, et al., "The Wellness Program of CIGNA Health Care Reduces Employee Health Risks," *American Journal of Health Promotion* 8, no. 5 (1994):388.

120. F. Alemi and P. Higley, "Reaction to 'Talking' Computers Assessing Health Risk," *Medical Care* 33, no. 3 (1995):227–232.

121. C. Petersen, "Sara Lee's Recipe for Wellness," *Managed Healthcare* 4, no. 2 (1994):18–22.

122. "Checkup Centers Take Health Assessments to a New Level," *Healthcare Demand Management* 2, no. 2 (1996):22–27.

123. "Computer System Quizzes Patients about Their Health Risks," *Inside Preventive Care* 1, no. 9 (1995):8.

124. R. Weiss, "Organizations Collaborate To Provide Wellness Programs to Area Businesses," *Health Progress* 76, no. 2 (1995):60, 61.

125. C. Arciti, et al., "Ten Years of Anti-Smoking Programs in Italy," *American Journal of Health Promotion* 9, no. 3 (1995):190–200.

126. E. Alberti and J. Sutton, "Improving Outcomes Reporting in a Senior Wellness Program," in *Clinical Practice Improvement,* eds. S. Horn & D. Hopkins (Washington, DC: Faulkner & Gray, 1994), 237–246.

127. "Patients at California Clinic Test New Internet Application," *Health Data Management* 5, no. 8 (1997):20.

128. "Profile Measures Health of Younger Population," *Inside Preventive Care* 3, no. 6 (1997):8.

129. L. Chapman, "Recognize Serial Feedback Model by Its Versatility," *Employee Health & Fitness* 17, no. 2 (1995):22–24.

130. L. Uttich and G. Dobbins, "The Database Difference," *MPR Exchange* 20, no. 3 (1994):4, 5.

131. "Assessment Program Counsels Patients To Make Lifestyle Improvements," *Inside Preventive Care* 3, no. 1 (1997):1–4.

132. "Survey by Kaiser," 1A, 12A.

133. "Honeywell Gets Preventive with Employee Incentives," *Wellness Program Management Advisor* 1, no. 3 (1996):8, 9.

134. "52 Ways To Lose a Pound a Week," *Prevention* 46, no. 3 (1994):65–73, 126, 127.

135. J. Sheeska and D. Woolcott, "An Evaluation of a Theory-Based Demonstration Worksite Nutrition Promotion Program," *American Journal of Health Promotion* 8, no. 4 (1994):263, 264, 253.

136. Gemson and Sloan, "Efficacy," 462–466.

137. "25 Trends," Special Edition.

138. R. Patterson, "Health Lifestyle Patterns of U.S. Adults," *Medical Benefits* 11, no. 19 (1994):11.

139. M. Campbell, "Preventive Habits Become Pacemaker for Healthy Hearts," *Managed Healthcare* 4, no. 5 (Special Supplement, May 1994):37–40.

140. "Lose Pound after Pound," *Prevention* 48, no. 1 (1996):65–71.

141. K. Glanz and T. Rogers, "Worksite Nutrition Program," *Health Promotion in the Workplace,* 2d ed., eds. M. O'Donnell & J. Harris (Albany, NY: Delmar, 1994), 271–299.

142. L. Breslow, et al., "Development of a Health Risk Appraisal for the Elderly (HRA-E)," *American Journal of Health Promotion* 17, no. 5 (1997):337–343.

143. G. Kaplan and V. Brinkman-Kaplan, "Worksite Weight Management," in *Health Promotion in the Workplace,* 2d ed., eds. M. O'Donnell & J. Harris (Albany, NY: Delmar, 1994), 300–342.

144. "These Seven Keys Can Lead to Successful Weight Loss," *Employee Health & Fitness* 17, no. 2 (1995):Supplement.

145. G.K. Goodrick and J. Foreyt, "Why Treatments for Obesity Don't Last," *Journal of the American Dietetic Association* 91, no. 10 (1991):1243–1247.

146. Kaplan and Brinkman-Kaplan, "Worksite Weight Management," 300–342.

147. E. Wogensen, "New Museum Educates Children about Health, Safety, and Environmental Issues," *Health Care Strategic Marketing* 13, no. 3 (1996):10.

148. Chapman, "Affecting Safety," 74–76.

149. E. Nelson and J. Wasson, "Using Patient-Based Information To Rapidly Redesign Care," *Healthcare Forum Journal* 37, no. 4 (1994):25–29.

150. Kaplan and Brinkman-Kaplan, "Worksite Weight Management," 300–342.

151. T. McGarrity, et al., "Results of a Television-Advertised Public Screening Program for Colo-Rectal Cancer," *Archives of Internal Medicine* 149, no. 1 (1989):140–144.

152. N. Carrera, "Mammographies Increasing, Help Cut Cost of Treating Cancer," *Denver Business Journal,* February 24–March 2, 1995, 3C.

153. "Osteoporosis Breaks with Tradition by Bringing Screening to Worksites," *Inside Preventive Care* 3, no. 5 (1997):1, 2.

154. J. Wechsler, "Employers Offer Breast Cancer Screening for Employees," *Managed Healthcare* 3, no. 11 (1993):50.

155. "Hospital System Hits the Streets for Wellness," *Employee Health & Fitness* 17, no. 9 (1995):102–104.

156. "Mall-Based Mammography Service Reaches Women," *Inside Preventive Care* 1, no. 11 (1996):7.

157. Goodrick and Foreyt, "Why Treatments," 1243–1247.

158. D. Scammons, et al., "The Role of 'Free' Mammograms in Motivating First-Time Screening," *Journal of Ambulatory Care Marketing* 6, no. 1 (1995):59–71.

159. D. King, "Non-Invasive Screening for Coronary Atherosclerosis," *The Next Generation of Health Promotion* (Boston, MA: Institute for International Research Conference, 1995).

160. Carrera, "Mammographies," 3C.

161. S. Hurley, et al., "Effectiveness, Costs and Cost-Effectiveness of Recruitment Strategies for a Mammographic Screening Program To Detect Breast Cancer," *Journal of the National Cancer Institute* 84, no. 11 (1992):855–863.

162. E. King, et al., "Promoting Mammography Use through Progressive Interventions: Is It Effective?" *American Journal of Public Health* 84, no. 1 (1994):104–106.

163. A. Peck, "Controversial Procedure," *Managed Healthcare* 3, no. 9 (1993):21.

164. Lynch, *Demand Management.*

165. C. Petersen, "Managed Care's 'Genetic Code,' " *Managed Healthcare* 4, no. 9 (1994):1, 20–25.

166. "OTA Says Preventive Care without Cost Sharing Does Not Save Money," *Business & Health* 12, no. 4 (1994):14.

167. "The Illogic of Health Care," *Modern Healthcare,* 17 May 1993, 68.

168. I. Gram and S. Slenker, "Cancer Anxiety and Attitudes toward Mammography among Screening Attendees, Non-Attendees and Women Not Invited," *American Journal of Public Health* 82, no. 2 (1992):249–251.

169. P. Eastman, "Breast Cancer Detection Becoming Easier," *AARP Bulletin* 8, no. 8 (1993):1, 20, 21.

170. D. Scannon, et al., "The Role of 'Free' Mammograms," 59–71.

171. K. Griffin, "The Life Savers: 8 Medical Tests You Shouldn't Ignore," *Health* 10, no. 3 (1996):107–112.

172. *Critical Success Factors for Mobile Mammography Services in a Mature Managed Care Environment* (Washington, DC: The Health Care Advisory Board, 1994).

173. "Shoppers Specials on Bone Scans," *Business & Health* 14, no. 7 (1996):8.

174. "Breast Self-Examination Project: Reaching Women Who Are Ignoring the Possibility," *Medical News Report* 3, no. 8 (1993):107–111.

175. *Critical Success Factors.*

176. Eastman, "Breast Cancer Detection," 1, 20, 21.

177. "Video Winner," *Modern Healthcare,* 13 July 1992, 92.

Health Improvement Vendors

American Corporate Health Programs
Exton, PA
— *Worksite Health Promotion,
Prevention*

BBP Center for Health Programs
Waterford, CT
— *Weight/Nutrition, Stress, Smoking*

Center for Advancement of Health
New York, NY

Customer Potential Management
E. Peoria, IL
— *HRAs*

Diet Improvement, Nutrition
Education System
Amherst, NY

"Dump Your Plump"
South Haven, MI
— *Weight Managment*

Employee Managed Care Corp.
[EMC²]
Seattle, WA
— *Lifestyle/Personal Health
Management*

ERS Healthcare Communications
Los Angeles, CA
— *Phone HRAs*

ERIS Survey Systems
Indianapolis, IN
— *HRAs*

Fitness Systems
Minneapolis, MN
— *Fitness Centers*

Greenstone Healthcare Solutions
Kalamazoo, MI
— *Internet HRAs*

Health Awareness, Inc.
Southfield, MI
— *Worksite Wellness*

Health Decisions, International
Golden, CO
— *Call Center Health Promotion*

Health Desk, Corp.
Berkeley, CA
— *HRA Software*

Health Enhancement Systems
Midland, MI
—*Health Promotion Packages*

HealthLine Systems
San Diego, CA
—*Call Center, HRAs, Info Tapes*

Health Management Corp.
Richmond, VA
—*Lifestyle Management*

Health Management Resources
Boston, MA

Health Marketing Solutions
Bainbridge Island, WA
— *"Wellness Challenge"*

Health Promotion Network
Elmhurst, IL

Healtheon Corp.
Palo Alto, CA
—*Software, Internet Information*

Healthtrac
Menlo Park, CA
—*Health Risk Reduction*

Healthtrax
Glastonbury, CT
—*Worksite Fitness, Health Risk Management*

Institute for Wellness Education
Wellesley, MA

Johnson & Johnson Health Care Systems, Health Management Services
Piscataway, NJ
— *"Life for Life," Comprehensive Health Improvement*

Lab One
Lenexa, KS
—*HRA, Screening Profiles*

Loyola University Medical Center
Maywood, IL
—*On-Site HRAs*

Mind/Body Institute
Boston, MA

Mosby Consumer Health
St. Louis, MO
—*Printed, Video Materials, HRAs*

National Center for Health Promotion
Southfield, MI

Optum Health
Golden Valley, MN

Performance & Health through Interactive Technologies
San Diego, CA

SmartTalk
Salt Lake City, UT
—*Call Center Software, Wellness Reminders*

StayWell Health Management Systems
St. Paul, MN
—*Health Promotion*

Summex Corp.
Indianapolis, IN
— *"Health Monitor" (HRA), "Comincents" Wellness Incentives, "Comprevent" Risk Reduction*

Unison Corp.
Denver, CO
—*HRAs, Phone Interventions*

United Healthcare Center for
    Corporate Health
Oakton, VA

Wellbridge Co.
Deerfield, IL
    —*Health & Wellness*

Wellness Councils of America
Omaha, NE

Wellness South
Birmingham, AL
    —*Health Promotion*

Wellsource
Clackamas, OR
    —*Managed Prevention Systems,
    HRAs, Wellness, Population
    Health Management, Health
    Promotion*

Whole Person Associates
Duluth, MN

Wyeth-Ayerst Healthcare Systems

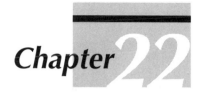

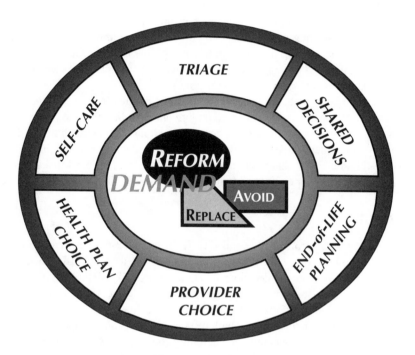

Chapter 22

TRIAGE

SELF-CARE

SHARED DECISIONS

REFORM

DEMAND

AVOID

REPLACE

HEALTH PLAN CHOICE

END-of-LIFE PLANNING

PROVIDER CHOICE

DECISION IMPROVEMENT

Where health improvement is intended to reduce the incidence and prevalence of disease and injury so as to prevent *need* for health care, decision improvement aims at encouraging and enabling consumers to make better *demand* decisions, to avoid avoidable demand, and to select the most appropriate types of unavoidable demand.

As defined in this book, there are six categories of interventions aimed at improving the decisions that consumers make with regard to their consumption of health care: (1) triage, (2) self-care, (3) shared decision making, (4) health plan choice, (5) provider choice, and (6) end-of-life planning. Each is an approach to changing prevailing ways that such decisions are being made.

In the case of triage and self-care, the purpose of interventions is to engage the views of professionals in the decisions consumers make, rather than have them rush or delay seeking care based on their own limited knowledge and skills. In shared decision making the purpose is virtually the opposite: to ensure that the views of consumers are engaged in what otherwise might be provider-dominated decisions that ignore the values of consumers.

In health plan choice, provider choice, and end-of-life planning, the challenge is to empower consumers by both encouraging and enabling them to make the best possible decisions in each of these critical situations. While much of the discussion in each of these three areas relates to reducing expenditures, this should be the hoped-for side effect rather than the explicit objective of such efforts. The aim is to improve consumer choices and cost savings will not always result.

TRIAGE

The term "triage" originally applied to decisions that providers made about who should receive priority in treatment. In this context it means using health care professionals to guide the decisions that consumers make about their own "emergency" situations. In many cases triage programs are what is referred to as managing demand.[1] Many efforts aimed at managing demand started with triage and have expanded to include other challenges, such as health risk identification and reduction (health improvement) and helping patients cope with chronic conditions (disease management), virtually any improvements that can be achieved through a telephone call center.[2]

In this book we define triage as specifically the phone information and counseling services that attempt to intervene in consumer responses to what they perceive as troubling symptoms. The purpose of triage phone programs is to enable consumers to make the best possible choice of what do under whatever circumstances bother them. In some cases the best choice may involve higher intensity and costs than consumers would have made unaided. In most cases it involves lower intensity/cost services, including taking care of the problem themselves.

Problems and Potential

The arguments made for inserting professional knowledge and perspectives into the consumer decision process is that consumers make some horrible decisions on their own. It has been argued that 25% to 50% of all ambulatory care visits made by consumers and 55% of all ED visits are unnecessary.[3] One study concluded that between 50% and 80% of callers to triage services do not need professional attention.[4] Another argued that between 70% and 90% of problems among seniors involved conditions that they themselves or another lay person caregiver could care for.[5] A staff HMO determined that 25% to 44% of all its clinic visits were unnecessary.[6]

Not all these unnecessary visits can be avoided. Some ED visits can only be rerouted to less intense forms of care. Where consumers feel themselves to be in such an emergency that they do not dare even delay the few minutes needed to get phone advice, they will rush to care instead. Where providers cannot be bothered doing careful analysis of a patient's problems, they may simply refer them to the ED. Where other, more appropriate options are simply not available or open to callers, they may still end up in the wrong place from a purely medical perspective. Nevertheless there is clearly plenty of room for improvement in this area of health care consumption.

Benefits to Payers

The vast majority of reports on results actually achieved describe the savings that sponsors have enjoyed as a result of triage programs. One vendor of triage services reports that 49% of callers initially intent on seeing a physician decided they could do without, and 78% decided against going to an ED. Among seniors, 38% decided they did not need to see a physician, and 74% avoided the ED.[7] One study found that only 3.5% of callers needed to go to an ED or urgent care provider, while 35% to 40% could wait for a normal clinic visit and the rest could take care of their own problem, with guidance and reassurance.[8]

A pediatric phone triage program found that 60% of callers took care of the problem themselves, where 75% had intended to go to an ED.[9] Another program produced a 20% drop in physician and ED visits.[10] An Internet triage program had its users indicating that they were able to avoid an ED visit 6% of the time and avoided a physician office visit 25% of the time.[11] Another program reduced physician office visits by 5% in the first six months.[12]

In terms of money saved, The Wisconsin Education Association Insurance Trust saved $1,157,831 by triaging employees and dependents, with a return on investment (ROI) ratio of $2.40:1.[13] An HMO estimated its savings at $174 per member per year.[14] The Norand Corporation cut its costs 20.6%.[15] One vendor claims savings average $70 to $100 per call.[16] A survey of multiple examples found ROI ratios ranging from $2:1 to $3:1; while a formal study found an average ROI ratio of $3.17:1.[17]

Benefits to Providers

Even for providers not at financial risk for the consumption and expenditures of their patients, triage programs can offer benefits. Triage/advice lines save physicians the time they would otherwise spend in handling patient "emergencies" after hours and the time their staff would spend dealing with concerned patients and parents.[18] The responsibility of covering patient needs after hours becomes far less onerous if only a small proportion of calls are referred to the covering physician. One physician group that developed its own triage program found that only 5% of calls needed the attention of a physician.[19]

Benefits to Consumers

Even more important, perhaps, are the benefits that triage services can bestow on consumers, and indirectly thereby, through higher satisfaction and retention, on employers, health plans, and providers. One HMO promotes its triage program as offering quicker referrals to specialists, without the need for primary physician "gatekeeper" approval; triage nurses can even make appointments with specialists, if appropriate, and can precertify the need for ED visits.[20] In general, consumers who use triage lines and are enabled to substitute self-care for professional services gain more immediate resolution of their problem and save travel and copayments.[21]

A triage professional is typically able to calm and reassure callers, even where they are referred to the same source of care they would have sought prior to calling.[22] Callers gain confidence in their own abilities to cope with the problem themselves, increasing self-efficacy.[23] When they call about chronic conditions, their coping skills and independence are reinforced.[24] Because of these benefits, triage programs can be promoted as gateways to needed care, rather than gatekeepers that get in the way of needed care.[25]

Applications

Many physician groups, including Cleveland Clinic[26] and Carle Clinic,[27] offer their own triage programs. A pediatric group uses its own registered nurses for after-hours triage.[28] Another group makes using its triage line comforting and easy as part of its appointment-making system.[29] The Harvard Community Health Plan offers its members a computer-based triage system.[30] One of the most interesting applications is the Robert Wood Johnson Foundation–sponsored community-wide triage program in Boise, Idaho, where providers and payers are cooperating in promoting more appropriate use of services by all residents.[31]

Perhaps the ultimate triage program involves a hospital's having a triage phone just outside its ED. Since the hospital is required by law to do a diagnostic workup on any patient who enters, it can use the phone to advise some callers that they can avoid the ED wait and costs through self-care or going to another, less intensive source.[32] Or an even later form of triage can be used by critical care specialists who take over for primary physicians when their patients come to the ED. They triage ED patients to observation versus admission or arrange home care so patients can avoid an inpatient stay.[33]

Limits and Concerns in Triage

One concern about triage is that it might end up promoting a lot of wasteful calls by the worried well, who would otherwise not have sought advice from any professional. This could add to costs without having any effect on utilization or savings.[34] Another is that physicians may not always agree with nurses' advice. Even within the ED, nurses and physicians often disagree on triage decisions, with physicians overriding nurse decisions.[35] The quality of advice may vary widely, depending on the training and experience of people answering triage phone calls.[36]

Triage by nurses can put providers and payers at risk. In one case a mother was advised to take her feverish child to a distant ED that was in the plan's network rather than a closer one. The jury awarded the parents $45 million when they concluded that the delay in care caused permanent brain damage to the child.[37] Although nurse counselors are supposed to be giving information and offering choices to callers, rather than giving advice, it is a distinction difficult to make and explain to juries.

Triage phone lines also expand the risks to patient privacy, introducing a new set of people and records about callers' conditions and concerns over and above their physicians. Patients or their physicians may object to having strangers become acquainted with intimate details about the lives of callers. Callers may be concerned that the sole purpose of triage is to interfere with their access to care so as to increase the profits of plans or providers.

Advice

The first essential in triage programs is to obtain the acceptance, cooperation, and support of physicians. They should be involved in deciding to offer a triage service and in developing the protocols or algorithms used by those who handle the calls.[38] Physicians will need to be taught, trained, and informed about their new roles as partners in empowering patients.[39] They should be included in deciding whether to use protocols or algorithms in dealing with specific problems.[40]

The personnel who will handle calls must be carefully selected, trained, and managed. They should stress the limitations of phone information, since they cannot examine the patient, offering information and options rather than recommendations and advice.[41] They should have well-developed computer software to facilitate and document each interaction.[42] Callers should be followed up to learn which options they chose and how it worked out.[43]

It is not enough to simply offer a triage program; it must be made attractive and convenient to consumers.[44] Fortunately consumers have indicated high levels of acceptance of such programs, primarily because of the usual 24-hour everyday availability of information.[45] If calling a triage service is made mandatory, it will likely be perceived as an onerous interference with access. If it is a voluntary option, it can be marketed as a benefit. Informing consumers about how their choices can affect their out-of-pocket costs provides some added benefit.[46] Allaying consumer anxiety and empowering them to handle their own problems are distinct and significant benefits. (See Exhibit 22–1.)

A triage program should be part of an integrated program aimed at empowering consumers and at improving their health and consumption of services.[47] It has been found, for example, that coupling the triage service with self-care guides, training, and education can significantly improve its effect.[48] In Wisconsin, it essentially doubled the ROI ratio from $2.40:1 to $4.75:1.[49]

Programs should be customized to particular consumer segments, such as children, seniors, and women.[50] Sponsors should learn the existing state of self-efficacy and orientation toward self-care in preparing to implement and market their programs. People seek professional attention or advice when they reach the limits of their self-efficacy, when their pain or anxiety levels are unacceptable.[51] They may well know what to do in most circumstances but may lack *confidence* in their own knowledge and abilities, needing only to be reassured.[52]

To promote triage call line use by consumers, sponsors may add special benefits over and above the "natural" benefits of anxiety relief and self-efficacy gains, for example. They may reduce the out-of-pocket obligation for callers who go through the triage process as opposed to rushing off on their own. The health plan's benefits and coverage should promote the use of triage.[53]

Make or Buy?

There are many vendors who offer phone triage packages. (See Appendix 22–A for a list.) On the other hand, many providers have long operated their own triage functions and may be perfectly comfortable adapting them to capitation payment realities. Hospitals may find they can easily convert physician referral/information services to triage use.

Vendors may have advantages in offering already developed and tested personnel, expertise, and computer systems, enabling sponsors to initiate programs immediately versus spend their own time and resources in development. Where populations at risk are relatively small, vendors can offer economies of scale, since they serve multiple sponsors and populations. Each sponsor should consider the particular advantages and disadvantages that apply in each case.

A key risk in taking the triage program in-house comes when internal performance is managed and evaluated in terms of cost savings, alone or primarily. This

Exhibit 22–1 Triage

PROBLEMS / POTENTIAL	x Many don't need professional services (25%–50% of ambulatory, 55% of ED calls) x Provider may be in a hurry & send consumers to wrong place x Dramatic reduction in ambulatory / ED visits often achieved x Customer satisfaction & plan retention increased x Provider gains added time to spend with patients with greater health care needs x Increases consumer self-efficacy & improves assessment of needed services x Consumers avoid hassle, time costs, out-of-pocket expense
EXAMPLES	x Provided by physician groups x Community services may be jointly provided by provider and insurers x ED may provide triage services while patients are waiting for care
CONCERNS	x Difference of opinion among professionals makes developing protocols difficult x Inaccurate advice or unheeded instructions may put providers & payers at risk x Risks to patient privacy increased
ADVICE	x Ensure physician buy-in & train personnel x Make the service attractive & convenient for callers x Integrate telephone triage services with other services x Customize the service to market segments

can put the sponsor at legal and reputation risk of being seen as interested solely in limiting access and enhancing profits. For providers who have a mix of fee-for-service (FFS) and capitation patients, a triage program may create a kind of split-personality problem, where some callers are to be encouraged to use services and specialists, while others are to be empowered to care for themselves or referred to their primary physician. Avoiding this split by treating all callers the same will damage either the FFS or capitation side of the business.

If a vendor is chosen over performing the triage function in house, methods of payment should be chosen carefully. While the most common fee system is per capita, matching the sponsor's risk, this may provide an incentive for the vendor not to promote use of the service, since every use represents cost. Paying based on savings would entail the same risk as using reductions in consumption and expenditures for managing the in-house function. Sponsors would be advised to set explicit objectives or standards for consumer satisfaction, perceived benefits, and similar nonfinancial outcomes as part of the vendor contract, if not the basis for payment.[54]

(Note: These same caveats and suggestions apply for all make-buy decisions and all issues related to payment of vendors.)

SELF-CARE

In one sense, self-care is an inherent part of triage, since triage includes informing callers about self-care opportunities and promoting their sense of self-efficacy. However, triage services can be sold and conducted without any specific self-care component, and self-care can be separately or independently sold and conducted.

Self-care is a critical component of disease management in the sense that people with acute or chronic conditions are empowered to do as much for themselves as possible and appropriate. This discussion will focus on self-care as a replacement alternative to professional attention for distressing symptoms that might drive unnecessary use of care for acute or chronic conditions, whether part of decision improvement or disease or disability management efforts. (See Exhibit 22–2.)

Problems and Potential

Whether triage or self-care, the problems and potential are similar. People tend to seek and consume professional services for conditions they could have easily handled on their own. In triage, self-care is one of many options for dealing with distressing symptoms; in self-care it is the only one of interest.

To indicate the problem and potential of self-care, consider that consumers are estimated to handle roughly 80% of all their health-threatening problems by themselves already. If they were to lose confidence or otherwise shift this proportion

Exhibit 22–2 Self-Care

Problems / Potential	✗ Self-care is often the most appropriate response to a vast number of symptoms ✗ Inappropriate utilization significantly reduced with appropriate self-care ✗ Provider gains added time to spend with patients with actual health care needs ✗ Consumer gains increased self-efficacy & better assessment of needs
Examples	✗ Self-care guides may be provided by health care providers or insurers ✗ Self-care "kits" may be provided to consumers ✗ On-site training expedites hospital stays by making patients & families able to care for recovery needs
Concerns	✗ Sponsors need to motivate & guide consumer to appropriate self-care ✗ Materials must be carefully selected for accuracy & accessibility ✗ Information may need to be tailored for individual populations
Advice	✗ Identify high-use targets for interventions instead of entire populations ✗ Integrate self-care initiatives into integrated program of health improvement

downward, say to 70%, that would increase their demands for attention by 50%, by insisting that professionals deal with 30% versus 20% of those problems. By the same token, if they could increase their reliance on self-care from 80% to 90%, they would cut their demand for attention by 50%.[55]

One analysis indicated that 23% of all encounters with physicians were for "time-limited acute symptoms" that would have gone away by themselves if ignored or treated with no more than rest and watchful waiting.[56] Another noted how often simple allergy symptoms are mistaken for something more serious, resulting in demands for attention.[57] Still another concluded that 40% to 70% of all physician visits could have been avoided.[58]

Self-care may be the most appropriate, or at least equally appropriate and least expensive option, for a vast number of symptoms. Studies have indicated that it is certainly by far the most common response to most symptoms, depending on how much the symptoms distress consumers and interfere with their normal activities. On the other hand, consumers may also delay or avoid seeking care when they should, overrelying on self-care.[59]

Self-care has aroused one of the highest interest levels among sponsors aiming to improve consumption of health services.[60] It has been described as a great opportunity by one of the foremost proponents of managing demand.[61] The challenge, as with triage, is to aim for improving, rather than merely reducing, the use of services, therefore making sure that self-care is chosen and employed effectively by consumers, as well as frequently.

Benefits to Payers

Employers, health plans, and at-risk providers should all gain when consumers use self-care appropriately. Outpatient/ambulatory care utilization can go down significantly, as in Wisconsin, where employees and dependents of the Education Association cut their use of care by 24.7% to 78.8% across four categories of outpatient services.[62] A program aimed at promoting self-care among the disadvantaged cut inappropriate ED usage by 68%.[63]

Blue Cross/Blue Shield of Pennsylvania achieved a reduction of 24.3% in outpatient claims.[64] Kaiser reduced ambulatory care visits by 17%, with a 35% reduction in minor visits.[65] The Air Force was able to reduce physician visits by 16% and ED visits by 34%.[66] FHP reported reductions of 15.4% in office visits for the top 10 problems and 32.8% for problems specifically targeted for self-care.[67]

The Florida Hospital Medical Center was able to cut its costs by $30,954 (among 365 employees responding to its survey) over just five months, or $203.53 per employee.[68] Delaware Power saw its costs go down 3.7% compared to a 21.4% increase in the prior year.[69] In a number of applications, one self-care guide achieved reported savings per employee ranging from $50 to $550, including savings from reduced lost work days.[70] Another reported savings ranging from $161 to $203 per employee, with ROI ratios as high as $55:1.[71]

Comparing the impact on health plan members with and without deductible/ copay incentives, one study found that self-care lowered health service use by 7.1%, where members had out-of-pocket obligations, and 24.9% where they had first-dollar coverage.[72] A pediatric clinic reduced fever visits by 35%,[73] while a Medicare HMO cut costs $36.65 per household, with a $2.19:1 ROI ratio.[74]

Benefits to Providers

In contrast to triage, which records the redirection of callers, it is difficult to measure the extent to which self-care reduces demands on providers, such as after-hours coverage by physicians. On the other hand, physicians are increasingly accepting the idea of promoting self-care. The proportions supporting the idea grew from 31% in 1979 to 61% in 1995, according to one study.[75]

Benefits to Consumers

Consumers gain from self-care as previously described under triage. They enjoy even more independence from providers, since they can turn to their self-care guides rather than having to call a triage counselor. Consumers supplied with self-care assistance report higher levels of satisfaction.[76] They assert higher levels of self-efficacy and confidence and better health.[77] Patients suffering from depression reported three times the level of improvement when given self-help materials compared to those given no materials.[78]

Applications

Self-care programs usually consist of a self-care guide, ranging from pamphlet size to large books. They may include special education and training in self-care techniques, especially when aimed at consumers with specific acute or chronic conditions. Self-care cold and flu kits are available for $2 to $3 each.[79] On-line self-help advice is available over the Internet.[80] Home testing kits for a variety of conditions are available.[81]

Inpatient "self-help" programs have operated for many years, enlisting the aid of family members as well as patients in enhancing the inpatient experience as well as reducing costs.[82] Parents trained in caring for sick and premature babies have enabled far earlier discharges from inpatient care, pleasing both parents and payers.[83] The growing Planetree movement is empowering patients and families to play a far more significant role in inpatient care and in managing their own conditions generally.[84]

Limits and Concerns

Self-care involves somewhat fewer risks than triage because sponsors do not directly insert themselves in consumer decision making. Consumers have complete control over whether they resort to self-care materials and employ what they find there. In fact, just as with triage, sponsors are likely to need to motivate consumers to use self-care, even where materials are readily available.[85]

Sponsors must still be careful in selecting or developing self-care materials and education programs to be sure they are offering guidance that can be defended in court as medically appropriate and beneficial to consumers, as opposed to a blatant attempt to discourage health care use. There are limits to what individual consumers may be able to understand and apply, as well as limits to what any consumer can do without medical training.[86]

Some who have employed self-care programs have found that it has little impact on some conditions. One study found no reductions in use of care for backache or headache, for example, and a realized savings of only $8 per consumer.[87] Another found that it actually increased visits by children for earaches, though it decreased visits for most other causes.[88] There is no guarantee that every self-care guide will work for every population, though the vast majority of experience has been highly positive, with significant results in the same year as initiation of the program and increasing ROI ratios over time.

Advice

One approach to improving the efficiency of self-care programs is to identify high risks rather than the entire population as targets for intervention. Records on use of physician visits and EDs for trivial conditions or for uncontrolled chronic conditions can enable sponsors to pick out promising targets for attention and let them focus attention on those whose consumption behavior most needs to be changed.[89] Combining self-care and triage produces significantly greater effect than either one alone.[90]

As with triage, self-care initiatives should be part of an integrated program of demand improvement rather than used on a stand-alone basis. Since both the idea and the materials may get old quickly, given the changeability of consumer attitudes, programs and materials should be varied over time to keep them fresh. The same is true for marketing efforts used to promote self-care.

Make or Buy

The make or buy decision is easier with self-care, since it does not need to involve an ongoing service. With the large variety of self-care guides available (see Appendix 22–A for list), sponsors are likely to find one that they and concerned physicians will accept. While one guide may serve for a number of years, updating is probably safer, and the costs of most guides, especially with volume discounts, are generally quite reasonable.

Outside vendors may also be used in introducing self-care to a population for the first time or in conducting education and training programs to supplement written materials. Where triage and self-care are to be used together, it makes sense to seek a vendor who supplies both services and materials, so that triage counselors will be thoroughly familiar and consistent with self-care materials and the two can work synergistically.

SHARED DECISION MAKING

The aim of shared decision-making (Exhibit 22–3) programs is to enable consumers to participate meaningfully in decisions related to high-cost treatments where there are significantly different options available. In effect, such programs aim to enable patients to be their own advocates, ensuring that their values are at least considered, if not dominant, in treatment choices.[91] Shared decision making is supposed to improve the quality of care and its outcomes, in addition to possibly reducing health care expenditures.[92]

The chief aim of shared decision making is to improve the quality of the decisions that are made. Vickery and Lynch defined the whole of managing demand as "the support of individuals so that they may make rational health and medical decisions based on consideration of benefits and risks."[93p.??] By combining expert opinion and objective data with consumer values and perspectives, decisions can be fostered that are best for all concerned.[94]

Problems and Potential

The nation's bill for unnecessary testing and medical and surgical procedures has been put as high as $200 billion a year, though some of the costs represent bureaucratic burdens, "defensive medicine," and other factors not directly related to consumer choices.[95] A more conservative Rand study concluded that 25% of all surgery was unnecessary, costing $50 billion a year.[96] Physicians' family members have been found to get significantly less surgery for many conditions, for example, than do unrelated consumers, suggesting that uninformed consumers are getting too much.[97]

The chief advantage sought by most sponsors is a reduction in higher-cost treatment options. The involvement of consumers is sought because experience has shown that they tend to be more conservative than providers when it comes to choosing treatments. Additional tests represent added trouble, inconvenience, and perhaps pain and discomfort. Getting more care is not what consumers necessarily want.[98]

Exhibit 22–3   Shared Decision Making

PROBLEMS / POTENTIAL	✗ May assist in reducing higher-cost treatment options ✗ May reduce risk of malpractice suits as patients understand the options & choose freely ✗ Reduces cost & produces savings as patients choose less expensive treatment options ✗ Under capitation, assists providers in cost containment ✗ Save provider time as patients come to the provider better informed ✗ Increase consumer self-efficacy & control over health care decisions ✗ Better informed consumer choices
EXAMPLES	✗ Interactive video programs assist in evaluating surgical options ✗ Internet systems offer professional & peer perspectives on treatment options ✗ Computer & video resource centers provide wide variety of information on conditions & options
CONCERNS	✗ Resignation to conditions may need to be overcome ✗ Used in areas where overtreatment was occurring; as becomes more prevalent may encounter diminishing returns ✗ Risk that patients will know "too much" about options & condition
ADVICE	✗ Ensure physician buy-in & train personnel ✗ Consumers should be coached in appropriate use of the materials ✗ Make sure programs are highly interactive to promote use ✗ Test consumer understanding ✗ Evaluate for cost & care effectiveness over the long term

With pharmaceutical companies increasingly advertising directly to consumers, the need for objective data to help consumers decide grows.[99] The average consumer is reluctant to get involved in medical decisions, even to question the physician or ask for a referral in order to get a second opinion.[100] When consumers are uninformed, the impact of their perceptions and preferences can be entirely in the wrong direction.[101] With the scandals and lawsuits attending so many efforts to control providers or demarket procedures by denying coverage, a program where consumers themselves reduce unnecessary and wasteful health care is much to be desired.[102]

Benefits to Payers

Shared decision-making programs have been shown to reduce the costs of care in a variety of ways[103] and produce savings for payers.[104] Kaiser was reported as saving $300,000 from the use of one procedure-specific video.[105] Where consumers chose the Ornish diet and exercise program instead of coronary bypass or angioplasty, for example, each saved $10,000 to $25,000.[106]

When applied across one population at risk, shared decision making produced a 10% drop in total hospital days.[107] Interactive videos on benign prostate hyperplasia reduced surgery for that problem by 59% to 61% in one study.[108] For a series of different procedures, another study found that, on average, informed consumers decided not to have surgery 47% of the time, 50% among seniors.[109] Health plans that have used shared decision making have found higher member satisfaction and retention.[110]

Benefits to Providers

Financial benefits to providers apply only under capitation, since consumers in shared decision making tend to opt more for no treatment or less aggressive and expensive options.[111] All providers stand to gain, however, when shared decisions reduce the risks of lawsuits. When patients play an active role in choosing treatment, they appear to be less likely to sue over less than perfect results.[112] Moreover, shared decision-making technologies can test consumer knowledge and demonstrate informed consent, reducing the risk of lawsuits on that question.[113]

Most shared decision initiatives include prepared information for consumers to use on their own. This will automatically save providers time and energy that they or their staff would otherwise spend informing patients. It may not actually reduce their operating costs, but it will give them opportunities to do something else with the time saved.

In spite of these benefits, many physicians have resisted sharing power with patients.[114] Some appear simply to hate the idea.[115] Others disagree over how much and what kinds of information consumers should get in order to participate in making decisions.[116] In general, it appears that acceptance is growing among physicians as they gain experience with it in practice.[117]

Benefits to Consumers

By definition, sharing in the making of medical decisions gives consumers greater control over their lives, a key benefit.[118] It is argued that active participation in treatment decisions is, by itself, a healing force.[119] Where it has been studied, greater involvement has promoted better clinical outcomes (both perceived and measured), higher patient satisfaction, lower pain severity, and better perceived health.[120]

Applications

The Shared Decision-Making Program at the Dartmouth Medical School uses videos on specific decisions, so that patients may consider the issues at their leisure.[121] CIGNA is working on videos for 30 different conditions.[122] The federal Agency for Health Care Policy & Research offers general advice on questions consumers should ask before deciding on surgery.[123]

Internet systems such as the CHESS program at the University of Wisconsin offer both professional and peer perspectives on treatment options (e.g., for AIDS/HIV and breast cancer).[124] Companion Health Care (South Carolina) uses videos in a three-step program, where patients first complete a questionnaire on their condition; watch an interactive video on a touch-screen television monitor in the physician's office, getting a customized printout reviewing treatment options; then discuss the video and options with the physician.[125]

A hospital uses a computer resource center to offer its patients information on their diagnosis and treatment options.[126] An employer added out-of-pocket obligation in its pharmacy benefit to get employees to actively consider generic drug options.[127] CD-ROM software is available to empower consumers to learn about their conditions and possible treatments.[128] Consumers can purchase a phone calling card entitling them to 30 minutes of phone conversation with selected expert physicians.[129]

Limits and Concerns

In some cases consumers may have to be encouraged to seek treatment. Studies have shown that many elderly patients resign themselves to living with readily correctable conditions because they feel the problem arises from old age.[130] Second surgical opinion programs as devices for improving decisions about surgery proved ineffective and have largely been abandoned.[131]

Shared decision initiatives have largely been applied to conditions where it was generally felt that providers were overusing testing or treatment procedures.[132] As initiatives add to the conditions they address, it is likely that they will encounter diminishing returns, finding fewer cases where consumers will differ from providers, or running into conditions where consumers will demand more treatment than providers would have chosen.

As with triage, shared decision initiatives open up the risks of many more people becoming acquainted with patient information that the patients would not want known.[133] Where providers themselves sponsor such initiatives, this may entail little added risk, but where employers or health plans are sponsors, there may arise problems among employees and members, and the number of participants in such initiatives may suffer as a result.[134]

Advice

As with triage and self-care, getting physicians involved in developing shared decision initiatives is essential in promoting their acceptance and cooperation.[135] Consumers should be offered choices as to the extent of their participation in decisions and a choice of ways to get good information.[136] They should be coached and helped in using complex information technologies.[137] Wherever possible, the information and decision-making experience should be customized to each patient, as well as to each condition and decision.[138]

The more interactive the method for conveying information, the better—it promotes involvement by and impact on consumers.[139] A variety of methods to suit individual preferences and multimedia technologies rather than reliance on a single medium is recommended.[140] Consumers with their own computers and Internet access can combine multimedia software, CD-ROM, and Internet possibilities. For patients lacking personal access, health plans, employers, and providers can offer their facilities.

Because treatment decisions may change over time, evaluation of impact should include long-term follow-up of patients who participate in shared decision initiatives. It may be that some, perhaps many, merely postpone treatment for chronic conditions or select one treatment, only to end up with another when the first one fails. The total cost and utilization over an entire episode should be tracked to evaluate total impact.[141]

HEALTH PLAN CHOICE

Everyone involved in improving consumer health and demand has an interest in influencing choices of health plan. Employers may feel that some plans offer lower costs to them or better employee health, productivity, and other side effects.

Health plans want some consumers to choose them, and others not to, though there are legal limits on what they can do to influence selection. Providers want consumers to choose plans that include them in their network or to select their own provider service organization plans, where they offer them (Exhibit 22–4).

Problems and Potential

It is clear that some plans perform better than others, though each employer must decide which performance factors are most important in selecting plans to offer employees. HMOs have frequently been found to be more efficient than indemnity plans, though they may also offer richer benefits and end up costing as much to employers. Some HMOs are as expensive as indemnity plans, or more so.[142]

The first challenge to employers is choosing the best plans to offer employees. For larger employers with plenty of market clout, it is rarely a problem getting available plans to bid for their business, though there may be limited numbers and types of plans available in specific locations. Even small employers have been able to save by forming or joining purchasing alliances and cooperatives. By offering larger numbers of covered lives, individual employers can gain clout in terms of coverage and services as well as price.[143]

Choosing the right plans is only half the job; getting employees to make the best selection among those available is equally important. By enabling and encouraging employees to choose lower cost health plans, employers and other payers can save significantly. One Medicaid program, for example, saved 13.8%, or $17 million a year by switching beneficiaries into a managed care plan.[144] Since Medicaid can simply direct beneficiaries, it enjoys an advantage over other payers, even Medicare. For them it is necessary to persuade or attract consumers to choose a particular plan.

We already know a great deal about the factors that influence consumer choices of health plan, so influencing choice would seem possible. One of the difficulties, however, is that what we know is often contradictory. Some surveys indicate that access to care is the key factor.[145] Others highlight consumers' past experience, information provided by plans, family, and friends.[146]

When asked to indicate what factor is most important to their choice, 37% of consumers in one study named "cost," 26% named "coverage," and 22% "choice of doctors."[147] Another study found consumers rating coverage as most important, followed by the plan's reputation and choice of providers.[148] Another found quality of physicians rated first, then coverage for the price and access to appointments.[149]

Variations in findings may simply reflect differences across different populations. Results may also vary because researchers asked questions differently or designed surveys with different intentions and biases. In any case it is almost always advisable to treat each population as idiosyncratic, learning what its consumers want in health

Exhibit 22–4 Health Plan Choice

PROBLEMS / POTENTIAL	
	✗ EMPLOYERS MUST DETERMINE WHICH PERFORMANCE FACTORS ARE MOST IMPORTANT IN PLAN CHOICE
	✗ EMPLOYER MUST ASSIST EMPLOYEES TO MAKE BEST SELECTION AMONG AVAILABLE CHOICES
	✗ WITH TAILORED PRODUCTS, COSTS CAN BE REDUCED WHILE EMPLOYEE SATISFACTION IS ENHANCED
	✗ WITH CAPITATION, PROVIDERS MAY GET BETTER MIX OF PATIENTS TO ENHANCE FINANCIAL STABILITY
	✗ INCREASED CHOICE ENABLES CONSUMERS TO FIND APPROPRIATE MIX OF PROVIDED SERVICES
EXAMPLES	
	✗ FINANCIAL INCENTIVES ASSIST IN GETTING EMPLOYEES TO SWITCH TO HMO
	✗ EMPOWERMENT THROUGH INFORMATION HELPS WITH CHOICE
	✗ ADVERTISING & TELEPHONE CAMPAIGNS CAN HELP GET INFORMATION TO CONSUMERS
CONCERNS	
	✗ THE YOUNG & HEALTHY MAY CHOOSE HMOs WHILE THOSE AT RISK RETAIN MORE EXPENSIVE PRODUCT
	✗ REPUTATION OF HMOs FOR SLUGGISH SERVICE & COST CUTTING MAY INCREASE RELUCTANCE TO CHANGE TO LOWER COST PROGRAMS
ADVICE	
	✗ INVOLVE CONSUMERS IN DESIGNING PROGRAMS & SELECTING PLANS
	✗ BUILD IN ENOUGH BENEFIT TO CONSUMERS SO THEY SHARE THE PREFERENCE
	✗ INCLUDE LARGE NUMBER OF PHYSICIANS IN THE PANEL SO CONSUMERS HAVE CHOICE

plans and what factors make the difference to them. Populations differ enough to make results derived from other groups of consumers unreliable.

Benefits to Payers

Selection of the right plans can save payers money, as already mentioned. Missouri public employees saved the state 32.5%, or $38 million, for example, by increasing the proportion of employees in managed care from 25% to 65%.[150] Southern California Edison saved $20 million by steering more of its 50,000 employees into its direct contract plan.[151] Xerox saved $115 per covered life by moving employees toward the lowest cost HMO.[152] On the other hand, Lockheed gave up pushing employees to join an HMO when it found no cost savings.[153]

Selection of whether to include an employee's working spouse on one employer's plan versus the other's is another choice of interest to employers. If one employer offers a better benefit package and/or premium obligation, it may find itself spending more while employers offering less do not incur any insurance costs where two working spouses are involved. Getting each employee to choose single coverage where there are no children, and balancing proportions who have family coverage can save dollars for employers.

Benefits to Providers

Providers under fee-for-service plans benefit whenever consumers choose health plans in which those providers are included. Under capitation, providers retain business when a current patient chooses a network that includes them, and can gain patients if someone else's or an unattached patient chooses them, so the more networks a provider is in, the greater the chance for keeping and gaining patients. With capitation, providers are also concerned about their mix of patients, since too many frail/unhealthy or high-risk patients can bankrupt them.

Benefit to Consumers

Consumers can benefit from lower-priced health plans whenever they have partial obligation for premiums. They can also lose where plans have low cost because they have high deductibles and copays, or low benefit coverage. They stand to be greatly affected by the extent to which health plans invest in and are successful at initiatives that improve their health and empower them to make the best decisions on treatments and providers.

A key factor in most consumer decisions regarding health plans is the extent to which they have choices. Being able to keep one's present physician, if desired, to use one's favorite hospital, to have a wide choice among therapies may not be as important as cost and benefits, but it comes close for many consumers. Having the information and skills to make the best choices is a separate, though related benefit. Having many choices of plans, as can happen when small employers join coops and alliances, is yet another benefit.

Though the extent to which employers and health plans share savings with consumers varies, the potential for consumers gaining financially from their choice of health plans is real and significant. One study estimated that the total savings from choosing managed care plans would be $383 billion in the United States 1990 to 2000. It estimated that the average worker took home an extra $228 to $356 and the average family $408 to $549 as the result of selecting managed care options, combining lower premium costs, out-of-pocket obigations, and increased wages.[154]

Applications

The challenge to payers and providers alike is to get consumers to make the right health plan choices. Plans need to market to consumers as well as employer and union clients to gain covered lives.[155] Employers need to market to employees and their families to promote getting more people in preferred plans.

The most common approach to guiding employee choices seems to be financial incentives. Xerox strove to double the proportion of its employees in HMOs from 40% to 80% by paying only the costs of the lowest priced plan in each market, requiring the employee to pay anything above that.[156] Southern California Edison used the same approach.[157] Empire Blue Cross/Blue Shield boosted premiums on individual indemnity coverage by 30% to 35% to encourage shifts to its HMO option.[158] IBM offered better coverage and lower deductibles/copays to encourage shifting.[159] GTE offers a 5% discount on premiums.[160]

Some employers have used even more explicit incentives. Boeing offered bonuses of $600 to all employees who switched to HMO coverage in the first year of its incentive program, $400 if they switched the second year, and $200 if the third.[161] Hershey offered a $150 bonus and waiver of the first year premium obligation to those who would switch to one of its managed care plans.[162] General Motors faced the problem that union agreements with the United Auto Workers (UAW) prohibited union employees' having to pay any portion of their premium, so it could only use incentives with its nonunion employees.[163]

Some aim to empower rather than entice their employees, offering performance information to help employees choose the best plans. Baxter gave its employees a *For Your Benefit* booklet to help employees choose; American Express supplied quality and cost information and got 70% of employees to choose HMOs. GTE published a consumers' guide to help its employees decide, while Wells Fargo used information in its employee newsletter, on posters, and in brochures.[164]

New York Citibank supplies employees with a personal computer (PC) disk three months before they make health plan decisions, plus video information and phone counseling.[165]

Business Consumer Guide offers information on HMOs nationwide via the Internet and even allows consumers to enroll on-line.[166]

Despite an inability to offer incentives, an employer coalition, working with health plans, was able to increase the proportion of retirees choosing HMO coverage from 6% to 10%.[167] The Medica HMO in Minnesota offered a 25% cut in premiums and increased its enrollment among state employees from 3,500 to 10,500 in one year.[168] Missouri required health plans to bid on a standardized benefit package and paid only the cost of the lowest price plan, increasing HMO enrollment from 25% to 65% of employees.[169]

Providers have worked hard to steer consumers to the "right" health plans. The University of North Carolina Hospitals undertook an extensive advertising and phone counseling campaign to help consumers choose plans that included its system in the provider network, and increased its enrollment by 10%.[170] Well-positioned, prestigious hospitals and medical groups can help health plans who include them in provider networks market to consumers.

Concerns and Issues

While many employers have had great initial success in promoting selection of managed care options, they are likely to run into the law of diminishing returns. Those unconverted employees may have particularly strong ties to their present plans and providers and may distrust HMOs and other managed care plans; hence the growing popularity of point of service (POS) plans as an intermediate option.[171] HMOs may have attracted more young, healthy consumers initially and find that as proportional enrollment increases, they get older, sicker members who drive their cost up.[172]

Those consumers unconvinced as to the advantages of HMOs are likely to be harder to convince than those already favorably predisposed, or at least open minded.[173] Managed care plans have frequently suffered from poor reputations on access to care, waits for appointments, and phone service.[174] One study found that new enrollees in an HMO had double the maternity utilization in their first year, significantly increasing the HMO's costs.[175]

There is some potential legal risk in steering consumers toward particular health plans, though perhaps not as great as steering them toward specific providers. As performance data on plans themselves and on the providers in their networks become more readily available, employers are likely to be at risk if they select and steer employees toward plans with poor performance. Only time will tell if they will be held liable for steering employees to merely average plans and providers; the risks in steering to clearly substandard plans, merely because they are cheaper, are already real. The one safe approach seems to be to give employees real choices, then let them decide.

Advice

One common suggestion to help influence consumer choice is to involve consumers in designing benefit programs and in selecting the health plans among which they must choose.[176] Standardizing benefits so that cost differences are clear is helpful whether or not financial incentives are used.[177] Obtaining performance data from all plans considered and supplying such data in understandable ways to consumers is also recommended with or without incentives.[178] National Commission for Quality Assurance (NCQA) accreditation and HEDIS measures are a start.[179]

To achieve the greatest success in steering consumers toward payer- or provider-preferred plans, it is advisable to build in enough benefit to consumers so that they share in the preference. Sharing the savings with them is one approach that employers can easily use.[180] Ensuring that their physicians are included in the provider network is another.[181] Perhaps the best benefit to build in is the full set of benefits available through health and demand improvement programs.[182]

PROVIDER CHOICE

Choosing providers is a challenge to consumers whether they are selecting a personal or family physician, a specialist for particular problems, or a provider of urgent, emergency, or convenience care. While family practitioners are especially trained to serve as first contact and care coordinators for entire families, internists for adults, and pediatricians for children, some physicians labeled as specialists may actually make the best primary physicians for some patients (Exhibit 22–5).

Women of childbearing age and beyond often demand to use their obstetrician as their primary physician. Consumers with chronic conditions may insist on and may be better off with specialists such as cardiologists for chronic heart problems, endocrinologists for diabetes, and allergists or pulmonary specialists for asthma, for example. Selecting the setting for care is the challenge in triage, while selecting the best treatment is the aim of shared decision making. Here we are talking about selecting the best individual provider.

Increasingly payers are offering consumers the option of selecting alternative medicine providers. While this option is often limited to providers to whom the consumer's primary physician refers, it is likely that the movement toward "open access" plan options, where consumers can bypass their gatekeepers and self-refer

Exhibit 22–5 Provider Choice

PROBLEMS / POTENTIAL	✗ PROVIDER VARIANCE IN COST, QUALITY & SERVICE ✗ NONPHYSICIAN PROVIDERS CAN TRIM COSTS WHILE INCREASING PATIENT SATISFACTION ✗ KNOWING WHEN SPECIALIST IS NEEDED VS. PHYSICIAN OR PHYSICIAN EXTENDER IS CRITICAL ✗ CUSTOMER SATISFACTION & PLAN RETENTION INCREASED AS SPONSORS ENSURED QUALITY OF PROVIDERS ✗ APPROPRIATE SELECTION HELPS PROVIDERS ENSURE THEY ARE PREFERRED, THUS INCREASING PATIENT SATISFACTION ✗ INCREASED CONSUMER SATISFACTION WITH PERSONAL INVOLVEMENT ✗ IMPROVED QUALITY OF CARE & OUTCOMES
EXAMPLES	✗ HOSPITALS CAN PROVIDE PHYSICIAN INFORMATION & REFERRAL SERVICES WITH INTERACTIVE MULTIMEDIA PRESENTATIONS ✗ CONSUMER GUIDEBOOKS AND INDEPENDENT INFORMATION SERVICES HELP CONSUMERS MAKE INFORMED CHOICE
CONCERNS	✗ HEALTH CARE CONSUMERS MAY NOT MAKE "RATIONAL" CHOICES ABOUT THEIR PROVIDERS ✗ CONVENTIONAL WISDOM MAY BE WRONG ✗ NEW PHYSICIANS OR PHYSICIANS WITH MINOR BLEMISH ON RECORD MAY NOT GET PATIENTS
ADVICE	✗ ENSURE REASON FOR SERVICE IS TO ENHANCE VALUE TO CONSUMERS NOT JUST REDUCE COST ✗ MAKE MEANINGFUL QUALITY & PERFORMANCE DATA AVAILABLE TO CONSUMERS ✗ GIVE CONSUMERS INCENTIVES AS WELL AS INFORMATION TO MOTIVATE BEST CHOICES

to specialists, will at some point include self-referral to selected categories of alternative care providers. Where consumers are demanding access to such providers, and cost of care by such providers is less than that for traditional medicine, payers have double the reasons for offering the option.

Problems and Potential

Different providers have been shown to have widely different performance in terms of cost, quality, and patient service performance. Programs such as the Pennsylvania Health Care Cost Containment Council and Greater Cleveland Health Care Quality Choice have long offered reports on variable performance among providers, both hospitals and physicians. It has been argued that by enabling consumers to "buy right," the performance of providers will improve as well as the health of consumers.[183]

Studies have shown that consumers are perfectly happy using nurse practitioners (NPs) and physician assistants for routine medical needs, for example. Since these nonphysician providers have also demonstrated their ability to manage the health and care needs of populations more inexpensively than physicians, which providers are chosen by consumers can make a big difference to overall demand and expenditures.[184]

Studies have suggested that getting care from a specialist can make a significant difference in mortality from heart attacks.[185] Physicians specializing in the care of AIDS patients do significantly better than ones who rarely treat them, though consultation can bring the performance of primary physicians up significantly.[186] The best hospitals have been shown to have significantly fewer deaths and complications than others.[187]

Advantages to Payers

Where NPs were used as primary care sources for Medicaid patients, the government saved an average of $41.20 per beneficiary per month in one example, thanks to fewer hospital days and ED visits, though more nurse visits.[188] By directing employees to Centers of Excellence for organ transplants, one health plan saved from 23% to 31% on various organs, though its costs for kidney transplants were 1% higher.[189]

Aetna found that its Centers of Excellence savings were so great they allowed paying for patient and family travel.[190] A birth center offered costs for maternity care 50% lower than hospitals.[191] Where consumers seek care from alternative providers, cost savings frequently occur. For patients with allergies, for example, treatment by herbalists with stinging nettles was 82% cheaper than with the most popular prescription drug.[192]

In many cases treatment by alternative care providers may prove less expensive than costs of traditional medicine. At the same time a large portion of alternative treatments and providers have never been tested by the kinds of rigorous scientific outcomes studies being advocated for traditional medicine. If alternative providers are to be included as options, and particularly if advocated for specific conditions, they should be evaluated and selected with the same care as are physicians. Plans and employers have both moral and legal obligations to ensure that they direct or empower consumers to make the best provider choices possible.

Benefits to Providers

In a somewhat indirect example of provider benefit, the program that offered information to consumers to help them select physicians kept a record of what information consumers accessed.[193] It supplied reports on what facts were proving important to consumers so that providers could improve their marketing to consumers—by expanding evening and weekend availability, for example.[194]

In general, providers at risk gain when consumers choose specialists who are in their chosen referral networks, because of lower prices, better quality, sharing risk, or whatever reasons lie behind their being chosen for the network. The same applies to consumer choices of hospital, home health care, complementary medicine provider, or any other therapist. Where consumers choose to obtain care from an inpatient hospitalist, primary physicians can save the time and energy required in managing inpatients.[195]

Benefits to Consumers

Consumers should also benefit whenever choice of provider improves the quality of care and its outcomes. Ideally they will also gain when the best choice means lower costs, through lower copayment or shared savings. Preferred provider networks in POS and PPO health plans are designed to give consumers a financial benefit if they choose providers within the network (e.g., a 10% or 20% copayment if they use in-network providers versus a 20% or 40% copayment for out-of-network providers).[196]

Consumers save in copayments if chosen providers' fees are lower, even in indemnity plans.[197] By informing consumers what prevailing (i.e., "usual, customary, and reasonable") fees are for specific services, Ryder encouraged its employees to select providers who charged no more than that or to negotiate lower fees if they did.[198]

Applications

Hospitals have long offered physician information and referral services by phone, though these have been aimed primarily at bringing in more patients to the hospital. Both providers and health plans have offered information kiosks in malls and other convenient locations to facilitate and guide consumer choices.[199] Touch-screen computer monitors permit consumers to use their own criteria in making selections.[200] HealthPartners HMO in Minnesota provides information on-line or on diskette for members with computers.[201] Cleveland Clinic offers its own published guide on physicians, counting on consumers to lean toward its physicians.[202]

There are growing numbers of consumers' guidebooks and information services offered independently, such as *Choice Tools*.[203] The Greater Cleveland Health Quality Choice program offers information on physicians and hospitals to help consumers choose the best.[204] As with health plans, employers have used a combination of incentives and information to urge employees to choose the "best" providers, offering information on prices to overcome consumers' reluctance to ask.[205]

Limits and Concerns

One of the problems in promoting better provider choices among consumers is that they may not make selections on what payers or providers would argue are rational grounds. One study found that only 18% consider prices in selecting providers; only 9% ask providers about fees.[206] Consumers may have emotional attachments to particular physicians and hospitals based on location, familiarity, or other factors unrelated to either quality or cost.[207]

Conventional wisdom regarding the best provider choices is occasionally wrong. The Veterans Affairs (VA) system offered sick veterans improved access to primary physicians, for example, and found that those veterans were hospitalized one third more than before.[208] A geriatric evaluation and management program specializing in elderly patients improved quality and satisfaction for its patients but had no impact on utilization or costs.[209]

There are definite risks in attempting to influence consumer decisions related to providers. Requirements that members of managed care plans choose a primary care "gatekeeper" who is at risk for the specialty services and hospital care they use can promote limiting access, consumer dissatisfaction, and litigation.[210] Steering consumers toward specific providers can put employers, health plans, and physicians at legal risk if those providers are clearly substandard.[211]

One serious risk of empowering consumers with more information about which are the best providers is that they will concentrate their demands on a few providers, creating access problems. Will any informed consumer choose surgeons performing their first operation or diagnosing their first patient? What happens to physicians with no track record to judge by or with one bad outcome in a small number of cases?

Advice

The best advice for anyone guiding consumer choice of providers is essentially the same as applies in triage, shared decisions, and health plan choices. First, aim the guidance at delivering a clear consumer benefit, rather than simply reducing expenditures. Document the criteria used in selecting providers for any restricted network or preferred list, and be sure the reasons stress quality.[212] In general, it is probably wiser for sponsors to select providers based on quality than to negotiate price, as opposed to choosing the lowest bidders and hoping their quality is okay. Patients who are able to retain the same physician for many years, for example, spend significantly less on medical care.[213]

This means that payers and providers at risk will have to have meaningful quality and performance data to make their choices.[214] Employers are increasingly demanding performance data from providers.[215] Fortunately such data return benefits to providers in their own quality improvement efforts, though they can also add significantly to provider costs.

Giving consumers incentives as well as information to motivate and enable them to make the best provider choices is also advised.[216] Making information accessible (e.g., through pharmacists) may help.[217] Paying them to choose the hospital preferred by the employer has been tried.[218] Helping providers chosen by sponsors for quality and cost reasons to make attractive and satisfying offers to consumers can help promote unified preference and consumer choice.[219] Alternatively, offering consumers the physicians and hospitals they already prefer, and working with popular providers on quality and cost can also work.

END-OF-LIFE PLANNING

Empowering consumers to make the best choices regarding the use of services at the end of their or their loved ones' lives is a particularly challenging aspect of improving demand. There are significant legal risks attending any involvement in such decisions. Sponsors are likely to be presumed to be in it for their own financial benefit and are subject to public reputation damage and retention problems as well as legal risk. Yet there is great room for improvement on all dimensions of what makes a good end-of-life decision (Exhibit 22–6).

Problems and Potential

Most attention is focused on the "excessive" expenditures for health care around the end of life. Futile and expensive efforts to preserve life of dubious quality have been attacked by a variety of journalists, policy analysts, and politicians. A Stanford medical study found that 13% of patients used 32% of resources for what researchers termed "potentially ineffective care."[220] It has been widely reported that 30% of all Medicare expenditures occur in the last year of beneficiaries' lives.[221]

Exhibit 22–6 End of Life Planning

PROBLEMS / POTENTIAL	✗ ADVANCE DIRECTIVES, LIVING WILLS & DURABLE POWERS OF ATTORNEY HELP GUARANTEE PEOPLE GET KIND OF CARE THEY DESIRE AT OFTEN A LOWER COST ✗ COST SAVINGS AS WELL AS INCREASED SATISFACTION & RETENTION FOR SPONSORS ✗ REDUCTION IN BURDEN OF MANAGING TERMINAL ILLNESS ✗ CAN SIGNIFICANTLY REDUCE RISK OF LITIGATION ✗ CONSUMERS GAIN SENSE OF CONTROL OVER THE PROCESS AS WELL AS EMOTIONAL, PSYCHOLOGICAL & SPIRITUAL BENEFITS
EXAMPLES	✗ PROVIDERS DEVELOP SPECIFIC PROGRAMS FOR END-OF-LIFE TREATMENT PLANNING
CONCERNS	✗ ENSURING INFORMATION IS TRANSFERRED FROM ONE PROVIDER TO ANOTHER IS DIFFICULT ✗ DIFFERENCE OF OPINION AMONG PROFESSIONALS MAKES DEVELOPING PROTOCOLS DIFFICULT ✗ DIFFERENCES OF VALUES AMONG PATIENTS, FAMILIES & PROFESSIONALS MAKE IMPLEMENTATION OF PROTOCOLS DIFFICULT ✗ GRIEVING MAY INHIBIT FAMILIES' ABILITY TO IMPLEMENT END-OF-LIFE PLANS
ADVICE	✗ PROMOTE CONSUMER RIGHTS & CONTROL ✗ WORK TO ENSURE THAT EVERYONE INVOLVED IN THE PROCESS IS INFORMED & CONSIDERED IN THE IMPLEMENTATION OF THE PLANS ✗ CUSTOMIZE THE SERVICE TO CONSUMER SEGMENTS

Where patients and families have prepared advance directives, living wills, or durable medical powers of attorney, significant reductions in end-of-life expenditures have been realized. One study found hospital charges averaging $31,200 for patients with advance directives versus $49,000 for those without.[222] In another study where patients and families planned the last illness, hospital costs averaged only $30,478, compared to an average of $90,305 for unplanned.[223] One account suggested that $60 billion could be saved each year through better management of terminal illnesses, though it admitted $10 billion was probably a more achievable savings.[224]

In addition to costs, there is evidence that people do not get the kind of care they wish at the end of their lives. Poor care and a poor match between expressed wishes and actual care experiences are the rule rather than the exception. Providers are often blamed as being part of a system that simply does not know when to stop.[225] Physicians have been found to rarely know patients' wishes or to consider them to be contrary to professional principles.[226]

When patients are transferred from one facility to another, advance directives are frequently lost. One study found that 74% of patients with do-not-resuscitate directives did not have that directive accompany them when they transferred from a nursing home to a hospital.[227] A study at Stanford indicated that 20% of hospital costs could be saved if ICU patients who showed no progress in their first five days were simply allowed to die.[228]

Cutting off care to patients is by no means a simple matter, however. Patients and their families can also be part of the problem. They often demand heroics when there is no hope of improving the patient's condition. They also decline care in many cases where significant improvement is possible.[229] While Medicare offers a hospice benefit to beneficiaries in the last six months of life, experience indicates that most patients enter a hospice too late, averaging only a month in the hospice program, with many dying within a week, not enough time to benefit from the psychological and spiritual support for them and their families.[230]

Benefits to Payers

Savings in expenditures are the obvious benefit for payers. For employers, a well-planned and managed terminal illness of family members can also benefit employees' morale, productivity, and retention. Futile care takes a lot out of family members as well as patients, and fighting with the system to make up for the lack of preplanning can make employed family members ineffective on the job.

Benefits to Providers

For physicians, advance planning and family agreement over care at the end of life can take away a lot of the burden of managing terminal illness. It can also significantly reduce the risk of litigation for overtreating or undertreating patients. For hospitals, it can eliminate the new phenomenon of "wrongful life" litigation, such as the case where a jury awarded a family $16.6 million because the hospital ignored patient and family wishes and insisted on keeping a patient on life support.[231]

Benefits to Consumers

Aside from the emotional, psychological, and spiritual benefits of well-managed end-of-life planning, consumers have much to gain in terms of a sense of control over what happens in their own and family members' lives versus what they often see as an uncaring and unresponsive health system. They may gain financially if everyone has agreed not to devote a family member's estate to futile care. The examples of Richard Nixon and Jackie Kennedy dying at home with their families showed the public what a well-managed death could be.[232]

Applications

The Health Care Partners Medical Group (Los Angeles) developed an Options program for end-of-life treatment planning, offering informed choices to patients and family on how they want to spend the rest of the life in question and offering support services to address clinical, social, and spiritual needs. Among those participating in the program, only 35% even went to the hospital during the final illness, and only 15% died there. The program achieved not only significant cost savings but great family support.[233]

Many consumer and community organizations have conducted public information programs regarding advance directives, living wills, and similar end-of-life planning documents. Physicians and lawyers are becoming more likely to bring up the subject with families. Even employers are including end-of-life planning programs in their employee assistance program activiites.

Limits and Concerns

In light of the legal, professional, and personal conflicts involved in end-of-life situations, it is no wonder that we have not solved this problem. The ideal answer is probably what is called "compression of morbidity," in which we live a high-quality life until the very end, then have everything break at once and reach the end quickly.[234] Failing that, we are faced with problems of defining "futile care" in general and deciding what it means in individual cases. Do patients have the right to demand futile care as well as refuse it; do physicians have the right to refuse to provide futile care when demanded?[235]

Well-managed end-of-life care does not necessarily produce cost savings. In one example no savings were found linked to having advance directives, though it was not clear if providers were informed of them.[236] In another study of four hospitals around the country, neither pain nor costs were found to be reduced by a carefully managed terminal illness support program.[237] Acceptance of end-of-life planning is high in principle but low in practice. One study found that 90% of patients and families for whom death occurrred in the hospital agreed with the care provided, preferring agressive intervention over dying at home or in a hospice. Another found that patients with serious illnesses would want aggressive treatment even if it prolonged their lives by as little as a week.[238]

Advice

For sponsors of end-of-life improvement initiatives, it is clear that program efforts should aim at promoting consumer rights and control, plus quality of life for patients and family rather than cost savings.[239] Programs should consciously aim to deliver benefits to consumers and should monitor patient and family perceptions to be sure benefits are felt. Incentives such as lower premiums for consumers who have signed advance directives might be considered.[240]

Substantial efforts are needed to promote not only public awareness of end-of-life issues but public action. Sponsors might do well to join with religious and community organizations in promoting initiatives rather than risk skepticism if they conduct their own.[241] One hospital was able to get 18.5% of discharged patients to complete an advanced directives form by writing to patients and including a pamphlet on the subject as well as offering a phone counseling line. Of those completing the directive form, 90% indicated preference for no heroics, while 3% insisted on everything being done to keep them alive.[242]

Above all, sponsors should work to ensure that everyone who might play a role in managing the end of life—for example, physicians, patients, family members, hospital, nursing home, clergy—is involved in, aware of, and understands what consumers decide. Achieving the specific consumer behaviors of interest—planning end of life and executing the necessary legal documents to guide providers—is only the first step in changing the way death is actually experienced.[243]

REFERENCES

1. "Demand Management Links Consumers, Information to Healthcare System," *Health Management Technology* 16, no. 9 (1995):8, 12.

2. J. Gemignani, "Demand Management: Dial-A-Nurse," *Business & Health* 14, no. 7 (1996):50.

3. D. Powell, "Cost Savings: The Economic Impact of Demand Management," in *Demand Management® for Health Care* (Chicago, IL: Strategic Research Institute, May 30, 1996).

4. J. Whalley-Hill and S. Mooney, "Aggressive Patient Education Program Reaps Cost Containment Rewards for Providers," *Capitation & Medical Practice* 2, no. 7 (1996):1–3.

5. E. Wogensen, "Demand Management Helps Patients Make More Appropriate Use of Medical Resources," *Strategic Health Care Marketing* 12, no. 8 (1995):4, 5.

6. L. Raposa, "Harvard's New 'Doc' Makes House Calls," *Boston Herald,* 27 June 1991, 1, 44.

7. Health Decisions, Inc., *Year-End Report* (Golden, CO: 1995).

8. "Health System Minnesota and the Minnesota Blues Partner for Telephone Medical Treatment Advice," *Health Care Strategic Management* 14, no. 3 (1996):5.

9. "Phone-Based Triage System Brings Bottom-Line Benefits to Pediatric Hospitals, Physicians," *Healthcare Demand Management* 1, no. 1 (1995):9–11.

10. D. Wise, "The Power of Education," *Business & Health* 12, no. 7 (1994):11.

11. E. Wogensen, "Ready or Not, Providers Will Be Communicating with Consumers On-Line," *Strategic Health Care Marketing* 12, no. 7 (1995):3, 4.

12. B. Zoller, "Member-Centered Managed Care and the New Media," in *Health and the New Media,* ed. L. Harris (Mahwah, NJ: Lawrence Erlbaum, 1995), 21–43.

13. "Insurer Gets Cost Savings from Demand Management," *Accountability News for Health Care Managers* 2, no. 8 (1995):2, 3.

14. " 'Demand Management': A New Frontier for Cost Reductions," *Physician's Managed Care Report* 3, no. 12 (1995):133–136.

15. J. Harrington and J. Wardle, "Employer's Perspective: Managing Self-Funded Healthcare," *The Alliance Bulletin,* August 1995, 4, 7.

16. "Telephone Service Aims To Cut Costs by Providing Care at Tight Place, Time," *St. Anthony's Managing Community Health and Wellness* 2, no. 2 (1995):5.

17. A. Barnett, "Is Knowledge Really Power for Patients?" *Business & Health* 11, no. 5 (1995):29–36.

18. "An 'Advice Nurse' Saves Your Patients—And You," *The Physicians Advisory* 94, no. 12 (1994):3, 4.

19. R. Sberna, "Nurses a Phone Call Away with Clinic Info Line," *Modern Healthcare,* 14 August 1995, 33.

20. D. Algeo, "Doctor Forecasts Triage Prelude to Medical Golden Age," *The Denver Post,* 16 March 1996, 1D, 2D.

21. "An 'Advice Nurse'," 3, 4.

22. M. Dickens, "Panicky Phone Calls Don't Faze Our Nurses," *Medical Economics* 68, no. 16 (1991):109–112.

23. Zoller, "Member-Centered Managed Care," 21–43.

24. Wogensen, "Ready or Not," 3, 4.

25. I. Lazarus, "Medical Call Centers," *Managed Healthcare* 5, no. 10 (1995):56–59.

26. Sberna, "Nurses a Phone Call Away," 33.

27. J. Pollard, "Patient Advisory Nurse—A Program That Works," *Group Practice Journal* 41, no. 5 (1992):14–16.

28. Dickens, "Panicky Phone Calls," 109–112.

29. B. Melville, "Profile: Minnesota Blue Cross and Blue Shield Shaves Health Care Costs," *Health Care Competition Week* 10, no. 15 (1993):6, 7.

30. T. Defino, "Patients Given More Responsibility for Their Care," *Managed Healthcare,* October 1993, 63, 64.

31. "Building a Better Patient," *Physician Referral Update* 9, no. 1 (1996):2, 3.

32. W. Lynch, *Demand Management in Healthcare* (Chicago, IL: Strategic Research Institute, May 30, 1996).

33. "Physician Triage Practice Reduces LOS, Saves HMO Dollars," *Healthcare Demand Management* 2, no. 6 (1996):88–90.

34. "Telephone Service," 5.

35. "Quality Watch," *Hospitals & Health Networks,* 5 June 1996, 10.

36. R. Rupp, et al., "Telephone Triage: Results of Adolescent Clinic Responses to a Mock Patient with Pelvic Pain," *Journal of Adolescent Health* 15 (1994):249–253.

37. K. Kearney, "Medical Call Centers and the Law," in *Demand Management® for Healthcare* (Chicago, IL: Strategic Research Institute, May 30–31, 1996).

38. W. Bell, "Telephone-Based Demand Management: What You Need To Know Now," *Health Care Strategic Management* 14, no. 3 (1995):6–8.

39. "Building a Better Patient," 2, 3.

40. B. Wolcott, "Managed Care's Driving Force; Demand Management," *InfoCare,* January–February 1996, 12–15.

41. "Call Notes," *Hospitals and Health Networks Pacesetters* (1997):28, 29.

42. "Demand Management Links Consumers," 8, 12.

43. A. Peck, "Phone Service Cuts Costs by Guiding Consumers through Health Care Maze," *Managed Healthcare* 4, no. 1 (1994):24–26.

44. I. Ritter, "HMO Employs Telemarketing for Modifying Member Behavior," *Strategic Health Care Marketing* 10, no. 2 (1993):9–11.

45. "Phoning In for Medical Advice," *Hospitals & Health Networks,* 5 February 1996, 16.

46. Peck, "Phone Service," 24–26.

47. "Telephone Service," 5.

48. Wogensen, "Demand Management," 4, 5.

49. "Insurer Gets Cost Savings," 2, 3.

50. Algeo, "Doctor Forecasts," 1D, 2D.

51. Lynch, *Demand Management in Healthcare.*

52. D. Neal, et al. "Telephone Service Reduces Demand for Medical Treatment," *Inside Preventive Care* 1, no. 5 (1995):1–3.

53. Lynch, *Demand Management in Healthcare.*

54. S. MacStravic, "Improving Health and Utilization: Can Vendors Help?" *Strategic Health Care Management* 14, no. 8 (1996).

55. D. Sobel, "Self-Care, Values Lead to Healthy Communities," *Health Progress* 75, no. 6 (1994):70–72, 79.

56. V. Elsenhaus, et al., "Use of Self-Care Manual Shifts Utilization Pattern," *HMO Practice* 9, no. 2 (1995):88–90.

57. "A Cough and a Wheeze Do Not a Cold Make," *Employee Health & Fitness, Health & Well-Being Supplement,* May 1994, 1.

58. M. Sims, "Healthy Workers Equal Healthy Bottom Line," *Denver Business Journal,* September 30–October 6, 1994, 9B.

59. E. Stoller, et al., "Self-Care Responses to Symptoms by Older People," *Medical Care* 31, no. 1 (1993):24–42.

60. P. Braus, "Selling Self-Help," *American Demographics* 14, no. 3 (1992):48–52.

61. D. Vickery and D. Iverson, "Medical Self-Care and Use of the Medical Care System," in *Health Promotion in the Workplace,* 2d ed., eds. M. O'Donnell and J. Harris (Albany, NY: Delmar, 1994), 367–389.

62. "An 'Advice Nurse,' " 3, 4.

63. "Self-Care Pilot Project Meets Expectations," *Health S.E.T. Helping* 8, no. 1 (1995):1, 4.

64. "Claims Data Analysis, Satisfaction Survey Show DM Program's Impact," *Healthcare Demand Management* 2, no. 1 (1996):10–12.

65. R. Coile, "Integrating the Patient into Healthcare Systems," *Hospital Strategy Report* 5, no. 5 (1993):2.

66. *Preliminary Report on United States Air Force "Take Care of Yourself Study* (Menlo Park, CA: Healthtrac, 1994), unpublished study.

67. G. Kamas, "Assessing the Value of DMS by MCOs," in *Demand Management Services* (Dallas, TX: International Business Communications, October 19–20, 1995).

68. "Continuum of Care," *Hospitals & Health Networks,* 5 June 1994, 20, 21.

69. F. Glasgow and D. Weiss, "Demand Management," in *Demand Management Services* (Dallas, TX: International Business Communications, October 19–20, 1995).

70. *HealthyLife® Self-Care Guide Evaluations* (Farmington Hills, MI: American Institute for Preventive Medicine, 1995).

71. D. Powell, "Cost Savings: The Economic Impact of Demand Management," in *Demand Management® for Healthcare* (Chicago, IL: Strategic Research Institute, May 30–31, 1996).

72. Barnett, "Is Knowledge Really Power?" 29–36.

73. J.S. Robinson, et al., "The Impact of Fever Health Education on Clinic Utilization," *AJDC* 143 (1989):698–704.

74. D. Vickery, et al., "The Effect of Self-Care Interventions on the Use of Medical Services with a Medicare Population," *Medical Care* 26, no. 6 (1988):580–588.

75. M. Mettler and S. Degenfelder, "The Empowering Clinic," in *Demand Management Services* (Dallas, TX: International Business Communications, October 19–20, 1995).

76. Wise, "The Power of Education," 11.

77. E. Wogensen, "Empowering Patients To Take Better Care of Themselves Can Cut Utilization of Medical Services," *Strategic Health Care Marketing* 11, no. 9 (1994):5, 6.

78. "Yes, Virginia, Self-Help Books Really Help," *Medical Self-Care* 54 (1990):14, 15.

79. R. Cohen, "Demand Management Takes One More Step," *Healthcare Marketing Report* 14, no. 4 (1996):15.

80. T. Ferguson, "Consumer Health Information," *Healthcare Forum Journal,* January/February 1995, 28–33.

81. "Testing Hits Home," *Prevention* 45, no. 11 (1993):22, 23.

82. M. Wann, "Patients' Kin Prove Adept as Adjunct Nurses," *Healthweek News* 5, no. 6 (1991):9.

83. J. Pickens, "Community Caring Project Focuses on 'Mothercraft,' " *Healthcare Marketing Report* 11, no. 2 (1993):6, 7.

84. D. Martin, et al., "The Planetree Model Hospital Project: An Example of the Patient as Partner," *Hospital & Health Services Administration* 35, no. 4 (1990):591–601.

85. M. Edlin, "Demand Management: Saving Money with Self-Help," *Managed Healthcare* 5, no. 8 (1995):28–30.

86. D. Vickery and A. Levinson, "The Limits of Self-Care," *Generations,* Fall 1993, 53–56.

87. P. Terry and A. Pheley, "The Effect of Self-Care Brochures on Use of Medical Services," *Journal of Occupational Medicine* 35, no. 4 (1993):422–426.

88. M. Sandberg, "Self-Care Programs Produce Immediate Results," *Managed Healthcare* 4, no. 7 (1994):33.

89. Elsenhaus and Bledsoe, "Use of Self-Care Manual," 88–90.

90. J. Otis and A. Jacobs, "Power to the Patient: How Demand Management Makes Consumers an Active Part of Healthcare Decisions," in *Demand Management Services* (Dallas, TX: International Business Communications, October 19–20, 1995).

91. L. Schiff and R. Service, "Empowered Patients Buy More Efficient Care," *Business & Health* 14, no. 6 (1996):35–42.

92. Barnett, "Is Knowledge Really Power?" 29–36.

93. D. Vickery and W. Lynch, "Demand Management: Enabling Patients To Use Medical Care More Appropriately," *JOEM* 37, no. 5 (1995):551–557.

94. "Empowerment, Education Cited as Keys to Effective Demand Management Program," *Healthcare Demand Management* 1, no. 2 (1995):30–32.

95. "Wasted Health Care Dollars," *Consumer Reports,* July 1992, 435–448.

96. P. Rubin, "When and How To Challenge Your Doctor," *U.S. News & World Report,* 10 May 1993, 63–68.

97. G. Dominghetti, et al., *International Journal of Technology Assessment in Health Care,* 9, no. 4 (1993):505.

98. M. Magee, "Information Empowerment of the Patient: The Next Payer/Provider Battlefield," *Journal of Outcomes Management* 2, no. 3 (1995):17–21.

99. C. Petersen, "Direct-to-Consumer Drug Ads Gain More Acceptance," *Managed Healthcare* 5, no. 9 (1995):S35.

100. "Consumers," *Hospitals & Health Networks,* 5 October 1995, 24–26.

101. W. Lynch, et al., "Predicting the Demand for Healthcare," *Healthcare Forum Journal* 39, no. 1 (1996):20–24.

102. "Technology Assessment: Public Access, Public Trust," *Health Technology Assessment News,* May–June 1994, 1–3.

103. A. Barron, "Cutting Out Unnecessary Surgery," *Risk & Benefits Management* 2, no. 6 (1987):25–27.

104. M. Battagliola, "Making Employees Better Health Care Consumers," *Business & Health* 10, no. 6 (1992):22–28.

105. "Videos Earn Kaiser Savings, High Satisfaction Marks," *Accountability News for Health Care Managers* 2, no. 10 (1995):2, 3.

106. M. McGarry, "Marketing Challenge for Ornish Heart Program," *Healthcare Marketing Report* 13, no. 12 (1995):7–9.

107. P. O'Donnell, "Managing Health Costs under a Fee-for-Service Plan," *Business & Health* 5, no. 3 (1987):38–40.

108. P. Gapen, "The Beginning of a Beautiful Friendship," *Managed Healthcare* 3, no. 10 (1993):65, 66.

109. *Year End Report 1995* (Golden, CO: Health Decisions, Inc., 1995).

110. B. Solberg, "Wisconsin Resource Center Integrates Educational Efforts," *Inside Preventive Care* 1, no. 10 (1996):1, 5.

111. D. Holzman, "Interactive Video Promotes Patient-Doctor Partnership," *Business & Health* 10, no. 4 (1992).

112. E. Wogensen, "Managed Care Expressing Intense Interest in New Patient Education Tool That May Cut Utilization: Not All Providers Thrilled," *Strategic Health Care Marketing* 10, no. 9 (1993):10, 11.

113. Wogensen, "Managed Care," 10, 11.

114. R. Winslow, "Videos, Questionnaires Aim To Expand Role of Patients in Treatment Decisions," *Wall Street Journal,* 25 February, 1992, A5.

115. A. Gramling, "Make Your Patients Better Health-Care Consumers," *Medical Economics* 71, no. 22 (1994):42A–42D.

116. Magee, "Information Empowerment," 17–21.

117. D. Borfitz, "Practice Guidelines Address Physician-Driven Demand for Care; Will Demand Management Go On-Line?" *Strategic Health Care Marketing* 13, no. 4 (1996):3–5.

118. Winslow, "Videos, Questionnaires," A5.

119. S. Marcus, "Preparing for the Impact of the Technologically-Empowered, Proactive Patient," *Multimedia Patient Education* (Phoenix, AZ: Institute for International Research, December 1, 2, 1994).

120. S. Kaplan, et al., "The Effects of a Joint Physician-Patient Intervention Program on Health Outcomes and Interpersonal Care," *Clinical Research* 41, no. 2 (1993):541A.

121. J. Cassidy, "Outcomes Data: Rational Utilization, Better Doctor-Patient Relations," *Health Progress* 73, no. 10 (1992):36.

122. "CIGNA Using Outcomes Video for Patient Decision-Making," *Accountability News for Health Care Managers* 1, no. 3 (1994):7.

123. "Consumers," *Hospitals & Health Networks,* 5 April 1996, 19.

124. K. Taylor, "Shopping for Surgery," *Hospitals & Health Networks,* 20 July 1993, 42–44.

125. "Interactive Video Program Empowers Breast Cancer Patients To Make Informed Decisions," *Healthcare Demand Management* 1, no. 2 (1995):24, 25.

126. "Easy Access," *Modern Healthcare,* 18–25 December 1995, 68.

127. "Employers Use Incentives To Steer Workers to Generic Drugs," *Business and Health* 11, no. 9 (1993):10.

128. G. Keizer, " 'Doc-in-Box' Always On Call," *The Denver Post,* 12 February 1996, 1C.

129. P. MacPherson, "Call for a Consult," *Hospitals & Health Networks,* 20 February 1996, 70.

130. Lynch, *Demand Management for Healthcare.*

131. J. Schiffman, "Revising Second-Opinion Health Plans," *The Wall Street Journal,* 24 May 1989, B1.

132. J. Wennberg, "Shared Decision Making and Multimedia," in *Health and the New Media,* ed. L. Harris (Mahwah, NJ: Lawrence Erlbaum, 1995), 109–126.

133. Winslow, "Videos, Questionnaires," A5.

134. D. Borfitz, "Medical Call Centers Serve Multiple Functions: For Now, Health Plans Taking the Lead," *Strategic Health Care Marketing* 13, no. 3 (1996):4–8.

135. Borfitz, "Medical Call Centers," 4–8.

136. M. Mettler and D. Kemper, "Shared Decisions," *HMO Magazine* 35, no. 5 (1994):73–76.

137. E. Mort, "Shared Decision-Making Programs: Helping the Patient Make Informed Medical Decisions," *The Picker Report* 3, no. 2 (1995):9.

138. P. O'Neill, "Tailoring Interactive Interfaces To Suit Patient Needs," in *Multimedia Patient Education* (Phoenix, AZ: Institute for International Research, December 1, 2, 1994).

139. A. Peck, "Doctor-Patient Consultation Goes Prime Time," *Managed Healthcare* 3, no. 11 (1993):62, 63.

140. "Patient Education Technology Enhances Satisfaction and Savings," *The Singer Report on Managed Care Systems & Technology* 16 (1993):1–5.

141. Peck, "Doctor-Patient Consultation," 62, 63.

142. "Study: HMO's Lower Costs Have a Price," *Hospitals & Health Networks,* 5 April 1995, 60.

143. S. Alt, "Xerox Wants at Least 89% of Its Employees in Selected HMOs," *Contract Healthcare,* September 1988, 40.

144. "Managed Care Costs Okla. Medicaid Less," *Hospitals & Health Networks,* 5 May 1996, 71.

145. G. Leavenworth, "Solutions for Small Businesses," *Business & Health* 11, no. 12 (1993):44–52.

146. H. Smith and R. Rogers, "Factors Influencing Consumers' Selection of Health Insurance Carriers," *Journal of Health Care Marketing* 6, no. 4 (1986):6–14.

147. A. Schrader, "Picking, Choosing Health Care," *The Denver Post,* 13 July 1996, 1B.

148. O. Mascarenhas, "Marketing Health Care to Employees," *Journal of Health Care Marketing* 13, no. 3 (1993):34–46.

149. D. Scotti, et al., "An Analysis of the Determinants of HMO Reenrollment Behavior," *Journal of Health Care Marketing* 6, no. 2 (1986):7–16.

150. D. Wise, "When One Purchaser Has the Clout of Many," *Business & Health* 13, no. 11 (1995):59.

151. J. Johnsson, "Direct Contracting: Hospitals Discover Its Risks and Rewards," *Hospitals,* 20 May 1990, 40–45.

152. M. Traska, "Xerox Reports HMOs Saving $115 Per Insured Over Fee-for-Service," *Managed Care Outlook* 5, no. 13 (1992):4.

153. D. Mayer, "Lockheed Ends First Ever Program Requiring 1-Year HMO Enrollment," *Health-Week,* 23 November 1987, 2, 41.

154. "Health Plans Cut Costs for Families, AAHP Study Shows," *Managed Healthcare* 7, no. 7 (1997):8.

155. R. Upton, "Targeting Health Care Consumers," *Hospitals & Health Networks,* 5 October 1995, 94.

156. Traska, "Xerox Reports HMOs," 4.

157. Johnsson, "Direct Contracting," 40–45.

158. "Empire Blue Cross/Blue Shield," *Hospitals & Health Networks,* 5 October 1993, 23.

159. J. Packer-Tursman, "IBM Seeks Savings in Push for HMO Enrollment," *Managed Healthcare* 4, no. 1 (1994):26.

160. K. DeMott, "Employers Use Survey Data To Steer Workers to 'Exceptional' Plans," *Report on Medical Guidelines and Outcomes Research* 5, no. 15 (1994):5, 6.

161. "Boeing To Give Cash for Managed Care Enrollment," *Business & Health* 14, no. 1 (1996):13.

162. J. Montague, "Low Fat, Low Cost," *Hospitals & Health Networks,* 5 August 1993, 76.

163. "A Double Decker Model," *Business & Health* 14, no. 2 (1996):48.

164. M. Edlin, "Cashing In on Communication," *Managed Healthcare* 5, no. 2 (1995):19–22.

165. S. Siegelman, "Health Plan Options: Inquiring Employees Want To Know," *Business & Health* 9, no. 1 (1991):14–22.

166. "Looking for an HMO? Let Your Mouse Do the Walking," *Modern Healthcare,* 5 February 1996, 40.

167. "Retiree Enrollment in Florida HMO Nears 10%," *Health Care Strategic Management* 13, no. 3 (1995):5, 6.

168. C. Sardinha, "Price Cuts Help Medica Win Market Share and Improve Risk Selection," *Managed Care Outlook* 8, no. 2 (1995):4.

169. Wise, "When One Purchaser," 59.

170. "Hospital Uses Telephone System To Capture Market," *Healthcare PR & Marketing News* 5, no. 6 (1996):4.

171. L. Kertesz, "United Blazes a Trail in Managed Care," *Modern Healthcare,* 8 April 1996, 46.

172. D. Lerner, et al., "GE Sheds Light on Managed Care's Impact on Health," *Business & Health* 11, no. 9 (1993):48–54.

173. W. Kuznar, "Convincing the Skeptics," *Managed Healthcare* 4, no. 4 (1994):1, 18, 19.

174. L. Lopez, "Choosing the Best HMO," *Business & Health* 13, no. 1 (1995):22–26.

175. J. Robinson, et al., "Health Plan Switching in Anticipation of Increased Medical Care Utilization," *Medical Care* 31, no. 1 (1993):43–51.

176. Siegelman, "Health Plan Options," 14–22.

177. R. Blankenau, "Confused Consumers," *Hospitals & Health Networks,* 5 July 1993, 31.

178. P. Fetsch, "Demonstrating Value to Purchasers of Managed Care Products," *The Academy Bulletin,* May 1994, 1, 2, 7.

179. "Choosing an HMO: A Difficult Task Becomes Easier as Standards Emerge," *Employee Health & Fitness* 18, no. 4 (1996):37–39.

180. "Employers Can Do More To Lower Health Costs, Says Expert," *Qual-Med Briefings* 2, no. 2 (1992):1, 3.

181. Johnsson, "Direct Contracting," 40–45.

182. Kuznar, "Convincing the Skeptics," 1, 18, 19.

183. W. McClure, "Buying Right: The Consequences of Glut," *Business & Health* 3, no. 9 (1985):43–46.

184. J. Kerekes, "Nurse-Managed Primary Care," *Nursing Management* 27, no. 2 (1996):44–47.

185. "Does a Heart Attack Demand More Than Primary Care?" *Business & Health* 14, no. 1 (1996):13.

186. L. Markson, et al., "Implications of Generalists' Slow Adoption of Zidovudine in Clinical Practice," *Archives of Internal Medicine* 154, no. 13 (1994):1497–1504.

187. "Quality Nursing Care Linked to Lower Mortality Rates," *American Journal of Health Promotion* 9, no. 3 (1995):186.

188. Kerekes, "Nurse-Managed Primary Care," 44–47.

189. K. Taylor, "Transplants Flourish under Managed Care," *Hospitals & Health Networks,* 20 March 1994, 64–66.

190. "Aetna Health Plans Forms National Cardiac Care Program," *Health Care Strategic Management* 13, no. 12 (1995):5.

191. "Birth Centers Offer Safe Alternative to In-Hospital Delivery," *Healthcare Demand Management* 2, no. 1 (1996):1–6.

192. C. Miller, "Major Health Care Marketers Endorse Alternative Treatment," *Marketing News* 31, no. 3 (1997):1, 6.

193. F. Joosi, "Twin Cities HMO Buys Into Interactive Kiosk Concept," *Strategic Health Care Marketing* 13, no. 2 (1996):5–7.

194. "Plan Puts Provider Quality Data On-Line To Create Competition, Conduct Research," *Accountability News for Health Care Managers* 2, no. 3 (1995):1, 8.

195. L. Kertesz, "Specialists Taking 'Gatekeeper' Role," *Modern Healthcare,* 13 May 1996, 47.

196. "Burger King's Hospital PPO Cut Costs 10%, To Save $2 Million," *Managed Care Week* 1, no. 27 (1991):1.

197. P. Kenkel, "Utah Employees' Health Plan Aims for Wiser, Thriftier Patients," *Modern Healthcare,* 30 August 1993, 68–70.

198. J. Charles and W.B. Latham, "Med Facts: How Ryder Helps Employees Make Smart Choices," in *Driving Down Health Care Costs* (New York, NY: Panel Publishers, 1991), 12-1–12-13.

199. Jossi, "Twin Cities HMO," 5–7.

200. C. Appleby, "Doc Shopping," *Hospitals & Health Networks,* 20 July 1995, 49, 50.

201. J. Morley, "Cleveland Health Quality Choice Project," *FAHS Review,* November–December 1990, 22–25.

202. C. Jensen, et al., "A Consumer Guide for Marketing Medical Services," *Quality Review Bulletin* 18, no. 5 (1992):164–171.

203. Taylor, "Transplants Flourish," 64–66.

204. Morley, "Cleveland Health," 22–25.

205. G. Leavenworth, "These Employees Light the Way to Lower Costs," *Business & Health* 14, no. 2 (1996):41–44.

206. "Consumer Attitudes toward Health-Care Purchases," *Health Care Strategic Management* 11, no. 3 (1993):5.

207. Taylor, "Transplants Flourish," 64–66.

208. Appleby, "Doc Shopping," 49, 50.

209. R. Toseland, et al., "Outpatient Geriatric and Management," *Medical Care* 34, no. 6 (1996):624–640.

210. R. Dubois and K. Blank, "Bringing Clinical Accuracy to Provider Profiling Systems," *Managed Care Quarterly* 3, no. 2 (1995):69–76.

211. "Managed Care and Mandatory Movies," *Journal of the American Medical Association* 276, no. 13 (1996):1023.

212. "Managed Care and Mandatory Movies," 1023.

213. "Currents—Consumers," *Hospitals & Health Networks,* 20 March 1997, 16.

214. Dubois and Blank, "Bringing Clinical Accuracy to Provider Profiling Systems," 69–76.

215. Leavenworth, "These Employees Light the Way to Lower Costs," 41–44.

216. Morley, "Cleveland Health," 22–25.

217. S. Szeinbach, "How Referral Networks Help Patients," *Medical Interface* 5, no. 1 (1992):40–44.

218. "Rewards Spur Employee Use of WI Provider," *Hospitals,* 20 September 1987, 60–62.

219. Taylor, "Transplants Flourish," 64–66.

220. L. Esserman, et al., "Potentially Ineffective Care," *Journal of the American Medical Association* 274, no. 19 (1995):1544–1551.

221. "Focus on Advance Directives To Bolster DM Efforts," *Healthcare Demand Management* 1, no. 8 (1995):113–116.

222. W. Weeks, "Advance Directives and the Cost of Terminal Hospitalization," *Archives of Internal Medicine* 154, September 26 (1994):2077–2083.

223. "Ethics," *Hospitals & Health Networks,* 5 May 1994, 16.

224. A. Lewis, "How Living Wills Could Save Billions," *Business & Health* 12, no. 9 (1994):68.

225. "Care for Dying Americans Needs Substantial Improvement, Say Researchers," *Health Care Strategic Management* 14, no. 1 (1996):9.

226. J. Greenwald, "Living Wills Present New Challenges," *Modern Healthcare,* 17 June 1996, 60, 62.

227. R. Morrison, et al., "The Inaccessibility of Advance Directives on Transfer from Ambulatory to Acute Care Settings," *Journal of the American Medical Association* 274, no. 6 (1995):478–482.

228. "When To Cut Off Care in the ICU," *Hospitals & Health Networks,* 20 December 1995, 14.

229. E. Friedman, "A Sense of Loss," *Healthcare Forum Journal* 38, no. 2 (1995):9–12.

230. C. Thompson, "Hospice Services Underused," *The Denver Post,* 18 July 1996, 8A.

231. "Large Award in Michigan Life-Support Care," *Modern Healthcare,* 26 February 1996, 14.

232. A. Lewis, "How Living Wills Could Save Billions," 68.

233. "Options Program Cuts Demand for Care While Improving Quality of Life for Terminally Ill Patients," *Healthcare Demand Management* 1, no. 1 (1995):13–16.

234. J. Fries, "Aging, Natural Death and the Compression of Morbidity," *New England Journal of Medicine* 303, no. 3 (1980):130–135.

235. "The Concept of Futility," *Health Progress* 74, no. 10 (1993):21–31.

236. "Ethics," 16.

237. "Care for Dying Americans Needs Substantial Improvement, Say Researchers," 9.

238. G. Kolata, "Dying Patients Want Aggressive Care, Study Finds," *The Denver Post,* 18 January 1997, 7A.

239. Kolata, "Dying Patients," 7A.

240. K. Miniclier, "Dignity in Death a Fervent Wish," *The Denver Post,* 12 March 1996, 1B, 4B.

241. J. Summers, "Take Patient Rights Seriously To Improve Patient Care and Lower Costs," *Health Care Management Review* 10, no. 4 (1985):55–62.

242. S. Rubin, et al., "Increasing the Completion of the Durable Power of Attorney for Health Care," *Journal of the American Medical Association* 271, no. 3 (1994):209–212.

243. J. Morrissey, "Communication Key in Life-or-Death Decisions," *Modern Healthcare,* 24 April 1995, 76.

Decision Improvement Vendors

Access Health
Rancho Cordova, CA
— *Call Centers "Ask-A-Nurse Advantage," "Personal Health Advisor"*

Aetna Health Plans
Hartford, CT
— *"Informed Health" Nurse Counselors*

The Alliance
Denver, CO
— *"Healthy Answers" Triage/ Information*

American Institute of Preventive Medicine
Farmington Hills, MI
— *Wellness/Self-Care Guides*

Cardinal Health, Medical Strategies Division
Dublin, OH
— *"Healthtouch" Information Kiosk*

CHESS Computer Network, U. Wisconsin
Madison, WI

Consumer Health Services
Boulder, CO
— *(Physician referral, education registration)*

Doctors, Inc.
Seattle, WA
— *Decision Counseling, Triage*

Employee Managed Care Corporation [EMC²]
Seattle, WA
— *Call Centers*

ERS Health Communications
Los Angeles, CA
— *Health Information*

Face Communications
Chicago, IL
— *(multimedia, interactive)*

First Help
Boulder, CO
— *Triage/Phone Counseling*

Greystone.Net
Atlanta, GA
— *(Internet, Website development)*

Health Decisions International
Golden, CO
—*Triage, Shared Decisions*

HealthDesk
Berkeley, CA
—*(Online health information)*

Healtheon
Palo Alto, CA
—*Internet Information for Plan Choice*

HealthLine Systems
San Diego, CA
—*Triage Software*

HealthSource, St. Joseph Hospital
Houston, TX
—*Call Centers*

Healthtrac
Menlo Park, CA
—*Self-Care Handbooks*

HealthWise
Boise, ID
—*Decision Counseling, Self-Care Handbooks*

Intracorp
Philadelphia, PA
—*"Smart Choices" Decision Counseling*

Johnson & Johnson Health Care
Systems, Health Management
Division
Piscataway, NJ
—*Self-Care Guides*

Micromass Communications
Raleigh, NC
—*(Communications software)*

Mosby Consumer Health
St. Louis, MO
—*(Self-care training, handbook)*

National Health Enhancement
Systems
Phoenix, AZ
—*"Centramax" Call Center*

Nurse On Call
Atlanta, GA
—*Triage, Counseling*

Online System Services
Denver, CO
—*(Internet connectivity)*

Optum Health
Golden Valley, MN
—*(Call centers)*

Problem Knowledge Couplers [PKC]
Burlington, VT
—*Triage, Information*

Strategic Systems, Inc.
Albuquerque, NM
—*"The Medical Information Line"*

Total Health Management Division,
Adventist Health Systems Sunbelt
Orlando, FL
—*Call Centers, Triage, Shared Decisions*

United Healthcare Center for
Corporate Health
—*"Taking Care Program" "Informed Care Service" Self-Care Books, "Personal Nurse Advisor"*

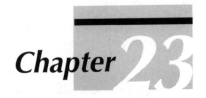
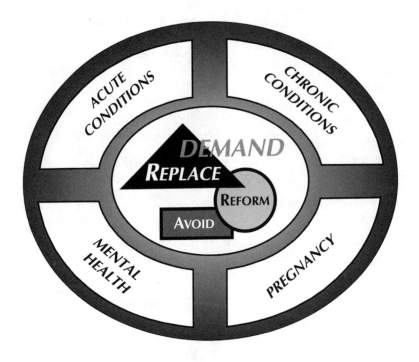

Chapter 23

DISEASE MANAGEMENT

In many, perhaps most discussions of disease management, the emphasis, even exclusive focus, is on providers of care rather than consumers. This may be a consequence of the term itself, since "disease" sounds like it ought to be managed by professionals. Where health and decision improvement have, by necessity, focused on consumers, the importance of consumers in disease management is only slowly being recognized and addressed.

Disease management (sometimes called "disease state management" or "disease prevention and management") applies to consumers who have specific diagnosed conditions. It would probably be better to use the label "condition self-management," since it addresses conditions (such as physical injuries and pregnancy) that are not diseases, and (in our treatment) focuses on consumer management of their own conditions, but disease management has become the accepted term.

In any case the intent of "condition self-management" is to improve the process and outcomes of care by enlisting the full and effective cooperation of patients and their family/friends as caregivers therein. The expectation of such management is that this will significantly reduce the costs of such conditions to consumers, payers, and providers at risk—and add greatly to consumer quality of life.

Some definitions of disease management go beyond managing diagnosed conditions. One defines it as "a comprehensive, integrated approach to care and reimbursement based on the natural course of a disease, with treatment designed to address the illness by maximizing the effectiveness and efficiency of care delivery. The emphasis is on preventing disease and/or managing it aggressively where intervention will have the greatest impact."[1(p.1)] Another refers to it as "a systematic, population-based approach to identifying those at risk, intervening using information from a growing field of evidence-based medicine, and measuring patient outcomes once an intervention is in effect."[2(p.3)]

These definitions go well beyond what we will discuss under this rubric. They include prevention and detection, which we have discussed under health improvement. They address primarily what providers do, more frequently as case management or continuum of care management, whereas we focus our discussion chiefly on what consumers do. Disease management is a partnership in any case, involving payers and providers, perhaps vendors, but primarily adding the efforts of consumers, optimizing their contributions to process and outcome improvement and cost reduction.

Like the rest of the four categories of demand improvement, disease management focuses on empowering consumers to behave in optimum ways, on "managing" patient and caregiver behaviors so as to achieve specific improvements. It includes four categories of conditions that have significant impact on consumer health and sponsor expenditures:

1. acute conditions,
2. chronic conditions,
3. mental/behavioral conditions, and
4. pregnancy and maternity.

While the last is certainly not a "disease," the aims and approaches to optimizing consumer self-management of pregnancy and infant care are essentially similar to those for the other three conditions.

Acute conditions cover all disease and injuries that have a limited course, a beginning, and an end with an episode of care that lasts a relatively short time.

Patients with acute conditions are "cured," are rehabilitated (where they have some remaining chronic limitations), or die. Chronic conditions are normally endured for the rest of one's lifetime, though some can be "cured" to the point where they need no further attention after lengthy treatment.

The reasons for separating acute and chronic conditions as categories for disease management are chiefly those related to the time frame involved. Acute patients and caregivers typically are asked to change their lifestyles and to engage in cooperative care efforts once or a few times for a short period. Chronic patients and their caregivers are usually asked to commit to permanent lifestyle changes and to frequently, often daily or more, repeat efforts over the patient's entire life.

The reason for mentioning acute conditions separately is strictly to ensure that sponsors considering investment in disease management, particularly providers, include acute as well as chronic conditions in their thinking. The basic challenges in improving consumer/caregiver self-management of acute and chronic conditions are essentially the same, and will be discussed together. Moreover the greatest of these challenges, noncompliance, is so frequently addressed without regard to whether consumers are not complying with instructions relative to acute or chronic conditions as to make separate discussion impossible.

We will discuss mental/behavioral conditions and pregnancy/parenting separately, however. These are sufficiently different from the general class of acute and chronic conditions as to make separate discussion more useful. They are also treated as unique challenges for disease management in practice, each with its own set of issues and recommendations.

The "behaviors" of patients with diagnosed conditions may, technically, include the choices they make of providers and procedures on their own or in shared decisions with providers. We have chosen to discuss these decisions under decision improvement, since they emphasize the mental process of making a decision (admittedly including acting upon it) rather than specific changes in behavior occasioned by their condition.

There are four principal aims in optimizing consumers' behavior when they are diagnosed as having specific conditions. Consumers are asked to (1) recognize and report symptoms and play a key role in planning or revising treatment; (2) comply with medications and other treatment instructions; (3) make specified changes in their lifestyles necessitated by their condition; and (4) keep to a schedule of appointments or contacts to monitor their condition and their compliance with treatment and lifestyle regimens. If they adopt and maintain appropriate regimens in all four, they are supposed to enjoy valuable benefits themselves as well as save sponsors significant expense. It is the challenge of disease management to see that they do.

ACUTE AND CHRONIC CONDITIONS

Problems and Potential

It has been shown that 5% of the population account for 60% of total health care expenditures, while 50% of the population account for only 3%.[3] Among Medicare populations, 1% of consumers account for 30% of expenditures.[4] While this suggests that concentrating disease management efforts on a relative few could save significant sums, it is not certain that the 5% of the general population and 1% of the Medicare population who account for such a large portion of total expenditures are the same people every year (Exhibit 23–1).

Among Medicare populations, those with chronic conditions represent a larger proportion of high care users and tend to be more consistently the high-risk group. Among younger populations, however, acute conditions account for a larger proportion, so there is far greater "turnover" among the high-risk group. The best predictive models, as discussed in Chapter 21, are able to identify *in advance* only the 30% of the population who account for 60% of expenditures, and these involve a mix of acute and chronic conditions.

Chronic conditions are typically given the greatest attention in disease management because the people who have them are more easily identified in advance and are subject to continuing expenditures over a long period. Consumers with acute conditions are identified when they contract such conditions, and they are typically the responsibility of providers. Consumers with chronic conditions are under the care of providers but are subject to attention from employers, health plans, and outside disease management services vendors as well.

Diabetes is frequently mentioned as a high-prevalence, expensive, chronic condition with a wide variety of complications, including kidney, eye, heart, and circulatory problems. It has been cited as the fourth leading cause of death and for accounting for annual US health care expenditures of between $92 billion and $112 billion a year.[5] Its prevalence grew from 11 million people to 16 million between 1983 and 1995.[6] Over 300,000 hospital admissions each year list diabetes as principal diagnosis, not counting cases where complications of diabetes were the causes.[7]

Costs to employers have been estimated at $47 billion in lost work days and productivity, over and above health care expenditures, representing $7,300 per year and 11.9 lost work days per employee with diabetes.[8] Out-of-pocket costs to diabetics are estimated at $12.3 billion a year.[9] Prevalence as much as twice the national average has been reported for Native Americans and other ethnic minorities.[10] And of the 16 million people with diabetes, only half have been diagnosed.[11]

Exhibit 23–1   Acute & Chronic Conditions

PROBLEMS / POTENTIAL	X HUGE SHARE OF TOTAL COSTS DUE TO SMALL NUMBER OF CONSUMERS
	X CHRONIC CONDITIONS LARGEST SHARE OF MEDICARE EXPENDITURES
	X COSTS TO EMPLOYERS INCLUDE LOWER PRODUCTIVITY, ABSENTEEISM
	X SIGNIFICANT SAVINGS ACHIEVED WITH MANY CHRONIC CONDITIONS
	X PATIENT / CAREGIVER INVOLVEMENT IN ACUTE CONDITIONS ALSO SAVES COSTS
EXAMPLES	X ORNISH HEART DISEASE REVERSAL PROGRAM GETS ROI RATIOS OF 5:1–20:1
	X CHESS COMPUTER NETWORK FOR AIDS REDUCES COSTS BY 1/3
	X PACE PROGRAM FOR SENIORS CUTS HOSPITAL DAYS BY 65%
	X ASTHMA PROGRAM REDUCES HOSPITAL ADMISSIONS BY 2/3
	X TIGHT SELF-MANAGEMENT OF DIABETES CUTS COMPLICATIONS 56%–76%
CONCERNS	X NOT ALWAYS POSSIBLE TO PREDICT HIGH-COST CONSUMERS IN ADVANCE
	X HIGH TURNOVER AMONG PATIENTS, PLAN MEMBERS & EMPLOYEES MAY REDUCE SPONSOR INTEREST IN INVESTMENTS WITH LONG-TERM PAYOFF
	X NOT ALL SPONSORS SUITABLE FOR PROMOTING DISEASE MANAGEMENT
ADVICE	X IDENTIFY HIGH-RISK / USE / COST CONSUMERS FOR GREATER ATTENTION
	X EXPLOIT MULTIPLE COMMUNICATIONS TECHNOLOGIES
	X EMPOWER BOTH PATIENTS & CAREGIVERS AS PARTNERS; SUPPORT WITH TRAINING, EQUIPMENT & COMMUNICATIONS
	X CLARIFY SHARING OF ROLES, COSTS & SAVINGS AMONG RISK SHARERS

Asthma is almost as high in prevalence, with 10 to 12 million cases estimated and mortality from asthma having increased by 40% from 1982 to 1991.[12] The annual costs of asthma are far less than for diabetes but still amount to $6.2 billion a year.[13] In one study 40% of avoidable hospitalizations for Medicaid beneficiaries were attributed to asthma.[14] The average health care costs for patients with severe asthma have been set at $30,000 each year.[15] Both prevalence and costs for asthma tend to be significantly higher among poor, inner-city, minority children.[16]

Ulcers are said to affect 500,000 new victims each year, adding to the 4.5 million already suffering. They are estimated to account for one million hospital admissions each year and cost $1.8 billion for hospital care, $125 million for physician visits, $50 million for medications, and $300 million in lost work days.[17] The combination of diabetes, asthma, and ulcers is said to account for one quarter of all employee health and lost productivity costs.[18]

Like diabetes, hypertension is a high-prevalence, high-cost, and high-complications condition. It affects 55 million Americans and costs $15 billion a year in direct expenditures.[19] Its indirect/complications costs are estimated at $110 billion.[20] Allergies are said to cost $10 billion.[21] Gastroesophogeal reflux disease (GERD) affects 17.5 million people.[22] Arthritis affects 32.6 million in one estimate,[23] 38 million in another, with growth to 59 million expected by the year 2020.[24]

Costs for medications, primarily for chronic conditions, cost Medicare beneficiaries $326 per person each year out of pocket, representing 26% of their personal health care cost obligations.[25] The costs to the nation for negative outcomes of treatment are estimated at $76.6 billion a year, including noncompliance and medications that are contraindicated.[26] Noncompliance with medications is estimated at 40% on average, much higher for some medications.[27] It is estimated that 11% of Medicare admissions are due to such noncompliance[28] and 3% to 5% of all hospital admissions.[29]

Examples of Disease Management Success

On the plus side, hundreds of success stories have been published noting the positive impacts on health and sponsor savings achieved through improving consumer behavior during acute and chronic conditions. The Ornish program of lifestyle changes to reverse heart disease has been estimated to have an ROI ratio of $5.55:1 when counting only surgery prevented and $20.00:1 when counting long-term costs and lost work days averted, in addition to avoiding the risks and discomforts of surgery.[30] When heart surgery could not be avoided, active participation by patient and family has helped reduce costs by 21% and length of stay by 19%.[31]

Disease management for arthritis reduced physician visits by 33% after 20 months and by 43% after 48 months in one example.[32] The Stanford Arthritis Program saved $702 in health care costs per patient with rheumatoid arthritis and $243 per patient with osteoarthritis, at an average cost per patient of $54.[33] Physician visits were reduced by 40%.[34]

The CHESS program of disease management by computer reduced costs for AIDS patients by 33% at a cost of only $60 per patient for computer time.[35] Mayo Clinics program for urinary tract infections saved $60,000 in six months.[36] Good Samaritan Hospital, Lebanon, Pennsylvania, reduced its congestive heart failure (CHF) readmission rate from 12% to 3% and saved $750,000 in the process.[37] The Harris Methodist Health System, Austin, Texas reduced inpatient admission by 44%, patient days by 57%, and ED visits by 67% through its sickle cell anemia program.[38]

Fallon Healthcare System, Worcester, Massachusetts, cut hospital days in its senior HMO by 65% through its Program for All-inclusive Care for the Elderly (PACE).[39] Sioux Valley Hospital, Sioux Falls, South Dakota, saved itself $1,260,000 in losses and cut patient days by 66% and ICU days by 96% through its community case management program for cerebral palsy patients.[40] A Veterans Administration clinic cut physician visits in half and costs by 28% by using frequent phone contacts between visits for its chronically ill patients.[41]

The National Jewish Center, Denver, Colorado, reduced hospitalization rates for the asthma patients it managed to 14.8% compared to unmanaged patients' 42.5%.[42] In an inner-city case, one nurse, working eight hours a week, reduced asthma admissions by 85% and ED visits by 79%, saving an estimated $100,000.[43] Harvard Community Health Plan reduced pediatric asthma admissions by 25%[44]; United Healthcare reduced them by 85% in three years.[45] Prime Care (Wisconsin HMO) saved $867,000 with costs of $32,000 for an ROI ratio of $27:1.[46]

The Diabetes Control and Complications Trial showed that eye complications could be reduced by 76%, kidney by 56%, and nerve by 69% through aggressive patient management of insulin-dependent diabetes.[47] The Chicago NBD bank system cut diabetic hospitalizations by 72%, bed days by 62%, ED visits by 71%, and lost work days by 63% in the first year of its program.[48] The Central States Southeast and Southwest Health & Welfare Fund reduced admissions by 20%, outpatient visits by 53%, ED visits by 23%, and physician visits by 14% in a voluntary program where 99% of eligible diabetic patients chose to participate.[49]

Sponsors have adopted a variety of approaches in managing conditions. Group Health of Puget Sound (Washington) uses "road maps" based on stages of readiness for 13,000 diabetic members of its plan.[50] Kaiser uses group sessions of up to 25 chronic patients at a time to reduce physician time required by 50%.[51] A community clinic provides phone triage and advice for AIDS patients.[52] Sharp Healthcare (San Diego) triages patients into those requiring routine or intensive monitoring or full case management.[53]

An Interstudy report indicated that 50.4% of HMOs had asthma programs, 45.4% diabetes, 15.6% AIDS/HIV, 14.5% cholesterol, 14.1% CHF, 11.5% hypertension, 9.9% cancer, 6.1% depression, 1.5% osteoporosis, 1.1% arthritis, and 23.7% one or more other chronic condition programs. Of those reporting outcomes, 74.0% achieved reduced ED use, 73.7% enjoyed fewer hospital admissions, 48.8% reduced specialist visits, 34.4% reported less diagnostic testing, 33.3% lowered their use of home health care, 28.2% reported fewer primary care physician (PCP) visits, and 25.2% lowered prescription drug use. Moreover 34.5% reported lower overall costs.[54]

While published reports are likely to reflect successful efforts and sponsors of unsuccessful efforts may be reticent about them, it is clear that a variety of sponsors have achieved significant success, often in a short time, through disease management. Many different technologies, from classroom education to computer networks, have been used to promote patient and family contributions and monitor compliance and conditions. Sponsors have many options as to which conditions, which patients, and which tactics to choose.

Concerns and Barriers

One of the greatest barriers to effective disease management, particularly for chronic conditions, is turnover. Patients who change jobs or otherwise change their health plan, who choose or are forced to change providers, represent a serious problem in coordination.[55] Where multiple agencies, including both payer and provider sponsors as well as vendors, community, and government organizations are involved, coordination to achieve both effective and efficient programs is equally problematic.[56]

Sponsors may see a large upfront investment to empower consumers to manage their own chronic conditions as a waste of resources if consumers change plans frequently. They may limit medication and provider choices in an effort to control expenses while seriously jeopardizing long-term outcomes for patients, as has been charged against HMOs relative to AIDS.[57] Payers and providers may not agree on what is best for managing patients or patients may not agree with either and not comply with treatment and advice.[58]

Some conditions may be beyond the capabilities of some sponsors. Achieving full success with treatment for TB, for example, requires compliance for a full year with prescribed medications. Compliance failures mean that treatment may have to be changed because of drug resistance caused by noncompliance, resulting in costs of $100,000 per patient. In one example, the full compliance rate was only 10%.[59]

Some components of disease management require significant upfront capital investments, in addition to training of patients and caregivers. Asthma peak flow meters and breathing support machines can cost hundreds of dollars[60]; new blood glucose testers that avoid the need for blood sticks in managing diabetes cost $400 and up.[61] Supply costs for insulin-dependent diabetics range from $1,200 to $2,500 each year.[62] A ThAIRapy vest to keep lungs clear and keep cystic fibrosis patients out of hospitals costs $15,900.[63]

There is a major question of responsibility in disease management: who should do it and who should incur the costs and share the savings? Since employers stand to gain savings in lost work days and productivity, should they take responsibility because they gain more? Should providers take it on because managing disease is their mission? Should health plans take it on because they have the numbers of patients with specific conditions needed to achieve economies and qualities of scale?

Outside vendors may seem a good choice. Many pharmaceutical firms have developed disease management offerings, though this threatens discontinuity with providers.[64] Will such firms retain an interest in disease management if sponsors push for prevention and lifestyle approaches to condition management as well as medication compliance, thereby reducing the market for medications?[65]

Some critics have argued that disease management has not yet proven itself.[66] Information systems are typically inadequate to monitor everything that is done for specific patients; hence we cannot be sure whether results are attributable to particular programs.[67] In some cases careful monitoring by patients has led to an increase in utilization, as patients detected more minor crises.[68]

Some have insisted that social conditions must be corrected before real success is achieved. The housing conditions and cockroach infestations that promote and aggravate asthma among inner-city children should be corrected.[69] Where indigent patients with diabetes do not have refrigerators, how are they to comply with insulin regimens?[70] With widespread illiteracy, how can patients understand what they are to do?[71]

Effective disease management may be complicated by health plan gatekeeper systems. Many studies have found primary physicians less effective than specialists for particular conditions. One found generally poor compliance among rural primary physicians with standards for managing diabetes, for example.[72] Should endocrinologists be primary physicians for diabetics, cardiologists for heart disease patients, nephrologists for kidney disease?[73] If providers take on disease management, will they fully empower patients or fight to preserve professional prerogatives?

It may be that disease management pays off for sponsors only when they focus on the higher risk, more serious cases. One study found an ROI ratio of $11.22:1 when addressing only severe asthma patients, for example, and a ratio of $.62:1— that is, a *loss*—when addressing everyone.[74] But consumers stand to gain whether high risk or not. Is saving money the only reason for empowering patients?

Laws and regulations present a particular problem relative to disease management. How can sponsors protect the privacy of consumers and confidentiality of sensitive information while coordinating the efforts of multiple providers and organizations?[75] How can they protect against the legal risks of violating patient privacy or antidiscrimination laws such as the Americans with Disabilities Act?[76] Clearly great care must be taken in selecting consumer targets and specific program tactics for disease management.

Suggestions

The first and often greatest challenge in disease management is the accurate and complete identification of those within a population who have a condition of interest. In practice, any combination of consumer surveys, medical records, claims data, prescription data, self-testing, and clinical testing may be needed to identify most consumers with a given condition.

Each of these data sources, individually, is likely to miss some, perhaps many of those with the condition. Type II diabetes (noninsulin-dependent diabetes mellitus, or NIDDM) is generally held to be a condition identified in only half of those afflicted, for example. Early identification of pregnancy is essential to early risk identification and prenatal care but relies on consumer action, including home self-testing in most cases. For each condition of interest, the best combination of detection techniques should be chosen to ensure the highest degree of identification.

The action recommendations we can make for successful disease management efforts fall neatly into the three components of the $I = MC^2$ model. The first requirement is to motivate patients and potential caregivers. Get them to commit to playing an effective role in managing their condition. Second, enhance their capability and identify and eliminate barriers to their carrying out their role. Third, prompt, remind, and promote their remembering what, where, when, and how to carry out that role.

Motivation

It might seem that the benefits available to consumers and their caregivers from effective disease management should be motivation enough. They gain control over their conditions, save deductibles and copays from avoided utilization, improve their health and quality of life, and generally enjoy better outcomes. Motivation may be enhanced by promoting consumer awareness of such benefits and confidence in achieving them. It may also take adding in some incentives, at least for some people.

Make sure patients and caregivers fully understand the benefits of playing their respective roles, of complying with medications and lifestyle changes, of reporting symptoms and side effects, and of keeping scheduled contacts—and what the risks are of not doing so.[77] Ask them if they know someone, a friend, acquaintance, or perhaps a celebrity, who had the same condition and enjoyed the benefits of compliance or the harm of noncompliance.[78] If not, supply a case example or invite them to discuss the condition with someone else who has it or to participate in a support group.

Invite patients and caregivers as partners in managing the condition. Try naming them as coinvestigators in a study to trace the effects of the planned treatment upon them, specifically.[79] A negotiated contract might be worked out, specifying the roles of patient, caregivers, and providers or sponsors involved, with patient and caregivers publicly and formally committing to their part.[80] Schedule specific actions, such as a change in lifestyle, series of appointments, or taking medications on the calendar at one time.[81]

Where patients are insufficiently motivated by the effects on their own lives of complying or not, enlist the support of their significant others—for example, spouses, children, friends, coworkers—to supply some peer pressure (along with support and reminders).[82] Make whatever behaviors they are to adopt as enjoyable as possible or at least reduce as many of the unenjoyable costs as possible.[83] Ask them what it would take to make them want to adopt and continue them or at least increase their willingness to do so.[84]

Each consumer and caregiver may perceive a different added value, based on each's value structure and priorities. Most should perceive and value the increase in control over the condition to be achieved. Some may think in terms of improved appearance, functioning, performance, energy, or other benefits from lifestyle changes. Those who comply with medications may gain a sense of accomplishment knowing how their behavior contributed to the outcomes achieved. Those who report symptoms appropriately and keep appointments may gain greater self-respect for their ability to keep promises and discipline themselves. Sponsors who understand the personal and cultural values of individual patients and plan accordingly are more likely to succeed.[85]

Extrinsic incentives may be added to intrinsic. A compliance contract may specify rewards consumers will give themselves or sponsors will give them after completing a course of treatment, making a lifestyle change, or achieving some health status parameter. Providers have used gifts or chances in a lottery for a big prize to patients who kept all appointments, for example.[86] Periodic rewards or recognition for continued "good behavior" can help where accomplishments are long term.

Potentially the best motivator for sponsors to use is promoting the highest levels of patient/caregiver satisfaction and trust. Make sure consumers are fully informed of side effects, costs, and risks of treatment as well as benefits and can call someone if they have questions or concerns.[87] Micromedex (Denver, Colorado) offers its Ultimedex program, for example, that prints out plain-English discussions of specific conditions and the benefits/risks of treatment that providers can use.[88] Make sure they understand that lapses are not failures and that they know what to do if they miss an appointment or dose of medication.[89] And make sure that they know what side effects might happen and that they should report them rather than decide to cease compliance.[90]

Key factors affecting the probability of consumer compliance with medical advice include complexity, triability, and observability. Complexity relates to how complicated the desired behavior is (e.g., how often a pill must be taken, whether multiple behaviors are involved). Triability involves whether consumers can try it and see (e.g., taking one pill versus agreeing to surgery). Observability reflects the extent to which others would see and support a change in behavior, as opposed to having no way of knowing if a consumer complied.

Anything that sponsors can do to reduce the complexity of a desired behavior change (e.g., package multiple medications into a single dose) will tend to improve compliance. If sponsors can make a behavior change triable, such as by offering a trial visit to a health club, consumers are likely to accept the trial versus commit to a long-term contract. By making a behavior change observable, perhaps through group activities or buddy systems, compliance can be improved.

Capability

Ask whatever consumers and caregivers can think of that might interfere with their fully playing their roles.[91] No sponsor is likely to be able to guess what these might be for particular cases, and asking shows a caring mode that will aid in motivation and maintaining relationships. Check if patients and caregivers can accurately describe what, when, where, and how they will behave (perhaps give a pop-quiz or ask them to repeat instructions given) to be sure they fully understand their parts.[92]

Make the desired behavior as easy as possible for consumers. Make appointments convenient for them versus having provider convenience dominate, for example.[93] Make lifestyle changes as simple as possible, with the least disruption to previous preferences and habits necessary to achieve the desired results.[94] Train consumers in the use of equipment and devices and have them demonstrate their skills to be sure they feel comfortable and confident about using them.[95] Provide simplifiers, such as unit doses or prepackaged medications that make them easier to use.[96]

Monitor compliance carefully and respond immediately to lapses. This will show that the sponsor cares about the consumer/caregiver contribution. It can also serve as a basis for discovering reasons for low motivation or barriers that can then be addressed. Asking for feedback about their experiences and feelings from patients and caregivers will also demonstrate sponsor concern and enable the identification of problems.[97]

Consciousness

For behaviors that are to be repeated frequently over a long period or that are complex, prompting consumers and caregivers to stimulate and maintain their awareness of what to do is likely to be essential. One study of medication compliance, for example, found that 14% of noncompliers never got around to filling their prescription, and 13% failed to even start taking it after getting it filled, while 29% stopped taking it too soon, and 22% did not take enough.[98] Among consumers who have to take only one medication once a day, compliance is 75% to 80%, where if multiple medications or multiple times a day, compliance falls to 35% to 40%.[99]

Even the most committed consumers with no significant barriers can simply forget a new behavior, appointment, dose, or symptom that is to be reported. Frequent prompts are likely to be more effective than one set of instructions given at the beginning of a regimen.[100] Diaries that consumers use to record their behaviors can help remind them—and when reviewed by sponsors, identify lapses to be addressed.[101]

There are automated phone reminder systems that sponsors can use to prompt consumers to take medications, remind them of lifestyle changes, ask about symptoms, or give them a chance to confirm or cancel an appointment.[102] Electronic pill dispensers page patients when their doses are due and record usage for physician or pharmacist review.[103] A home health manager is available that not only reminds patients when a medication or treatment is due, but reports to providers if the patient does not comply.[104]

Pharmacists can check if patients refill prescriptions on time and can enlist physicians and even drug companies in promoting compliance.[105] Special efforts, including more frequent reminders, can be used for patients who express concerns over remembering or who are found to be poor at compliance. Obtaining feedback from consumers about reasons for lapses and suggestions for effective reminders can enhance their commitment as well as provide useful ideas.[106]

New technologies can be enlisted in prompting compliance. HealthPartners, a Minnesota HMO, provides telemedicine monitoring devices to selected patients that can transmit vital signs, voice, and pictures at the instigation of patient or provider.[107] Health Desk Corporation, Berkeley, California, offers software to help patients remember behaviors and symptoms to be reported and prepare for visits. It also monitors health indicators.[108]

The more personalized and customized prompting communications are, the more effect they are likely to have. With many technologies available to customize messages, there is no need to fall back on mass boilerplate for consumers who wish to be seen, respected, and treated as individuals.[109] Generally the more sources for reminders, the more media use and different messages employed, the greater the effect.[110]

MENTAL/BEHAVIORAL HEALTH CONDITIONS

Conditions reflecting problems with mental health, often referred to as behavioral and sometimes emotional health, are treated separately by most health insurance plans and have their own set of providers in most cases. They are of special interest in disease management because, like some medical conditions, such as diabetes and hypertension, they are associated with a wide range of "complications" that add to their overall costs to consumers, payers, and society (Exhibit 23–2).

Mood and behavior problems are associated with 25% of medical visits, for example, and are rarely diagnosed or treated as part of the problem by primary physicians, resulting in significant suffering and disability among consumers.[111] Treatment for diagnosed mental illness cost $40 billion in 1990 and was estimated to account for a total of $273 billion, counting all its effects.[112] Estimates are that 19% of US adults, 29 million people, meet criteria for mental illness at least once in any six-month period with anywhere from 9% to 35% of medical problems linked to mental health problems.

Another source estimates that 11 million people are, at any one time, affected by some mental illness problem, and that one person in eight will be at some time.[113] Depression is one of the most common and treatable problems, but only one third of those with this problem are said to *ever* be diagnosed and treated. Some estimate that 22% of the population is affected by some form of depression each year, costing society $43.7 billion each year.[114] It costs employers $11.7 billion in days of lost work and $12.7 billion in diminished performance, as well as $8.3 billion in hospital costs, $2.9 billion in outpatient care, and $1.2 billion in medications.[115]

Substance abuse, a separate behavioral health problem, is estimated to cost $25 billion to government and taxpayers alone.[116] It has been tied to one fifth of all Medicaid hospital days.[117] It is a serious danger to pregnant women, with an estimated 11% of all babies born to mothers who used alcohol or drugs and 100,000 "crack babies" a year and costs of $20 billion.[118] Workers with substance abuse problems cost employers five times more in workers' compensation expense and 2.5 times more in medical benefits each year.[119] Alcohol abuse has high prevalence among the elderly, with an estimated 3 million alcoholics over 60 years of age, poorly diagnosed, yet with high success rates when treated.[120]

Examples of Successful Programs

The Employee Assistance Program Professional Association cites ROI ratios of $5.00:1 to $7.00:1 for behavioral health interventions, including drops in absenteeism of 66% and sick leave reductions of 37%.[121] Substance abuse programs produce returns of from $5.00:1 to $16.00:1 counting savings in all categories of employee costs.[122]

Exhibit 23–2 Mental/Behavioral Conditions

PROBLEMS / POTENTIAL	✗ DEPRESSION & OTHER MENTAL ILLNESS OFTEN NOT DIAGNOSED, LEAD TO SIGNIFICANT MEDICAL CARE USE / EXPENSE ✗ SUBSTANCE ABUSE A SERIOUS SOCIAL PROBLEM AS WELL AS CAUSE OF ILLNESS, INJURY, HEALTH CARE USE & EXPENSE ✗ MENTAL ILLNESS ESTIMATED COSTS OVER $240 BILLION / YR.
EXAMPLES	✗ EAP PROGRAMS REDUCE ABSENTEEISM UP TO 2/3, SICK LEAVE COSTS BY 1/3 ✗ TREATING MENTAL HEALTH PROBLEMS CUTS MEDICAL VISITS BY 1/3 ✗ SUBSTANCE ABUSE PROGRAM CUTS ED VISITS BY 1/3
CONCERNS	✗ INSURANCE COVERAGE FOR MENTAL / BEHAVIORAL CARE OFTEN INADEQUATE ✗ DEFINITIONS & SUBJECTIVE DIAGNOSES MAY PROMOTE ABUSE OF SYSTEM BY CONSUMERS & PROVIDERS ✗ CONSUMERS OFTEN RETICENT ABOUT MENTAL / BEHAVIORAL PROBLEMS ✗ PRIMARY CARE PHYSICIANS OFTEN MISS MENTAL / BEHAVIORAL CONDITIONS
ADVICE	✗ LOOK FOR COMMUNITY ORGANIZATIONS AS PARTNERS IN ADDITION TO RISK SHARERS ✗ EMPHASIZE PREVENTION & EARLY DETECTION FOR MENTAL AS WELL AS PHYSICAL CONDITIONS ✗ ENLIST FAMILIES IN TREATMENT, SELF-MANAGEMENT & SUPPORT

Harvard Community Health Plan used a series of six weekly sessions lasting 90 to 120 minutes for members suffering stress-related problems and cut their medical visits by 50%.[123] Group Health of Puget Sound uses local community health center networks, enlisting patients and family to sign contracts committing to their roles.[124] A series of studies found that successful treatment of mental health problems decreased medical visits from 10% to 33%, improved medical and surgical outcomes, and reduced hospital stays.[125]

Kaiser used a behavioral health approach to pain management, teaching patients and families coping skills and promoting general fitness to reduce outpatient visits by 40%.[126] One substance abuse treatment program achieved a 33% reduction in ED visits and expenditures, with a $7.00 ROI ratio.[127] A family confrontation approach to alcohol problems succeeded in getting 90% of alcoholics into treatment.(128) An employer-sponsored "drink wise" program cut alcohol use by 75% among moderate to problem drinkers.[129] Drug education efforts in junior high schools found participants 49% less likely to use drugs and 66% less likely to use multiple drugs.[130]

Concerns and Barriers

It has been argued that payers tend to shortchange mental health problems and patients, insisting on short periods of treatment for all patients, even the most severe, and penalizing providers who do not adhere to restrictions.[131] Many health plans fail to adequately cover behavioral health problems, shifting costs to the medical side.[132] Social advocacy campaigns are well meant, but often poorly targeted, with the wrong audiences, wrong appeals, and poor relevance.[133]

Payers are concerned because the definitions and parameters of mental and behavioral illness are seen as vague and subjective, putting them at risk for unlimited liability. Unlike illegal drugs, alcohol is widely felt to have some benefits for health, so that its abuse must be controlled, rather than its use avoided, requiring careful definition of what constitutes abuse.[134]

Suggestions

Because mental/behavioral problems typically have social as well as personal causes and consequences, it makes sense to partner with community organizations in a general approach to dealing with problems, in addition to specific sponsor efforts.[135] Substance abuse problems are better approached via prevention and at early ages in schools, requiring community-wide cooperation. Teaching young people how to cope with peer pressures and life problems and promoting self-esteem and self-efficacy seem to help.[136]

Greater effort is needed in identifying people with behavioral health problems and in getting them into treatment as soon as possible. Enlisting the family in treatment is usually helpful. Using peers to describe their experiences and successes or failures, as spokespersons or in support groups seems to achieve greater credibility and effect. "Remarketing" desirable behavior rather than focusing exclusively on "demarketing" undesirable behavior has particular application with substance abuse.[137]

Since the proper use of alcohol has benefits, providing education and guidelines on how to do it properly is advised.[138] Healthy drinking can be promoted in the workplace, with training and rehearsal in refusing another drink acceptably and general promotion of self-esteem and self-efficacy.[139]

MATERNITY

Empowering women to achieve healthy pregnancies and have healthy babies represents one of the greatest opportunities for "disease," or condition, management. The estimated cost of preventable birth defects range from $100,000 to $500,000 per case.[140] CIGNA found that a normal, full-term baby cost an average of $11,209 in its first 18 months, whereas a normal premature baby cost $36,134 and an abnormal premature baby cost $89,426[141] (Exhibit 23-3).

Infant mortality in the United States is near the worst among developed nations and our ranking is getting worse. Rates for minorities are frequently twice that of whites.[142] Fully 8% of all births are premature or immature, accounting for 85% of all maternity-related expenses.[143] Complications of drinking and drug use during pregnancy, as well as pregnant women with diabetes, have already been mentioned.

Examples of Successful Programs

The use of a doula, or birth counselor, during pregnancy and delivery has been shown to reduce Caesarean birth rates from 18% to 8%; to reduce the use of epidural anesthesia from 55% to 8%; and to reduce birth induction by drugs from 44% to 17% of cases. The average length of labor was 7.4 hours with a doula, compared to 9.4 without; only 10% of babies needed to be kept in the hospital over 48 hours, compared to 24% when no doula was involved. All this occurred at a cost of $200 per mother.[144]

In general, programs to reduce the rate of prematurity among babies born have reported ROI ratios of from $3.00:1 to $10.00:1.[145] Roughly half of women at high risk of having premature babies can be identified through screening and counseling, with high success in achieving full-term births under proper pregnancy management.[146] On average, each premature birth averted saves $21,000.[147] And in most cases, success in such programs can be achieved in a short time, a year or two, compared to the longer term payoff of many other conditions.

CIGNA uses incentives of maternity gifts to encourage women to complete a maternity risk survey and enroll in its pregnancy management program if high

Exhibit 23–3 Maternity

PROBLEMS / POTENTIAL	✗ HUGE POTENTIAL FOR COST SAVINGS & QUALITY-OF-LIFE IMPROVEMENT ✗ US INFANT MORTALITY & IMMATURITY RATES AMONG WORST FOR DEVELOPED COUNTRIES ✗ PROBLEMS FAR WORSE FOR MINORITIES & POOR
EXAMPLES	✗ "DOULA" BIRTH COUNSELORS IMPROVE OUTCOMES, REDUCE COSTS DRAMATICALLY ✗ PRENATAL CARE PROGRAMS ACHIEVE ROI RATIOS OF 3:1–10:1 ✗ HMOs COLLABORATE IN PRENATAL CARE, GET IMMATURITY RATES 28% BETTER THAN NATIONAL AVERAGE ✗ WORKPLACE HEALTHY PREGNANCY PROGRAM INCREASES HEALTHY BABY PERCENTAGE FROM 69% TO 93%
CONCERNS	✗ WOMEN MAY HIDE PREGNANCY TO PROTECT JOBS, WORKPLACE STATUS ✗ ELIMINATING FINANCIAL BARRIERS NOT SUFFICIENT TO ACHIEVE DESIRED PRENATAL CARE ✗ SOME MATERNITY PROGRAMS CONTROVERSIAL DUE TO LINKS TO CONTRACEPTION & ABORTION ✗ NOT POSSIBLE TO IDENTIFY ALL POTENTIALLY HIGH-RISK MOTHERS
ADVICE	✗ IDENTIFY & FOCUS ON HIGH RISKS BUT WATCH LOW RISKS AS WELL ✗ CUSTOMIZE PROGRAMS TO NEEDS & WISHES OF PARTICULAR POPULATIONS ✗ USE VARIETY OF COMMUNICATIONS CHANNELS TO MAINTAIN CONTACT THROUGHOUT PREGNANCY

risk. It reduced Caesarean section rates from 26% to 14% and average lengths of stay from 3.1 to 2.4 days at a total cost of $5,177 for 77 participants.[148] Biggs Supermarkets waived all maternity deductibles and copays if women completed all prenatal care, while Haggar covered all costs if women initiated care in the first trimester. American Title Insurance achieved an ROI ratio of $6.70:1 with its program.[149]

The Hannaford Bros. grocery chain required women to initiate care in the first trimester or lose all maternity benefits. It achieved rates of premature birth half the national average and estimated savings of $200,000 a year.[150] Blue Cross of Virginia used Health Management Corporation's Baby Benefits program to save $73,843 on 1,390 cases, counting only medical costs in the first four months postpartum.[151] The Chesapeake Health Plan's (Baltimore, Maryland) Medicaid HMO cut its sick baby rate from 5.7% to 2.7%.[152]

Healthdyne Management's "Baby Steps" program (Marietta, Georgia) used home prenatal visits, phone monitoring, and high-risk management to reduce NICU admissions by 24% and days by 21%. Moreover it saved $3 million in an HMO with 560,000 covered lives.[153] Six HMOs with 1.3 million covered lives collaborated in a program that achieved 87% success in getting women to initiate care in the first trimester compared to the average of 76% and achieved a low birthweight rate of 5% compared to the US average of 7%.[154]

In Atlanta, Georgia, Egleston Children's Hospital at Emory University collaborated with the Georgia Chamber of Commerce to promote healthy pregnancies in the workplace, increasing the proportion of well babies born from 69% to 93%.[155] In Rhode Island, a program offering pregnant teens a chance in a lottery if they sought prenatal care increased participation by 30%.[156] A prenatal care coordinator program for Medicaid mothers reduced costs per delivery by an average of $873 per case.[157] To reach pregnant teens living on the street, one public health program gave them a voice mail service so their friends could reach them, and so could their nurse counselor.[158]

Concerns and Barriers

Some women postpone telling anyone they are pregnant for fear of damage to their career or job security.[159] The self-selection that biases the mix of women who participate in pregnancy management programs makes scientific conclusions as to their efficacy difficult.[160] Medicaid coverage by itself has not improved birth outcomes for uninsured women.[161] Getting them financial access to care and a provider who will care for them is not enough.[162]

Programs related to maternity tend to be controversial in many cases. Should teen pregnancies be prevented via abstinence or contraception; should abortion be available where prevention is unsuccessful? Can the best pregnancy outcomes be achieved without significant investment in curing social problems?[163] While pregnancy management programs identify high-risk mothers, half of all adverse fetal outcomes arise from lower risk pregnancies.[164] While great successes have been achieved through pregnancy management efforts, not everyone responds. Shall women be penalized if they fail to behave correctly while pregnant?

Suggestions

Sponsors would be wise not to leave pregnancy management entirely to providers. Physicians have been found to spend an average of less than two hours per pregnancy in contact with mothers. Employers and health plans as well as hospitals can significantly supplement what pregnant women learn from and are motivated to do by their physicians. Pregnancy management should begin before conception, for example, with genetic counseling to identify risks, with immunization against rubella (saves $350,000 per case of congenital rubella syndrome averted), and with nutrition counseling.[165]

Pregnancy management programs have to be customized to the populations addressed. Medicaid mothers are unsuited for phone-based monitoring and counseling programs, for example, when up to 40% of them have no phones. They may be far less receptive to self-reporting of symptoms and subject to a unique set of risk factors such as domestic violence.[166] For other women, phone programs have proven highly successful.[167]

In addition to programs aimed at specific high-risk populations, general community awareness of the risks of pregnancy and the potential of pregnancy management can promote healthier outcomes for everyone.[168] Reminders to providers as well as to mothers as to what each should do can maintain higher levels of compliance and improve outcomes.[169]

REFERENCES

1. K. Southwick, "Disease Management Broadens Focus of Care from Episodic to Long-Range," *Strategies for Healthcare Excellence* 8, no. 6 (1995):1–9.

2. R. Epstein and M. McGlynn, "Disease Management: What Is It," *Disease Management & Health Outcomes* 1, no. 1 (1997):3–10.

3. D. Johnson, "Disease Management Brings Major Challenges," *Health Care Strategic Management* 13, no. 5 (1995):2, 3.

4. "Study Shows 1% of Americans Use 30% of Health Expenditures," *Business & Health* 11, no. 12 (1993):10.

5. C. Caruthers, "Tallying the Costs of Diabetes," *Business & Health* 14, no. 1 (Special Supplement A, January 1996):8–13.

6. "HMO's Diabetes Program Tests New Model of Behavior Change," *Healthcare Demand Management* 1, no. 4 (1995):60–64.

7. "Experts Declare Most Admissions among Diabetics Are Avoidable," *Healthcare Demand Management* 1, no. 8 (1995):124, 125.

8. D. Anderson, "What Employers Need To Know about Diabetes," *Business & Health* 14, no. 1 (Special Supplement A, January 1996):22–24.

9. D. Anderson, "Managed Care Meets the Diabetes Management Challenge," *Business & Health* 14, no. 1 (Special Supplement A, January 1996):19–21.

10. "Impact of Diabetes," *USA Today,* 31 May–2 June 1996, 1A.

11. "New Approaches to Managing Diabetes," *Business & Health* 14, no. 1 (Special Supplement A, January 1996):6–8.

12. "Asthma," *Mayo Clinic Health Letter,* Medical Essay Supplement, February 1996, 1–8.

13. K. Southwick, "Strategies for Managing Asthma," *Managed Healthcare* 4, no. 10 (1994):S13–S19.

14. *Colorado Medicaid Primary Care Physician Initiative and Ambulatory Care Sensitive Hospitalizations* (Denver, CO: Colorado Health Data Commission, 1995).

15. "Asthma Study Identifies Better Outcomes in Comprehensive Treatment Approach," *Report on Medical Guidelines and Outcomes Research* 5, no. 4 (1994):1–3.

16. P. Lozano, et al., "Use of Health Services by African-American Children with Asthma on Medicaid," *Journal of the American Medical Association* 274, no. 6 (1995):469–473.

17. C. Grahl, "New Thought on Ulcer Causes Paves the Way for Successful Disease State Management," *Managed Healthcare* 2, no. 4 (1992):50–52.

18. J. Mandelker, "Managing Chronic Disease," *Business & Health* 12, no. 11 (1994):45–50.

19. S. McBride, "Taking a Long-Term View of Hypertension," *Managed Healthcare* 5, no. 1 (1995):S19–S21.

20. M. Smith and W. McGhan, "More Bang for the Buck in Managing High Blood Pressure," *Business & Health* 14, no. 5 (1996):44–47.

21. L. Meszaros, "Allergy: Old Nemesis, New Approaches," *Managed Healthcare* 6, no. 4 (1996): S32–S34.

22. "New Short-Term Treatment Option for GI Disorders," *Disease State Management* 1, no. 3 (1995):33, 34.

23. *Annual Report* (Golden, CO: Health Decisions, International, 1995).

24. W. Kuznar, "A Future Epidemic in Need of Better Therapy," *Managed Healthcare* 4, no. 11 (1994):S34, S35.

25. R. Porper, "The Elderly, Prescription Drugs, and Medicare Managed Care," *Medical Interface* 5, no. 3 (1992):64–66.

26. "New Disease Management Device Targets Prescription Drug Noncompliance," *Healthcare Demand Management* 1, no. 8 (1995):117–119.

27. Anderson, "What Employers Need," 22–24.

28. *Basic Statistics about Home Care 1991* (Washington, DC: National Association for Home Care, 1991), 3.

29. L. Scott, "Providers Push for Remedies to Costly Drug Noncompliance," *Modern Healthcare,* 15 April 1996, 44–50.

30. "Alternative Treatment of Heart Disease Pays Dividends," *INC.* 18, no. 11 (Advertising Supplement, August 1996).

31. M. Buser, "Pre-Established Care Guides Patients to Recovery," *California Hospitals* 7, no. 4 (1993):10–12.

32. *Annual Report.*

33. S. Mazzuca, "Economic Evaluation of Arthritis Patient Education," *Bulletin on the Rheumatic Diseases* 43, no. 5 (1994):6–8.

34. K. Lorig, "Arthritis Self-Help Course," *HMO Practice* 9, no. 2 (1995):60, 61.

35. M. Kennedy, "A Tool for Patient Education," *Health Data Management* 4, no. 2 (1996):61–65.

36. "Mayo Clinic Develops Disease Management Strategy To Handle Capitation," *Capitation & Medical Practice* 1, no. 10 (1995):6–8.

37. "Demand Management Holds Key to Prepaid Profits," *Capitation Management Report* 2, no. 3 (1995):33–37.

38. "Make Pain Management a Part of Your Care Continuum," *Healthcare Demand Management* 2, no. 3 (1996):33–36.

39. "PACE Program Reins in Demand for Hospitalization, Nursing Home Care Among the Frail Elderly," *Healthcare Demand Management* 1, no. 2 (1995):25–27.

40. K. Taylor, "Community Case Management: Moving Beyond the Hospital Walls," *Hospitals & Health Networks,* 5 August, 1994, 182.

41. J. Wasson, et al., "Telephone Care as a Substitute for Routine Clinic Follow-Up," *Journal of the American Medical Association* 267, no. 13 (1992):1788–1793.

42. "Asthma Program Slashes Hospitalization Costs," *Disease State Management* 1, no. 3 (1995): 31–33.

43. M. Bricklin, "The Power of Proactive Prevention," *Prevention* 46, no. 2 (1994):45, 46, 116.

44. K. Terry, "Disease Management: Continuous Health-Care Improvement," *Business & Health* 13, no. 4 (1995):64–72.

45. T. Troy, "Asthma Monographs Give MCOs the Tools Necessary To Battle a Costly Disease," *Managed Healthcare* 5, no. 5 (1995):12.

46. J. Montague, et al., "How To Save Big Bucks," *Hospitals & Health Networks,* 5 May 1996, 18–24.

47. D. Anderson, "A Conceptual Revolution in Diabetes Care," *Business & Health* 14, no. 1 (Special Supplement A, January 1996):14–17.

48. Caruthers, "Tallying the Costs," 8–13.

49. "Narrow the Scope To Widen the Savings," *Business & Health* 14, no. 4 (Supplement B Special Report, April 1996):6.

50. "Diabetes Team Attacks Eye Disease, Foot Ulcers," *Disease State Management* 1, no. 3 (1995):30.

51. "HMOs Trade Individual Office Visits for Group Visits," *Physician's Managed Care Report* 4, no. 3 (1996):31, 32.

52. S. Henry, et al., "A Computer-Based Approach to Quality Improvement for Telephone Triage in a Community AIDS Clinic," *Nursing Administration Quarterly* 18, no. 2 (Winter 1994):65–73.

53. "How One Large Health System Is Gearing Up for a Capitated Future," *Capitation Management Report* 1, no. 1 (1995):13–16.

54. "HMOs Aggressively Developing Disease Management Programs: Cost Reductions Reported," *Healthcare Demand & Disease Management* 3, no. 6 (1997):94–96.

55. D. Berwick, "Seeking Systemness," *Healthcare Forum Journal* 35, no. 2 (1992):22–28.

56. M. Conklin, "Disease Management Stealing Patients from Health Systems," *Health Care Strategic Management* 13, no. 2 (1995):1, 23.

57. "Do HMOs Shortchange AIDS, Psychiatric Patients? *Health Progress* 77, no. 2 (1996):59.

58. L. Scott, "Disease Management Faces Obstacles," *Modern Healthcare,* 12 June 1995, 30–33.

59. J. Smith, "Can Managed Care Do It All?" *Health Systems Review,* November/December 1994, 34–37.

60. "Early Discharge Planning Is Key to Lower LOS, Experts Say," *Managed Care Outlook* 8, no. 1 (1995):3.

61. "Companies Race To Develop Pain-Free Tests for Diabetes," *The Denver Post,* 10 March 1996, 19A.

62. Caruthers, "Tallying the Costs," 8–13.

63. P. Gerber, "Penny Wise and Pound Foolish," *Managed Healthcare* 6, no. 1 (1996):29, 30.

64. Conklin, "Disease Management," 1, 23.

65. "Managing Chronic Diseases through Alliances between Pharmaceutical Companies and Health Plans," *TrendWatch* 5, no. 2 (1995):2, 6.

66. "Successful Disease State Management Requires Collaboration, Documented Results," *Health Care Strategic Management* 13, no. 9 (1995):5.

67. Terry, "Disease Management," 64–72.

68. S. Watson, "Patient, Heal Thyself," *Computerworld Health Care Journal,* April 1996, H8.

69. D. Haney, "Roach Is No. 1 Urban Asthma Culprit," *The Denver Post,* 16 June 1996, 24A.

70. J. Ziegler, "Improving Diabetes Management through Employer/Provider Partnerships," *Business & Health* 14, no. 1, Special Supplement (1996):25–28.

71. "Consumers," *Hospitals & Health Networks,* 5 January 1996, 16, 17.

72. R. Zoorob and A. Mainous, "Practice Patterns of Rural Family Physicians Based on the American Diabetes Association Standards of Care," *Journal of Community Health* 21, no. 3 (1996): 175–182.

73. "Specialist Gatekeeper Model Aimed at Cutting Demand among Chronically Ill," *Healthcare Demand Management* 1, no. 2 (1995):22, 23.

74. M. Krahn, "Issues in the Cost-Effectiveness of Asthma Education," *Chest* 106, no. 4 (1994): 264S–269S.

75. M. Hurley, "Case Management: Communicating Real Savings," *Business & Health* 14, no. 3 (1996):29–36.

76. "Industry Leaders Share Insights at Disease Management Conference," *Health Management Technology* 16, no. 10 (1995):12.

77. R. Bachman, "Better Compliance: Physicians Making It Happen," *American Family Physician* 48, no. 5 (1993):717, 718.

78. D. Murray, "Proven Ways To Win Patient Compliance," *Medical Economics* 72, no. 17 (1995):82–97.

79. E. Frank, et al, "Alliance, Not Compliance," *Journal of Clinical Psychiatry* 56, Supplement 1 (1995):11–17.

80. Bachman, "Better Compliance," 717, 718.

81. A. Bernstein, "Booking Multiple Appointments Encourages Completed Cases," *Practice Builder Monthly Briefing,* September 1994, 8, 9.

82. T. DeLoughry, "Improving Quality through Mutual Patient and Provider Responsibilities," *The Next Generation of Health Promotion* (Boston, MA: Institute for International Research, September 18–19, 1995).

83. D. Milner, "Reducing the No-Show Rate in Medical Practice," *Journal of Medical Practice Management* 7, no. 4 (1992):260–262.

84. "One of a Kind: Patients Need Individualized Treatment," in *Talk about Prescriptions 1995 Planning Guide* (Washington, DC: National Council on Patient Information and Education, 1995), 3–6.

85. P. Sanchez, "The Potential for Marketing in the Clinical Services Area," *Health Marketing Quarterly* 10, no. 1/2 (1992):59–67.

86. A. Bean and J. Talaga, "Appointment Breaking: Causes and Solutions," *Journal of Health Care Marketing* 12, no. 4 (1992):14–25.

87. "One of a Kind," 3–6.

88. D. Algeo, "Medical Databases Save Lives," *The Denver Post,* 12 February 1996, 1C, 5C.

89. "Advancing Medicine Communications and Compliance: Putting the Patient First," in *Talk about Prescriptions 1995 Planning Guide* (Washington, DC: National Council on Patient Information and Education, 1995), 1–3.

90. "Advancing Medicine," 1–3.

91. "One of a Kind," 3–6.

92. "Let's All Talk: Medicine Education Is a Team Effort," in *Talk about Prescriptions 1993 Planning Guide* (Washington, DC: National Council on Patient Information and Education, 1993), 1–13.

93. Milner, "Reducing the No-Show Rate," 260–262.

94. Bean and Talaga, "Appointment Breaking," 14–25.

95. "Advancing Medicine," 1–3.

96. K. Southwick, "Noncompliance: The Other Side," *Managed Healthcare* 3, no. 4 (1993):92–95.

97. "Let's All Talk," 1–13.

98. Anderson, "What Employers Need To Know," 22–24.

99. Southwick, "Noncompliance," 92–95.

100. P. Elliott, "How I Keep My Patients on the Road I Mapped for Them," *Medical Economics* 68, no. 13 (1991):63–67.

101. M. O'Brien, et al., "Adherence to Medication Regimens," *Medical Care Review* 49, no. 4 (Winter 1992):435–454.

102. V. Leirer, et al., "Automated Telephone Reminders for Improving Ambulatory Care Service," *Journal of Ambulatory Care Management* 15, no. 4 (1992):54–62.

103. Scott, "Providers Push," 44–50.

104. B. Smith, "Entrepreneur Addresses 'Other Drug Problem,'" *The Denver Business Journal,* 22–28 September 1995, 46A.

105. S. Neibart, "An Innovative Drug Compliance Program," *Medical Interface* 5, no. 5 (1992):29, 30.

106. "One of a Kind," 3–6.

107. Bachman, "Better Compliance," 717, 718.

108. P. Schuchman, "Minn. HMO Finds Telemedicine Technology Cuts Costs and Visits," *Managed Home Care Report* 2, no. 12 (1995):9–12.

109. "Tailored Disease Management Communications," *Inside Preventive Care* 2, no. 2 (1996):4.

110. Bachman, "Better Compliance," 717, 718.

111. A. Epstein, et al., "Behavioral Disorders," *HMO Practice* 9, no. 2 (1995):53–56.

112. J. Ficken, "The Use of Psychological Screeners for Containing Costs and Improving Outcomes," *Health Care Strategic Management* 14, no. 3 (1996):6–8.

113. "Mental Health Screen Boosts Primary Care Detection of Hidden Behavioral Problems," *Healthcare Demand Management* 1, no. 7 (1995):108–110.

114. E. Meszaros, "Skies Overcast, Therapies Variable," *Managed Healthcare* 5, no. 10 (1995):S16–S20, S36.

115. "Study Shows Social Costs of Depression on Par with Costs of Heart Disease," *Managed Healthcare* 4, no. 1 (1994):S13.

116. K. Pallarito, "Financial Toll of Substance Abuse Studied," *Modern Healthcare,* 20 February 1995, 18.

117. K. Pallarito, "20% of Medicaid's Hospital-Care Costs Traced to Substance Abuse," *Modern Healthcare,* 19 July 1993, 8.

118. L. Wagner, "Costs of Maternal Drug Abuse Drawing Notice," *Modern Healthcare,* 20 March 1990, 21.

119. "Wellness Quick Stats . . . On Substance Abuse," *Wellness Program Management Advisor* 1, no. 3 (1996):4.

120. "Alcoholism in the Elderly," *Hospitals & Health Networks,* 20 October 1995, 12.

121. "When 'Warm Fuzzies' Don't Work: Use Hard Facts To Prove Your Value," *Wellness Program Management Advisor* 1, no. 3 (1996):4, 5.

122. "Wellness Quick Stats," 4.

123. H. Burnes, "Personal Health Improvement Program," *HMO Practice* 9, no. 2 (1995):59, 60.

124. "Form Alliances with Community Mental Health Programs," *Healthcare Demand Management* 1, no. 9 (1995):129–132.

125. E. Mumford, et al., "The Cost-Offset Effect of Mental Health Treatments on Medical Utilization," *American Journal of Psychiatry* 141 (1984):1145–1158.

126. S. Tulkin, "Behavior Intervention Programs That Work," *HMO Practice* 9, no. 2 (1995):57, 58.

127. "Substance Abuse Treatment Pays Off," *Business & Health* 12, no. 10 (1994):17.

128. M. Lance, "Either Get Treatment for Your Drinking, or Leave This Family," *Medical Self-Care* 54 (1990):28, 33, 72, 73.

129. "Program Helps Moderate Drinkers To Cut Back," *Employee Health & Fitness* 17, no. 8 (1995):91–93.

130. G. Botvin, et al., "Long-Term Follow-Up Results of a Randomized Drug Abuse Prevention Trial in a White Middle-Class Population," *Journal of the American Medical Association* 273, no. 14 (1995):1106–1112.

131. "Do HMOs Shortchange," 59.

132. D. Garnick, et al., "Finding Coverage That Fits," *Business & Health* 13, no. 12 (1995):29–33.

133. B. Cutler and E. Thomas, "This Is Your Brain on Drugs," *Health Marketing Quarterly* 11, no. 3/4 (1994):9–26.

134. "Alcohol: Spirit of Health," *Consumer Reports on Health* 8, no. 4 (1996):37, 39, 40.

135. "Form Alliances," 129–132.

136. T. Backer, et al., *Designing Health Communications Campaigns: What Works?* (Newbury Park, CA: Sage, 1992).

137. L. Donohew, et al., "Attention, Need for Sensation and Health Communication Campaigns," *American Behavioral Scientist* 38, no. 2 (1994):310–322.

138. " 'By the Numbers' Program Targets Alcohol Use," *Employee Health & Fitness* 17, no. 1 (1995):5–10.

139. N. Kishchuk, et al., "Formative and Effectiveness Evaluation of a Worksite Program Promoting Healthy Alcohol Consumption," *American Journal of Health Promotion* 8, no. 5 (1994):353–362.

140. "Addressing the High Costs of Birth Defects," *Business & Health* 13, no. 11 (1995):16.

141. M. Cameron, "Prenatal Care: A Small Investment Begets a Big Return," *Business & Health* 11, no. 6 (1993):50–53.

142. C. Kent, "Slow Progress against Infant Mortality," *Medicine & Health,* 11 May 1992, 1–4.

143. G. Kenworthy and N. Gospo, "Development of an Effective Utilization Management Program at Celtic Life Insurance Company," *Quality Review Bulletin* 16, no. 4 (1990):138–142.

144. J. Kennel, et al., "The Effect of Continuous Emotional Support during Labor," *Journal of the American Medical Association* 265 (1991):2197–2201.

145. C. Elliott and T. Varon, "Containing Health Care Costs: The Effects of an Infant Wellness Program," *Health Marketing Quarterly* 12, no. 4 (1995):63–74.

146. Kenworthy and Gospo, "Development of an Effective Utilization Management Program," 138–142.

147. J. Packer-Tursman, "A Growing Priority," *Managed Healthcare News* 3, no. 9 (1993):57, 58.

148. L. Boudreau, "Evaluation of the Use of Incentives To Increase Participation in Prenatal Education and the Effect on Cesarean Section Rate and Length of Stay," *American Journal of Health Promotion* 8, no. 5 (1994):388–389.

149. Cameron, "Prenatal Care," 50–53.

150. G. Leavenworth, "How a Store Owner Became a Savvy Shopper," *Business & Health* 13, no. 4 (1995):23–25.

151. Elliott and Varon, "Containing Health Care Costs," 63–74.

152. M. Conklin, "HMO Cuts Premature Baby Rate in Half," *Health Care Strategic Management* 13, no. 2 (1995):9.

153. "Information Technology Helps Slash Maternity Costs," *Healthcare Demand Management* 1, no. 3 (1995):33–37.

154. "HMOs Earn High Marks for Prenatal Care," *Managed Care Competitive Network,* Spring/Summer 1994, 8.

155. "Public-Private Partnership Drives Wellness Programs at Small and Midsized Companies," *Employee Health & Fitness* 16, no. 10 (1994):125–128.

156. L. Smith, "Getting Junkies To Clean Up," *Fortune,* 6 May 1991, 103–108.

157. B. Solberg, "Wisconsin Prenatal Care Coordination Proves Its Worth," *Inside Preventive Care* 2, no. 3 (1996):1, 5, 6.

158. D. Weiss, "Demand Management: Using Information Technology To Improve Healthcare Delivery," *Demand Management® for Healthcare* (Chicago, IL: Strategic Research Institute, May 30–31, 1996).

159. Cameron, "Prenatal Care," 50–53.

160. K. Fiscell, "Does Prenatal Care Improve Birth Outcomes? A Critical Review," *Medical Benefits,* 30 March 1995, 4.

161. "Medicaid Managed Care for Prenatals?" *Health Care Strategic Management* 11, no. 3 (1993):4.

162. J. Morrissey, "Oregon Plan Covering Medicaid Patients Is Off to a Rough Start," *Modern Healthcare,* 4 September 1995, 90–92.

163. T. Sowell, "Health-Care Cure Could Be Worse Than 'Crisis,' " *Rocky Mountain News,* 24 March 1993, 47.

164. United Healthcare, "Mother Child Connection 'Bright Futures' Program," *Demand Management® for Healthcare* (Chicago, IL: Strategic Research Institute, May 30–31, 1996).

165. M. McKnight, "4 Ways to Improve Your Prenatal Program," *Business & Health* 12, no. 5 (1994):47–50.

166. "Medica Tailors Pregnancy Intervention to Medicaid," *Inside Preventive Care* 2, no. 2 (1996):5, 6.

167. United Healthcare, "Mother Child Connection."

168. C. Schultz and K. Schultz, "Poverty and Prenatal Health Care in America: Trends, Costs and Recommendations," *Journal of Ambulatory Care Marketing* 5, no. 2 (1994):149–159.

169. P. Taulbee, "Prenatal Care Study Offers Lessons for Improvement to HMOs," *Report on Medical Guidelines & Outcomes Research* 5, no. 2 (1994):10, 12.

Disease Management Vendors

Accordant Health Services, Inc.
Greensboro, NC
— *"Unusual" Diseases*

Accountable Oncology
Alexandria, VA
— *Cancers*

Air Logix
Dallas, TX
— *Asthma, COPD*

American Health Corp.
San Antonio, TX

APACHE Medical Systems, Inc.
McLean, VA

Capitated Disease Management
Services
Montclair, NJ

Cardiac Solutions
Buffalo Grove, IL
— *CHF, Coronary Artery Disease*

CHESS Computer Network, U.
Wisconsin
Madison, WI
— *Support Groups for AIDS, Breast
Cancer, Others*

City of Hope Oncology Network
Duarte, CA
— *Cancers*

Control Diabetes Services
Dallas, TX

Disease Management Purchasing
Consortium & Advisory Council
Boston, MA
— *Broker for buyers rather than
vendor*

Diabetes Treatment Centers of
America
Nashville, TN

Eidetics, Inc.
Watertown, MA

Employee Managed Care Corp.
[EMC²]
Seattle, WA
— *Pregnancy, Chronic and
Catastrophic Conditions*

Green Spring Health Services
Columbia, MD
— *Behavioral Health, EAP*

Greenstone Health Solutions
Kalamazoo, MI

Hastings Healthcare Group
Pennington, NJ

Health Decisions International
Golden, CO
—*Pregnancy, Chronic Conditions*

HealthLine Systems
San Diego, CA
—*Call Center Software for*
Pregnancy, Chronic Conditions

Health Management Corp.
Richmond, VA
—*Chronic Conditions "Better*
Prepared," Pregnancy "Baby
Benefits"

Health Desk Corp.
Berkeley, CA
—*Software*

Healthtrac
Menlo Park, CA
— *"Babytrac" Pregnancy, Chronic*
Conditions

Integrated Therapeutics Group
(Schering Plough)

Johnson & Johnson Health Care
System, Health Management
Division
Piscataway, NJ

Matria Healthcare
Marietta, GA
—*Maternity*

Meditrac
Southfield, MI
—*Medications Compliance*

Mosby Consumer Health
St. Louis, MO

National Respiratory Centers
Lexington, KY
—*Asthma, COPD*

Nidus Information Services
New York, NY
— *"Well Connected" Information*

Olsten Health Services
Melville, NY
—*(Home Health)*

Optum Health
Golden Valley, MN
— *"Human Health Risk*
Management"

Paidos Health Management
Deerfield, IL
—*Neonatal, NICU babies*

PCS Health Systems (Eli Lilly)
Scottsdale, AZ

Preventive Medicine Research
Institute
Sausalito, CA
—*Dean Ornish's Heart Disease*
Reversal Program

Problem Knowledge Coupler [PKC]
Burlington, VT
—*Chronic Conditions*

Quantum Health Resources
— *"Chronicare"*

Renaissance Health Care, Inc.
Lexington, MA
—*ESRD*

Salick Healthcare
Los Angeles, CA
—*Cancers*

San Vita
McHenry, IL
— *Pregnancy*

Specialty Care Systems
Lake Forest, IL
— *Cardiovascular*

Spectrascan Health Services
Windsor, CT
— *Breast Cancer*

Stuart Disease Management Services
Wilmington, DE
— *"Multi-Disease Analysis
Program" for selecting which
disease(s) to manage*

Total Health Management Division of
  Adventist Health Services Sunbelt
Orlando, FL

Unison
Denver, CO
— *"Personal Advantage" for
Seniors*

Universal Self Care
Roanoke, VA
— *Diabetes, Other*

Value Health/Value Behavioral
  Health, Value Rx
Avon, CT

Vivra Specialty Partners
San Mateo, CA
— *Multiple Common Conditions*

Wellsource
Clackamas, OR
— *Chronic Conditions*

In addition, most of the large pharmaceutical firms, including Bristol Myers Squibb, Glaxo Wellcome, Merck Medco, Parke Davis, Pfizer, Searle, Smith Kline Beecham, Stuart, and Upjohn, have divisions or programs devoted to disease management or pharmacy benefit management. Some own one or more of the vendors listed above.

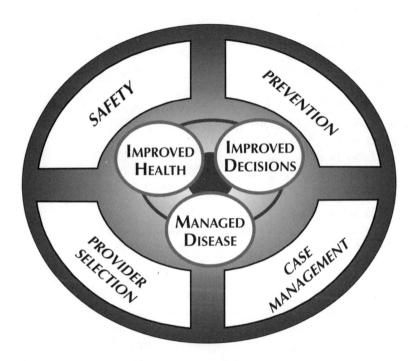

Chapter 24

DISABILITY MANAGEMENT

PROBLEM AND POTENTIAL

Concern has grown about the dramatic growth in disability costs, counting workers' compensation (WC), short-term disability (STD), and long-term disability (LTD) expenditures. Such growth had been overshadowed by the larger national health care expenditures but was even more dramatic and currently rivals the "health care crisis" in the eyes of employers.[1]

It has been estimated that job-related injuries and illnesses cost more than AIDS or Alzheimer's disease and as much as cancer or heart disease, with injuries accounting for 6,500 deaths and 13.2 million workers affected, and illnesses responsible for over 60,000 deaths and 860,000 affected workers. Direct costs for health care were estimated at $65 billion with indirect costs for lost wages and productivity $106 billion for a total of $171 billion in the United States in 1992.[2]

Recent estimates call for expenditures for workers' compensation medical costs alone to reach $150 billion by the year 2000. Since STD and LTD employee payments have always exceeded medical costs, which typically make up roughly 40% of the total, overall disability costs could easily reach $400 billion by that time.[3] And that does not count the costs of worker absenteeism and replacement.

One report estimated that 780,000 workers a year are out of work for five or more months.[4] A Louis Harris poll found 56% of workers were out sick at least one day a year, averaging three days' absence apiece, with at least 18 million employees debilitated by chronic or episodic pain. This poll found that benefit managers tend to greatly underestimate the extent of such debilitation while overestimating its impact on absenteeism.[5]

Disability is a special concern because of the additional costs created by the workers' compensation system, litigation, fraud, and abuse.[6] Workers who are injured often ask their physicians to extend their disability so as to enjoy more time off with pay.[7] Studies have found that medical costs and reported pain levels are higher and disability longer when there is potential litigation involved.[8] Risks of litigation have to be addressed by employers in addition to the medical and disability costs of occupational illness and injury.[9]

When medical conditions are treated under workers' compensation insurance, they tend to cost much more than when the same conditions are treated under employee health insurance. When treated under WC insurance, one study found workers were more than twice as likely to be hospitalized (14.4% versus 6.6% of cases) and spend more than four times as long "disabled" (206.6 days versus 51.0) as when health insurance covers the case.[10] Another study found costs 43% higher under WC than under health insurance.[11] (See Exhibit 24–1.)

Because WC insurance is normally based on "first-dollar" coverage, with no deductible or copay, employees have an incentive to report as work-related even conditions that are minor and offer no promise of disability benefits. And once under WC insurance, employees have no reason to worry about the costs of treatment.[12] Despite this many argue that occupational illnesses and injuries covered under WC insurance actually understate the extent of the problem, since many workers and/or physicians fail to see the connection to workplace factors.[13]

Even as we move away from the dominance of manufacturing, with its high risks of injury, to service and white collar industries, which are normally safer, we are finding a host of new problems. Carpal tunnel syndrome and other repetitive

Exhibit 24–1 Disability Management

PROBLEMS / POTENTIAL	CONCERNS
✗ COSTS FOR WORKERS' COMP & DISABILITY PAYMENTS GROWING EXPLOSIVELY ✗ MAJORITY OF WORKERS ABSENT AT LEAST ONE DAY EACH YEAR ✗ COSTS FOR TREATMENT UNDER WORKERS' COMP HIGHER THAN FOR OFF-THE-JOB CONDITIONS ✗ PREVENTION OF OCCUPATIONAL ILLNESS & INJURY MOST COST-EFFECTIVE	✗ WORKERS MAY FEEL ENTITLED TO SICK LEAVE ABSENCES EVEN WHEN NOT SICK ✗ ILL & INJURED WORKERS MAY "GAME THE SYSTEM" TO ENJOY DISABILITY PAYMENTS RATHER THAN WORK ✗ LITIGATION POTENTIAL MAY PROMOTE DELAYS IN TREATMENT ✗ SHIFT TO WHITE COLLAR EMPLOYMENT INTRODUCING NEW TYPES OF INJURY ✗ STATE LAWS VARY, BUT GREATLY AFFECT WHAT EMPLOYERS CAN DO ✗ FEDERAL LAWS, INCLUDING ADA, MAY COMPLICATE OR RESTRICT PROGRAMS

stress/cumulative trauma conditions are exploding across the country, increasing at an average rate of 20% a year in the entire labor force and over 90% a year on average among office workers in one study.[14] Costs of such injuries are estimated at $21 billion a year.[15]

Occupational asthma is the most common pulmonary illness caused by workplace conditions, representing an estimated 2% to 15% of all asthma.[16] As growing numbers of workers retire earlier, they are leaving employers with more younger workers whose wages and salaries may be lower but whose absenteeism and injury risk is higher.[17] Teenagers in service industries are particularly high risks.[18]

The burden of disability costs is not shared equally by all. Some industries, such as construction, resources extraction (e.g., mining, timber), and manufacturing have notoriously high injury costs, while others, such as financial institutions, have extremely low costs. Yet even within the same industry, there is wide variability in annual costs per worker.[19] Employers with well-managed disability programs were found to have average costs per case of $23,733 in one study, compared to $43,300 for employers lacking such programs. At least 50% of all disability costs are felt to be controllable.[20]

CONTROL PROGRAMS

Disability management has three basic categories of control programs corresponding to health and decision improvement and disease management in controlling conventional health costs. The first line of defense is prevention and safety, with environmental risk management, ergonomic furniture, tools, and equipment. Next come choices by employers and employees regarding the providers and procedures that will be used to treat a problem that was not prevented. Finally comes case management, in which providers and workers determine the length and costs of disability, whether and when employees return to work.

Safety/Prevention

As is true with health care utilization and costs in the group insurance area, moving "upstream" to prevent or to minimize disease and injury in the first place is generally regarded as the most cost-effective approach to disability management. Many safety and prevention efforts are entirely in the hands of employers—creating safer work environments, tools, and equipment. Creative Windows of Elkhart, Indiana, downsized tools to fit the hands of women workers, redesigned equipment and rotated work assignments, and cut its carpal tunnel injuries in half[21] (Exhibit 24–2).

Most safety programs require the involvement of employees, however. Educating them on safe practices and work processes can be effective if employers actu-

Exhibit 24–2 Safety/Prevention

EXAMPLES	✗ "MARKETING" SAFE BEHAVIOR REDUCES INJURIES BY 89% ✗ ANALYZING & CORRECTING CAUSES OF PAST INJURIES REDUCE INCIDENCE BY 43%, LOST WORK DAYS BY 71% ✗ STATE & FEDERAL GOVERNMENTS CAN OFFER SUPPORT & ASSISTANCE AS WELL AS REGULATION
ADVICE	✗ ENLIST EMPLOYEES IN ADDRESSING OWN RISKY BEHAVIOR & PREVENTION POTENTIAL ✗ LOOK FOR ENVIRONMENTAL, EQUIPMENT & SYSTEM CHANGES AS WELL AS EMPLOYEE BEHAVIOR CHANGES TO REDUCE ILLNESS & INJURY ✗ IDENTIFY HIGH-RISK EMPLOYEES FOR EXTRA ATTENTION ✗ PROMOTE IMPROVED FITNESS AS GENERAL PREVENTIVE ✗ SHARE SAVINGS IN SOME WAY WITH EMPLOYEES

ally change their behavior accordingly. Making complementary changes in equipment, such as wrist pads to help reduce carpal tunnel conditions among computer operators, may also help.[22] One employer used an internal advertising and marketing effort to promote safe behavior, reducing its injuries from 18 a year to 12 to 8 to 2 and saving $250,000 in WC claims.[23]

Providing safety equipment such as weight-lift support belts is one thing; getting employees to wear them may be another; and only wearing them will make a difference.[24] Just as in nonwork settings, identifying and paying special attention to high-risk employees may prove more cost-effective than aiming at everyone.[25]

Work-site fitness and exercise programs are frequently successful in reducing injuries, as well as in promoting productivity and morale. The Westinghouse Electric Assembly plant in College Station, Texas, promoted a daily 10-minute strength and flexibility exercise program that achieved 97% to 100% worker participation. Seeing one's peers all engaged in the program and knowing that each worker is in sight of the others promotes peer conformity.[26] Short, frequent exercise breaks have proven advantageous. Hon Furniture Company used a program of five-minute breaks every hour to cut its number of injuries by 67%.[27]

DETECTIVE WORK

Identifying the causes of past injuries and illnesses is something every employer should include in its disability management program. The A.T. Cross pen company analyzed its history of injuries to find common causes and reduced its incidence of injuries by 43% and its lost work days by 71%.[28] Lacks Enterprises (Michigan) eliminated hazards and reduced accident rates by 34%, severity by 42%.[29] Portland Glass (Westbrook, Maine) identified its safety problems and reduced its costs by 65% over five years.[30]

GETTING HELP

There are many sources of help for employers interested in prevention. Their insurance company will most often have safety programs available that it will want to try to reduce its risk. In addition, even government agencies such as the Occupational Safety and Health Administration (OSHA) can help. In Maine, OSHA achieved a 47% reduction in WC claims among employers participating in its accident/injury prevention program over three years.[31]

State governments may also provide support. Oregon provides safety consultants who work with employers to identify and reduce risks. They have reduced the rate of worker injuries by 2 per 1,000 workers and cut WC premiums for employers by 34%.[32] The University of Washington (Seattle) has provided work-site safety advice and consultation to employers for 30 years and keeps premiums 40% lower than in other states.[33]

The best source of help, however, is likely to be employees themselves. Except for angry and embittered employees aiming to harm their employer, workers do not want to become ill or injured and have a natural desire to protect their own health. If they are encouraged and enabled to identify and reduce risks, they can be more effective than many outside helpers, since they know the workplace much better.

Employee safety committees have proven effective in Michigan's Lacks Enterprises.[34] Involving union representatives and employees in a team approach with management can increase the number of people working toward solutions.[35] Regular safety meetings helped Portland Glass achieve its significant savings.[36]

If the natural desire to protect one's safety and health is insufficient, employers can offer incentives to encourage employee involvement. Medical Plastics Laboratory (Gatesville, Texas) pays $25 quarterly bonuses to individuals free of injury and distributes savings from its injury risk pool every year. It reduced annual lost work days from over 500 to just 35 in four years, paying as much as $600 per employee from the risk pool.[37] On the other hand, Portland Glass found that offering financial incentives tended to promote underreporting of injuries.[38]

PROVIDER SELECTION

One of the most popular approaches among employers seeking to reduce their disability costs is to turn to managed care providers. One study found WC medical costs 38.5% lower in managed care capitation providers as compared to fee-for-service (FFS) providers.[39] Another found that costs in HMOs were 54% lower, while costs in PPOs were 13% lower. As a generalization, managed care is held to save between 10% and 40% on WC costs[40] (Exhibit 24–3).

Managed care organizations are finding receptivity among employers and are increasingly extending their marketing efforts into workers' compensation and disability management. In one survey 51% of HMOs already offered a WC product, and of those who did not, 61% indicated they were planning to do so.[41] Another, more recent survey found 72% of managed care organizations in the WC business, though PPO plans were by far the most popular, with 81% of the market, compared to 14% for HMOs and 4% for EPOs.[42]

In some cases insurers do their own provider selection for injured workers. ITT Hartford's Catastrophic Injuries Management Program selects Centers of Excellence such as Craig Rehabilitation Center (Denver), Gaylord (Connecticut), and Baylor (Texas) for rehabilitation of quadriplegia and paraplegia patients, reducing costs 23% thereby.[43] Kaiser has developed its own occupational medicine clinics

Exhibit 24–3 Plan/Provider Selection

EXAMPLES	X Managed care provider systems can save 10%–40% on costs X Centers of Excellence for high-cost injuries & treatments can reduce costs X HMOs & providers offering specialized occupational health services X On-site providers offer easy access & coordination of care, minimize lost time from work
ADVICE	X Be wary of possible backlash if restricting employee choices X Enlist employees in plan & provider selection process to promote their cooperation & acceptance X Watch for state laws governing employee choices X Share savings from changing / restricting plans / providers with employees

in California, offering its own physicians as disability management providers.[44] Some hospitals are taking on risk as WC medical care providers.[45]

Another approach is for employers to provide medical care on site. A large number of employers, from Coors Brewing Company (Denver, Colorado) to John Deere (Moline, Illinois) to L.L. Bean (Freeport, Maine) offer on-site medical providers, sometimes as their employees or contractors or through contracts with medical groups such as Mayo Clinic. On-site medical centers can screen employees for problems, including drug abuse, and can promote prevention and early treatment, as well.

Not all employers are relying on physicians. Many employers are using on-site nurse practitioners and occupational health nurses to both prevent problems and treat them promptly when they arise. Physicians provide back-up support, but the nurses carry the day-to-day responsibility. The US Sugar Corporation (Clewiston, Florida) uses its nurses in case management as well. Hewlett Packard (Palo Alto, California) used such an approach to cut its WC costs by 19%.[46]

It has been argued that steering workers to the right provider is second only to preventing injury in the first place as a way to reduce employer costs.[47] However, not all employers have the legal right to direct injured employees to specific providers; it depends on state workers' compensation laws. In Colorado, where a change in state law gave employers the right to choose providers for their employees, critics have argued that choices are dictated entirely by the desire to save money, that physicians "cave in" to employer preferences when treating patients, and that the employees suffer the consequences. Though WC rates have gone down by 22% in five years and employers have saved an estimated $2 billion, the greatly reduced liability that employers bear has reduced their motivation to prevent injury, adding to the negative impact on workers.[48]

CASE MANAGEMENT

It seems to be generally agreed that the best beginning for effective management of individual cases of occupational illness or injury is immediate beginning of treatment. Employers who lack on-site capabilities are urged to make arrangements with nearby medical providers and hospital EDs so that injured workers can be seen as soon as possible. Rather than leave it entirely up to the employee, employers are urged to take over with transportation arrangements, appointments, and whatever else it takes to ensure that workers are seen immediately.[49]

The L.L. Bean Co. offers on-site physical therapy to workers with mild injuries such as carpal tunnel syndrome, so they do not have to lose work days. Their program resulted in an increase in claims (10%) but a far larger decrease in claims costs (40%).[50] (See Exhibit 24–4.)

For all but clearly minor, short-term problems, employers are urged to begin case planning and management immediately, setting specific goals for the dura-

Exhibit 24–4 Case Management

EXAMPLES	✗ ON-SITE TREATMENT & REHABILITATION SAVES LOST DAYS AT WORK
	✗ SPORTS MEDICINE APPROACH OF IMMEDIATE REHABILITATION MAY PREVENT PERMANENT DISABILITY
	✗ WORK HARDENING & JOB ADJUSTMENT MAY ENABLE EARLIER RETURN
ADVICE	✗ INITIATE CASE MANAGEMENT PLAN IMMEDIATELY & MAINTAIN CONTACT WITH EMPLOYEE THROUGHOUT CARE EPISODE
	✗ ENLIST FAMILY MEMBERS IN SUPPORTING EMPLOYEE, REMINDING OF APPOINTMENTS & SELF-CARE
	✗ ENLIST IMMEDIATE SUPERVISORS IN SUPPORTING CASE MANAGEMENT & PROMPT RETURN TO WORK
	✗ SHARE SAVINGS WITH EMPLOYEE IN SOME WAY

tion of disability and scheduling a specific date for return to work.[51] Duration guidelines can be used to both guide providers in managing treatment and remind workers and their family members that the employer confidently expects the employee to promptly return to work.[52]

Employers are advised to integrate WC, STD, and LTD programs so that they can manage their entire disability program in a coordinated fashion.[53] They should work to empower employees to return to work as soon as possible, encouraging them through treatment and rehabilitation, maintaining contact throughout the duration of disability. Often psychological more than physical factors inhibit injured workers from early return. Fears that they will be unable to function as they once did, and simply getting out of the habit of going to work every day, can be powerful barriers.[54] In one case of successful case management, a worker with a herniated disk returned to work two months earlier than normal, with $8,000 saved in medical costs and $63,000 in disability expense.[55]

Some providers recommend a "sports medicine" approach—initiating rehabilitative treatment as soon as the employee can stand it so that workers "get back in the game" before they lose their skills and confidence. Studies have shown that 50% of workers who are disabled and out of work for six months return to work; if one year, the proportion goes down to 25%; and after two years, hardly any return.[56]

Prompt return may not mean returning to the same job. Though work-hardening may be used to prepare for return to the same activities after a serious injury or illness, offering alternative employment on a temporary or permanent basis is often effective. Weyerhaeuser Corporation uses a "task bank" of activities suitable for recovering workers so they can return to work even if not quite ready for their regular job.[57] Chrysler Corporation combined return-to-work and disability protocols with light duty assignments to reduce its disability costs by 24%.[58]

Maintaining contact with injured workers throughout their treatment and rehabilitation is recommended for a variety of reasons. It shows workers the employer's continuing interest in their welfare, sustaining worker loyalty and reducing litigation risks.[59] Employers, including teams of the injured employee's coworkers, supervisor, and case managers can enlist the employee and family members in a coordinated effort to promote early return to work.[60]

Instead of virtually abandoning injured workers until they prove they are fit to return, employers are finding that partnering with employees in a common effort to promote fast and effective treatment, coordinated rehabilitation, and planned return is far more effective in controlling disability costs. Helping workers with physician's appointments and claims forms, setting goals for recovery and return, and helping employees achieve them has proven more cost-effective.[61]

There is a special challenge in disability management related to pregnancy. Pregnant workers must be evaluated to determine when they should go on maternity leave or have their duties revised in light of their pregnancy. Special arrangements may be made to enable them to work up to close to their scheduled delivery, if they so wish.[62] After delivery, providing on-site breastfeeding facilities has been shown to significantly reduce maternity leave time and absenteeism due to caring for a sick baby.

RECOMMENDATIONS

Based on the experience of employers and insurers in disability management, there seem to be some general themes running through successful efforts that can be translated into recommendations:

- Try including WC/disability "performance" in the criteria used to judge business unit and manager performance. The number of employees should be large enough to minimize chance variation, and the performance measures should be truly subject to the managers' control. This seems to work better than holding only corporate human resources or insurance/risk management staff responsible.
- Try integrating WC/disability and health insurance cost management (i.e., all the demand improvement categories), recognizing that there is a lot of overlap across them, with synergies and economies available through combining them, since they all aim at the same people, employees.
- Try aligning incentives of all who participate in managing WC/disability and health insurance costs (e.g., via capitation financing mechanisms, or performance incentives tied to specific results in reducing injuries and illness, or use of and expenditures for services and prompt return to work).
- Try integrating employees, both individually and collectively, in specific disability management efforts—in safety/prevention, provider and treatment selection, rehabilitation, and return. Much more will be accomplished with employees as enthusiastic and effective partners than as adversaries.
- Try incorporating employees' family members in specific efforts. They have a great interest in preventing disability, in effective treatment and rehabilitation, and in prompt return to work, and they can provide both caregiver and moral support.
- Try sharing the savings that will result from successful disability management with employees, both individually and collectively. Aside from the motivational effects of dollar incentives, such sharing has symbolic value in demonstrating and reinforcing a partnership relationship and common effort.

REFERENCES

1. M. Lipowski, "Big Benefits in a Fertile Ground," *Managed Healthcare* 5, no. 9 (1995):42–44, 52.
2. B. Coleman, "Workplace Injuries More Costly Than AIDS," *The Denver Post,* 28 July 1997, 1A, 11A.

3. L. Kertesz, "HMOs Mine Workers' Comp Market," *Modern Healthcare,* 25 September 1995, 66, 71.

4. K. Robbins, "The Growing Costs of Disability," *Business & Health Special Report: The Advantages of Managed Disability,* 1993, 8, 9.

5. M.L. Hurley, "The High Price of Pain," *Business & Health* 14, no. 6 (1996):31–33.

6. F. Cerne, "Lowering the Boom on Workers' Comp," *Hospitals & Health Networks,* 20 August 1994, 50–52.

7. "Doc, Can't You Give Me a Few More Weeks Off?" *Business & Health* 13, no. 9 (1995):11.

8. C. Brigham, et al., "The Changing Role of Rehab: Focus on Function," *Patient Care* 30, no. 3 (1996):144–159.

9. "Employers Can Reduce Costs for Job-Related Injuries through HMOs, Survey Says," *Business & Health* 11, no. 9 (1993):12.

10. "Proven Managed Care Techniques Urgently Needed in Workers' Compensation Area," *Managed Care Resource Guide* 2, no. 1 (Special Edition 1995):4.

11. "Back Injury Costs More If It's Job-Related," *Business & Health* 14, no. 5 (1996):11, 12.

12. "Workers Compensation Is Killing Business," *Marketing to Doctors* 5, no. 6 (1992):4.

13. J. Pearson, et al., "We're All Practicing Occupational Medicine," *Patient Care* 30, no. 3 (1996):42–67.

14. B. Dimmit, "Repetitive Stress Injuries: Relieving Pain at the Bottom Line," *Business & Health* 13, no. 5 (1995):21–24.

15. "Carpal Tunnel Isn't the Only Route to Repetitive Stress," *Business & Health* 14, no. 5 (1996):12.

16. E. Bardena, et al., "Occupational Asthma: Breathing Easier on the Job," *Patient Care* 30, no. 3 (1996):100–117.

17. "Acute Illness and Older Workers: Dispelling the Myth," *Medical Benefits,* 30 December 1991, 4.

18. T. Chester, et al., "Caution: Work Can Be Hazardous to Your Health," *Patient Care* 30, no. 3 (1996):70–98.

19. R. Habeck, "Employer Factors Related to Workers' Compensation Claims and Disability Management," *Rehabilitation Counseling Bulletin* 34, no. 3 (1991):210–226.

20. L. Brenner, "A Workplace Armageddon," *Corporate Finance,* March/April 1993, 18–22.

21. Dimmitt, "Repetitive Stress Injuries," 21–24.

22. "How Companies Manage Disability Costs Successfully," *Business & Health Special Report: Advantages of Managed Disability,* 1993, 10–17.

23. "Making Safety Pay," *Profiles in Health Care Marketing,* January/February 1993, 2–5.

24. L. Driscoll, "Compensating for Workers' Comp Costs," *Business Week,* 3 February 1992, 72.

25. M. Fruen, "Disability Management Focuses on Prevention," *Business & Health* 10, no. 12 (1992):24–29.

26. S. Pronk, et al., "Impact of Daily 10-Minute Strength and Flexibility Program in a Manufacturing Plant," *American Journal of Health Promotion* 9, no. 3 (1995):175–178.

27. Driscoll, "Compensating," 72.

28. "Workers Compensation," 4.

29. N. Varettoni, "Creative Management Helps Cut Employee Disability Costs," *Business & Health* 11, no. 12 (1993):57–61.

30. "Safety Programs Pay Off," *INC.* 18, no. 6 (1996):114.

31. D. Wise, "An OSHA You Could Love," *Business & Health* 14, no. 2 (1996):27–30.

32. Brenner, "A Workplace Armageddon," 18–22.

33. "Boosting Safety in Small Business," *CenterScope Challenge* (University of Minnesota, Minneapolis) 1, no. 2 (1996):1, 2.

34. Varettoni, "Creative Management," 57–61.

35. Habeck, "Employer Factors," 210–226.

36. "Safety Programs," 114.

37. "Savings through Self-Funded Workers' Comp?" *Employee Health & Fitness* 17, no. 6 (1995):66, 67.

38. Habeck, "Employer Factors," 210–226.

39. "An Insider's Look at Workers' Compensation," *Business & Health* 11, no. 9 (1993):12.

40. "HMOs Make a Move on Workers' Comp," *Business & Health* 14, no. 1 (1996):56.

41. Kertesz, "HMOs Mine Workers' Comp," 66, 71.

42. "HMOs Make a Move," 56.

43. J. Smith, "The Best Care Not Cheapest Pays Off," *Health Systems Review* 28, no. 2 (1995):50–52.

44. M. Edlin, "Kaiser OM Clinics Help Curb Calif. WC Costs," *Managed Healthcare* 4, no. 10 (1994):16.

45. "Hospitals Practice Using 'Shadow HMOs,' " *Health Care Strategic Management* 13, no. 7 (1995):17.

46. C. Petersen, "On-Site Alternatives," *Managed Healthcare* 2, no. 9 (1993):61, 62.

47. Brenner, "A Workplace Armageddon," 18–22.

48. S. Steers, "Still Hurting," *Westword* 19, no. 31 (1996):14–21.

49. Habeck, "Employer Factors," 210–226.

50. Wise, "An OSHA You Could Love," 27–30.

51. "How Companies Manage," 10–17.

52. G. Leavenworth, "Setting Standards for Workers' Comp," *Business & Health* 12, no. 10 (1994):49–54.

53. Fruen, "Disability Management," 24–29.

54. "The Value of a Partnership Approach," *Business & Health Special Report: The Advantages of Managing Disability,* 1993, 20–22.

55. Fruen, "Disability Management," 24–29.

56. Brigham, et al., "The Changing Role of Rehab," 144–159.

57. "Workers Compensation," 4.

58. "How Companies Manage," 10–17.

59. "An Insider's Look," 12.

60. "Aetna Finds Success with In-House Integrated Disability Program," *St. Anthony's Managing Community Health & Wellness* 2, no. 7 (1996):5, 7.

61. "Many Physicians Lack Essential Knowledge of Pregnant Employees' Working Conditions," *Occupational Health Management* 2, no. 10 (1995):145, 146.

62. "Lactation Services Lower Claims Costs, Boost Morale, Reduce Absenteeism," *Employee Health & Fitness* 17, no. 10 (1995):109–114.

Disability Management Vendors

Integrated Health Management
  Associates
www.ihma-inc.com

Johnson & Johnson Health Care
  Systems, Health Management
  Division
Piscataway, NJ
  —*Fitness, Safety*

Mosby Consumer Health
St. Louis, MO
  — *"Wellness at Work," EAP*

Towers Perrin
www.towers.com

Value Health
Avon, CT
  —*Workers Compensation, Provider
  Networks*

In addition, most large workers' compensation and disability insurance companies, as well as occupational health providers, are likely to offer some types of programs to reduce disease and injury and promote choice of the best providers, as well as prompt recovery and return to work.

Chapter 25

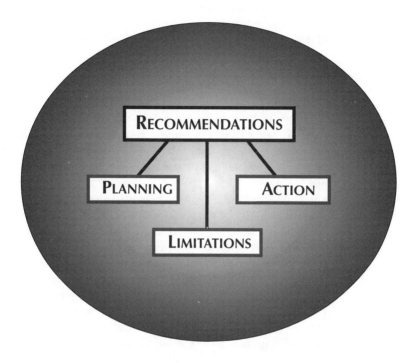

FINAL COMMENTS

After a thorough consideration of the concept of demand improvement and an examination of the hundreds of practical examples described in previous chapters, we feel some final comments are both possible and in order. First, we will summarize the major concepts and strategic options available for planning demand improvement efforts. Then we will make some general action recommendations to those considering and engaging in demand management initiatives.

PLANNING RECOMMENDATIONS

We have introduced four categories, or domains, of demand improvement initiatives, differing by their consumer targets, intentions, and methods. We recommend that these be used as a foundation for planning health and demand improvement strategies and initiatives. A recap of the four domains follows.

The Four Domains

We have presented health improvement, decision improvement, disease (self-) management, and disability (self-) management as offering significant promise to potential sponsors and as being equally worthy of consideration as categorical approaches to improving demand. Sponsors should consider the full set of domains in examining whether, where, and how many investments and initiatives would be worthwhile.

We also recommend that vendors, most of whom started with one or a few product or service offerings in one of the four domains, look at expanding their offerings to other domains. It appears that many are doing so already, as call center vendors expand from their initial focus on physician referral, for example, to triage and decision counseling within decision improvement, then to health risk behavior assessment and reduction (health improvement) and supporting self-management of chronic conditions and reminding of appointments (disease self-management). It is likely that as sponsors expand their investment in demand improvement, they will seek to limit the number of vendors they deal with, so vendors with multiple offerings would have an advantage.

The Set of Effects

We have described seven categories of effects that have been used by sponsors in reporting what they have achieved: changes in consumer program participation, mind-states, behavior, health status, health services utilization, expenditures, and a range of value added to consumers, employers, health plans, and providers. These effects can be used in both strategic and tactical planning, in managing and monitoring specific initiatives, and in evaluating the results of those initiatives.

The most immediate of these effects (i.e., participation, mind-states, perhaps behavior) are useful in monitoring the early impact of initiatives though are difficult measures to put a dollar value upon. The intermediate effects (i.e., behavior, health status, and utilization quality) are likely to be the most appropriate basis for setting goals and objectives and the greatest *source* of value to the variety of stakeholders affected. The utilization quantity and expenditure effects are best treated as the deserved rewards for successful demand improvement initiatives, though they are also sources of added value to stakeholders.

The relationship among these effects is as important as each one is individually. In some cases there may be a simple and linear cause-and-effect relationship that can be used to promote one effect with confidence that it will end up producing the desired results in another. In other cases the relationship may be complex and nonlinear, requiring greater sophistication in planning and greater care in evaluation of efforts. We recommend that sponsors consider each one of these effects in every case. By tracking the full set of effects, sponsors can build the strongest basis for attribution of success to their own efforts.

Stages of Change

We consider Prochaska's stages of change or stages of readiness model as the most useful and thoroughly tested published model for planning specific changes in consumer behavior. It is useful in identifying which consumers need to be addressed and which are most promising as targets for initiatives. It is helpful in designing interventions tailored to specific segments of consumers and in increasing the effectiveness and efficiency of such interventions.

This model has already proven itself in a wide range of applications, though primarily for health risk and prevention/early detection behaviors (health improvement). We recommend that sponsors use it in planning decision improvement and disease and disability management initiatives as well. Its history suggests it has the most promising potential specific to changing behavior and to health-related behavior in particular.

Composite Behavior Change Model ($I = MC^2$)

Our review of published behavior models and of specific examples of demand improvement initiatives has led us to conclude that the three operational or manageable factors most useful in changing consumer behavior are motivation, capability, and consciousness. We feel the $I = MC^2$ model will help sponsors in understanding first why consumers are not already behaving in a manner sponsors desire. Barriers seem always to be some combination of lack of motivation, capability or confidence therein (self-efficacy), and lack of consciousness (awareness or remembering).

This model also suggests categories for specific interventions that can move targeted consumers from one stage of change to the next and ultimately entire populations to an improved pattern of health and demand behaviors. Learning about consumer mind-state changes in levels of motivation, capability, or consciousness can provide early indications of the impact of initiatives. We recommend that all three factors be addressed in planning, implementing, and monitoring specific behavior change initiatives in conjunction with the stages of change.

ACTION RECOMMENDATIONS

Demand versus Supply Focus

We recommend that sponsors consider consumer-focused demand improvement along with or instead of provider-focused supply restrictions when seeking ways to manage their risks, reduce expenditures, and improve their performance. We cannot promise that demand improvement in general, nor any one domain or category of initiative, will make sense for all sponsors, nor for all situations. The uniqueness of each sponsor and population precludes any such generalization, but experience indicates that the potential for demand improvement should always be included in sponsors' overall risk management.

The vast majority of published examples of demand improvement initiatives have shown success and, where reported, positive and admirable return on investment, with ROI ratios typically 2:1 or greater. We suspect, however, that there may be many unsuccessful efforts whose sponsors chose not to publish their failure. We know from published cases that sponsors often report effort before anything but anecdotal indications of results have been noted and often report results such as participation, mind-state, or behavior changes whose value is impossible to estimate.

Where sponsors choose to engage in provider-focused supply control as well as consumer-focused demand improvement, we believe that it is essential that they coordinate, if not integrate, such efforts. Providers are key elements in most demand improvement initiatives, and sponsors who aim to control providers' delivery of services should consider the impact of control initiatives on their relationship with providers and on providers' enthusiasm for cooperating in demand improvement efforts.

We recognize that sponsors have a significant dilemma under capitation financing systems: should they aim to attract mostly healthy, low-utilization populations in the first place or convert the populations they do attract to healthier and lower demand behaviors after enrollment? Sponsors who attract only or mostly healthy, low-utilization consumers (as employees, enrollees, or patients) will have little or no need for demand improvement.

It is difficult to achieve and maintain success through attraction of healthy consumers alone, however. Government legislation and regulation seriously hamper any effort to screen out higher risks, and since healthy, low-demand consumers are desirable for all sponsors at risk, the competition is fierce. Moreover, even consumers who are healthy and low-demand types at the time of enrollment will get older and become worse risks over time. They are also more likely to shift health plan and provider loyalties, since their good health and low demand mean they derive less benefit from their relationships.

We are convinced that all sponsors are likely to be better off, at some point, if they acquire and demonstrate demand improvement capabilities. This can entail its own risk, of course, if they end up attracting sicker, higher use consumers because of success in improving the health and demand of such consumers, as discussed in Chapter 23. On the other hand, a balanced strategy of initiatives across all domains and benefiting all members of the population should help control this risk over time.

Sponsor Contributions

We recommend that sponsors look first to themselves as past contributors to their current problems or failures in demand improvement. How many employers have had limited success in achieving participation among their employees in health screening or work-site safety educational programs because they have failed to give employees time off to participate? How many health plans have limited success in achieving high levels of immunization or early detection because they fail to cover such services as insured benefits? How many providers have limited success in promoting healthier behavior, better patient choices, or management of chronic conditions because they insisted on their own privileges as professionals rather than enlisting patients as partners or recognizing their independent capabilities?

When looking at motivational, capability, or consciousness barriers to improving consumer behavior, sponsors should look carefully at themselves and aggressively invite constructive criticism by employees, enrollees, and patients. Given the reluctance of most consumers to criticize, special effort will be needed to overcome natural reticence. Partnering sponsors may invite criticism of their partners, for example, so that consumers do not have to criticize a given sponsor directly. Ask consumers to report on what they hear from others or on what they believe others think if they prove unwilling to criticize or identify problems as their own.

Being open to criticism and suggestions from consumers is a way of overcoming the blinders that sponsors might have regarding the extent to which they are part of the problem, rather than part of the solution. By being truly open and welcoming of criticism and suggestions, sponsors stand to learn a great deal of which they might otherwise remain ignorant. In addition, such a stance will stimulate trust and better working relations with consumers.

Capitation Payments

Virtually all capitation payment systems adjust for age and sex characteristics of covered populations, recognizing that these factors make a significant difference to a population's use and costs of heath care. Unfortunately the factor that makes the greatest difference in use and costs, namely the health status of individuals, is typically not an adjustment factor. At one level this may seem only fair, preserving the community rating ideal and not discriminating against the chronically ill or disabled.

However, such nondiscrimination can end up by penalizing health plans and provider systems that are most successful in treating people with chronic conditions. As described in Chapter 23, plans and providers successful in disease management could end up with a higher proportion of people with chronic conditions. As a result, their financial viability would be jeopardized, hardly a fitting reward for such success. The only way to prevent this from happening is to adjust capitation payments based on health status so that people with chronic conditions would warrant higher payments, thereby encouraging plans and providers to enroll them and manage their health and demand.[1]

This is already done in Medicaid populations, where beneficiaries in different eligibility categories, such as disabled versus Aid to Families with Dependent Children, bring different capitation payments to HMOs. It can easily be done with Medicare populations in a budget-neutral manner, since all beneficiaries are paid for by the federal government. Among employed, commercially insured populations, such adjustment can be problematic, though at least there are relatively fewer with chronic conditions than among Medicare members.

Having to pay more for employees with chronic conditions would necessarily provide an incentive to employers to avoid hiring and keeping employees with chronic conditions. However, this incentive already applies to self-insured and experience-rated employers, which represents by far the largest proportion of employees. Paying plans and providers higher amounts for sick enrollees will at least encourage both to engage in disease management efforts for such populations, which can deliver significant value to those enrollees as well as save sponsors money.

If employers reduce payments to plans and plans to providers after each success in reducing use and costs among chronically ill members of a covered population, the beneficial effects of health status adjustment diminish. In effect, such reductions would mean plans and providers are forced to shoot for a continuously moving target, with each success in reducing expenditures followed by "punishment" in the form of reduced payment. An equitable sharing of savings should be part of every demand improvement effort.

It would be patently unfair for plans and providers to continuously enjoy the financial fruits of demand improvement success while employers continue paying the same rates. As with so many other issues in improving demand, it makes sense for both payers and providers to share such savings, with annual splitting of the difference between national average-cost-adjusted rates and actual costs of serving such populations. Sharing savings with the chronically ill for their part in producing cost savings makes equally good sense.

Partnership with Consumers

We believe that by far the best approach to improving health and demand behavior is an active partnership with consumers. This means first that sponsors should be open, honest, and thorough in discussing their reasons for seeking particular behavior changes. Especially where consumer trust of a sponsor is low, such candor may be the only way to achieve consumer cooperation. In any case, candor will tend to promote trust and enhance long-term relations with consumers, where secrecy or manipulative approaches will damage them.

Being open will also help ensure that sponsors include clear and significant consumer benefit as an essential if not primary focus for demand improvement initiatives. Explicit consumer benefit will help balance the sponsor benefits desired and thereby help avoid the scandals and negative public responses that have characterized so many supply-focused efforts. It will also promote the achievement of added sponsor performance value such as employee loyalty and morale, member and patient retention, and their value-adding effects.

Perhaps the surest way to ensure that consumer benefits are a major focus of demand improvement initiatives is to ensure that consumers are empowered to make informed choices. Communicating "report cards" on health plans, providers, procedures, and behavior changes based on the benefits they have delivered to consumers will enable consumers to make their own choices about which benefits they value most. Giving consumers choices and enabling them to choose well may be one of the most powerful benefits sponsors can offer. It can not only promote improved behavior but also strengthen consumers' trust in and relationships with sponsors.

As consumers make better choices and improve their health and demands, sponsors should report to those consumers the continuing benefits they have gained to promote their awareness and appreciation thereof. Surveying consumers on the psychosocial benefits they perceive will also heighten their awareness. This in turn should enhance their continuing improvement and participation.

Because of clear consumer benefit, sponsors will be in a position to invite direct consumer involvement in planning specific initiatives. Consumers may advise and inform sponsor planning through sample surveys, advisory panels, focus groups, pilot testing, and many other forms of involvement to help sponsors improve the effectiveness and efficiency of their efforts. Such involvement, by itself, will also help promote trust and lasting relationships.

By being open about their own benefit, sponsors open themselves up to possible consumer insistence on sharing in sponsor gains. Where this is the case, sponsors must consider the added cost of gainsharing and the effect it will have on their net gains. They should also consider how such sharing will perhaps add to consumer motivation and further strengthen long-term relationships. Reporting and sharing what they gain from consumers' own efforts in demand improvement should go a long way toward restoring and enhancing trust.

Choice

One key aspect of successful demand improvement programs appears to be *choice*. Unlike "management" approaches, where the choice is between obey and disobey, consumers seem to respond better to having real options and being able to exercise choice. The lack of a reasonable range of choices in health plans or providers has kept many consumers from enrolling in managed care plans, even when encouraged by employers and governments to do so. The lack of a choice other than abstinence scuttled a teen pregnancy prevention effort in California.[2]

Choice is one way to avoid charges of coercion or manipulation of consumers and to ensure that they perceive enough value in hoped-for changes of behavior to choose to make them. It will help address the confounding variability and changeability that characterize consumers, where a single option would fail. Choice may be one way to preserve the future of managed care, though it may be too late, according to at least one author.[3]

Targeting versus Self-Selection

Ample evidence in published studies of demand improvement efforts indicates that consumers who volunteer to participate in specific initiatives tend to be those at the low-risk end of the spectrum. It is equally clear that many sponsors fail to discriminate when offering programs to consumers, allowing those with the most interest to select themselves, thereby promoting the likelihood that lower risk consumers participate in greater numbers.

While "discrimination" in many ways is dangerous and illegal, indiscriminate recruitment of participants has two negative impacts on particular initiatives. First, it tends to result in fewer higher risk–higher potential consumers participating in programs, therefore less impact than might have occurred if even the same proportion of high-risk consumers participated as there are in the population of interest. Second, it tends to bias evaluations of initiatives by making behaviors, health status, utilization, and expenditure measures for self-selected participants artificially low compared to the population as a whole.

Unless sponsors devote enough effort to recruiting at least the same proportion of high-risk as low-risk consumers to participate in interventions as there are in the population, they are in danger of overestimating the impact of the interventions. At the same time they will most likely achieve less impact in fact than they would have with as many high risks as low risks or, preferably, more high risks than proportionate representation would require. Thus they will overestimate the value of their efforts while underachieving in terms of real value.

This is not to say that sponsors should go after high risks just because they are more serious problems and would produce higher value results if their behavior were improved. Their *probability* of improvement, considering where they are along the stages of change and what motivation, capability, and consciousness factors need to be changed to achieve specific improvements, is as important as the *value* of such improvement. The point is that sponsors would be better advised to make deliberate choices about who they will target for specific initiatives, rather than letting consumers select themselves.

Management Information Systems

In addition to the specific investments required for particular demand improvement initiatives, sponsors need to make significant added investments in information systems. Few sponsors already enjoy the kinds of information systems that enable them to conduct a fully informed analysis of where the most serious health and demand problems are, where the most promising opportunities for intervention are, who the most promising consumer targets for attention are.

Without solid information, sponsors may target the wrong consumers, aim for improvements in the wrong behavior, or expect the wrong results. When this occurs, not only are they likely to be disappointed in the outcomes they achieve, but also they are prone to throw out the baby with the bathwater and deny themselves what they could gain from well-planned, evidence-based interventions.

Both strategic and tactical planning of demand improvement interventions call for comprehensive, accurate, and up-to-date population-based data. So do the implementation, monitoring, and ongoing management of such interventions. Perhaps most critical, an informed evaluation of specific initiatives should include an informed look at the entire population of interest, those affected by the intervention as well as those unaffected, and the full range of effects.

Information systems will most often have to be built sequentially, as some pieces of information are needed in order to decide what to collect next. Health risk assessments, for example, may be needed to determine which consumers are the most appropriate and promising subjects for further information gathering. Claims and utilization data may be needed to identify the most promising subjects for clinical testing and attitude surveys.

Information systems capable of collecting, storing, and reporting comprehensive and timely health and demand characteristics of entire populations of interest are virtually nonexistent and will be expensive to develop. On the other hand, without such information, sponsors are largely flying blind into what may prove to be expensive and dubious investment or certainly suboptimal results. There may be many opportunities for successful initiatives while information systems are still in the developmental stage, but at some point, such systems are likely to be essential.

Communications Technology

Because of the rapid pace of development and change in communications technologies, it is difficult to be specific regarding how sponsors ought to use them. On the other hand, developing technologies in computer software and CD-ROM capabilities; interactive video disks; software and television; the Internet and World Wide Web sites; and e-mail, for example, offer significant potential for reaching a large and growing segment of the population.

New interactive communications technologies seem especially promising for improving consumer health and demand behaviors. Video disks, computer software, and television all provide opportunities for interaction. Sponsors would be well advised to become familiar with these new technologies. On the other hand, traditional communications methods involving written materials, phone, and fax, for example, should not be ignored. It is likely that a mix of technologies will be needed to reach and have the desired impact on diverse populations.

Like the choice of any demand improvement targets and objective, decisions regarding communications technologies should be made in light of what populations are to be reached, what objectives achieved, and what value outcomes are achievable. Some may be worthwhile enough to justify investing in placing cable modems, two-way monitors, even computers in selected consumers' homes, for example, when such technologies promise cost-effective and valuable results.

While we cannot recommend a specific communications technology investment to any particular sponsor without knowing a great deal about each sponsor's population and intentions, we strongly recommend that sponsors become thoroughly familiar with these new technologies and with convergent technologies combining phone, computers, and television, for example, in a single appliance. Many of these technologies are likely to prove among the best ways to achieve particular demand improvement and relationship building objectives. Sponsors who fail to keep up are likely to find themselves surpassed by competitors.

Strategic Approach

While most of the demand improvement initiatives we have reviewed were developed incrementally, perhaps later coordinated through an emergent strategy, we recommend that sponsors newly considering demand improvement investments develop a comprehensive strategic approach. This requires the kind of management information system previously described, though sponsors lacking such a system should not postpone investment in demand improvement until a complete system is in place.

All sponsors are likely to be under pressure to deliver short-term performance results to please shareholders or trustees and protect existing jobs. The natural response to such pressure is to emphasize actions with short-term payoff. Only a wide-ranging, strategic approach is likely to be able to balance short-term with long-term payoffs and to achieve a balanced pattern of investment. Only a strategic approach is likely to recognize the full range of systems dynamics affecting demand improvement.

Sponsors may well begin their involvement in demand improvement by choosing the first promising investment they become confident in, and focusing initially on short-term results. If they stay with a piecemeal or incremental mode, however, they risk seeing their competitors achieve the advantages that strategic thinking and investment offer. We recommend that as soon as possible sponsors develop demand improvement capabilities as part of their core competencies. This will require long-term commitment at the highest levels of the organization.

Whatever domains are chosen, consumers targeted, and behavior change objectives formulated, we recommend that demand improvement be thought of as a continuous challenge, part of continuous quality and performance improvement, rather than looking for 100% conversion to a desired behavior in a short time. Setting expectations as high as perfect behavior across an entire population simply invites frustration and promotes disappointment.

Experience clearly indicates that many members of a population will be readily convertible to the desired behavior, as they are well along in stages of change and have only modest barriers of motivation, capability, or consciousness preventing their conversion. At the same time, many others will be highly resistant to change, dogmatically convinced that their current behavior is fine, that they have a constitutional right to be foolish, that external factors make all the difference, or that they are not responsible. Improving behavior among such people will likely take years and may never be achieved.

Evaluation

From reported examples of demand improvement initiatives by various sponsors, we have concluded that we have a long way to go in the sophistication of evaluation methods being used. Perhaps because of the exploding interest in improving health and demand in general, there are abundant opportunities to publish reports of specific programs in newsletters, vendor reports, and annual reports, as well as in a wide variety of journals. However, the quality control over what kinds of results are reported and over the rigor of evaluation employed is often lax.

We have seen many reports of initiatives that get into print as soon as they are initiated, before any systematic results are even possible. As reported in Chapter 5, there are large numbers of initiatives whose success has been reported in terms of numbers of participants and in changes in awareness or attitudes, with no evidence of behavior changes that could at least lead to some improvement in health status, utilization, or expenditures and thereby demonstrate value and show real impact. Even reported changes in behavior, while often worthwhile accomplishments, fall short if they do not look at health status, service use, and expenditure effects, plus value-adding effects attributable thereto.

Many sponsors and vendors seem all too anxious to get reports of results into print as soon as possible, often before a full picture of results and value derived could conceivably be discovered. We have seen reports of results at three, five, six, eight, and nine months extrapolated to produce estimates of longer periods rather than waiting for a full year, for example. We have found all too few reports covering multiple years' results and thereby indicating whether initiatives encounter diminishing or increasing returns, costs, or both.

The use of comparison groups—of comparable populations at minimum or preferably experiment versus control groups so that the impact of a specific initiative can be isolated and results confidently attributed to that initiative—is all too rare. Many reports involve self-selected participants who must be suspected of being more motivated, capable, and conscious relative to changing behavior and perhaps already evidencing healthier behavior and better demand than nonparticipants. Without random or controlled selection, before and after as well as ongoing comparisons, many of the results reported must be suspect.

We are worried that a kind of Gresham's Law may apply—that bad evaluations flooding publications will make readers and potential sponsors wary of all evaluations and drive out truly rigorous and reliable evaluations. We recommend that both evaluators and publishers greatly enhance the sophistication and rigor of evaluations with longer time frames, more careful comparisons, and measures of as many of the set of effects as possible, particularly those reflecting value. In addition to providing a sounder basis for evaluation, the set of effects, if demonstrated to have occurred as intended, greatly strengthens confidence in attribution of results to interventions.

To determine the full value of interventions, their extended, indirect, and systems effects must be sought and examined. This includes the added value that ALL stakeholders, from consumers to payers to providers, enjoy. It includes all attributable impact, such as improved recruitment and retention of employees for businesses and improved image and member retention for health plans, for example. Only where such added-value effects are looked for and planned for are they likely to be both discovered and confidently attributed to specific interventions or overall strategies.

The American Journal of Health Promotion has established an enviable record of publishing rigorous evaluations of health improvement initiatives. Thus far it has no equivalent counterpart in decision improvement or disease and disability management. We challenge these latter disciplines to develop journals of equal value and to promote rigorous and reliable evaluations to at least compete with anecdotal bragging and selling.

Selecting Partners

We recommend that sponsors look carefully for and at opportunities to enlist partners in their demand improvement planning and in specific initiatives. Among risk-sharing partners, one stakeholder group is likely to be best suited for some consumers, some behaviors, some domains or initiatives, and some tactics, while other partners are better suited for others of each. Involving all partners in strategic planning and in actual initiatives will keep all tuned in to the importance and potential of demand improvement.

Involving partners automatically raises issues of sharing costs and gains, though these are present in any case. Having such issues raised and settled at the outset provides the possibility of sharing results and returns based on contributions to specific initiatives and to the value obtained by each partner, rather than power politics after the fact. Up-front planning can promote continuing, mutually beneficial working relationships among partners in strategic and tactical efforts.

Looking for community partners beyond the scope of financial risk sharing is worth considering in most cases, as well. Many behavior changes can probably be achieved only through community-wide efforts; many others may prove more effective or efficient if carried out by a large number of organizations and focused on a larger population, a "community of solution" that is different from the at-risk population of concern to any one sponsor.

This is not to say that partnerships should automatically be preferred and pursued in every case. There are likely to be many situations in which a single sponsor is able to do more, to achieve more faster by working alone than by partnering with anyone (other than consumers, of course). Many communities may lack the infrastructures and willingness to work together that have characterized the community efforts reported in Chapter 19. We merely recommend that sponsors *consider* the advantages and disadvantages of partnership approaches, as opposed to striking out on their own without such consideration.

It appears likely that some stakeholders in community efforts are paying less than their fair share of the costs of such efforts, leaving others to pay more than their share. A study of hospital-sponsored poison control centers (these are specialized triage services), for example, found that such centers were clearly cost-effective, saving $175 in medical expense per call at a cost of only $28. However, hospitals paid roughly 45% of the costs of such centers, while enjoying only 15% of the savings. Private payers enjoyed 36% of the savings, but paid only 11% of the costs.[4]

Gainsharing

While demand improvement should focus first on improving consumer health and quality of life as well as clinical outcomes, it will mostly be used with the expectation of savings in health care expenditures for populations of interest. There will necessarily arise an issue of who shall share in the savings that are achieved. We recommend a full and equitable sharing among all who participate in demand improvement efforts, including consumers.

This is in sharp contrast to the pattern of nonsharing that has often been the focus of criticisms of managed care. It has been argued that employers and other payers do not gain from savings achieved by managed care, only the managed care organizations themselves.[5] There is little evidence that consumers have gained from such savings or have even been discussed as possible participants in sharing.

Self-insured employers who achieve savings on their own through on-site wellness efforts could share these savings with employees in the form of lower out-of-pocket premiums, deductibles, or copays; incentives; and bonuses. Health plans that achieve savings will likely be forced by market realities to share some of their savings with employers but could share them with members through improved service or benefits.

When providers are risk-sharing partners in demand improvement strategies and programs, they will naturally share in any savings achieved under global capitation. Specific shares will depend on contract arrangements among hospitals, primary physicians, and specialists. Undoubtedly conflicts will arise as to who deserves what share based on their contribution to savings, but these can be worked out among the partners.

The trickiest sharing issue is likely to be how to deal with continued savings. Demand improvement initiatives that have achieved significant reductions in avoidable morbidity and replaceable demand and that have reformed demand so as to reduce costs have continuing effect and are likely to require continuing effort to maintain low levels of expenditures. Yet market forces may insist that payments be reduced to the health plans or providers responsible for the reductions.

In Chapter 1 we outlined a purely hypothetical example where a combination of avoided morbidity and replaced and reformed demand cut total health care costs per person by half. If such a reduction were accomplished in fact, what should payment levels be to plans and providers? If their payments are cut by the same percentage, they will in effect be "punished" for achieving the reduction. Moreover, there may not be enough money in the reduced payment to permit investment in continuing demand improvement efforts needed to keep expenditures low.

In effect, payers would enjoy continued savings over what their expenditures would have been without the demand improvement effort, while plans and providers enjoy only the one-time benefit of reduced expense when payment levels were based on unimproved demand. Employers dealing with health plans and plans dealing with providers may undermine motivation and even capability to engage in effective demand improvement if they insist on enjoying the continuing benefits thereof while other partners are limited to one-time benefit.

We recommend that risk-sharing partners move toward long-term contracts that spell out long-term sharing from their demand improvement efforts and successes. Long-term contracts, per se, will facilitate investment in demand improvement initiatives with longer term payoff, helping to balance what might otherwise be an exclusive focus on short-term initiatives. They will also enable a more equitable sharing of savings among all partners, including consumers.

National Clearinghouse

Because demand improvement is still a relatively new idea, and particularly because comprehensive, strategic approaches have been rare, we believe that a national clearinghouse should be established to promote, receive, analyze, and report on particular strategies and initiatives so that all sponsors and all communities can learn what works best. Since there is no mandate to engage in demand improvement nor standard regulations governing how to do so, every sponsor and community can be seen as a natural experiment and possible benchmark for everyone else.

Foundations may be sources of support for such a clearinghouse. The Robert Wood Johnson Foundation has already sponsored community-wide initiatives in the Boise, Idaho, region. The American Association of Health Plans may find that sponsoring such a clearinghouse will help promote more positive attitudes toward health plans. Just as collecting, analyzing, and reporting results of medical treatments is essential to improving the process and outcomes of medical care, so should the same approach be applied to demand improvement.

This is not to assert that what works in one situation, with one set of sponsors, consumer targets, behavior objectives, and tactics will necessarily work everywhere else. This is another reason why rigorous evaluation is essential—otherwise flawed evaluations may promote mindless repetition of whatever worked best anywhere, without considering why or how unique circumstances limit inference from one situation to another.

Medical treatment trials have the advantage of focusing on physiological outcomes primarily and construct their samples to represent the population having the condition of interest. (They have had an unfortunate tendency to rely on samples of males and to extrapolate results to females, however.) When rigorous methods of experiment and analysis are employed, the results are usually generalizable to other populations.

The same is not true with health and demand improvement initiatives, however. The "treatments" that are applied have to work in a context of physical, psychological, social, and spiritual factors that may not apply to other populations. Rarely are systematic analyses made of why initiatives worked or did not; the results are simply reported as experienced. In any given instance it will be impossible to be sure whether unique characteristics about the population targeted, the specific tactics employed, the precise behavior changes aimed for, or some mix of these factors made the difference between success and failure.

Generalizing from published results to any other population is necessarily speculative. If circumstances are similar enough and there have been a large number of past successes, sponsors may feel more confidence in their speculations, but they can only be sure a given intervention will work when it has worked.

The general public and the health care system need the ability to share in what can be learned from each demand improvement experience. If a clearinghouse for medical outcomes to help identify the best treatment for specific conditions is worthwhile, so will be a clearinghouse to help identify the best ways to enlist consumers in improving their health and demand. It can be used to weed out unqualified and unsuccessful vendors from the growing numbers claiming expertise and vying for a piece of the exploding market for demand improvement assistance.

Such a clearinghouse should be collaboratively developed and financed by the full range of sponsors at risk, as well as by foundations and community organizations committed to better health and health care. It should promote and assist in improving the quality of planning and evaluation, as well as being a repository of information and examples. It would probably be able to contribute to its own financing by charging for specific studies and reports, using such partial dependence to ensure it is meeting the needs of its constituents. The Health Enhancement and Research Organization (HERO), Birmingham, Alabama, with support from over 25 organizations, is an example of a clearinghouse operation.[6] The American Productivity and Quality Center, Houston, Texas, is already engaged in studying the effects of health on productivity and could be a possible participant.[7] The Coalition for Healthier Cities and Communities has promised to report case studies, success stories, and best practices information.[8]

The federal Agency for Health Care Policy and Research (AHCPR) has promoted and funded 12 designated centers across the United States and Canada for the improvement of medical care through its Evidence-Based Practice program.

These centers review published research and conduct their own to identify best practices and technologies that AHCPR then publishes as benchmark examples for all to go by.[9] We urge a similar approach for demand improvement, with private or public sponsorship.

The discipline of demand improvement is just beginning and has a long way to go before its potential and limitations are fully realized. All who are involved in or affected by efforts to improve the health and demand behaviors of at-risk and community populations should be willing to make a common cause in furthering the development of the discipline and improving the effectiveness and efficiency of interventions. This may well be counter to traditional notions of corporate secrecy, but we believe that all will gain much more by working together than by protecting mutual ignorance.

CONCERNS AND LIMITATIONS

While this book has championed the idea of improving demand, we are not unaware of nor insensitive to concerns and limitations related thereto. There is real risk that we may impose ideas of what is "sanitarily correct" in ways similar to what is politically correct.[10] Sponsors may, even unconsciously, define and attempt to promote desirable behavior in terms of their own values, ignoring the values of consumers. There have been indications that this has already occurred in regard to hysterectomies.[11] We feel that the best guard against unwarranted and uninvited sponsor intrusion is to empower consumers to make the best choices in light of their own values. Otherwise demand improvement efforts may become manipulative or coercive rather than of benefit to consumers.

Because information about the health and demand behaviors of populations and individual consumers is indispensable to demand improvement, there is great risk to personal privacy and to the confidentiality of such information. As program sponsors work with partners, community organizations, and vendors to plan, implement, and evaluate specific initiatives, many people will have access to sensitive information. It is essential that privacy and confidentiality be maintained *at levels that consumers expect* to preserve consumer trust and the long-term success of health and demand improvement efforts.

We feel that the kinds of demand improvement interventions described in this book have extraordinary potential for solving, or at least greatly reducing sponsors' and society's problems with respect to health care. And in stark contrast to past attempts to restrict consumer access and control provider behaviors, demand improvement promises great value to consumers as well. Care will have to be taken by sponsors to keep an eye on long-term as well as short-term effects, on individual as well as population impact, and on consumer as well as their own financial interests, but such care should be well worth the caring.

REFERENCES

1. G. Church, "Twin Cities' Friendly Plans," *TIME,* 14 April 1997, 36–39.

2. T. Jameson, "Calif. Abstinence-Only Effort with Teens a Failure, Study Shows," *The Denver Post,* 9 August 1997, 21A.

3. R. Herzlinger, *Market-Driven Health Care—Who Wins, Who Loses in the Transformation of America's Largest Service Industry* (Reading, MA: Addison-Wesley, 1997).

4. "Hospitals Are Paying for Poison Control Centers, But Not Reaping the Benefits," *Health Care Strategic Management* 15, no. 3 (1997):7, 8.

5. D. Drake, "Managed Care: A Product of Market Dynamics," *Journal of the American Medical Association* 277, no. 7 (1997):560–563.

6. R.W. Whitner and M. Dundon, "The Health Enhancement Research Organization (HERO)," *American Journal of Health Promotion* 11, no. 6 (1997):388–393.

7. "Currents—Human Resources," *Hospitals & Health Networks,* 5 July 1997, 13.

8. "National Coalition Forms," *Inside Preventive Care* 3, no. 4 (1997):6.

9. "AHCPR Announces 12 Evidence-Based Practice Centers," *Health Care Strategic Management* 15, no. 8 (1997):6.

10. B. Paulsen, "Against Health Correctness," *Health* 10, no. 7 (1996):10.

11. R. Rubin, "Politically Incorrect Surgery," *Health* 10, no. 7 (1996):104–112.

Index

D

About the Authors

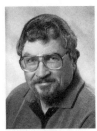 **Scott MacStravic** is the owner of Demand Engineering in Golden, Colorado, an organization that consults with employers, providers, health plans and vendors on health promotion, demand reform, and disease management. He is also a faculty member at the University of Colorado in Denver. The author of nine books in health care marketing, he is also a prolific author of more than 150 articles on health care strategy and marketing, and demand improvement.

Dr. MacStravic completed his undergraduate studies at Harvard University, followed by graduate studies in public affairs and hospital administration at the University of Minnesota, where he obtained his doctoral degree. His 25-year career as a health care strategist and marketer includes administrative and consulting positions at Michigan Blue Cross (Detroit), the American Rehabilitation Foundation (Minneapolis), the Minnesota State Planning Agency (St. Paul), and the U.S. Public Health Service as well as positions as marketing vice-president at Health and Hospital Services Corporation (Bellevue, WA—now Peach Health) and Provenant Health Partners (Denver, CO—now Centura Health Corporation). His mostly concurrent 24-year teaching career includes positions on the faculty at the Medical College of Virginia (Richmond) and the University of Washington (Seattle) in addition to the University of Colorado.

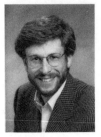 **Gary Montrose** is founder and president of Ashby • Montrose & Co., a Denver-based healthcare consulting practice specializing in ambulatory care, health, disease and demand management matters for providers, health plans and information technology vendors.

Mr. Montrose has led program planning, strategy and business development engagements for over 100 clients. He began his consulting practice after completing graduate studies in healthcare policy and economics at the University of Wisconsin-Madison. Over the past fifteen years, he has helped bring to market some of the most innovative products and strategic business consortiums in the emerging demand management industry. His healthcare engagements have included work for AT&T, USWest, Microsoft, United Airlines, MCI, PacifiCare (formerly FHP), Healthwise, InforMedical, Jones Intercable, Florida Hospital and the care management divisions of Merck, Pfizer and Upjohn Pharmaceuticals.

Montrose is an honors graduate from the University of California at Berkley in Political Science and Communications and Public Policy. He has been named to several industry publication editorial boards, has taught healthcare strategic planning as Adjunct Faculty at Denver University, and has been twice recognized as one of the top 20 consultants in the field of integrated delivery systems by the Washington D.C.-based Health Care Advisory Board. He can be reached at (303) 753-0708 in Denver, Colorado.